Outcomes for Children and Youth with Emotional and Behavioral Disorders and Their Families

Outcomes for Children and Youth with Emotional and Behavioral Disorders and Their Families

Programs and Evaluation Best Practices

SECOND EDITION

Edited by

Michael H. Epstein
Krista Kutash
Albert J. Duchnowski

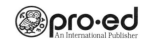
An International Publisher

8700 Shoal Creek Boulevard
Austin, Texas 78757-6897
800/897-3202   Fax 800/397-7633
www.proedinc.com

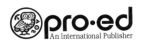

© 2005 by PRO-ED, Inc.
8700 Shoal Creek Boulevard
Austin, Texas 78757-6897
800/897-3202   Fax 800/397-7633
www.proedinc.com

Library of Congress Cataloging-in-Publication Data

Outcomes for children and youth with emotional and behavioral disorders and their
    families : programs and evaluations, best practices / edited by Michael H. Epstein, Krista
    Kutash, Albert Duchnowski.—2nd ed.
        p. cm.
    Includes bibliographical references and index.
    ISBN 0-89079-989-X (sc. : alk. paper)
    1. Behavior disorders in children.   2. Adolescent psychopathology.   I. Epstein, Michael
H.   II. Kutash, Krista.   III. Duchnowski, Albert J.

RJ506.B44098 2004
618.92'89—dc22

                                                                        2004044232

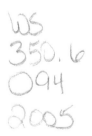

Art Director: Jason Crosier
Designer: Nancy McKinney-Point
This book is designed in Gill Sans and Minion.

Printed in the United States of America

1 2 3 4 5 6 7 8 9 10   06 05 04 03 02

Contents

Preface to the Second Edition

In the 6 years since the publication of the first edition of *Outcomes,* there has been significant activity in the multiple arenas that affect children who have emotional disturbances and their families. For the first time, the Surgeon General of the United States issued a report on the status of the nation's mental health. The report contained a major section devoted to children, and a national conference was held to develop an action agenda to implement the report's recommendations. President George W. Bush signed into law the No Child Left Behind Education Act, which has extensive implications for all children, including those with emotional disturbances. The legislation holds schools accountable for the educational performance—reading, arithmetic, and written expression—of all children, including those with special needs. Most recently, the President's New Freedom Commission on Mental Health issued its report addressing issues related to America's citizens who have mental illness. This commission had a subcommittee devoted specifically to assessing the mental health needs of children and developing recommendations for improving services for them and their families.

The mental health needs of children have gained the attention of policymakers and planners at the local, state, and federal levels. The expanse of activity is evident in policy, advocacy, research, and practice. In particular, the federal role in improving outcomes for children who have emotional disturbances and their families continues to grow. The Departments of Education and Health and Human Services continue to advance research and program development through various grant initiatives, and several chapters in this edition contain reports on projects supported by these agencies. Of particular note is the growth in the number of demonstration projects supported by the Comprehensive Children's Mental Health Services Program, administered by the Center for Mental Health Services. There are now more than 60 communities across the country that have received support to develop comprehensive systems of care affecting more than 60,000 children and their families. Several chapters in this edition report on evaluations of this important initiative at both the local and national levels.

The last few years have witnessed a major increase in the use of evidence-based practices in human services systems. Programs that serve children who have emotional disturbances are being evaluated more rigorously than ever as to their efficacy and their effectiveness in the field. Many authors of chapters in this edition will be recognized as leaders in the research on and evaluation of evidence-based practices. In addition, several chapters in this edition address issues specifically related to methodology and models of evaluation aimed at supplying empirical evidence supporting the effectiveness of mental health services delivered to children and their families.

As with the first edition, we hope this book will be useful to a variety of audiences associated with this extensive field. We continue to believe that progress in the field will be most effectively accomplished through a partnership of researchers, families, practitioners, advocates, and policymakers.

Michael H. Epstein
Krista Kutash
Albert J. Duchnowski

Contributors

Beth Jordan Armstrong, MS
Kentucky Department for Mental
  Health and Mental Retardation
Children and Youth Services Branch
100 Fair Oaks Lane, 4W-C
Frankfort, KY 40621

Steven M. Banks, PhD
The Bristol Observatory
521 Hewitt Road
Bristol, VT 05443

Kelli Y. Beard Jordan, PhD
University of Oregon
Institute on Violence and Destructive
  Behavior
Eugene, OR 97403-1265

Leonard Bickman, PhD
Vanderbilt University
Center for Mental Health Policy
1207 18th Avenue South
Nashville, TN 37212

Cindy Booth, BA
Oregon Youth Authority
530 Center Street NE,
Suite 200
Salem, OR 97301-3765

Eric J. Bruns, PhD
University of Maryland School
  of Medicine
Department of Psychiatry
701 W. Pratt Street, Suite 430
Baltimore, MD 21201

Michael Bullis, PhD
University of Oregon
Institute on Violence and Destructive
  Behavior
Eugene, OR 97403

John D. Burchard, PhD
University of Vermont
Department of Psychology
226 Dewey Hall
Burlington, VT 05405

Jane Burke, MS
University of Illinois at Chicago
Mental Health Services Research
  Program
104 S. Michigan Avenue, Suite 900
Chicago, IL 60603

Barbara J. Burns, PhD
Duke University School of Medicine
Department of Psychiatry and
  Behavioral Sciences
Box 3454
Durham, NC 27710

Patricia Chamberlain, PhD
Oregon Social Learning Center
160 East 4th Street
Eugene, OR 97401

Annie Chung, PhD
Ohana Clinical Care, Inc.
PO Box 715
Kapaa, HI 96746

Tim Connor, MA, MS
Wisconsin Bureau of Community
    Mental Health
1 West Wilson Street, Room 455
Madison, WI 53707

Judith A. Cook, PhD
University of Illinois at Chicago
Mental Health Services Research
    Program
104 S. Michigan Avenue,
Suite 900
Chicago, IL 60603

E. Jane Costello, PhD
Duke University School of Medicine
Department of Psychiatry and
    Behavioral Sciences
Box 3454
Durham, NC 27710

Celeste Dickey
Bethel School District
Clear Lake Elementary School
4646 Barger Drive
Eugene, OR 97402

Albert J. Duchnowski, PhD
University of South Florida
Florida Mental Health Institute
Research and Training Center for
    Children's Mental Health
13301 Bruce B. Downs Boulevard
Tampa, FL 33612-3899

J. Mark Eddy, PhD
Oregon Social Learning Center
160 East 4th Street
Eugene, OR 97401

Michael H. Epstein, EdD
University of Nebraska
Department of Special Education
202 Barkley Memorial Center
Lincoln, NE 68583-0732

Elizabeth M. Z. Farmer, PhD
Duke University School of Medicine
Department of Psychiatry and
    Behavioral Sciences
Box 3454
Durham, NC 27710

Edward G. Feil, PhD
University of Oregon
Institute on Violence and Destructive
    Behavior
Eugene, OR 97403-1265

Rebecca Ann Fetrow
Oregon Social Learning Center
160 East 4th Street
Eugene, OR 97401

Genevieve Fitzgibbon, BA
University of Illinois at Chicago
Mental Health Services Research
    Program
104 South Michigan Avenue,
Suite 900
Chicago, IL 60603

Michelle D. Force, MA
University of Vermont
Department of Psychology
266 Dewey Hall
Burlington, VT 05405

E. Michael Foster, PhD
Pennsylvania State University
Department of Health Policy
    and Administration
116 North Henderson Building
University Park, PA 16802-6500

Robert M. Friedman, PhD
University of South Florida
Florida Mental Health Institute
Child and Family Studies
13301 Bruce B. Downs Boulevard
Tampa, FL 33612-3899

Barbara J. Friesen, PhD
Portland State University
Regional Research Institute
Research and Training Center on Family
    Support and Children's Mental Health
PO Box 751
Portland, OR 97207-0751

Michael J. Furlong, PhD
University of California, Santa Barbara
Gevirtz Graduate School of Education
Santa Barbara, CA 93106

Stephen A. Gilbertson, MS
Wraparound Milwaukee
Milwaukee County Behavioral Health
    Division, Child and Adolescent Branch
9201 Watertown Plank Road
Milwaukee, WI 53226

Annemieke M. Golly, PhD
University of Oregon
Institute on Violence and Destructive
    Behavior
Eugene, OR 97403-1265

Jorge Gonzalez, PhD
Texas A&M University
Department of Educational Psychology
704 Harrington Tower
College Station, TX 77843-4225

Paul Greenbaum, PhD
University of South Florida
Florida Mental Health Institute
Child and Family Studies
13301 Bruce B. Downs Boulevard
Tampa, FL 33612-3899

Colleen A. Halliday-Boykins, PhD
Department of Psychiatry and
    Behavioral Sciences
Medical University of South Carolina
67 President Street, CPP/243
Charleston, SC 29425

Mark K. Harniss, PhD
University of Washington
Center on Human Development
    and Disability
Box 357920
Seattle, WA 98195-7920

Craig Anne Heflinger, PhD
Vanderbilt University
Mayborn Building, Room 203
Magnolia Circle
Nashville, TN 37232

Kimberly Hoagwood, PhD
Columbia University
Department of Child Psychiatry
1051 Riverside Drive, #78
New York, NY 10032

E. Wayne Holden, PhD
ORC Macro
3 Corporate Square, Suite 370
Atlanta, GA 30329

Sarah McCue Horwitz, PhD
Yale University School of Medicine
Department of Epidemiology and
    Public Health
60 College Street, Room 310
New Haven, CT 06520

Christina Hoven, PhD
Columbia University
1051 Riverside Drive,
Unit 43
New York, NY 10032

Bruce Kamradt, MSW
Wraparound Milwaukee
Milwaukee County Behavioral Health
    Division, Child and Adolescent
    Branch
9201 Watertown Plank Road
Milwaukee, WI 53226

Kelly Kelleher, MD
University of Pittsburgh
School of Medicine
3510 Fifth Avenue, Suite 1
Pittsburgh, PA 15213

Nancy M. Koroloff, PhD
Portland State University
Regional Research Institute
Research and Training Center on Family
    Support and Children's Mental Health
PO Box 751
Portland, OR 97207-0751

Krista Kutash, PhD
University of South Florida
Florida Mental Health Institute
Research and Training Center
    for Children's Mental Health
13301 Bruce B. Downs Boulevard
Tampa, FL 33612-3899

Margaret Lathrop
Bethel School District
Clear Lake Elementary School
4646 Barger Drive
Eugene, OR 97402

Qinghong Liao, MS
ORC Macro
3 Corporate Square, Suite 370
Atlanta, GA 30329

Nancy Lynn, MSPH
University of South Florida
Florida Mental Health Institute
Research and Training Center
    for Children's Mental Health
13301 Bruce B. Downs Boulevard
Tampa, FL 33612-3899

Nancy Marchand-Martella, PhD
Eastern Washington University
Department of Counseling, Educational,
    and Developmental Psychology
MS 92, 141 B Martin Hall
Cheney, WA 99004

Ronald C. Martella, PhD
Eastern Washington University
Department of Counseling, Educational,
    and Developmental Psychology
MS 92, 141 C Martin Hall
Cheney, WA 99004

Paul Mooney, PhD
Louisiana State University
Department of Curriculum and
    Instruction
219A Peabody Hall
Baton Rouge, LA 70803

Sarah A. Mustillo, PhD
Duke University School of Medicine
Department of Psychiatry and
    Behavioral Sciences
Box 3454
Durham, NC 27710

Nancy J. Nagel, MA
Colorado Mental Health Services
3824 West Princeton Circle
Denver, CO 80236

J. Ron Nelson, PhD
University of Nebraska
Department of Special Education
202 Barkley Memorial Center
Lincoln, NE 68583-0732

Hoang Nguyen, BS
ORC Macro
3 Corporate Square, Suite 370
Atlanta, GA 30329

John A. Pandiani, PhD
Vermont Department of Developmental
    and Mental Health Services
103 South Main Street
Waterbury, VT 05671-1601

Robert Paulson, PhD
University of South Florida
Florida Mental Health Institute
13301 Bruce B. Downs Boulevard
Tampa, FL 33612-3899

John Pendergrass
Oregon Department of Education
Youth Corrections Education Program
255 Capitol Street NE
Salem, OR 97310-0203

Kindle Anne Perkins-Rowe, PhD
University of Oregon
Institute on Violence and Destructive
    Behavior
Eugene, OR 97403-1265

Michael Pullmann, MS
Portland State University
Regional Research Institute
Research and Training Center on Family
    Support and Children's Mental Health
PO Box 751
Portland, OR 97207-0751

Theresa Rea, BS
Portland State University
Regional Research Institute
Research and Training Center on Family
    Support and Children's Mental Health
PO Box 751
Portland, OR 97207-0751

Stephanie Reich, BA
Vanderbilt University
Center for Mental Health Policy
1207 18th Avenue South
Nashville, TN 37212

John B. Reid, PhD
Oregon Social Learning Center
160 East 4th Street
Eugene, OR 97401

M. Jamila Reid, PhD
University of Washington
305 University District Building
Box 354801
Seattle, WA 98195

Vestena Robbins, PhD
Kentucky Department for Mental Health
    and Mental Retardation
Children and Youth Services Branch
100 Fair Oaks Lane, 4W-C
Frankfort, KY 40621

Abram Rosenblatt, PhD
University of California, San Francisco
Department of Psychiatry
44 Montgomery Street,
Suite 1450
San Francisco, CA 94104

Melisa D. Rowland, MD
Medical University of South Carolina
Department of Psychiatry and
    Behavioral Sciences
67 President Street, CPP/243
Charleston, SC 29425

Sonja K. Schoenwald, PhD
Medical University of South Carolina
Department of Psychiatry and
    Behavioral Sciences
67 President Street, CPP/243
Charleston, SC 29425

Bonita M. Seibert, LCSW, MSW
University of Oregon
Institute on Violence and Destructive
    Behavior
Eugene, OR 97403-1265

Herbert H. Severson, PhD
University of Oregon
Institute on Violence and Destructive
    Behavior
Eugene, OR 97403-1265

Stephanie A. Shepard, MA
Oregon Social Learning Center
160 East 4th Street
Eugene, OR 97401

Monica M. Simon, MS
Vermont Department of Developmental
  and Mental Health Services
103 South Main Street
Waterbury, VT 05671-1601

Nirbhay N. Singh, PhD
ONE Research Institute
PO Box 4657
Midlothian, VA 23112

Todd Sosna, PhD
3788 Brenner Drive
Santa Barbara, CA 93105

Jeffrey R. Sprague, PhD
University of Oregon
Institute on Violence and Destructive
  Behavior
Eugene, OR 97403-1265

Al Stein-Serousi, PhD
PIRE Chapel Hill Center
1229 East Franklin Street, 2nd Floor
Chapel Hill, NC 27514

Robert L. Stephens, PhD, MPH
ORC Macro
3 Corporate Square,
Suite 370
Atlanta, GA 30329

Arlene Rubin Stiffman, PhD
Washington University
George Warren Brown School
  of Social Work
Campus Box 1196
One Brookings Drive
St. Louis, MO 63130

Jesse C. Suter, MA
University of Vermont
Department of Psychology
266 Dewey Hall
Burlington, VT 05405

Alexandra L. Trout, PhD
University of Iowa
College of Education
N459 Linquist Center
Iowa City, IA 52242-1529

Deanne Unruh, PhD
University of Oregon
Institute on Violence and Destructive
  Behavior
Eugene, OR 97403-1265

Hill M. Walker, PhD
University of Oregon
Institute on Violence and Destructive
  Behavior
Eugene, OR 97403-1265

Christine Walrath, PhD
ORC Macro
116 John Street, 8th Floor
New York, NY 10038

Melissa Williams, MEd
6430 North Glenwood
Chicago, IL 60626

Carolyn H. Webster-Stratton, PhD
University of Washington
305 University District Building
Box 354801
Seattle, WA 98195

Michelle W. Woodbridge, PhD
University of California, Santa Barbara
Campus Outreach Initiatives
1503 South Hall
Santa Barbara, CA 93106

Descriptions of Children, Families, and Service Utilization

The System of Care 20 Years Later

CHAPTER 1

Krista Kutash, Albert J. Duchnowski, and Robert M. Friedman

In the first edition of this text, the opening chapter was titled "Community-Based Systems of Care: From Advocacy to Outcomes" (Lourie, Stroul, & Friedman, 1998). In that chapter the authors traced the history of the children's mental health services field, discussed the emergence of the system-of-care model (Stroul & Friedman, 1986, 1996), and examined its impact on the delivery of children's mental health services and outcomes for the children served and their families. They concluded that "the system-of-care model has already had a major impact on the children's mental health field; however, the full potential of this model to contribute to improving outcomes for children and their families is still to be realized" (Lourie et al., 1998, p. 17). Six years later our conclusion is not very different. The good news is that there have been some significant advances in the children's mental health services field that have enhanced the effectiveness of the system-of-care approach. Several chapters in this edition illustrate this point and document the refinements and improvements in meeting the needs of a very complex group of youth and their families.

The purpose of this chapter is to discuss the current impact and relevancy of the system-of-care model for the children's mental health services system. After almost 20 years, is the system of care a viable program model? From a policy perspective the answer appears to be "yes." In the landmark report on the mental health of the nation by the Surgeon General (U.S. Department of Health and Human Services, 1999), the section on children's mental health recommended the continued development of systems of care. The report concluded, "The multiple problems associated with 'serious emotional disturbance' in children and adolescents are best addressed with a 'systems' approach in which multiple service sectors work in an organized collective way" (p. 193). More recently, a report on the recommendations from special commissions created by states to examine mental health services issues proposed, as the first recommendation, that there be a continued focus on the values and principles of systems of care for children (Friedman, 2002). Although the support of policymakers is clear, the response from the research community is more complicated and reveals some conflict.

This chapter begins with a brief review of the context that led to the development of systems of care nationally. This is followed by an examination of recent empirical advances that have been made in understanding the number of youth who have serious emotional disorders, components within the system of care, and outcomes of systems of care. Some findings describing the costs of services for mental health care and the future of public mental health services for this group of youths and their families are also discussed, along with recommended next steps for systems-of-care research.

PUBLIC POLICY AND THE SYSTEM OF CARE

In 1984 the National Institute of Mental Health (NIMH) initiated the Child and Adolescent Service System Program (CASSP), with the goal of assisting states and communities in developing systems of care for children with serious emotional disorders and their families (Day & Roberts, 1991). At that time, the conceptualization of a system of care was based on a policy decision to focus on the population of children with a serious emotional disturbance and their families. This was defined as a diagnosable mental disorder of at least 6 months' duration requiring services from at least two systems. An increased emphasis was put on the functional impairment associated with the disorder (Stroul & Friedman, 1986). There was recognition that children with such serious emotional disturbances were involved in many systems in addition to mental health, especially education, child welfare, and juvenile justice, although there were only general data describing the number and characteristics of children needing mental health care, the nature of the service delivery system, and outcomes for youth with serious emotional disorders. Since then, research on children's mental health services has made significant strides in both the number of studies conducted and the quality of the work.

A framework for the system of care was published as a monograph by Stroul and Friedman (1986) and became a blueprint for states and communities in their efforts to improve children's mental health services. This framework was based on a combination of the best available data on effective services and systems and a set of values and principles that was derived through input from representatives of various stakeholder groups. The overall system-of-care initiative owed much to intense national advocacy. *Unclaimed Children* (Knitzer, 1982), a study conducted by Jane Knitzer for the Children's Defense Fund, is often cited as a watershed event in the children's mental health field (Duchnowski, Kutash, & Friedman, 2002); it served as a major catalyst of reform.

While Knitzer (1982) reported on the results from the previous two decades of neglect by the public sector for children who needed mental health services, there were some initiatives during that period aimed at improving mental health services. For example, in 1969 the Joint Commission on Mental Health of Children published its report on an intensive study of the status of mental health care for children. The recommendations in the report were very progressive and are still relevant today. There was an emphasis on early intervention, collaboration, and the development of an integrated service delivery system. However, the report was largely ignored by Congress. In the 1970s, short-lived and minimally funded initiatives were passed to address the mental health needs of children. For example, in 1972 a provision was added to the Community Mental Health Center Act to make funds available to train staff who worked with children, and the Most in Need Program was funded in 1979.

During the Carter administration, an emphasis on mental health led to the passage of the Mental Health Systems Act. This act included children and recommended collaboration among the major agencies serving children and their families. However, the act was repealed in 1981 when Ronald Reagan took office as president. Reagan's "New Federalism" consolidated federal programs for mental health and alcohol abuse into block grants to the states. However, the budgets for the block grants were cut significantly, leaving the states with reduced resources for these populations.

Unclaimed Children (Knitzer, 1982) presented powerful case studies revealing the lack of a systematic and responsible presence by public agencies in meeting the needs of children who were in need of mental health services. Knitzer particularly emphasized the failure of child-serving systems to work collaboratively and accept responsibility for serving children with emotional disturbances, as well as the absence of continua of care, which resulted in excessive use of restrictive residential placements. The report served as a rallying point for advocates and was a contributing factor in the funding of CASSP. Although CASSP was a very modestly funded program (states received $150,000 a year for 5 years), it achieved a level of success that was probably not anticipated by even its most ardent supporters (Day & Roberts, 1991). Private foundations joined the federal government in supporting the development of community-based programs for children's mental health services. In 1988, the Robert Wood Johnson Foundation funded its Mental Health Services Program for Youth, awarding grants to eight communities to develop local systems of care. In 1992, the Annie E. Casey Foundation began its Urban Child Mental Health Initiative, funding four inner-city communities to develop service delivery programs for the mental health needs of children.

Also in 1992, the federal Center for Mental Health Services (CMHS), part of the newly created Substance Abuse and Mental Health Services Administration (SAMHSA), received funding for the largest federal program to date that targeted children's mental health services. Through the Comprehensive Community Mental Health Services for Children and Their Families Program, Congress appropriated an initial allocation of $5 million, which has since grown to $90 million. CMHS awards as much as $5 million to local communities to support their efforts, and almost 70 grants have been awarded to date. Many of the programs described in subsequent chapters in this text have been supported by these grants.

Important policies affecting children who have emotional disorders also have been initiated by the education sector. The first was the Education for All Handicapped Children Act of 1975, reauthorized in 1990 as the Individuals with Disabilities Education Act (IDEA). These acts ensured the right to a free, appropriate education for all children, including those with disabilities.

Through the provisions of these acts, children who have emotional disorders are entitled to be educated in the least restrictive setting possible with the related services needed to achieve maximum educational outcomes. In 2002, President George W. Bush signed the No Child Left Behind Act into law. This initiative emphasizes school reform and accountability to improve academic outcomes for all children. The impact on children who have emotional disorders is yet to be evaluated but is expected to be substantial.

The final component of the context influencing the system of care is financing. During the 1990s there were two significant changes. Initially, mental health services for children were financed largely through state funds and through a fee-for-service mechanism. In the early 1990s states began to expand their funding by relying on federal funds through the Medicaid program (Friedman, 2002). However, as the costs grew, states and the federal government used managed-care mechanisms to contain the costs of all health care, including mental health. Although managed care has had some positive impact on systems of care—for example, restrictive hospital placements have been reduced—this system has not adequately supported the broad range of services characteristic of systems of care.

In summary, this has been a brief description of the advocacy, policies, and funding mechanisms that compose the context in which systems of care have been developing for almost two decades. The development is ongoing, and there is much support at the policy level to warrant continued efforts aimed at achieving the full potential of the system of care.

SYSTEM-OF-CARE PRINCIPLES

Several excellent sources contain detailed descriptions of the values, principles, and components of the system of care (see, e.g., Lourie et al., 1998). The values and principles that serve as the foundation of the model were influenced by the report of the Joint Commission on the Mental Health of Children (1969) and the findings from Jane Knitzer's study (1982). In particular, these studies criticized the overreliance on residential placement, the failure to recognize families as important partners in helping their children, and the disregard of the culture of the child and family. Addressing these criticisms, Stroul and Friedman (1986) proposed as core values of the system of care the need to be child centered and family focused, community based, and culturally competent. In addition, they proposed 10 guiding principles that emphasize individualized services, family participation, early intervention, and adequate transition services. These values and principles are to be incorporated into the operations of all child-serving agencies that participate in developing integrated, collaborative systems of care that achieve the best possible benefit for children and families.

In addition to influencing the manner in which services are provided to children and their families, the system of care has served as a framework for investigating important issues in the children's mental health field. The complex problems of determining reliable prevalence estimates and a systematic description of the characteristics of the children who are served in the system are two important issues that have been examined in the system-of-care framework.

HOW MANY CHILDREN?

The system-of-care framework was developed to meet the multiple and complex needs of children and adolescents with severe emotional disturbances and their families. Although the terms *severe emotional disturbances* and *seriously emotionally disturbed* are not diagnostic terms, they are used to describe youth whose problems are so severe as to require long-term intervention from the mental health sector as well as other child-serving agencies. Focusing systems of care on this group of youth was intentional, as this group was seen as being underidentified and inappropriately served, needing an array of services at varying levels of intensity. Mental health services alone were not enough to meet the needs of these youth. "Children with severe emotional disturbances almost universally manifest problems in many spheres including home, school and community. As a result, they require the intervention of other agencies and systems to provide special education, child welfare, health, vocational and, often, juvenile justice services" (Stroul & Friedman, 1986, p. xxi). This definition of serious emotional disturbances was further codified by SAMHSA's Center for Mental Health Services in 1993 (see Table 1.1).

A federal task force convened by the Center for Mental Health Services reviewed the research on prevalence and concluded that about 1 in 5, or 20%, of children have a diagnosable mental disorder, and about 1 in 10 children, or 10%, have a serious emotional disturbance (Friedman, Katz-Leavy, Manderscheid, & Sondheimer, 1996). A child with a serious emotional disturbance not only has a diagnosable disorder but also demonstrates substantial impairment in functioning at home, in school, or in the community because of the disorder. Two more recent reviews of the literature also indicated that the prevalence of diagnosable disorders is approximately 20% (Costello, Gordon, Keeler, & Angold, 2001; Roberts, Attkisson, & Rosenblatt, 1998). Additionally, an analysis of data from the 1997 National Survey of American Families found a 21% prevalence rate (Kataoka, Zang, & Wells, 2002). Although there is less information about prevalence in young children than there is for children between 9 and 17 years of age, the research that is available indicates that the prevalence rate is not very different than it is for older children (Lavigne et al., 1996).

In an investigation to determine if levels of problem behaviors in children have increased over time, Achenbach, Dumenci, and Rescorla (2003) collected ratings of problem behaviors and competences from three national samples in 1976, 1989, and 1999. Approximately 20% of the 1999 sample scored within a range indicating the presence of mental health problems. Furthermore, results from the three groups of youths indicate that levels of

TABLE 1.1

Definition of Children with a Serious Emotional Disturbance

Pursuant to section 1912(c) of the Public Health Service Act, as amended by Public Law 102-321, "children with a serious emotional disturbance" are persons

- from birth up to age 18,[a]
- who currently or at any time during the past year,[b]
- have a diagnosable mental, behavioral, or emotional disorder of sufficient duration to meet diagnostic criteria specified with *DSM–III–R*,[c]
- that resulted in functional impairment that sufficiently interferes with or limits the child's role of functioning in family, school, or community activities.[d]

These disorders include any mental disorder (including those of biological etiology) listed in *DSM–III–R* or their ICD–9–CM equivalent (and subsequent revisions), with the exception of *DSM–III–R* "V" codes, substance use, and developmental disorders, which are excluded, unless they co-occur with another diagnosable serious emotional disturbance. All these disorders have episodic, recurrent, or persistent features; however, they vary in terms of severity and disability effects.

Functional impairment is defined as difficulties that substantially interfere with or limit a child or adolescent from achieving or maintaining one or more developmentally appropriate social, behavioral, cognitive, communicative, or adaptive skills. Functional impairment criteria during the referenced year without the benefit of treatment or other support services are included in this definition.

Note. From *Federal Register,* May 20, 1993, p. 29425.

[a] The definition of serious emotional disturbance in children is restricted to persons up to age 18. However, it is recognized that some states extend this age range to persons under 22 years. To accommodate this variability, states using an extended age range for children's services should provide separate estimates for persons below age 18 and for persons aged 18 to 22 within block grant applications.

[b] This reference year in each of the definitions refers to a continuous 12-month period because this is a frequently used interval in epidemiological research and because it relates closely to commonly used planning cycles.

[c] The *Diagnostic and Statistical Manual of Mental Disorders (DSM)* is a publication of the American Psychiatric Association, while the *International Classification of Diseases,* 10th revision (ICD–10) is a publication of the World Health Organization. Both of these publications will be updated periodically, and the revised nomenclatures are likely to affect both the language of mental disorders and the types of disorders currently included in or excluded from these definitions. As appropriate, the definitions will be updated by the Center for Mental Health Services accordingly.

[d] Functional impairment that "substantially interferes" will be operationally defined as part of the process of developing standardized methods for estimation.

problems increased from 1976 to 1989 and then decreased from 1989 to 1999. Levels of problems and competence were at their worst in 1989, and although both levels improved in 1999, problem levels were still somewhat higher than they were in 1976.

Although no national epidemiological study has been conducted to document the prevalence of children with mental health problems in the United States, the numerous local and regional studies that have been conducted have consistently estimated the prevalence of mental health disorders in children to be approximately 20%. These data support the overall premise of the system of care that there are many children in need of mental health services and that service systems need to be organized in a way that will address problems that occur in multiple domains and severity levels. What remain less clear are the prevalence of serious and persistent mental health problems in children and how child-serving agencies can be best organized to meet the needs of these children. The next section describes the research on the characteristics of youth with serious emotional disturbances and the services agencies use to serve them.

CHARACTERISTICS OF YOUTH WITH SERIOUS EMOTIONAL DISTURBANCES

When the system-of-care philosophy was developed, it was based not only on the premise that there was a significant number of children with serious emotional problems but also that the needs of these children were largely unmet. The few services available were excessively restrictive, consisting typically of residential care. The system of care further asserted that these children had mental or emotional disturbances of a long-term nature and that the persistence and severity of the condition resulted in impaired functioning in a variety of domains (i.e., school, home, community) that would require a range of services that cut across the responsibilities of child-serving agencies. Research has indicated that although many of the milder mental health disorders are short term in nature and do not have a major effect on functioning in school, at home, or in the community, youth with serious emotional disturbances typically tend to have a long history of emotional problems resulting in multiple diagnoses and behaviors that affect functioning (Friedman, Kutash, & Duchnowski, 1996).

Persistence

A cornerstone in the definition of serious emotional disturbance is that the condition will persist over time. Unlike many of the milder mental health conditions, serious emotional disturbances are thought to begin early in a child's life and to persist. Thus, development is disrupted in social, academic, and community functioning. Multiple studies have begun to document the persistence of serious emotional disturbances. In four different studies that focused on adolescents with serious emotional disturbances, the results were consistent. Parents first noticed emotional or behavioral difficulties in their child during early childhood (Duchnowski, Johnson, Hall, Kutash, & Friedman, 1993; Kutash & Duchnowski, 2004; Kutash et al., 2000; Silver et al., 1992; see Table 1.2). Furthermore, services for these children did not begin until approximately 2 years after the problems were first noticed. These results are further validated from two studies of a nationally representative sample of

TABLE 1.2
Age of Onset and First Service for Youth
with Serious Emotional Disturbances

| Study | N | Average Age | | |
		Entry into Study	Of Onset[a]	First Service
Silver et al., 1992	800	13.1	6.3	7.9
Duchnowski et al., 1993	87	14.2	6.9	10.9
Kutash et al., 2000	116	11.6	4.6	6.7
Kutash & Duchnowski, 2004	158	11.8	5.4	6.9
Wagner et al., 2003	255[b]	15–17	7.4	9.5
Wagner et al., 2003	535[b]	13–16	6.5	8.5

[a] Parent report.
[b] National representative sample.

adolescent youths who were in special education due to emotional or behavioral problems. In 1987 and again in 2001, Wagner, Cameto, and Newman (2003) found that parents reported their children were first identified as having a disability at 7.4 years and 6.5 years of age, respectively, and services began at 9.5 years and 8.5 years of age, respectively. These studies document the early onset of emotional and behavior problems in children and the persistence of the problems over time. Additionally, these results point to a gap between onset and delivery of services that indicates a need for better-coordinated early intervention efforts.

Severity of Impairment

An area in which the research has not kept pace with other developments in the children's mental health field is the measurement of functional impairment. Although legislation has required that a youth with a serious emotional disorder be identified with a disorder and that this disorder must result in functional impairment, this requirement has not been accompanied by recommended procedures and suggestions for specific measures of functional impairment (Canino, Costello, & Angold, 1999). The concept of functional impairment has moved to the forefront as an important issue for clinicians and researchers, but the empirical base for the measurement of the construct is in need of attention.

Canino et al. (1999) have outlined several challenges to the field in terms of operationally defining the construct of functional impairment. First is the need to clarify the distinction between psychiatric disorders and functional impairment, as it is difficult to ascertain which aspects of daily living are affected by a disorder. Another aspect that needs increased conceptual clarity is the distinction among the terms *functioning, competence, social adaptation,* and *impairment.* These terms reflect the fact that the concept of functioning runs along a continuum ranging from the positive notion of competence to the negative notion of impairment. A challenge specific to children is that the assessment of their functioning must take into consideration their developmental stage as well as the culture in which they were raised. Another issue is the specificity with which the concept should be measured. Currently, the field has instruments that assess functioning in a range of settings (i.e., domain-specific measures) as well as global measures. Given these numerous challenges facing the field, the lack of progress in this area is understandable. However, given the importance of this topic to both clinicians and researchers, it is unfortunate that more progress has not been made.

Even with the challenges in measuring functioning, the research field has provided ample documentation of the extensive impairment in multiple domains for youths with serious emotional disorders and the negative outcomes resulting from this impairment. Using statewide data collected on children receiving services from public mental health agencies, Hodges and Wotring (2000) documented that these youths experience impairments across multiple settings. For the 4,758 youths assessed on intake into services, 26% and 19% were rated as having a severe impairment in the school/work and home domains, respectively, whereas 38% and 37% of the youths had moderate levels of impairment in the behavior toward others and moods/emotions domains, respectively. Similar results were obtained from the first 31 communities receiving funding through the Center for Mental Health's (1999) Comprehensive Community Mental Health Services for Children and Their Families Program. These communities, funded specifically to serve youths with severe emotional disorders, reported that of the approximately 40,000 youths at entry, 69% had either moderate or severe levels of impairment in their school role, while 61% and 29% had either moderate or severe levels of impairment in their home role and community role, respectively. Clearly, these data support the system-of-care concept that youths with severe emotional disorders have needs that cross a variety of settings and that service systems should be designed to meet these multiple needs.

Another advancement in the research field has been the documentation of the role functional impairment plays in understanding the outcomes for children with mental health needs. For youths participating in the Great Smoky Mountains Study, children with both a diagnosis and functional impairment were almost four times as likely to have a negative outcome over a 4-year period (e.g., be arrested, drop out of school) as children with only a diagnosis (Canino et al., 1999). Likewise, Armstrong, Dedrick, and Greenbaum (2003) found the best longitudinal predictor of positive outcomes for youth with severe emotional disturbances was their initial level of functional impairment. These results highlight the predictive utility of measuring impaired functioning in children and the need to integrate the concept into service systems and clinical treatments.

SERVICE ACCESS AND UTILIZATION

One of the greatest advances over the last several years has been the growth in using national databases to gain a better understanding of how families access and utilize children's mental health services. In an analysis of 10 sources, including national household surveys and databases reflecting managed mental health specialty health-care claims, private insurance claims, and hospital inpatient and outpatient care records, the National Institute of Mental Health (2001) has produced the first national estimates of mental health utilization for children. Data from three national surveys indicate that between 5% and 7% of all children use mental health specialty services in a year, at a cost of $11.75 billion, or $173 per child. Across service types, outpatient services account for 57% of the cost, whereas residential inpatient costs account for 33% (see Table 1.3 for key findings). These results point to the disparities across racial and ethnic groups, with Black and Hispanic youths having lower rates of service use while having the highest rates of need. Results also indicate that a substantial amount of mental health care is provided in primary care settings (e.g., primary care physicians) and that the ability to access mental health services appears to be related to insurance status. That is, uninsured youths are less likely to receive mental health care; however, youths with public insurance (e.g., Medicaid) have higher rates of use than privately insured children.

Research is being conducted to document the critical role of the educational system in providing mental health services to children. Using data provided by the National Longitudinal Study of Adolescent Health (Add Health), Slade (2002) examined the use of school-based mental health services. The Add Health data set contains information on a nationally representative sample of adolescents attending Grades 7 through 12 in 132 geographically, ethnically, and economically diverse middle and high schools. The Add Health data set includes information from school administrators regarding the availability of school-based mental health counseling services as well as data from students ($N = 18,475$) and their parents. Results show that on-site mental health counseling is available for approximately three out of every five adolescents (i.e., 58%) who attend school. However, among all adolescents, school-based mental health services are used less frequently than non–school-based mental health services (4.4% vs. 8.8%). Slade reported that when mental health programs were available at school, students were significantly more likely to have seen a counselor during the past year. Students at schools identified as offering on-site mental health counseling reported greater usage than students at schools not offering school-based counseling (5.4% vs. 3.2%). This suggests that students may receive informal counseling from teachers, school nurses, school coaches, and other school staff who are not paid to provide counseling. Finally, Slade found that access to school-based counseling did not differ significantly by race.

Recently, two studies have been launched to examine the characteristics and the longitudinal outcomes of a nationally representative sample of youths with disabilities serviced in special educational environments, including youths identified as having emotional disturbances (ED). These two studies, the

TABLE 1.3

Key Findings from *Blueprint for Change:*
Research on Child and Adolescent Mental Health

- Based on three national surveys fielded between 1996 and 1998, between 5% to 7% of all children use any mental health specialty services in a year. This average rate is similar to the rate among adults, but it obscures major differences across age groups. Only 1% to 2% of preschoolers use any services, but 6% to 8% of the 6- to 11-year age group and 8% to 9% of the 12- to 17-year age group use any services.

- There is substantial variation in mental health service utilization by type of insurance, ranging from 8.4% for Medicaid enrollees to 4.0% for the uninsured. The intensity of outpatient care (number of visits) also differs. Children on Medicaid are estimated to have more than 1,300 specialty visits per 1,000 children per year, compared with 462 specialty visits per 1,000 children with private insurance, 391 visits per 1,000 children with other types of insurance, and 366 visits per 1,000 children with no insurance.

- Mental health utilization varies across racial/ethnic groups. Latinos are the least likely of all groups to access specialty care (5.0%), even though they and Black children have the highest rates of need (10.5%) based on measures in the National Health Interview Survey (NHIS). Approximately 7% of families with a child with need (based on NHIS measures) claimed financial barriers as the reason for not getting any mental health care.

- More than half of all outpatient specialty mental health services provided to children with private insurance are out-of-plan. The education sector likely provides a substantial portion of these services. Regarding inpatient mental health care, between 0.2% and 0.3% of children aged 1 to 17 use inpatient mental health services in community hospitals. This rate is much lower than the rate for adults (0.6%). Across all insurance types, adults and adolescents have greater inpatient days per 1,000 population than young children. Among the privately insured and the uninsured, adolescents have higher inpatient service use than adults. In contrast, among the publicly insured, inpatient days per 1,000 population are significantly higher for adults than for adolescents.

- Approximately 4.3% of children received psychotropic medication, and utilization is concentrated among older children: 5.0% of 6- to 11-year-olds and 5.6% of adolescents are on psychotropic medication, whereas only 0.7% of children ages 1 to 5 used such medication.

- Total treatment expenditures for children in 1998 are estimated to be approximately $11.75 billion, or about $173 per child. Adolescents (12–17) account for 59% of the total and also have the highest expenditures per child at $291; children 6 to 11 account for 34% of the total at $165 per child; children 1 to 5 account for 7% at $39 per child.

- Across service types, outpatient services account for 57% of the total ($6.7 billion), inpatient for 33% ($3.9 billion), psychotropic medications for 9% ($1.1 billion), and other services for 1% ($0.07 billion).

- Across children's insurance status, children with private insurance account for 47% ($5.5 billion), Medicaid enrollees for 24% ($2.8 billion), children with other public insurance for 3% ($0.4 billion), and the uninsured for 5% ($0.6 billion). We could not allocate state/local expenditures (21%, or $2.5 billion) by child insurance status. The majority of these services were provided to children with private insurance coverage or Medicaid, but they were not paid by insurance.

- Total expenditures on psychotropic medications for children in 1998 are estimated to be $1.1 billion. The largest proportion of expenditures was for stimulants, which accounted for slightly more than 40% of the total. Antidepressant costs was the second largest category, accounting for 33% of the total.

Note. From *Blueprint for Change: Research on Child and Adolescent Mental Health,* by National Institute of Health, 2001, Washington, DC: The National Advisory Mental Health Workgroup on Child and Mental Health Intervention Development and Deployment.

Special Education Elementary Longitudinal Study (SEELS) and the National Longitudinal Transition Study–2 (NLTS–2), are collecting data through interviews with parents and school staff. The initial findings reveal that school staff reported that a variety of services are provided to youths with emotional disturbances. For students receiving special education for emotional disturbances, 44% of the students in elementary or middle schools and 69% of the high school students received mental health services from the school. Additionally, mental health services and case management are provided at rates higher for students with emotional disturbances than for students in other disabilities categories. Parents of these students, however, are less likely to agree that schools are meeting their children's needs or that the services their children receive are enough when compared to reports of parents of students in other disability categories. Consequently, parents of students with emotional disturbances are less likely to be very satisfied with these services than parents of students with disabilities as a whole, and they are more likely to report that it took "a lot of effort" to obtain services (Wagner, 2003). However, there is evidence that mental health service delivery in schools has improved over the past decade. In 1987, only 5% of a nationally representative sample of transition-aged students with ED reported receiving mental health services in the school. This percentage increased to 34% in 2001 (Wagner et al., 2003).

EVALUATING OUTCOMES OF THE SYSTEM OF CARE

As the foregoing discussion indicates, children who receive services in community-based systems of care are a heterogeneous group of youths who display symptoms that are severe, who have problems that are complex, and whose impairment affects multiple domains of functioning. This heterogeneity presents challenges for providing effective services and may contribute to the difficulty researchers have encountered in efforts to produce empirical findings that link comprehensive systems of care to improved outcomes for youths who are served in these systems.

As Knapp (1995) has noted, evaluating complex systems that provide mental health services to children and their families is a process that is probably best approached by a series of investigations, beginning with intensive case studies to describe the programs and progressing to more rigorous experimental designs. The field may still be in need of more systematic description and efforts to clearly articulate and operationalize the components of the system of care. However, the urgent need to assess the impact of the system of care, including child- and family-level outcomes, has led to efforts to examine the system of care at both system and client levels, despite the absence of clear operational definitions for all of the values and principles of systems of care and well-developed measures of fidelity to a system-of-care model.

Hoagwood, Jensen, Petti, and Burns (1996) proposed a framework of five outcome domains that could be used to assess the evidence of impact for service delivery programs. The domains are organized in a hierarchical series reflecting widening spheres of influence: symptoms and diagnoses; functioning in home, school, and community; consumer perspectives such as satisfaction with services and family burden; stability of the child's environments; and systems (e.g., restrictiveness of services, organizational relationships, and costs). In general, the evaluation studies that have been completed have focused on the latter domains, especially systems issues, with fewer investigations reporting client-level findings (Duchnowski, Kutash, & Friedman, 2002; Rosenblatt, 1998).

What Have We Learned?

Most of the studies evaluating systems-of-care outcomes have used pre–post designs, with only a few comparison group studies and very little use of fidelity measures at either the system or practice levels (Duchnowski et al., 2002). Nevertheless, the literature base resulting from more than 20 studies of systems of care indicates a fairly consistent pattern of system-level outcomes supporting the system-of-care model. These findings include an increase in access to services, greater interagency collaboration, increased satisfaction by families, reductions in restrictive psychiatric placements, reduction in costs, and cost avoidance in other service systems (Duchnowski et al., 2002; Rosenblatt, 1998). An interesting system-level outcome was investigated by Foster (1998), who found that children served in a system of care received better and more timely follow-up services after being discharged from inpatient placements than similar children receiving traditional services at a comparison site.

The current literature does not contain any studies using rigorous experimental designs that have shown systems of care to be unequivocally superior to traditional care in improving clinical outcomes for children who have serious emotional disturbances. However, data from nonexperimental studies have produced encouraging findings. Rosenblatt (1998) reported positive results for the system of care in 8 of 9 studies evaluating the clinical status of participants and in 10 of 11 studies evaluating functional impairment. Hodges, Doucette-Gates, and Liao (1999) examined changes in functional impairment in children served in system-of-care programs. They reported significant decreases in scores on the *Child and Adolescent Functional Assessment Scale* (CAFAS) after 6 months of service. Their findings were from 873 youths who had varied backgrounds in terms of custodial status, history of psychiatric hospitalization, school performance, diagnosis, and legal involvement. None of these factors were related to improvement in functioning.

Three major comparison group studies have been conducted to examine the impact of the system-of-care model. The first is the Fort Bragg experiment conducted by Leonard Bickman and his colleagues (see, e.g., Bickman et al., 1995). Bickman and his colleagues examined the effects of a system-of-care model implemented at Fort Bragg and compared the outcomes to those of standard practice at a comparable army installation. The second study (the Stark County study), also conducted by Bickman and his colleagues (Bickman,

Noser, & Summerfelt, 1999), compared two randomly assigned groups of children, one served in a system of care and one served in traditional care. The third investigation is the comparison study of the national evaluation of the Comprehensive Community Mental Health Services for Children and Their Families Program (CCMHS), conducted by ORC Macro (see Chapter 22, by Stephens, Connor, Nguyen, Holden, Greenbaum, and Foster). Descriptions of the methodology and results of these studies have now been extensively published. Among the many references to the Fort Bragg study are Bickman et al.'s (1995) *Evaluating Managed Mental Health Services;* a special issue of the *Journal of Mental Health Administration* (1966, Vol. 23); and several journal articles (see Duchnowski et al., 2002, for a summary). In addition to the chapter in this text, the OCR Macro study is described in a special issue of the *Journal of Emotional and Behavioral Disorders* (2001, vol. 9).

Briefly stated, Bickman and his colleagues (1995) concluded that the system-of-care model implemented in both Fort Bragg and Stark County showed no significant differences in clinical or functional outcomes for youth when compared to outcomes for youth from standard practice communities. Furthermore, no significant differences were revealed after a 5-year follow-up of the Fort Bragg and standard practice participants (Bickman, Lambert, Andrade, & Penaloza, 2000). The conclusions reached by the authors of the Fort Bragg study have generated much controversy (Friedman & Burns, 1996). The study has been criticized for not implementing a system-of-service delivery that sufficiently incorporated the values and principles proposed by Stroul and Friedman (1986) as characteristic of a system of care. For example, there was a low level of family involvement, and children who did not have serious emotional disturbances were included in the study (Friedman & Burns, 1996). When analyses were conducted on the most impaired children, the results were more favorable to the system of care. Nonetheless, there is general agreement that the Fort Bragg and Stark County studies have brought about an important focus on the practice level. When systems of care are implemented in communities, it is assumed that an array of effective services will be available to individuals. However, there has been very little quality control of the individual practices in terms of measuring fidelity or adherence to program models. Consequently, investigations of the effectiveness of systems of care have resulted in a critical examination of the constraints that exist at the practice level. Systems of care will be effective in achieving positive outcomes at the child and family levels only if the individual services that compose the systems are effective; this is an important consideration for future research.

The longitudinal comparison study of the CMHS program is extensively described in Chapter 22 by Stephens et al. This study illustrates the complexity involved in evaluating a multisite system of care designed to address the needs of children who have serious emotional disabilities. Briefly stated, the results are mixed. Once again, systems-level outcomes generally favor system-of-care sites, while individual client-level outcomes are more equivocal. Stephens et al. also point to the need for better evaluation of the quality of individual services at the practice level as essential to any study of the effectiveness of a system-of-care service delivery program.

SUMMARY AND FUTURE STEPS

After almost two decades of development, a comprehensive and integrated system of care for children who have serious emotional disturbances and their families has been shown to result in an increase in access to and use of services. Families report more satisfaction with services received through a system of care, restrictive inpatient hospitalization is reduced, and better follow-up care is available when hospitalization does occur. While the question of the cost of a system of care compared to traditional services is not as clear, there is mounting evidence that systems of care, under specific operating conditions (see Chapter 10, by Foster and Connor), do not cost more. Furthermore, agencies other than the mental health system may experience significant cost avoidance for children served through a valid system of mental health services.

The research evaluating clinical and functional outcomes for children served in a system of care has not been as clear. Several studies using pre–post designs have shown improved outcomes in these domains for children served in a system of care, whereas more rigorous studies using randomized clinical trials and quasi-experimental designs have not shown such results. However, there is much controversy in the field about these later studies (i.e., Fort Bragg and Stark County) that challenges the results and conclusions offered by the authors. These studies have been criticized for not implementing a system of care that adheres to the values and principles proposed by the model's developers (Friedman & Burns, 1996). It would appear that a rejection of the program theory of the system of care is premature. What is needed, perhaps, is an increased focus on the theory of change for systems of care, the implementation of systems with fidelity to the model, and interventions at the individual services level.

There is no controversy concerning the urgent need to improve the mental health system for children. The President's New Freedom Commission on Mental Health, established in April 2002, reported that America's mental health service delivery system is "in shambles" (Hogan, 2002) and that "the mental health maze is more complex and more inadequate for children" (p. 5). In January 2002, a conference was convened to examine reports from mental health commissions in 13 states. The most important theme in these reports was a serious dissatisfaction with the adequacy of efforts to address the mental health needs of children, adolescents, and their families.

Since the release of the Surgeon General's report on the nation's mental health (U.S. Department of Health and Human Services, 1999), there has been renewed energy focused on children's mental health. Two themes that have implications for the system of care are present in the current reform initiatives that have originated at the federal level. The first is an emphasis on mental health as a public health challenge and a call to adopt public health strategies to meet this challenge. This is particularly true for children. Two senior members of the Centers for Disease Control and Prevention have listed children's emotional health and development as the third highest challenge in their list of the country's 10 most pressing health challenges (Koplan & Fleming,

2000). They point out how vaccinations and other health advances have made infancy and childhood less perilous and call for similar advances that will permit each child to achieve his or her full potential. The President's Commission on Excellence in Special Education (2002) has also called for the adoption of the public health model to assist children who have disabilities, including emotional disturbances. The commission proposed a new emphasis on identifying risk factors, universal designs aimed at prevention, and early intervention strategies. This is an opportunity for linkage between the children's mental health system and the education system, two systems that have not achieved a level of collaboration in the system of care necessary to significantly improve outcomes for children (Kutash & Duchnowski, 1997). Systems-of-care researchers have, for the most part, emphasized studies of the most seriously disturbed children and youth who have a long history of involvement in the system. Whereas a guiding principle of the system of care is prevention, early identification, and intervention, it is clear that this type of research must be greatly increased.

The second theme that has important implications for the future of the system of care is the renewed emphasis on evidence-based interventions at the practice level. As noted, the Fort Bragg, Stark County, and longitudinal comparison studies of the CMHS Program all have concluded that a lack of high-quality individual services greatly impedes the achievement of positive outcomes for children currently served in systems of care. At the federal level, the call for accountability by the education and social services agencies is directing attention to evidence-based practice. For example, in the No Child Left Behind Act (U.S. Department of Education, Office of Elementary and Secondary Education, 2002), the major piece of legislation aimed at school reform, evidence-based practice is referred to 110 times. The President's Commission on Excellence in Special Education (2002) has called for a change from a culture of process to a culture of results in special education. This message is relevant for the system of care. The good news is that there are evidence-based practices in the children's mental health field, some with extensive experimental support and others with emerging support (Burns, 2002). In their review of evidence-based community interventions, Burns and Hoagwood (2002) presented several evidence-based practices that are feasible for use in comprehensive, community-based programs for children who have serious emotional disturbances. Examples of these interventions include multisystemic therapy, treatment foster care, case management, and parent education and support (Burns, 2002). The challenge for system-of-care researchers is to identify systems that incorporate these features in their efforts to evaluate the effectiveness of systems of care. Of course, the researchers will have to be assisted by policymakers, planners, and the training community to ensure that there is the capacity and the infrastructure necessary to implement evidence-based practices on a scale that will achieve meaningful impact.

Training professionals to implement evidence-based practices is a formidable but achievable task. Practitioners may have to assume new roles and learn new skills to function effectively in a system of care that uses evidence-based practice. For example, if multisystemic therapy is implemented in community mental health center where office-based practice was the dominant treatment, staff may have to assume the role of a therapist who works in the home, the school, and perhaps at a playground or recreation center. System-of-care researchers, advocates, and administrators will need to collaborate to enhance the use of evidence-based practices in the field.

There is a third recommendation for the future that is more micro and more immediate. In the opening paragraph in the section on outcomes, we mentioned the heterogeneity of the children served in systems of care as a source of challenge to finding positive outcomes in the study. For example, the statistical variance produced by factors such as multiple diagnoses, variable service histories, and multiple risk factors may be preventing the emergence of group differences that are detectable through traditional data analysis models such as analysis of variance. Recently, growth mixture modeling with latent trajectory classes (Muthén & Muthén, 2000) has proved beneficial in demonstrating the effectiveness of alcohol abuse programs with varied populations and is being used in studies of children who have emotional disturbances (Greenbaum & Dedrick, 2003). It may be that the analysis of latent variables such as age of onset, comorbidity, and others may reveal improved outcomes for subclasses of participants in systems of care. This is a step that is emerging in the field, and we look forward to more work in this direction.

In a presentation to the President's New Freedom Commission on Mental Health, Friedman (2002) indicated that although there has been great expansion in systems of care, there was also an increasing recognition of the complexity of developing and implementing effective systems for children with serious emotional disturbances and their families. He called for an expanded framework for systems of care, including an increased emphasis on implementation issues, such as governance, financing, performance measurement and continuous quality improvement, theories of change, the development of an expanded provider network, human resource development, planning, and management information systems. He also pointed out that the increased focus on family partnerships, family choice of services and providers, cultural competence, strengths-based approaches, and individualized care at the practice level represent enormous departures from more traditional service delivery models and require further time for development and implementation. Although systems of care have been discussed for 20 years now, this represents a relatively modest amount of time in terms of the dramatic changes at the system level and the practice level that systems of care represent.

It has been said that the legacy of CASSP may be the nurturing of a strong family advocacy movement as well as the implementation of interventions that value families as equal partners (Lourie et al., 1998). In the same vein, the demand for effective outcomes and high-quality services by families served in systems of care may be the force that triggers the level of change necessary to demonstrate improved outcomes in the clinical and functional domains.

REFERENCES

Achenbach, T. M., Dumenci, L., & Rescorla, L. A. (2003). Are America's children's problems still getting worse? *Journal of Emotional and Behavioral Disorders, 10*(4), 194–203.

Armstrong, K. H., Dedrick, R. F., & Greenbaum, P. E. (2003). Factors associated with community adjustment of young adults with serious emotional disturbance: A longitudinal analysis. *Journal of Emotional and Behavioral Disorders, 11*(2), 66–76.

Bickman, L., Guthrie, P. R., Foster, E. M., Lambert, E. W., Summerfelt, W. T., Breda, C. S., et al. (1995). *Evaluating managed mental health services: The Fort Bragg experiment.* New York: Plenum Press.

Bickman, L., Lambert, E. W., Andrade, A. R., & Penaloza, R. V. (2000). The Fort Bragg continuum of care for children and adolescents: Mental health outcomes over 5 years. *Journal of Consulting and Clinical Psychology, 68*(4), 710–716.

Bickman, L., Noser, K., & Summerfelt, W. T. (1999). Long-term effects of a system of care on children and adolescents. *Journal of Behavioral Health Services and Research, 26,* 185–202.

Burns, B. J. (2002). Reasons for hope for children and families: A perspective and overview. In B. J. Burns & K. Hoagwood (Eds.), *Community treatment for youth: Evidence-based interventions for severe emotional and behavioral disorders* (pp. 3–15). New York: Oxford University Press.

Burns, B. J., & Hoagwood, K. (2002). *Community treatment for youth: Evidence-based interventions for severe emotional and behavioral disorders.* New York: Oxford University Press.

Canino, G., Costello, E. J., & Angold, A. (1999). Assessing functional impairment and social adaptation for child mental health services research: A review of measures. *Mental Health Services Research, 1,* 93–108.

Center for Mental Health Services. (1999). *Annual report to Congress on the evaluation of the Comprehensive Community Mental Health Services for Children and Their Families Program, 1999.* Atlanta: ORC Macro.

Costello, E. J., Gordon, P., Keeler, M. S., & Angold, A. (2001). Poverty, race/ethnicity, and psychatric disorder: A study of rural children. *American Journal of Public Health, 91*(1), 1494–1498.

Day, C., & Roberts, M. (1991). Activities of the child and adolescent service system program for improving mental health services for children and families. *Journal of Clinical Child Psychology, 20,* 340–350.

Duchnowski, A. J., Johnson, M. K., Hall, K. S., Kutash, K., & Friedman, R. M. (1993). The alternatives to residential treatment study: Initial findings. *Journal of Emotional and Behavioral Disorders, 1,* 17–26.

Duchnowski, A. J., Kutash, K., & Friedman, R. M. (2002). Community-based interventions in a system of care and outcomes framework. In B. J. Burns & K. Hoagwood (Eds.), *Community treatment for youth: Evidence-based interventions for severe emotional and behavioral disorders* (pp. 16–37). New York: Oxford University Press.

Foster, E. M. (1998). Does the continuum of care improve the timing of follow-up services? *Journal of the American Academy of Child and Adolescent Psychiatry, 37*(8), 805–814.

Friedman, R. M. (2002, July). *Children's mental health: A status report and call to action.* Paper presented to the President's New Freedom Commission on Mental Health, Washington, DC.

Friedman, R. M., & Burns, B. J. (1996). The evaluation of the Fort Bragg demonstration project: An alternative interpretation of the findings. *Journal of Mental Health Administration, 23,* 128–136.

Friedman, R. M., Katz-Leavy, J. W., Manderscheid, R. W., & Sondheimer, D. L. (1996). Prevalence of serious emotional disturbance in children and adolescents. In R. W. Manderscheid & M. A. Sonnenschein (Eds.), *Mental health, United States, 1996* (pp. 71–89). Rockville, MD: Substance Abuse and Mental Health Services Administration.

Friedman, R. M., Kutash, K., & Duchnowski, A. J. (1996). The population of concern: Defining the issues. In B. A. Stroul (Ed.), *Children's mental health: Creating systems of care in a changing society* (pp. 69–96). Baltimore: Brookes.

Greenbaum, P. E., & Dedrick, R. F. (2003). *Developmental trajectories of substance use and substance services among adolescents with serious emotional disturbance: Parallel processes of growth mixture modeling.* Paper presented at the 11th annual meeting of the Society for Prevention Research, Washington, DC.

Hoagwood, K., Jensen, P. S., Petti, T., & Burns, B. J. (1996). Outcomes of mental health care for children and adolescents: I. A comprehensive conceptual model. *Journal of the American Academy of Child and Adolescent Psychiatry, 35*(8), 1055–1063.

Hodges, K., Doucette-Gates, A., & Liao, Q. (1999). The relationship between the Child and Adolescent Functional Assessment Scale (CAFAS) and indicators of functioning. *Journal of Child and Family Studies, 8,* 109–122.

Hodges, K., & Wotring, J. (2000). Client typology based on functioning across domains using the CAFAS: Implications for service planning. *Journal of Behavioral Health Services and Research, 27,* 257–270.

Hogan, M. (2002). Foreword. *Interim report to the president.* Washington, DC: President's New Freedom Commission on Mental Health.

Joint Commission on the Mental Health of Children. (1969). *Crisis in child mental health: Challenge for the 1970s.* New York: Harper & Row.

Kataoka, S. H., Zang, L., & Wells, K.B. (2002). Unmet need for mental health care among U.S. children: Variations by ethnicity and insurance status. *American Journal of Psychiatry, 159,* 1549–1555.

Knapp, M. S. (1995). How shall we study comprehensive, collaborative services for children and families? *Educational Researcher, 24*(4), 5–16.

Knitzer, J. (1982). *Unclaimed children: The failure of public responsibility to children and adolescents in need of mental health services.* Washington, DC: The Children's Defense Fund.

Koplan, J. P., & Fleming, D. W. (2000). Current and future public health challenges. *Journal of the American Medical Association, 284,* 1696–1698.

Kutash, K., & Duchnowski, A. J. (1997). Creating comprehensive and collaborative systems. *Journal of Emotional and Behavioral Disorders, 5,* 66–75.

Kutash, K., & Duchnowski, A. J. (2004). The mental health needs of youth with emotional and behavioral disabilities placed in special education programs in urban schools. *Journal of Child and Family Studies, 13*(2), 235–248.

Kutash, K., Duchnowski, A. J., Robbins, V., Calvanese, P. K., Oliveira, B., Black, M., et al. (2000). The school and community study: Characteristics of students who have emotional and behavioral disabilities served in restructuring public schools. *Journal of Child and Family Studies, 9*(2), 175–190.

Lavigne, J. V., Gibbons, R. D., Christoffel, K. K., Arend, R., Rosenbaum, D., Binns, H., et al. (1996). Prevalence rates and correlates of psychiatric disorders among preschool children. *Journal of the American Academy of Child and Adolescent Psychiatry, 35*(2), 204–214.

Lourie, I., Stroul, B., & Friedman, R. M. (1998). Principles of a community-based system of care. In M. Epstein, K. Kutash, & A. Duchnowski (Eds.), *Outcomes for children and youth with emotional and behavioral disorders and their families: Programs and evaluation best practices* (pp. 3–20). Austin, TX: PRO-ED.

Muthén, B., & Muthén, L. (2000). Integrating person-centered and variable-centered analyses: Growth mixture modeling with latent trajectory classes. *Alcoholism: Clinical and Experimental Research, 24,* 882–891.

National Institute of Mental Health. (2001). *Blueprint for change: Research on child and adolescent mental health.* Washington, DC: The National Advisory Mental Health Council Workgroup on Child and Mental Health Intervention Development and Deployment.

President's Commission on Excellence in Special Education. (2002). *A new era: Revitalizing special education for children and their families.* Jessup, MD: ED Publications.

Roberts R. E, Attkisson C., & Rosenblatt, A. (1998). Prevalence of psychopathology among children and adolescents. *American Journal of Psychiatry, 155,* 715–725.

Rosenblatt, A. (1998). Assessing the child and family outcomes of systems of care for youth with serious emotional disturbance. In M. H. Epstein, K. Kutash, & A. J. Duchnowski (Eds.), *Outcomes for children and youth with behavioral and emotional disorders and their families* (pp. 329–362). Austin, TX: PRO-ED.

Silver, S. E., Duchnowski, A. J., Kutash, K., Friedman, R. M., Eisen, M., Prange, M. E., et al. (1992). A comparison of children with serious emotional disturbance served in residential and school settings. *Journal of Child and Family Studies, 1,* 43–59.

Slade, E. P. (2002). Effects of school-based mental health programs on mental health service use by adolescents at school and in the community. *Mental Health Services Research, 4*(3), 151–166.

Stroul B. A., & Friedman, R. M. (1986). *A system of care for children and youth with severe emotional disturbances.* Washington, DC: Georgetown University Child Development Center.

Stroul, B. A., & Friedman, R. M. (1996). The system of care concept and philosophy. In B. A. Stroul (Ed.), *Children's mental health: Creating systems of care in a changing society* (pp. 3–22). Baltimore: Brookes.

U.S. Department of Education, Office of Elementary and Secondary Education. (2002). *No child left behind: A desktop reference.* Washington, DC: Author.

U.S. Department of Health and Human Services. (1999). A report of the Surgeon General. Rockville, MD: U.S. Public Health Service.

Wagner, M. (2003). *A national view of students with emotional disturbances.* Paper presented at the 16th annual research and training center conference, Tampa.

Wagner, M., Cameto, R., & Newman, L. (2003). *Youth with disabilities: A changing population. A report of findings from the National Longitudinal Transition Study (NLTS) and the National Longitudinal Transition Study–2 (NLTS–2).* Menlo Park, CA: SRI International.

The Epidemiology of Mental Health Problems and Service Use in Youth

CHAPTER 2

Results from the Great Smoky Mountains Study

Elizabeth M. Z. Farmer, Sarah A. Mustillo, Barbara J. Burns, and E. Jane Costello

The current volume focuses on knowledge of best practices and outcomes for treating children with emotional and behavioral disorders. Most chapters focus on interventions and findings from innovative, state-of-the art approaches to meeting the needs of children and their families. This chapter sets the context for such work by examining the prevalence of emotional and behavioral disorders in the general population and patterns of service use among children with such problems.

This chapter focuses primarily on data from the Great Smoky Mountains Study (GSMS), an ongoing epidemiologic study of mental health problems and service use (Burns et al., 1995; Costello, Angold, Burns, Erkanli, et al., 1996; Costello, Angold, Burns, Stangl, et al., 1996). There is a paucity of data on the prevalence of mental health problems among children and a particularly conspicuous absence of studies that include detailed longitudinal data on both mental health problems and interventions intended to treat such problems. Data on the 1,420 children included in the Great Smoky Mountains Study provide an excellent opportunity to examine prevalence, continuity of disorder, comorbidity, functional impairment, sequences and patterns of service use, and naturalistic data on the effectiveness of "usual" care. Such information provides the context for studies of effective care and best practices, suggests key mediating and moderating factors, and supplies essential data for policy. It helps to place service-related findings in the context of all children with problems—those who make their way into various types of treatment as well as those who do not.

THE GREAT SMOKY MOUNTAINS STUDY

The GSMS, which began a decade ago, is being conducted in an 11-county area in the mountainous western region of North Carolina. This area was selected for several reasons. It represents an understudied section of the United

States—rural areas of the South and the Southeast. The population is nearly evenly divided between an urban center (Asheville) and dispersed rural small towns and individual homes. Nearly all children in the area attend public schools (which, as will be discussed below, provided the sampling frame for the study). In addition, the region includes the Qualla Boundary Reservation, home to the Eastern Band of the Cherokee Nation. Hence, it provides opportunities to explore psychiatric problems and service use among a representative sample of children and a unique chance to explore issues related to an understudied rural area and minority group.

Methodology

The GSMS was designed to (a) understand the developmental pathways of a large sample of children with a high need for mental health care; (b) estimate prevalence of disorders and risk factors in the population; (c) map the identified cases onto the general population; and (d) explore patterns of service use and outcomes among a representative sample of children (Costello, Angold, Burns, Stangl, et al., 1996).

Sample

Details of the sampling approach can be found elsewhere (Costello, Angold, Burns, Stangl, et al., 1996). The study used a two-stage sampling design. Briefly, children aged 9, 11, and 13 were randomly selected ($N = 4{,}500$) from a list generated from the school districts' management information systems (MIS) in the participating 11 counties. Parents completed a telephone screening questionnaire based upon externalizing items from the *Child Behavior Checklist* (Achenbach & Edelbrock, 1981, 1983). All children who scored above a predetermined cutoff were recruited into the study, as well as a 10% sample of children with lower scores. The cutoff was determined through pilot testing on clinical and general population children to provide adequate sensitivity and specificity for both service use and psychiatric diagnoses. This screen identified 1,346 eligible children, of whom 1,070 (79%) participated in the study.

As noted above, the geographic region included the Qualla Boundary. Some members of the Cherokee Nation attended public schools in the surrounding counties and were identified on the MIS. Others, however, attended school on the reservation. Therefore, a parallel study in the same geographic region included all 9-, 11-, and 13-year-old American Indians, regardless of where they attended school or their screen score. This sample contained 350 children (81% of eligibles).

To bring these samples together and to properly reflect population rates from the complex screening and sampling process, weights were attached to each respondent's data. Weights were inversely proportional to the sampling probability for children selected via the two-stage sampling and reflected the known population proportion of American Indians in the 11-county region. Throughout the chapter, we report percentages rather than actual numbers of respondents. These percentages have been weighted to reflect the total population from which the sample was recruited.

The sampling approach permits an accelerated cohort design. This means that the sample provides population-based estimates of mental health problems and service use for children aged 9 through 16, using multiple cohorts of youth at most ages to provide more robust estimates of rates. Questions about lifetime service use permit analyses of treatment trajectories that began prior to the GSMS study period.

The weighted sample reflects the composition of the area's youth population. It is nearly evenly divided between males (51%) and females (49%) and is predominantly White (90%). As noted above, American Indians were oversampled for the study. When weighted back to their population rate, American Indians account for approximately 4% of the region's population. An additional 7% of children are African American. At baseline, 24% of families were living below the federal poverty line, and 35% of children came from families in which the parent had not completed high school. Seventy-three percent of the children were covered by private health insurance, 14% were covered by public insurance (predominantly Medicaid or Indian Health Service coverage), and 13% were uninsured. Overall, on most variables, this sample appears to be quite representative of the United States and, more particularly, of the southeastern portion of the country. The only exception is the relatively few African American children in this region of the state.

Data Collection

Each child and a parent (the biological mother in 84% of cases) were interviewed at baseline and annually thereafter. Interviews were conducted with parent and child separately by different interviewers, and each interview lasted 2 to 3 hours. In addition, parents were contacted every 3 months between annual waves (by telephone where possible) to provide updated information on service use.

Measures

Analyses centered on three primary measures: the *Child and Adolescent Psychiatric Assessment* (CAPA; Angold & Fisher, 1999, Angold et al., 1995), the *Child and Adolescent Services Assessment* (CASA; Ascher, Farmer, Burns, & Angold, 1996; Farmer, Angold, Burns, & Costello, 1994), and *The Child and Adolescent Burden Assessment* (CABA; Messer, Angold, Costello, & Burns, 1996).

The CAPA gathers information on psychiatric symptomotology and associated functional impairment (Angold & Costello, 1995; Angold et al., 1995). It also collects data on a variety of domains (e.g., family composition, problems, and interactions; school attendance and performance; behavior in the home, community, and school). Computer algorithms have been developed to operationalize *DSM–III–R* and *DSM–IV* diagnoses. Test–retest reliability of CAPA diagnoses is comparable to that of other highly structured child psychiatric interviews (Angold & Costello, 1995; Angold & Fisher, 1999). All references to diagnoses in the current chapter are based on research-generated diagnoses from the CAPA and associated diagnostic algorithms.

The CASA gathers information from parents and children about services the children have received to address behavioral, emotional, or substance use problems (Ascher et al., 1996; Farmer et al., 1994). Service use is conceptualized broadly to include services delivered in a variety of settings and from a range of providers. For each type of service the respondent indicates whether the child has ever used that service and, if so, whether he or she has used the service in the 3 months preceding the interview. For most analyses, services are categorized into service sectors: specialty mental health (including inpatient and outpatient), education, child welfare, juvenile justice, and general medicine. The CASA has good to excellent test–retest reliability (Ascher et al., 1996; Farmer et al., 1994) and high concordance with provider records (Ascher et al., 1996; Bussing, Mason, Leon, & Sinha, 2003). Psychometrics are similar to other self- and parent reports of service use (Horwitz et al., 2001).

The CABA asks parents about possible impacts of the child's problems on the family. As with other measures of family impact (sometimes referred to as "burden"), the CABA covers both objective and subjective types of impact. Domains include financial impacts, effects on family relationships (both immediate and extended family), restriction of activities, stigma, and intrapersonal effects on the parent (e.g., worries, health problems, lack of confidence to handle problems). The measure has acceptable psychometrics and has been shown in previous work to be related to service use (Angold et al., 1998; Farmer, Burns, Angold, & Costello, 1997; Messer et al., 1996).

Analytic Approach

The complex sampling approach and repeated waves of data collection require statistical techniques that can account for autocorrelation across waves and design effects. Hence, as mentioned above, all results reported here refer to weighted percentages. Such percentages reflect estimates of rates, patterns, and relationships in the general population from which the sample was drawn. Statistical tests were performed using GENMOD within SAS, defining the type of correlation as unstructured, and using the generalized estimation equation (GEE) option with a logistic link function. We also used the robust variance estimates (i.e., sandwich type estimates), together with sampling weights to adjust standard errors of parameters to account for the two-phase sampling design. The use of multiwave data with appropriate sample weights capitalized on the multiple observation points over time while controlling for the effect on variance estimates of repeated measures.

Prevalence of Mental Health Problems

Background

A variety of studies during recent decades have attempted to estimate prevalence of psychiatric disorders among children (Anderson, Williams, McGee, & Silva, 1987; Cohen et al., 1993; McGee et al., 1990; Offord et al., 1987; Romano, Tremblay, Vitaro, Zoccolillo, & Pagani, 2001). Although there is variation in such estimates in terms of age range, sampling frames, respondents, measures, criteria for identifying disorder, time frame, and so forth, there has been an evolving consensus that approximately 20% of children in the general population meet criteria for some psychiatric disorder (Burns, Hoagwood, & Mrazek, 1999; Costello & Angold, 1995; U.S. Department of Health and Human Services, 1999).

Estimates of the prevalence of serious emotional disturbance (SED, defined as psychiatric diagnosis plus functional impairment) have varied in terms of the impairment criteria used. Friedman and colleagues (Friedman, Katz-Leavy, Manderscheid, & Sondheimer, 1996) estimated that 5% to 9% of the child population meet criteria for the most severe problems (psychiatric diagnosis plus extreme functional impairment) and 9% to 13% meet criteria if a less extreme definition of impairment is utilized. These findings are similar to those of an analysis of multiple studies by Costello and colleagues (Costello, Messer, Reinherz, Cohen, & Bird, 1998), who found rates of SED ranging from 5.4% to 7.4% with global impairment and 5.5% to 16.9% with domain-specific impairment.

For longitudinal studies with diagnostic information across time, cross-sectional prevalence of disorder increases as children age (8% among preschoolers, 12% for preadolescents, 15% for adolescents; Roberts, Attkisson, & Rosenblatt, 1998). There is substantial continuity of disorder across time. Using reports from published longitudinal studies, Costello and Angold (1995) showed 40% to 60% continuity of diagnoses (i.e., proportion of children who met diagnostic criteria at Wave 1 who continue to meet criteria at Wave 2).

GSMS Findings

Initial cross-sectional analyses of GSMS data supported the overall prevalence rate of approximately 20% for any diagnosis (overall rate of 20.3%; Costello, Angold, Burns, Erkanli, et al., 1996). These figures were based on initial interviews with parents and children, so they referred to children aged 9, 11, and 13 and covered symptoms evident in the 3 months preceding the interview. Emotional disorders (e.g., affective and anxiety disorders) were evident in 6.8% of the population, and behavioral disorders (e.g., conduct, oppositional, and attentional disorders) were seen in 6.6%. "Other" disorders (e.g., encopresis, enuresis, tics, Tourette's syndrome, obsessive compulsive disorder, bulimia, trichotillomania) were evident in 10.5% of the population, with considerably higher rates in boys than girls (14.96% vs. 5.87%). Comorbidity was substantial: 53% of children with depression, 38% of children with behavioral disorders, and 28% of children with anxiety disorders met criteria for additional diagnoses.

The GSMS data also have indicated the potential importance of recognizing functional impairment as an important element of categorizing and treating mental health problems among children. In cross-sectional analyses from Wave 1, 7.4% of children met criteria for both diagnosis and impairment (i.e., SED); 11.5% met criteria for a diagnosis but did not display significant functional impairment; and 14.2% showed significant impairment without meeting criteria for any diagnosis (Angold, Costello, Farmer, Burns, & Erkanli, 1999). In many studies, this final group of children would not be included as children with "problems," and in treatment settings they may not meet diagnostic criteria to justify treatment and/or payment. However, when children in this "impaired but undiagnosed" group are compared to children in the other groups on a number of dimensions (e.g., use of specialty mental health services, family impact, parent or child perception that the child has a problem or needs help), they are second to children with SED in all dimensions. For example, approximately 20% of children with SED, 10% of children with impairment only, and fewer than 5% of children with diagnosis only received specialty mental health services. For nearly 60% of children with SED, parent or child perceived that the child had a problem or needed help. This was true for approximately 30% of children with impairment only and for fewer than 20% of children with diagnosis only.

Current data from the GSMS sample include data on all children from age 9 through age 16. These cumulative data suggest that the widely used point prevalence estimate of 20% may downplay the magnitude of the number of children who are affected by psychiatric disorders. As Table 2.1 shows, cumulative rates of disorder suggest a substantially higher prevalence. Overall, 36.7% of children met criteria for some disorder between ages 9 and 16 (42.3% of boys and 31% of girls; Costello, Mustillo, Keeler, & Angold, 2003).

This recent work on the GSMS data has also provided new insights on continuity of disorder. Children who met criteria for a diagnosis at a given wave were more than three times more likely to have a diagnosis at a subsequent wave than children who had no previous disorder (Costello et al., 2003). Continuity (both within a given disorder and across disorders) was significantly higher in girls than in boys (Costello et al., 2003).

Data from the GSMS suggest a slightly different age-specific prevalence than that identified by Roberts et al. (1998), who found that increased age was associated with increased prevalence. Instead, as illustrated in Figure 2.1, longitudinal data from the GSMS showed that cross-sectional (i.e., 3-month) prevalence for any disorder was highest among 9- to 10-year-olds, dipped to its lowest level at ages 12 and 13, and then rose but remained relatively stable through age 16.

TABLE 2.1
Predictive Cumulative Prevalence of Psychiatric Disorders by Age 16

Disorder	Total % (SE)	Female % (SE)	Male % (SE)
Any disorder	36.7 (2.7)	31.0 (2.3)	42.3 (3.1)
Serious emotional disturbance	13.4 (1.8)	11.2 (1.7)	15.6 (1.8)
Any emotional disorder	15.0 (1.7)	17.1 (1.7)	13.0 (1.6)
Any anxiety disorder	9.9 (1.5)	12.1 (1.5)	7.7 (1.4)
Any depressive disorder	9.5 (1.1)	11.7 (1.2)	7.3 (1.0)
Any behavioral disorder	23.0 (1.7)	16.1 (1.2)	29.9 (2.2)

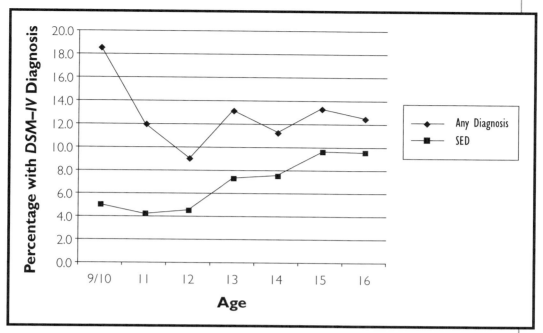

FIGURE 2.1. Three-month prevalence of any diagnosis and serious emotional disturbance (SED), by age.

Data on prevalence of SED across time followed quite a different trend from overall diagnoses. Cumulatively, 13% of children met criteria for SED at some point between ages 9 and 16. As shown in Figure 2.1, cross-sectional prevalence of SED increased with age and nearly doubled (from 4% to 7%) between ages 12 and 13. Although it was more common among boys than girls at all ages, the increased prevalence of SED with age was parallel for both genders.

Figure 2.1 shows that age 12 was a turning point in prevalence of disorder in several ways. As noted above, point prevalence of any diagnosis was lowest at this age. Costello et al. (2003) have suggested that at this developmental point, the prominent disorders of childhood (e.g., attention-deficit/hyperactivity disorder [ADHD], separation anxiety, enuresis, encopresis, tics) have subsided and the disorders more common in adolescence (e.g., depression, social phobia, drug abuse and dependence) have not yet appeared. It also signals a turning point in the likelihood that a child with a diagnosis will display significant functional impairment. Prior to age 12, the majority of children with a diagnosis did not meet criteria for SED. Beginning at 13, and becoming more pronounced as adolescence progressed, children were less likely to meet diagnostic criteria without also displaying substantial functional impairment.

Rates and Patterns of Service Use

Background
With increasing recognition of the number of children who have significant mental health problems, there has been corresponding interest in services

children receive to address such problems. There has been long-standing concern that many children who need mental health services do not receive them and that those who do receive them may be served in overly restrictive placements (Burns, 1991; Knitzer, 1982). Federal focus on this combination of issues resulted in development and dissemination of the Child and Adolescent Service System Program (CASSP; Stroul, 1993; Stroul & Friedman, 1986). CASSP provided guiding principles and technical assistance for states and communities throughout the nation to develop a continuum of services that would assist child-serving agencies to work together in a system of care to meet the multiple needs of children and their families. These initiatives have modified contemporary views of appropriate care for children with mental health problems (particularly children who are served via the public system), and available evidence suggests that they may improve access to services, range of services, and coordination of services (e.g., Burns, Farmer, Angold, Costello, & Behar, 1996; Stroul, 1993).

However, recent large-scale studies have all continued to show a substantial gap between the number of children with mental health problems and the number of children receiving mental health services (Burns et al., 1995; Kataoka, Zhang, & Wells, 2002; Ringel & Sturm, 2001; Verhulst & van der Ende, 1997). Recent meta-analyses from three large-scale studies (the National Health Interview Survey, the National Survey of American Families, and the Community Tracking Survey) show that 6% to 7.5% of children ages 6 to 17 received mental health services during the preceding year (Kataoka et al., 2002). Assuming even the conservative estimate of 20% of children with a mental health problem, there appears to be substantial underserving of children with problems.

GSMS Findings

The GSMS provides invaluable data on this front. At each annual wave, the CASA was used to ask parents and children about services the children used to address behavioral, emotional, or substance use problems. Data were collected for the past 3 months as well as for any use during the child's lifetime. These data provide a unique contribution to the literature in two ways. First, they include longitudinal data on service use across time. Second, they expand the definition of mental health services beyond the specialty mental health sector (i.e., inpatient and outpatient services provided by professionals within the mental health sector [psychologists, psychiatrists, clinical social workers]) to include services received from the broad system of care that serves children (Stroul & Friedman, 1986). Therefore, service use can be examined across time and from a wide range of providers. In addition, the rich data on psychiatric problems and family and child factors may be incorporated into analyses to explore factors that drive service use.

Overall Rates of Service Use

Early cross-sectional analyses of the GSMS data from the baseline wave (i.e., for children who were 9, 11, and 13) showed rates of use similar to those found in other cross-sectional studies (e.g., Verhulst & van der Ende, 1997). Approximately 20% of the general population met criteria for a psychiatric diagnosis, but only 4% of the population had used mental health services in the preceding 3 months. However, these initial analyses suggested a pattern of service use that laid important ground work for subsequent thinking and analyses. Although only 4% of children had received services from the specialty mental health sector, 16% had received services from some source to address a relevant problem (Burns et al., 1995). This higher prevalence of use included services provided by schools, juvenile justice, child welfare, and general medicine. More specifically, these analyses suggested the central role of schools in providing care for children.

These analyses also modified the picture of unmet need. Other studies have suggested that 75% to 80% of children with mental health problems do not receive any treatment (Kataoka et al., 2002; Ringel & Sturm, 2001). The cross-sectional analyses of GSMS data support at least this figure. Twenty percent of youth with SED and 12% of youth with a diagnosis (but without meeting criteria for SED) had received treatment within the mental health sector during the preceding 3 months. However, when the definition of *service* was expanded to include other sectors, 52% of youth with SED and 36% of youth with diagnosis (but not SED) had received services from some source (Burns et al., 1995).

Service Use by Sectors

These results suggest the importance of examining the full range of services that parents of children may utilize to address mental health problems. Data from the GSMS show that by age 16, more than half of the sample (62%) had used some type of service to address a mental health problem. As shown in Table 2.2, the most common provider of such services was the educational system (47%). Although some children received services via special education

TABLE 2.2
Service Use Point Prevalence, 3 Months and Lifetime (Through Age 16)

Service	3 Months			Lifetime
	Total Sample	Diagnosis Only	Diagnosis with Impairment (SED)	Total Sample
Any services	19%	36%	52%	62%
Specialty mental health	6%	12%	20%	29%
Education	9%	22%	22%	47%
General medicine	3%	7%	10%	17%
Social services	1%	2%	5%	8%
Juvenile justice	2%	2%	8%	5%

Note. SED = serious emotional disturbance.

within schools, the majority of the school-based care was provided by counselors, psychologists, and social workers within the school setting.

The specialty mental health sector was the second most commonly used service sector. It provided services to approximately 6% of the population during any given 3-month period and to 29% of the population by the time they reached age 16. Various analyses have shown what appears to be appropriate triaging of services, so that children with more severe psychiatric problems are more likely to be served within the mental health specialty sector (Burns et al., 1995; Farmer, Stangl, Burns, Costello, & Angold, 1999). As noted above, during each 3-month reporting period, 20% of children with SED had received services from the specialty mental health sector, compared to 12% of children with a diagnosis (but not SED).

General medicine was the third most common provider of services for children's mental health problems. Approximately 3% of the population received services from a pediatrician or family doctor during any given 3-month period, and 17% received such services at some point in their lives.

Relatively few youth received services for a mental health problem from either the social services sector or from juvenile justice. Approximately 1% to 2% received each of these types of services within any given reporting period, and 5% to 8% of the population received such services during their lifetime (up to age 16).

Patterns of Service Use Across Time

Analyses of service use across time began with examination of where children entered services. These analyses included data on where children entered the service system for children who entered services prior to the GSMS data collection period (i.e., before they were 9, 11, or 13) as well as for those who first entered services during the study period (Farmer, Burns, Phillips, Angold, & Costello, 2003). Therefore, for all youth, the term *sector of entry* refers to the first service a youth received in his or her life.

The education sector provided the point of entry for 60% of service users. Specialty mental health was the point of entry for approximately one-quarter of service users (27.3%), and general medicine provided the first service for approximately 13% of users. As expected, given the few children who used such services, child welfare and juvenile justice provided the point of entry for very few children (6.5% and 2.5%, respectively). These percentages sum to more than 100% because for approximately 9% of children, entry into services involved multiple services within a single episode of care, and it was not possible to determine a primary sector of entry.

Although education was the most common point of entry for children, it was also the sector that was least likely to lead to subsequent use of other services. Only 31% of children who entered services via the education sector went on to receive services elsewhere. This contrasts markedly with children who entered services via specialty mental health. For such children, fully 62% subsequently received services from at least one other child-serving sector (Farmer et al., 2003).

Service Use by Age

Given shifting rates of disorder across time, it is important to know whether services show corresponding variations in provision of services. As noted above, 3-month point prevalence of disorder was highest among 9- to 10-year-olds, dropped to a low around age 12, and then increased to a new relatively stable rate during adolescence. SED, in contrast, showed a progressive increase in point prevalence as children aged.

Figure 2.2 shows prevalence of service use by children of different ages. Patterns of any service use and use of specialty mental health services both showed a decrease at age 12 that mirrored the shifts in diagnosis. From ages 13 through 16, use of specialty mental health services increased, perhaps reflecting increasing rates of SED. Services via the education sector, in contrast, showed a relatively linear decline as children aged.

Factors Related to Service Use

Background

Use of mental health services may be driven by a wide range of factors. These may include characteristics of the child, his or her family, the surrounding social system, and the service system (e.g., Aday & Andersen, 1974; Andersen, 1995; Costello, Pescosolido, Angold, & Burns, 1998). As noted above, substantial numbers of children with mental health problems do not receive any care for such problems, and many children who do receive care receive it outside

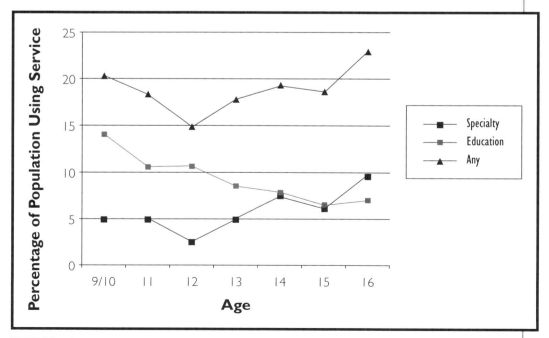

FIGURE 2.2. Three-month prevalence of service use by age.

of the specialty mental health sector. This section examines factors that influenced use of mental health services from a range of providers.

GSMS data have provided a wealth of information about factors that drive service use. These analyses have been based on cross-sectional snapshots or on short-term follow-ups. Such analyses have provided important information about service use, but they have not utilized the overlapping cohort design and large sample size to examine factors related to service use across the full range and sample of 9- to 16-year-olds.

Analyses include a set of explanatory variables that have been shown, in previous analyses of the GSMS data and other data sets, to be related to service use. These include severity or type of mental health problems (e.g., Cohen, Kasen, Brooks, & Stuening, 1991; Farmer et al., 1999; Leaf et al., 1996); demographic characteristics of the children (age, gender, race; e.g., Angold et al., 2002; Canino, Gould, Prupis, & Shaffer, 1986; Kataoka et al., 2002); characteristics of families (parental psychopathology, parental education, poverty; e.g., Hoberman, 1992; Verhulst & van der Ende, 1997); insurance coverage (e.g., Burns et al., 1995; Kataoka et al., 2002); and impact of the child's problems on the family (e.g., Angold et al., 1998; Farmer et al., 1997). Given the common geographic area and service system available to included children, system-level factors were not considered in these analyses.

The above description of service use by sectors and across time has included lifetime service use. Although these analyses are useful for describing patterns of service use across time, predictor variables are available only for the period between ages 9 and 16, while children and parents were completing annual GSMS interviews. Therefore, the following analyses on factors related to service use focus on service use during the primary reporting periods of the GSMS data collection. Analyses thus reflect predictors and service use during the 3-month period preceding each interview. This approach makes it possible to use all of the available data across years to examine relationships between concurrent psychiatric problems and other predictors and service use.

GSMS Findings

Analyses began with examination of bivariate relationships between predictor variables and service use (see Table 2.3). Figures in each column indicate the percentage of children in that category who used the indicated service (e.g., 19% of boys used any service; 6% used specialty mental health services).

These bivariate relationships show that boys and girls displayed quite similar types of service use. Significant differences were noted only for juvenile justice, a sector that was utilized by very few children.

Findings on race, in these bivariate analyses, showed relatively small absolute differences in service use across racial groups (i.e., Whites, African Americans, American Indians). When differences were evident, these figures suggest that prevalence of service use was disproportionately higher among minorities than Whites. For African Americans, this effect was significant only for services from child welfare. For American Indians, it held true for any services, education, juvenile justice, and use of multiple sectors.

TABLE 2.3

Bivariate Statistics of Independent Variables and 3-Month Service Use

Independent Variables	Any Service Use	Specialty Mental Health	Education	Social Services	General Medical	Justice	Multiple Sectors
			Dependent Variables [a]				
Gender							
Male	19	6	9	2	3	2**	16
Female	18	6	8	1	3	1	15
Race							
White	18	6	8	1	3	1	15
African American	22	8	12	6**	3	4	20
American Indian	22*	5	13**	1	3	4**	19*
Psychiatric disorder							
Any diagnosis	44**	16**	22**	4**	9**	4**	38**
SED	52**	20**	22**	5**	10**	8**	43**
Any diagnosis except SED	36**	12**	22**	2	7**	1*	32**
Parent's education							
<High school	23**	7	11**	2**	4	3**	20**
>High school	16	5	7	1	3	1	13
Parent's psychological state							
Parental mental illness	29**	11**	13**	2*	4*	2	25**
No parental mental illness	13	3	6	1	3	1	11
Poverty							
Poor	28**	8**	16**	3**	3	3**	23**
Not poor	16	5	7	1	3	1	13
Insurance							
Public	33**	14**	17**	5**	5*	5**	30**
Private	15**	5**	7**	0**	3*	1**	13**
Family impact							
Two or more	60**	27**	25**	6**	14**	7**	54**
One or none	14	3	7	1	2	1	11

[a] Numbers indicate percentage of youth in category who used service. SED = serious emotional disturbance.

*p < .05. **p < .01.

As expected, psychiatric problems were related to increased prevalence of service use (compared to children who did not meet criteria for a specific disorder) for all types of services. Children with SED were significantly more likely than children with a diagnosis (but not SED) to use any services, multiple services, specialty mental health, and juvenile justice services.

Parental and family factors (included here as low parental education, parental history of psychiatric problems, living in poverty, family impact) were related to increased use of a variety of services. A history of parental psychopathology was related to increased use of all services except juvenile justice. Low levels of parental education were associated with increased use of all services except specialty mental health and general medicine. Children living below the federal poverty line were more likely to use all services except general medicine. Children whose parents perceived a substantial negative impact on the family because of the child's problems were also more likely to receive services across all sectors.

Data on health insurance coverage showed a predictable hierarchical pattern across all service sectors (Burns et al., 1995). Children without insurance showed the lowest rates of service use, children with private insurance displayed mid-level use across all sectors, and children with public insurance showed the highest rates of use.

The above analyses suggest differential service use based on characteristics of children, families, and available resources. These bivariate relationships provide a portrait of which children are most likely to be receiving services (i.e., poor minority children with a psychiatric diagnosis [particularly SED] whose parents have low levels of education and a history of psychiatric problems and who are covered by public insurance). These associations, however, do not indicate which of these factors may be driving service use and which are spuriously related to it.

The following analyses include multivariate models to examine which factors predict service use, net of other factors. Models included all of the predictors discussed in the bivariate tables. Information on psychiatric problems was included in two ways—whether the child met criteria for any *DSM–IV* diagnosis during the relevant interval and, in a separate model, whether the child met criteria for SED versus a diagnosis (but not SED). Analyses were conducted for four dependent variables to examine factors related to different types of services. Dependent variables focused on use of any services (i.e., whether the child received services during the period from any provider), specialty mental health services, educational services, and services from multiple providers (within the designated 3-month period). Separate models were not run for services received via social services, general medicine, or juvenile justice sectors due to the relatively few children who received services in these sectors. All coefficients in Table 2.4 are odds ratios, with standard errors in parentheses. An odds ratio indicates the increased (or decreased) likelihood that a youth has of displaying the focal outcome in comparison to youth in the reference category.

Across all examined types of service use, the child's psychiatric problems were a primary explanatory factor. In all cases, children with a diagnosis

TABLE 2.4

Predicting 3-Month Service Use for Full Sample—Odds Ratios and (Robust Standard Errors)

	Any Services		Specialty Mental Health		Education		Multiple Sectors	
Male	0.98 (.02)	0.98 (.02)	0.99 (.01)	0.99 (.01)	0.99 (.01)	0.99 (.01)	0.99 (02)	1.00 (.02)
Age (years)	1.00 (.00)	1.00 (.00)	1.01 (.00)**	1.01 (.00)**	0.99 (.00)	0.99 (.00)**	1.00 (.00)	1.00 (.00)
Race: African American	0.99 (.04)	0.99 (.04)	0.99 (.02)	0.99 (.02)	1.02 (.04)	1.02 (.04)	1.00 (.04)	1.00 (.04)
Race: American Indian	0.98 (.02)	0.98 (.02)	0.95 (.01)**	0.95 (.01)**	1.00 (.02)	1.01 (.02)	0.97 (.02)	0.97 (.02)
Diagnosis (any)	1.18 (.03)**		1.05 (.01)**		1.09 (.03)**		1.14 (.04)**	
Diagnosis (without SED)		1.17 (.05)**		1.05 (.02)*		1.12 (.04)**		1.16 (.05)**
Diagnosis + impairment (SED)		1.18 (.04)**		1.05 (.03)*		1.06 (.03)*		1.11 (.04)**
Poverty	1.03 (.02)	1.03 (.02)	0.99 (.01)	0.98 (.01)	1.03 (.02)	1.03 (.02)	1.00 (.02)	1.00 (.02)
Parent education	1.02 (.02)	1.02 (.02)	1.00 (.01)	1.00 (.01)	1.01 (.01)	1.01 (.01)	1.03 (.02)	1.02 (.03)
Parent psychiatric history	1.10 (.02)**	1.10 (.02)**	1.05 (.01)**	1.05 (.01)**	1.04 (.01)**	1.04 (.01)**	1.08 (.02)**	1.08 (.02)**
Insurance: public	1.09 (.03)**	1.09 (.03)**	1.11 (.03)**	1.11 (.03)**	1.02 (.03)	1.02 (.03)	1.12 (.03)**	1.12 (.03)**
Insurance: private	1.00 (.02)	1.00 (.02)	1.02 (.01)	1.02 (.01)	0.99 (.02)	0.98 (.02)	1.01 (.02)	1.01 (.02)
Family impact (continuous)	1.08 (.01)**	1.08 (.01)***	1.05 (.01)**	1.05 (.01)**	1.04 (.01)**	1.04 (.01)**	1.08 (.01)**	1.08 (.01)**

Note. SED = serious emotional disturbance.

*$p < .05$. **$p < .01$.

were more likely to receive services than children who did not meet diagnostic criteria. These results suggest that once other factors are accounted for, children with SED and children with a diagnosis but not SED are approximately equally likely to receive services across sectors.

Two other factors were significant across all models, and both suggest the importance of family factors in service delivery to children. Regardless of type of service, children whose parents had experienced psychiatric problems in their own lives were more likely to receive services. And, across all services, children whose parents reported greater impact of the child's problems on the family were more likely to receive services.

Child's age provides additional explanatory value in two of the models, but in different directions. Controlling for other factors, older children were more likely to use specialty mental health services and less likely to receive educational services.

Recall that in the bivariate analyses, minority children were somewhat more likely to receive a variety of services. The multivariate models suggest that these findings emerged because of the correlation between race and other factors that lead to service use. Once other factors were held constant, American Indian children were significantly less likely to receive specialty mental health services and services from multiple providers.

Insurance played a role in receipt of services, except for services provided by the education sector. For any services, specialty mental health services, and multiple services, children with public insurance were more likely to receive services than were children with no insurance. Children with private insurance were indistinguishable from uninsured children in their patterns of service use.

SUMMARY AND DISCUSSION

Summary of Key Findings

This chapter has presented findings on psychiatric disorder and service use among a general population sample of children. Primary data collection covers ages 9 to 16. Therefore, results have focused on diagnoses and service use during these years. Retrospective data on onset of service use also make it possible to examine pathways into services, even for service users who entered services prior to study entry.

Cross-sectional analyses and the GSMS data support other widely published point prevalence estimates suggesting that approximately 20% of children meet criteria for a psychiatric diagnosis at any point in time. However, between ages 9 and 16, GSMS data show substantially higher cumulative rates of disorder of 31% for girls and 42% for boys, for an overall rate of 37%.

Prior work has also suggested substantial gaps between the number of children with diagnoses and the number of children who receive services. Current published estimates suggest that as many as 80% of children who need services do not receive any. The current analyses of lifetime service use (up through age 16) and point prevalence (for 3-month intervals) continue to suggest substantial unmet need. However, the magnitude of the gap depends heavily on definitions of both service use and need.

As noted above, the education sector plays a primary role in children's mental health services—both as the most common provider of services and as the point of entry for many children. The educational sector, however, differs from other sectors in various potentially important ways. For example, although it is the most common portal of entry for children, it is also the entry point that is least likely to lead to subsequent services from other sectors. Unlike most other sectors, it is also relatively nonhierarchical in its treatment of children—children with SED were no more likely to receive services within education than were children with just a diagnosis. Finally, in contrast to increasing prevalence of disorder across time and increasing use of specialty mental health services as children age, the education sector was most involved with younger children and less involved with adolescents.

Bivariate and multivariate analyses examined factors related to receipt of services. The bivariate analyses painted a familiar picture of children who receive services—poor, minority children from troubled families who are covered by public insurance. In support of previous findings and in line with appropriate provision of services, multivariate analyses suggest that, controlling for other factors, severity of a child's problems was a significant predictor of service use. These models also showed that parental psychopathology and family impact were related to all examined types of service use. Children who were covered by public insurance showed increased use of all services, except education, where services are nearly always provided without a fee to the family. Despite bivariate analyses showing higher than expected proportions of minorities (particularly American Indians) among service users, multivariate models suggested that, controlling for other factors, American Indians were less likely to receive services, particularly in specialty mental health settings.

Limitations

Findings reported here focus on children from a single geographic area. Although this area is representative of large sections of the United States and provides a view of an understudied region, findings may be influenced by this context. The counties included in this study are served by a relatively well-developed public mental health system for children. Therefore, findings on rates of service use may be somewhat higher than for other, less developed, areas in the same region.

The included counties provide a rare opportunity to examine psychopathology and service use in a relatively large American Indian population. In contrast, the region has a small African American population. Findings from additional work in another region of North Carolina (Angold et al., 2002) suggest that findings from the current study on minority and majority children are similar for American Indians and African Americans. That is, minority and majority children show similar rates of psychiatric disorder but minority children show lower rates of services (controlling for other factors). The GSMS findings, though, cannot provide robust estimates for African Americans.

Rates of psychiatric problems and service use are likely to be conservative estimates for a number of reasons. First, diagnostic and impairment data and detailed data on service use are available only for 3-month windows during the GSMS interview period. This means that detailed information is available only for children ages 9 to 16. Within these years, the most complete data are available for the 3-month primary period of each annual interview. Data on rates of disorder, therefore, refer to children who met criteria during one or more of these focal periods. Services data are also most complete for these focal periods during GSMS collection. However, retrospective and telephone data have been included to examine patterns of service use prior to the GSMS period (i.e., services prior to ages 9, 11, or 13, depending on age at entry) and for the 9-month period between data collections. Therefore, estimates of lifetime service use should reflect all received services (allowing, of course, for errors in recall), whereas multivariate models of predicting service use reflected such use only during the focal annual windows.

The Great Smoky Mountains Study is an ongoing longitudinal study. Data in the current chapter have covered children up through age 16. Data on what happens to these children, both in terms of psychiatric problems and service use, as they leave adolescence and move into adulthood will be available in coming years. All findings, therefore, should be regarded as a work in progress. At present, the GSMS data provide one of the best opportunities to study psychopathology and associated service use among a representative cohort of children and adolescents within the contemporary United States.

Implications and Future Directions

The results presented here begin to bring together data on mental health problems and service use during a substantial portion of childhood and adolescence for a representative cohort of children. They reinforce and expand the idea that psychiatric disorders affect a substantial number of children in our society, and substantially more than are identified by frequently cited point prevalence estimates. They also show that more than half of the children in this representative sample had some contact with services designed to address a behavioral, emotional, or substance use problem.

Data on service use suggest appropriate triaging of care. Regardless of how analyses were run, most sectors were differentially treating children based on level of need. Children with SED were at increased likelihood of receiving services via specialty mental health and from multiple sectors within the child-serving system. Multivariate analyses suggest that a substantial portion of this triaging may be responding to factors associated with family issues (e.g., family impact, parental mental health problems).

As expected, the education sector served the broadest range of children. This more equilateral coverage is expected because the educational system is the only child-serving system that has contact with this broad range of children. However, all else being equal, entry to services via education was least likely to result in subsequent services from any other sector. Such services were also most commonly provided in the elementary grades and declined as children aged. This may suggest that education does a good job of providing minimal services for a wide range of children early in life but is not, perhaps, responsive to and supportive of the service needs of more severely affected children. Additional inquiry is necessary to determine why school-based services are relatively isolated and what approaches may be successful to encourage greater integration of the educational system into a system of care.

These findings reinforce the importance of recognizing family-related issues when serving children. For all types of services, children whose parent had experienced mental health problems and whose parent reported that the child's problems were creating a greater negative impact on the family were more likely to receive services. As discussed before, both of these factors suggest the importance of understanding the role of parents in help-seeking and service delivery for children (Costello, Pescosolido, et al., 1998). Additional work is necessary to more fully understand these findings. It is possible that both of these factors serve as signals for families who are confronting multiple challenges. It is also possible that families' perceived impact of problems may be an important indicator of the need for services, one that should be considered in future discussions of need and unmet need.

These findings also further confirm the potentially influential role of insurance in providing mental health care for children. For all services except education (which provides services free of charge to all children), children with public insurance were significantly more likely than uninsured or privately insured children to receive treatment. Public debate and policy initiatives have focused on increasing coverage and availability of services for uninsured children. This is clearly a necessary step. However, these results suggest the need to broaden the discussion and policy to support increased access for children with private insurance.

Finally, these findings suggest the importance of recognizing mental health problems and service use in the developmental pathways of children. Longitudinal data suggest that mental health problems—rather than being rare conditions or events—affect more than one-third of all children, that more than one-quarter of the population receives some type of intervention from the specialty mental health sector, and that nearly half of children in the general population have some contact with services via the education sector. These findings on high rates of both problems and treatment have potential impacts on a number of levels. Increased dissemination of this information may help reduce the stigma of mental health problems and help-seeking by portraying the former as a common and almost "normative" aspect of development. From developmental, theoretical, and research perspectives, these findings suggest that mental health problems and service use are common and potentially influential components of the developmental pathways of children that should be taken into account in studies of typical development, as well as in studies focused on psychopathology and treatment outcomes.

REFERENCES

Achenbach, T. M., & Edelbrock, C. S. (1981). Behavorial problems and competencies reported by parents of normal and disturbed children aged 4 through 16. *Monographs of the Society for Research in Child Development, 46*(1), 1–82.

Achenbach, T. M., & Edelbrock, C. S. (1983). *Manual for the Child Behavior Checklist and Child Behavior Profile.* Burlington: University of Vermont.

Aday, L., & Andersen, R. (1974). A framework for the study of access to medical care. *Health Services Research, 9*(3), 208–220.

Andersen, R. M. (1995). Revisiting the behavioral model and access to medical care: Does it matter? *Journal of Health and Social Behavior, 36,* 1–10.

Anderson, J. C., Williams, S., McGee, R., & Silva, P. A. (1987). DSM–III disorders in preadolescent children: Prevalence in a large sample from the general population. *Archives of General Psychiatry, 44,* 69–77.

Angold, A., & Costello, E. J. (1995). Developmental epidemiology. In D. Cicchetti & D. J. Cohen (Eds.), *Developmental psychopathology: Vol. 1. Theory and methods* (pp. 23–56). New York: Wiley.

Angold, A., Costello, E. J., Farmer, E. M., Burns, B. J., & Erkanli, A. (1999). Impaired but undiagnosed. *Journal of the American Academy of Child and Adolescent Psychiatry, 38*(2), 129–137.

Angold, A., Erkanli, A., Farmer, E., Fairbank, J., Burns, B., Keeler, G., et al. (2002). Psychiatric disorder, impairment, and service use in rural African American and White youth. *Archives of General Psychiatry, 59,* 893–901.

Angold, A., & Fisher, P. (1999). Interviewer-based interviews. In D. S. M. Rutter, C. P. Lucas, & J. E. Richters (Eds.), *Diagnostic assessment in child and adolescent psychopathology* (pp. 34–64). New York: Guilford Press.

Angold, A., Messer, S. C., Stangl, D., Farmer, E. M. Z., Costello, E. J., & Burns, B. J. (1998). Perceived parental burden and service use for child and adolescent psychiatric disorders. *American Journal of Public Health, 88*(1), 75–80.

Angold, A., Prendergast, M., Cox, A., Harrington, R., Simonoff, E., & Rutter, M. (1995). The Child and Adolescent Psychiatric Assessment (CAPA). *Psychological Medicine, 25,* 739–753.

Ascher, B. H., Farmer, E. M. Z., Burns, B. J., & Angold, A. (1996). The Child and Adolescent Services Assessment (CASA): Description and psychometrics. *Journal of Emotional and Behavioral Disorders, 4*(1), 12–20.

Burns, B. J. (1991). Mental health service use by adolescents in the 1970s and 1980s. *Journal of the American Academy of Child and Adolescent Psychiatry, 30,* 144–150.

Burns, B. J., Costello, E. J., Angold, A., Tweed, D., Stangl, D., Farmer, E. M. Z., et al. (1995). Children's mental health service use across service sectors. *Health Affairs, 14,* 147–159.

Burns, B. J., Farmer, E. M. Z., Angold, A., Costello, E. J., & Behar, L. B. (1996). A randomized trial of case management for youths with serious emotional disturbance. *Journal of Clinical Child Psychology, 25*(4), 476–486.

Burns, B. J., Hoagwood, K., & Mrazek, P. J. (1999). Effective treatment for mental disorders in children and adolescents. *Clinical Child and Family Psychology Review, 2*(4), 199–254.

Bussing, R., Mason, D. M., Leon, C., & Sinha, K. (2003). Agreement between CASA parent reports and provider records of children's ADHD services. *Journal of Behavioral Health Services and Research, 30*(4), 462–469.

Canino, I. A., Gould, M. S., Prupis, S., & Shaffer, D. (1986). A comparison of symptoms and diagnoses in Hispanic and black children in an outpatient mental health clinic. *Journal of the American Academy of Child Psychiatry, 25,* 254–259.

Cohen, P., Cohen, J., Kasen, S., Velez, C. N., Hartmark, C., Johnson, J., et al. (1993). An epidemiological study of disorders in late childhood and adolescence: 1. Age- and gender-specific prevalence. *Journal of Child Psychology and Psychiatry and Allied Disciplines, 34*(6), 851–867.

Cohen, P., Kasen, S., Brooks, J. S., & Stuening, E. L. (1991). Diagnostic predictors of treatment patterns in a cohort of adolescents. *Journal of the American Academy of Child and Adolescent Psychiatry, 30*(6), 989–993.

Costello, E. J., & Angold, A. (1995). Developmental epidemiology. In D. Cicchetti & D. Cohen (Eds.), *Developmental psychopathology* (Vol. 1, pp. 23–56). New York: Wiley.

Costello, E. J., Angold, A., Burns, B. J., Erkanli, A., Stangl, D. K., & Tweed, D. L. (1996). The Great Smoky Mountains Study of Youth: Functional impairment and severe emotional disturbance. *Archives of General Psychiatry, 53*(12), 1137–1143.

Costello, E. J., Angold, A., Burns, B. J., Stangl, D. K., Tweed, D. L., Erkanli, A., et al. (1996). The Great Smoky Mountains Study of Youth: Goals, designs, methods, and the prevalence of DSM–III–R disorders. *Archives of General Psychiatry, 53*(12), 1129–1136.

Costello, E. J., Messer, S. C., Reinherz, H. Z., Cohen, P., & Bird, H. R. (1998). The prevalence of serious emotional disturbance: A re-analysis of community studies. *Journal of Child and Family Studies, 7,* 411–432.

Costello, E. J., Mustillo, S., Erkanli, A., Keeler, G., & Angold, A. (2003). Prevalence and development of psychiatric disorders in childhood and adolescence. *Archives of General Psychiatry, 60*(8), 837–844.

Costello, E. J., Pescosolido, B. A., Angold, A., & Burns, B. J. (1998). A family network-based model of access to child mental health services. In J. Morrissey (Ed.), *Research in community mental health* (Vol. 9, pp. 165–190). Greenwich, CT: JAI.

Farmer, E. M. Z., Angold, A., Burns, B. J., & Costello, E. J. (1994). Reliabilitiy of self-reported service use: Test–retest consistency of children's responses to the Child and Adolescent Services Assessment. *Journal of Child and Family Studies, 3,* 307–325.

Farmer, E. M. Z, Burns, B. J., Angold, A., & Costello, E. (1997). Impact of children's mental health problems on families: Relationships with service use. *Journal of Emotional and Behavioral Disorders, 5*(4), 230–238.

Farmer, E. M. Z., Burns, B. J., Phillips, S. D., Angold, A., & Costello, E. J. (2003). Pathways into and through care: Mental health services for children and adolescents. *Psychiatric Services, 54*(1), 60–66.

Farmer, E. M. Z., Stangl, D. K., Burns, B. J., Costello, E. J., & Angold, A. (1999). Service use for children's mental health across 1 year: Patterns and predictors of use. *Journal of Community Mental Health, 35*(1), 31–46.

Friedman, R. M., Katz-Leavy, J. W., Manderscheid, R. W., & Sondheimer, D. L. (1996). Prevalence of serious emotional disturbance in children and adolescents. In R. W. Manderscheid & M. A. Sonnenschein (Eds.), *Center for Mental Health Services: Mental health, United States, 1996* (Vol. Pub. No. [SMA] 96-3098, pp. 71–89). Washington, DC: Superintendent of Documents, U.S. Government Printing Office.

Hoberman, H. M. (1992). Ethnic minority status and adolescent mental health services utilization. *Journal of Mental Health Administration, 19*(3), 246–267.

Horwitz, S. M., Hoagwood, K., Stiffman, A. R., Summerfeld, T., Weisz, J. R., Costello, E. J., et al. (2001). Reliability of the services assessment for children and adolescents. *Psychiatric Services, 52*(8), 1088–1094.

Kataoka, S., Zhang, L., & Wells, K. (2002). Unmet need for mental health care among U.S. children: Variation by ethnicity and insurance status. *American Journal of Psychiatry, 159,* 1548–1555.

Knitzer, J. (1982). *Unclaimed children.* Washington, DC: Children's Defense Fund.

Leaf, P., Alegria, M. P. C., Goodman, S., Horwitz, S., Hoven, C., et al. (1996). Mental health service use in the community and schools: Results from the four-community MECA study. *Journal of the American Academy of Child and Adolescent Psychiatry, 35,* 889–897.

McGee, R., Feehan, M., Williams, S., Partridge, F., Silva, P. A., & Kelly, J. (1990). DSM–III disorders in a large sample of adolescents. *Journal of the American Academy of Child and Adolescent Psychiatry, 29*(4), 611–619.

Messer, S. C., Angold, A., Costello, E. J., & Burns, B. J. (1996). The Child and Adolescent Burden Assessment (CABA): Measuring the family impact of emotional and behavioral problems. *International Journal of Methods in Psychiatric Research, 6,* 261–284.

Offord, D. R., Boyle, M. H., Szatmari, P., Rae-Grant, N. I., Links, P. S., Cadman, D. T., et al. (1987). Ontario child health study: II. Six-month prevalence of disorder and rates of service utilization. *Archives of General Psychiatry, 44,* 832–836.

Ringel, J. S., & Sturm, R. (2001). National estimates of mental health utilization and expenditures for children in 1998. *Journal of Behavioral Health Services and Research, 28,* 319–333.

Roberts, R., Attkisson, C., & Rosenblatt, A. (1998). Prevalence of psychopathology among children and adolescents. *American Journal of Psychiatry, 155,* 715–725.

Romano, E., Tremblay, R. E., Vitaro, F., Zoccolillo, M., & Pagani, L. (2001). Prevalence of psychiatric diagnoses and the role of perceived impairment: Findings from an adolescent community sample. *Journal of Child Psychology and Psychiatry, 42*(4), 451–461.

Stroul, B. A. (1993). *Systems of care in children with severe emotional disturbance: What are the results?* Washington, DC: Georgetown University Child Development Center, CASSP Technical Center.

Stroul, B. A., & Friedman, R. (1986). *A system of care for severely emotionally disturbed children and youth.* Washington, DC: Georgetown University Child Development Center, CASSP Technical Assistance Center.

U.S. Department of Health and Human Services. (1999). *Mental health: A report of the Surgeon General.* Rockville, MD: U.S. Department of Health and Human Services, Substance Abuse and Mental Health Services Administration, Center for Mental Health Services, National Institutes of Health, National Institute of Mental Health.

Verhulst, F., & van der Ende, J. (1997). Factors associated with child mental health service use in the community. *Journal of the American Academy of Child and Adolescent Psychiatry, 36,* 901–909.

The Clinical and Psychosocial Characteristics of Children with Serious Emotional Disturbance Entering System-of-Care Services

CHAPTER 3

Christine Walrath and Qinghong Liao

The advent of the Comprehensive Community Mental Health Services for Children and Their Families Program in 1993 marked the beginning of a new phase in national efforts to serve children with mental health problems. The extensive network of system-of-care grant communities created by this program provides a foundation on which to develop and refine emerging strategies for responding to the issues raised in the Surgeon General's National Action Agenda and other national efforts (U.S. Department of Health and Human Services, 1999).

The program is administered by the Child, Adolescent and Family Branch within the Center for Mental Health Services (CMHS), Substance Abuse and Mental Health Services Administration (SAMHSA), U.S. Department of Health and Human Services. It uses as its guidepost the system-of-care approach (Stroul & Friedman, 1986) and is built on federal-, foundation-, and state-level initiatives, beginning with the Child and Adolescent Service System Program (CASSP) in 1984 and augmented by other federal and state initiatives in subsequent years. The system-of-care approach calls for a comprehensive spectrum of mental health services and other support services that are guided by a set of principles. The principles specify that services and supports should be individualized, family focused, and culturally competent. They should be community based and accessible, provided in the least restrictive environment possible, and offered through a collaborative, coordinated interagency network. The CMHS program funded four grant communities in 1993. By 2002, the initial investment of $5 million had grown to over $650 million, the largest federal investment ever in community-based mental health services for children and their families. There have been four cohorts of communities funded since 1993. The first cohort consisted of 22 communities funded in 1993 and 1994; the second contained 23 communities funded in 1997 and 1998; the third was 22 communities funded in 1999 and 2000; and the fourth consisted of the 25 communities funded in 2002. These funded cohorts total to 92 grants of 5 to 6 years awarded in 46 states and two territories, with more than 55,000 children and their families referred for system-of-care services.

The program's authorizing legislation (P.L. 102-321) calls for an annual evaluation to (a) describe the children and families served by the system-of-care initiative; (b) assess how systems of care develop and what factors impede or enhance their development; (c) measure whether children served through the program experience improvement in clinical and functional outcomes and whether those improvements endure over time and if so, why; (d) determine whether the consumers are satisfied with the services they receive; and (e) measure the costs associated with the implementation of a system of care and determine its cost-effectiveness. To date, the evaluation has been initiated with grant communities funded over the period from 1993 to 2000. Information in this chapter is based on data that were collected to describe the children and families served by the system-of-care initiative in the 67 communities funded between 1993 and 2000.

THE DEMOGRAPHIC CHARACTERISTICS (1993–2000)

As described in the previous section, there were three funded cohorts of communities between 1993 and 2000. The existence of a common set of basic descriptive variables across these three cohorts provides a unique opportunity to examine the gender, age, race/ethnicity, family income, custody status, and referral source profiles of more than 47,000 children served in the 67 funded communities across the United States.

For the communities in the second and third cohorts, funding for the 1997-funded communities ended in October 2003, and funding for the 2000-funded communities will end in 2006. In contrast, funding for the communities in the first cohort ended in 1998. Initially, descriptive analyses included all communities funded over the 1993–2000 period, but they were also performed separately for those communities in Cohort 1 as compared to those in Cohorts 2 and 3.

Children referred into system-of-care service communities between 1993 and 2000 were most often referred from the mental health system. They were predominantly boys and were often in their early adolescence at the time of referral. More than half of the children referred into service were Caucasian, and more than half were living in households with incomes below the poverty level. Table 3.1 details the descriptive profiles with and across cohorts.

The patterns for the descriptive profiles across Cohorts 2 and 3 are fairly consistent, with several exceptions. Although the average age of children referred is comparable between the 1993–1994 and 1997–2000 communities, a larger percentage of children were in the youngest (10.8%) and oldest (40.8%) age groups in the communities funded for 1993–1994 (Cohort 1) as compared

TABLE 3.1

Demographic Characteristics of Children Referred into Services in Communities
Funded in 1993–1994, 1997–2000, and Across All Funded Communities

	Previously Funded Communities[a] (Funded 1993–1994)	Currently Funded Communities[b] (Funded 1997–2000)	All Communities[c]
Gender	($n = 28,218$)	($n = 9,554$)	($n = 37,771$)
Male	60.0%	67.7%	62.0%
Female	40.0%	32.3%	38.0%
Age	($n = 28,190$)	($n = 94,933$)	($n = 37,683$)
Birth to 6 years	10.8%	6.4%	9.7%
7 to 11 years	23.4%	27.6%	24.5%
12 to 14 years	25.0%	33.2%	27.1%
15 years or older	40.8%	32.8%	38.8%
M (SD)	12.47 (3.54)	12.47 (4.06)	12.47 (3.94)
Race/ethnicity	($n = 38,201$)	($n = 9,024$)	($n = 47,225$)
White	54.7%	52.3%	54.2%
African American	14.7%	24.6%	16.6%
Hispanic/Latino	24.5%	1.6%	20.1%
Native American	1.8%	7.2%	2.9%
Other[d]	4.3%	14.3%	6.2%
Family income	($n = 8,142$)	($n = 7,861$)	($n = 16,003$)
Less than $15,000 per year	60.4%	46.6%	53.6%
$15,000/year or more	39.6%	53.4%	46.4%
Custody status	($n = 34,785$)	($n = 9,230$)	($n = 19,085$)
Both parents	25.9%	24.8%	25.4%
Single parent	52.9%	48.7%	50.9%
Not in custody of parents[e]	21.2%	26.4%	23.8%
Referral source	($n = 33,941$)	($n = 9,074$)	($n = 19,773$)
Justice	13.7%	17.5%	15.4%
Education	20.5%	19.9%	20.2%
Mental health	23.2%	22.8%	23.0%
Child welfare	14.5%	14.5%	14.5%
Family	16.0%	11.1%	13.7%
Other[f]	12.2%	14.2%	13.1%

Note. Percentages and means (M) are based on available data for each respective variable.
[a] Includes 22 funded communities.
[b] Includes 45 funded communities.
[c] Includes 67 funded communities.
[d] Due to the small number of cases, Other Race/Ethnicity includes children of Asian, Pacific Island, Native Alaskan, Hawaiian, multiple races, and other backgrounds.
[e] Not in Custody of Parents includes children in custody of relatives, friends, guardians, the state, and others.
[f] Other referral source includes child referred from health professionals, substance abuse professionals, and other sources.

to those in the communities funded for 1997–2000 (Cohorts 2 and 3; 6.4% and 32.8%, respectively). A much larger percentage of Hispanic children were referred into the Cohort 1 funded communities than into the Cohorts 2 and 3 funded communities (24.5% vs. 1.6%). In contrast, a larger percentage of

African American children (26.6% vs. 14.7%) and Native American children (7.2% vs. 1.8%) were referred into the 1997–2000 funded communities. These race, ethnicity, and age differences are likely a function of the geographic locations and target population definitions for those communities.

Although the custody status profiles were comparable for the 1993–1994 and 1997–2000 funded community analyses, a larger percentage of children were living in families with incomes less than $15,000 per year in the 1993–1994 funded communities (60.4% vs. 46.6%). Finally, although the mental health and education systems accounted for the largest percentage of referrals, respectively, into the 1993–1994 and 1997–1998 funded communities, a larger percentage of children were family referred (16.0% vs. 11.1%) and a smaller percentage were justice referred (13.7% vs. 17.5%) in 1993–1994 funded communities. Again, these slight differences may be indicative of collaboration and target population.

In summary, children have been referred into system-of-care programs over the last 10 years from multiple public agencies and private sources. The majority are boys, in their early adolescence, non-Hispanic White, and living in the custody of their parent(s) and in homes with family incomes under the poverty level. Although some variation in profile exists for children referred into the various cohorts of funded communities, these differences are most likely a function of the geographic location and target populations of these programs.

DEMOGRAPHIC CHARACTERISTICS (1997–2000)

Variation in the demographic and psychosocial characteristics of children with serious emotional disturbance (SED) referred into services has been well documented (e.g., Liao, Mantueffel, Paulic, & Sondheimer, 2001; Rosenblatt, Robertson, Wood, Furlong, & Sosna, 1998; Walrath et al., 2001). Specifically, characteristics such as basic demographics, child and family risk factors, referral source, reason for referral, and diagnosis have been shown to vary, and it has been argued that understanding the variation in these characteristics is critical to service planning and understanding changes in child clinical and functional outcomes over time.

Data collected so far from the system-of-care communities funded in 1997–2000 were analyzed to provide information on children's clinical profiles as a function of their demographic characteristics. Child age, gender, and race/ethnicity groups were created for the purpose of comparing child clinical and psychosocial characteristics. Specifically, presenting problems, diagnoses, child and family risk factors, and living arrangement at the time of referral into service were analyzed as a function of age, gender, and race/ethnicity. Similarly, delinquent behavior and school behavior, performance, and attendance in the 6 months prior to system-of-care service referral were also analyzed by these three primary demographic characteristics. Additional information on the variables and sample descriptives is provided in Table 3.2.

Analytic Techniques

In an effort to describe the clinical and psychosocial characteristics of the children and families and investigate demographic subgroup variation, each of the clinical and psychosocial variables was analyzed independently as a function of each demographic characteristic. These analyses were performed independently for each psychosocial and demographic characteristic. Logistic regression analysis, appropriate for assessing the relationship between a set of predictors (continuous or categorical) and a dichotomous dependent variable, was used for all binary (yes/no) clinical and psychosocial characteristics. Logistic regression analysis results in an odds ratio for each predictor variable or level of a categorical predictor variable. The odds ratio estimates the change in the odds of membership in the target group associated with a one-unit change in the predictor. For example, in Table 3.3, an odds ratio of 1.69 was reported for 7- to 11-year-old children presenting for services with an academic problem. Given that the birth to 6-year-old age group served as the reference category, this would be interpreted as follows: *Children in the 7- to 11-year-old age group are 1.69 times as likely as those in the birth to 6-year-old age group to be presented for system-of-care services due to an academic problem.* In addition, an odds ratio of .66 was reported for children 7 to 11 years old presenting for service with hyperactive or compulsive problems. This odds ratio would be interpreted as follows: *Children in the 7- to 11-year-old age group are 1.52 less likely than those in the birth to 6-year-old age group to be presented for system-of-care services due to hyperactive/compulsive problems.* Chi-square analyses, which assess the independence of two or more nominal variables by comparing expected frequencies with observed frequencies, were performed for the psychosocial variables with more than two categories.

Age Differences in Clinical and Psychosocial Characteristics

As described earlier, although the average age of children referred into service communities funded in 1997–2000 was 12.47 years, approximately one-third of the referred youth were ages 12–14 years; one-third were 15 years and older, slightly more than one-quarter were 7 to 11 years old, and the remaining youth (9%) were birth to 6 years old. As detailed in Table 3.3, there were significant age differences associated with presenting problems, diagnoses, child and family risk factors, delinquent behavior, and school behavior and performance.

An analysis of variance indicated significant age group differences in the number of presenting problems, $F(3, 8501) = 4.75$, $p < .01$, so number of

(*text continues on p. 53*)

TABLE 3.2
Variable Information: Child Clinical and Psychosocial Characteristics

Variable	Description	Descriptive Statistics
Presenting problem	At the time of intake into service the caregiver was asked to report on the presenting problems of the youth. Children can be presented with various and multiple problems.	Number of problems Range: 1–29 $M = 5.47$ $SD = 4.68$ Five most prevalent presenting problems categories used in the analysis were Noncompliance (45.3%) Physical aggression (42.4%) Academic problems (35.6%) Hyperactivity or impulsivity (31.5%) Attention difficulties (29.7%)
Diagnosis	Diagnostic information was abstracted from clinical records. Children referred into service have varied and multiple diagnoses.	Five most prevalent diagnostic categories used in the analysis were (these categories are not mutually exclusive) Conduct disorders (12.0%) Attention-deficit disorders (39.0%) Oppositional-defiant disorders (27.5%) Adjustment disorders (12.6%) Mood disorders (29%)
Child and family risk factors	Child and family risk factors consist of previous experiences of the child and the biological family that may be related to serious emotional disturbance. Lifetime risk factor information is obtained from the caregiver at the child's intake into service. Caregivers were asked to provide binary (yes/no) responses to questions about the lifetime history of child psychiatric hospitalization, physical abuse, sexual abuse, running away, suicide attempts, substance use, and sexual abusiveness to others; and lifetime family history of domestic violence, mental illness, and substance abuse among biological family members, as well as felony conviction of biological parents.	Number of risk factors (these categories are not mutually exclusive) Range: 1–3 $M = 4.04$ $SD = 2.58$ Lifetime child history of Psychiatric hospitalization (30.5%) Physical abuse (28%) Sexual abuse (22.3%) Running away (34.6%) Suicide attempts (16.1%)

(continues)

TABLE 3.2 *Continued.*
Variable Information: Child Clinical and Psychosocial Characteristics

Variable	Description	Descriptive Statistics

Child and family (*continued*)		Lifetime child history (*continued*)
		  Substance use (22.9%)
		  Sexual abusiveness to others (7.8%)
		Lifetime family history of
		  Domestic violence (50%)
		  Mental illness in biological family (54.7%)
		  Substance abuse in biological family (66.3%)
		  Felony conviction of biological parents (46.5%)

Living arrangement	The living arrangements of children referred into system-of-care services varied from less to more restrictive. Caregiver-reported child living arrangements were categorized into two groups: (a) Nonrestrictive placement includes the child living independently, with one or both biological parents, or in some other home living environment, such as an adoptive home, and (b) restrictive placement includes foster care, group home, residential treatment, and jail.	Number of placements in the 6 months prior to system of care service referral
		  Range: 1–5
		  $M = 1.90$
		  $SD = 1.56$
		Type of placement:
		  Restrictive placement (17.7%)

Delinquency	Children and youth age 11 years and older self-reported (yes/no) on lifetime arrest and arrest in the last 6 months.	Arrest:
		  Ever arrested (44.9%)
		  Arrested in the last 6 months (39.7%)

School performance	Caregivers also reported on their child's school behavior, performance, and attendance at the time of service intake. Specifically, caregivers provided binary responses (yes/no) to whether the child had been suspended or expelled in the last 6 months. In addition, caregivers were asked whether the child had attended school less than 50% of the days, between 50% and 75% of the days, or more than 75% of the days in the last 6 months, and whether he or she was failing all or most classes or had below-average, average, or above-average grades in the last 6 months.	School performance in the last 6 months:
		  Expelled (8.1%)
		  Suspended (44.7%)
		  Average or above-average attendance (59.8%)
		  Regular attendance: 75% of days or more (66%)

TABLE 3.3

Significant Age Differences in Clinical and Psychosocial Characteristics
of Children Referred into Services in Communities Funded in 1997–2000

Characteristic	Age at Time of Referral[a]			
	Birth to 6 Years	7 to 11 Years	12 to 14 Years	15 Years and Older
Logistic Regression Analyses				
Five most prevalent presenting problems[b]				
Noncompliance		*ns*	*ns*	*ns*
Physical aggression	Reference	*ns*	.62	.34
Academic problems		1.69	1.98	1.55
Hyperactive-impulsive		.66	.34	.18
Attention difficulties		.65	.35	.16
Five most prevalent diagnoses[c]				
Conduct disorder		*ns*	2.80	6.21
Attention-deficit disorder	Reference	1.42	.75	.34
Oppositional-defiant disorder		1.93	1.82	*ns*
Adjustment disorder		.54	.43	.33
Mood disorder		2.79	4.81	5.04
Lifetime child risk factor history[d]				
Psychiatric hospitalization		2.14	2.51	2.52
Physical abuse		*ns*	*ns*	*ns*
Sexual abuse	Reference	*ns*	*ns*	*ns*
Running away from home		1.42	2.95	5.13
Suicide attempt		2.04	3.96	4.94
Substance use		*ns*	7.80	31.07
Sexually abusive		*ns*	*ns*	.53
Lifetime family risk factor history[d]				
Domestic violence		*ns*	.54	.35
Biological family mental illness		*ns*	.70	.44
Felony conviction of biological parent	Reference	*ns*	.60	.44
Substance abuse in biological family		.71	.61	.44
Living arrangement at time of referral[e]				
Restrictive placement	Reference	*ns*	*ns*	1.67
Delinquent behavior[f]				
Ever arrested	Excluded	Reference	2.71	6.99
Arrested in the last 6 months			*ns*	*ns*
School behavior[f]				
Suspended in the last 6 months	Excluded	Reference	1.96	*ns*
Expelled in the last 6 months			1.87	2.18
Chi-Square Analyses				
School performance[g]				
Failing all or most classes		18.1%	32.1%	30.7%
Below average	Excluded	14.4%	13.6%	13.1%
Average		33.5%	30.6%	27.4%
Above average		34.0%	23.7%	28.9%

(continues)

TABLE 3.3 *Continued.*

Significant Age Differences in Clinical and Psychosocial Characteristics
of Children Referred into Services in Communities Funded in 1997–2000

	Age at Time of Referral[a]			
	Birth to 6 Years	7 to 11 Years	12 to 14 Years	15 Years and Older
Chi-Square Analyses (*continued*)				
School attendance[g]				
Attended less than 50% of days		6.0%	16.9%	23.2%
Attended between 50% and 75% of days	Excluded	12.9%	21.5%	22.1%
Attended more than 75% of days		81.0%	61.7%	54.7%

Note. Due to the large sample size and in an effort to report only meaningful differences, only those odds ratios that were significant at the $p < .01$ level or lower are considered significant.

[a] Birth to 6 years of age was used as the reference category for the logistic regressions.

[b] A child can be referred for more than one presenting problem; therefore, problem categories are not mutually exclusive. The number of presenting problems differed significantly by age group; therefore, it was covaried in all presenting problem analyses.

[c] A child can have more than one diagnosis; therefore, diagnostic categories are not mutually exclusive.

[d] The combined number of child and family risk factors differed significantly by age group; therefore, total number of risk factors was covaried in all child and family risk factor analyses.

[e] The number of living arrangements the child had in the 6 months prior to referral differed significantly by age group; therefore, number of living arrangements was covaried in the current living arrangement analysis. Restrictive placements included foster care/home shelter, group home/emergency shelter, residential treatment center, and jail.

[f] Children in the birth to 6-year category were excluded from school- and delinquency-related analyses, and the 7- to 11-year-old category served as the reference category for logistic regressions.

[g] Children in the birth to 6-year category were excluded; a chi-square analysis was performed and percentages are presented.

presenting problems was covaried in the presenting problem analyses. After controlling for the number of presenting problems, there were no differences in the odds of being referred for noncompliance as a function of age. However, children aged 7 to 11 years, 12 to 14 years, and 15 years and older were significantly less likely to be referred for hyperactivity/impulsivity and attention difficulties than children in the birth to 6-year-old age group; and children in the latter two age groups were less likely to be referred for physical aggression. Alternatively, and not surprisingly, all three older age groups were more likely to be referred for academic problems than the birth to 6-year-old group. At the time of entering system-of-care services, older children were much more likely to be diagnosed with conduct and mood disorders and less likely to be diagnosed with attention-deficit disorder compared to children in the youngest age group.

The combined number of child and family risk factors differed significantly as a function of age group, $F(3, 9039) = 39.81, p < .0001$, and were entered as a covariate into all child and family risk factor logistic regression models. As expected, after controlling for number of risk factors, children in the three older age groups, as compared to those in the birth to 6-year group, were significantly more likely to have reported lifetime experiences of psychiatric hospitalization, running away, suicide attempts, and substance use, with higher odds ratios being associated with older age groups. For example, although children in the 7- to 11-year group were 1.42 times as likely to run away from home as compared to the birth to 6-year group; children in the 12- to 14-year and 15-year and older groups were 2.95 and 5.13 times as likely, respectively. Similarly, the odds of suicide attempt increased across the three older age groups compared to the youngest, as did the odds of substance use. While children in the 12- to 14-year-old group were nearly eight times as likely to have used substances compared to the birth to 6-year-olds, children in the 15-year and older group were over 30 times as likely.

Inversely, children in the older age groups, particularly the 12- to 14-year and 15-year and older groups, were less likely to have reports of lifetime experience of family risks. This pattern was true for all of the family risk factors, but it was most dramatic for children in the 15-year and older group, which was .35 times as likely to have experienced domestic violence and .44 times as likely to have experienced family mental illness, substance abuse, and felony conviction. These relationships may suggest that different indicators and thresholds are used to make a younger child's referral into comprehensive services. For example, younger children (i.e., birth to 6 years) have had far less time for personal exposure to the child-level experiences, so it may be that the family risk experience is more often used to make referrals.

After controlling for the age differences in the number of living arrangements in the 6 months prior to system-of-care service intake, $F(3, 4624) = 52.80, p < .0001$, children aged 15 years and older were 1.67 times more likely to be living in a restrictive setting at the time of intake compared to children in the birth to 6-year group.

Children in the birth to 6-year group were excluded from all delinquency and school related analyses, and the 7- to 11-year-old age group was used as the reference category. Older children were much more likely to have a lifetime history of arrest as compared to children in the 7- to 11-year-old group; however, there were no differences in their odds of being arrested in the 6 months preceding service entry. In addition, children aged 12 to 14 years were nearly twice as likely as those aged 7 to 11 years to have been suspended or expelled in the 6 months prior to service intake, and children 15 years and older were also more likely to have been expelled.

There were significant age differences associated with both school performance, $\chi^2(6, N = 3,628) = 81.07, p < .0001$, and attendance, $\chi^2(4, N = 3,298) = 190.14, p < .0001$. Specifically, larger percentages of children aged 12 to 14 years and children 15 years and older were reported to be failing in school and smaller percentages were reported to be performing above average, as compared to children aged 7 to 11 years. Similarly, larger percentages of older children were irregularly attending school and smaller percentages were attending regularly, as compared to younger children.

Thus, with few exceptions (such as family risk factors and presenting problems), it appears that the clinical and psychosocial profiles of children deteriorate as they age. For example, older children are more likely to have engaged in risky behavior (e.g., running away from home, substance use), attempted suicide or been arrested, attended school infrequently, and lived in a restrictive living environment. Although the analyses of clinical and psychosocial characteristics were performed independently from one another, a pattern does emerge that illustrates the increasing likelihood of exposure to child risk factors, delinquency and school problems, and mood and conduct disorders for older children. More clarity will be gained from investigations into the relationships between and among these characteristics and how they relate to age.

Gender Differences in Clinical and Psychosocial Characteristics

As indicated earlier, more than two-thirds of the children referred into systems of care funded in 1997–2000 were boys. Table 3.4 includes information on the significant gender differences in clinical and psychosocial characteristics. Boys were used as the reference group for all logistic regression analyses. An investigation into the five most prevalent problems indicated that girls were less likely than boys to be referred for problems of physical aggression, academics, hyperactivity/impulsivity, or attention. In addition, although girls were less likely to be diagnosed with conduct, attention-deficit, and oppositional-defiant disorders, they were over 1.6 times as likely to be diagnosed with adjustment and mood disorders.

There were far fewer gender differences than there were age differences in child and family risk factors. After controlling for number of risk factors, girls were 2.77 times as likely to have a reported history of sexual abuse and were more likely to have run away from home and attempted suicide. However, they were less likely to have reports of being sexually abusive to others. The gender profiles of family risk factors were, for the most part, comparable.

The odds of living in a restrictive placement did not vary as a function of the child's gender; however, girls were less likely than boys to have a reported history of lifetime arrest or suspension and expulsion in the 6 months prior to service intake. Finally, there was no relationship between gender and academic performance; however, a larger percentage of girls were reported to attend school regularly and a smaller percentage were reported to attend school less than 50% of the days, $\chi^2(2, N = 3,503) = 22.70, p < .0001$.

Thus, although relatively fewer clinical and psychosocial differences are indicated as a function of gender, those that do exist are critical to recognize. The primary gender differences appear to be related to internal versus external diagnoses and behaviors. Girls referred into service appear to have a lower likelihood of presenting with externalizing problems and diagnoses and a greater likelihood of presenting with more internalizing diagnoses. In addition, the external psychosocial indictors of functioning in school and the community indicate fewer problems for girls, whereas the risk factors often associated with internal problems (e.g., suicide attempt, sexual abuse, running away) were

TABLE 3.4

Significant Gender and Race/Ethnicity Differences in
Clinical and Psychosocial Characteristics of Children Referred
into Services in Communities Funded in 1997–2000

	Gender[a]		Race/Ethnicity[a]	
	Boys	Girls	Nonminority	Minority
Logistic Regression Analyses				
Five most prevalent presenting problems[b]				
Noncompliance		*ns*		*ns*
Physical agression		.65		*ns*
Academic problems	Reference	.79	Reference	*ns*
Hyperactivity		.55		*ns*
Attention difficulties		.59		*ns*
Five most prevelant diagnoses[c]				
Conduct disorder		.40		1.95
Attention-deficit disorder		.37		.73
Oppositional-defiant disorder	Reference	.84	Reference	*ns*
Adjustment disorder		1.69		*ns*
Mood disorder		1.65		.80
Lifetime child risk factor history[d]				
Psychiatric hospitalization		*ns*		.77
Physical abuse		*ns*		.75
Sexual abuse	Reference	2.77	Reference	.72
Running away from home		1.44		1.24
Suicide attempt		1.75		*ns*
Substance use		*ns*		1.35
Sexually abusive		.43		*ns*
Lifetime family risk factor history[d]				
Domestic violence		*ns*		*ns*
Biological family mental illness	Reference	*ns*	Reference	.52
Psychiatric hospitalization of				
biological parent		*ns*		*ns*
Felony conviction of biological parent		.73		1.51
Substance abuse in biological family		*ns*		*ns*
Living arrangement at time of referral[e]				
Restrictive placement	Reference	*ns*	Reference	1.48
Delinquent behavior				
Ever arrested	Reference	.67	Reference	1.66
Arrested in the last 6 months		*ns*		1.71
School behavior				
Suspended in the last 6 months	Reference	.68	Reference	1.45
Expelled in the last 6 months		.64		1.39

(*continues*)

TABLE 3.4 *Continued.*

Significant Gender and Race/Ethnicity Differences in
Clinical and Psychosocial Characteristics of Children Referred
into Services in Communities Funded in 1997–2000

	Gender[a]		Race/Ethnicity[a]	
	Boys	Girls	Nonminority	Minority
Chi-Square Analyses				
School performance				
Failing all or most classes			29.5%	24.2%
Below average	*ns*	*ns*	13.8%	13.4%
Average			31.0%	30.7%
Above average			25.6%	32.8%
School attendance				
Attended less than 50% of days	13.8%	16.6%	*ns*	*ns*
Attended between 50% and 75% of days	16.7%	21.9%		
Attended more than 75% of days	69.5%	61.5%		

Note. Due to the large sample size and in an effort to report only meaningful differences, only those findings that were significant at the $p < .01$ level or lower are considered significant.

[a] Boys were used as the reference category for gender logistic regressions and nonminorities were used as the reference category for race/ethnicity logistic regressions.

[b] A child can be referred for more than one presenting problem; therefore, problem categories are not mutually exclusive. The number of presenting problems differed significantly by race/ethnicity; therefore, number of problems was covaried in the race/ethnicity presenting problem analyses.

[c] A child can have more than one diagnosis; therefore, diagnostic categories are not mutually exclusive.

[d] The combined number of child and family risk factors differed significantly by gender and by race/ethnicity; therefore, total number of risk factors was covaried in gender and race/ethnicity risk factor analyses, respectively.

[e] The number of living arrangements the child had in the 6 months prior to referral differed significantly by gender; therefore, number of living arrangements was covaried in the gender current living arrangement analyses. Restrictive placements included foster care/home shelter, group home/emergency shelter, residential treatment center, and jail.

more common for girls. These gender profiles seem to indicate that girls referred into system-of-care service environments tend to be accompanied by more internal indicators as compared to their male contemporaries.

Race and Ethnicity Differences in Clinical and Psychosocial Characteristics

As described earlier, the majority (52.3%) of children referred into system-of-care services in communities funded in 1997–2000 were non-Hispanic White. For the purposes of race/ethnicity analyses, nonminority children (i.e., non-Hispanic Whites) were compared to minority children. This decision was made for two primary reasons: (a) The Hispanic/Latino and Native American race and ethnicity categories included too few children to generate meaningful analyses and interpretation, and (b) there was no conceptual reason to create three race/ethnicity groups to compare nonminority to African American minority to non–African American minority children. Table 3.4 includes information on the significant race/ethnicity differences in clinical and psychosocial characteristics.

Overall, the clinical and psychosocial differences associated with race/ethnicity were small relative to those found for age and gender. However, after controlling for the number of presenting problems, there were no race/ethnicity differences in the type of presenting problem. Minority children were 1.95 times as likely to be diagnosed with conduct disorders and slightly less likely to be diagnosed with attention-deficit or mood disorder when compared to nonminority children. After controlling for the number of risk factors, small but significant race/ethnicity differences were found for several of the child and family risk factors. Most notably, children of a minority background were 1.5 times more likely to have a family member with a felony conviction and .52 times as likely to have a family member with a mental illness.

Similarly small but significant differences were found for living arrangement at the time of referral into service, delinquent behavior, and school behavior in the 6 months prior to referral. Specifically, minority children were between 1.4 and 1.7 times more likely to have lived in a restrictive setting at the time of intake into service, to have been arrested, and to have been suspended or expelled in the 6 months prior to service referral. However, despite these differences suggesting a slight increase in the odds of school problems for minority children, a higher percentage of minority children were performing above average and a lower percentage were failing most or all of their classes as compared to nonminority children, $\chi^2(3, N = 3,514) = 25.35, p < .0001$.

Thus, although the differences associated with minority status appear small relative to those associated with gender and age, there is some indication that children of minority racial and ethnic backgrounds have higher odds of behavioral problems (e.g., conduct disorder diagnosis, school problems, delinquency) when compared to nonminority children. Although consistent with other reports (Reid et al., 2000), these differences may be due to the geographic locale or target populations of the funded communities and should be interpreted in the context of relatively small odds ratios and a heterogeneous minority group.

Conclusions: Age, Race/Ethnicity, and Gender-Specific Profiles

In the above-reported analyses, the most dramatic clinical and psychosocial differences among children with serious emotional disturbance referred into system-of-care services were found with relation to age, fewer were found with relation to gender, and even fewer with relation to race and ethnicity. Interestingly, in the prevalence literature, a similar pattern has been demonstrated (Costello, Messer, Bird, Cohen, & Reinherz, 1998). Specifically, although a higher prevalence of serious emotional disturbance has been found among older children, gender and race/ethnicity differences in prevalence are minimal.

Much more research is required to understand the age, gender, and race/ethnicity differences in the prevalence literature as they relate to the clinical and psychosocial characteristic differences in the system-of-care literature. However, it appears that the same factors that affect the prevalence rates of serious emotional disturbance in a representative population sample may also be those that best distinguish the characteristics among children with serious emotional disturbance.

In addition, the demographic subgroup variations identified via these analyses are consistent with and expand upon earlier research focusing on children with serious emotional disturbance (e.g., Landrum, Singh, Nemil, Ellis, & Best, 1995; Liao, Mantueffel, Paulic, & Sondheimer, 2001; Rosenblatt et al., 1998; Walrath et al., 2001).

PATTERNS OF PRESENTING PROBLEMS (1997–2000)

Earlier analyses indicated that children enrolled in system-of-care programs were referred for multiple and varied problems, including both internalizing and externalizing problems. Understanding the patterns and mix of these presenting problems across children informs service planning, appropriate triaging, and resource allocation.

To examine different patterns of presenting problems, a latent class analysis (LCA) was conducted, and presenting problems were used as indicators to derive class membership. LCA is a statistical method for finding subtypes of related cases (latent classes) from multivariate categorical data. For example, it can be used to identify (a) distinct diagnostic categories given the presence/absence of several symptoms, (b) types of attitude structures from survey responses, (c) consumer segments from demographic and preference variables, or (d) subpopulations from their answers to test items. The results of LCA can also be used to classify cases to their most likely latent class.

Once the class membership was determined, the differential probabilities of having a particular problem within each class were examined. This probability is referred to as *conditional probability*—the probability of having a particular problem given class membership. For the purpose of interpreting the LCA results, the probability of .5 (50%) was used as the cutoff for indicating whether children in a particular class had a high probability of having a particular problem, and the probability of .3 (30%) was used to indicate a moderate probability. The LCA results indicated that a 10-class solution best fit the data, suggesting 10 distinct subgroups of children with different patterns of presenting problems. Table 3.5 summarizes the characteristics of each class.

The demographic characteristics across classes were compared. Although there were significant differences in areas such as age, gender, and referrals, most of them were not surprising given the class membership. For

TABLE 3.5

Characteristics of the 10 Classes of Presenting Problems

Class Membership	Label	Characteristics
Class 1 ($n = 1,026$)	Attention-deficit/ hyperactivity disorder (ADHD)	Moderate probabilities of noncompliance, academic problems, and poor peer interaction
Class 2 ($n = 892$)	Mildly delinquent	Police contacts and noncompliance Moderate probabilities of alcohol or substance abuse, truancy, and academic problems No ADHD
Class 3 ($n = 371$)	Delinquent with substance abuse	Aggressive, co-occurring substance abuse problems with police contacts and academic problems Moderately suicidal, attention difficulties Highest probability of police contact and alcohol or substance abuse compared to other classes
Class 4 ($n = 2,317$)	Low problem	Low probability on all presenting problems
Class 5 ($n = 1,000$)	Aggressive and noncompliant	Aggressive and noncompliant; low probability on all other presenting problems
Class 6 ($n = 268$)	Depressed with ADHD	Depressed and ADHD, noncompliant, problems at school Low self-esteem and social problems with adults
Class 7 ($n = 213$)	Suicidal	Highest probability in suicide ideation and suicide attempts among all classes
Class 8 ($n = 643$)	Depressed with aggression	Depressed with moderately aggressive behaviors and somatic complaints
Class 9 ($n = 516$)	Aggressive with ADHD	Aggressive and ADHD, noncompliant, academic and peer problems
Class 10 ($n = 421$)	Multiple severe problems	Severe problems in all areas Low probability of alcohol or substance abuse and truancy

example, boys had a higher probability to be in all classes except for Class 7, the suicidal group, where girls were more likely to be, $\chi^2(9, N = 7,665) = 263.28$, $p < .001$. Age differences were also in the direction that one would expect. On average, children in Classes 3 and 2 were the oldest, followed by children in Class 7, $F(9, 7597) = 107.90, p < .001$. Children in Class 1 were the youngest. This is likely related to the fact that children in Classes 3 and 2 had the highest probabilities of having alcohol/substance abuse problems, whereas children in Class 1 had the lowest probability.

In addition to demographic characteristics, previous service utilization was examined to determine whether children differed, with regard to their prior service use, across the 10 presenting problem groups. Significant differences across the classes were found in both the number of services and types of services received prior to their entry into system-of-care programs. As one might expect, the average number of services was the highest (2.5) among children in Class 10 and the lowest (1.3) among children in Class 4, $F(9, 7657)$ = 51.157, $p < .001$. In addition, children in Class 10 were more likely than children in any other class to have received prior services, with the exception of alcohol or substance abuse therapy. Although Class 4 was the "low-problem" class, for four of the five prior service categories (outpatient, school-based services, residential treatment, and alcohol or substance abuse therapy), children in Class 4 did not have the lowest probability of reporting having received them. This was particularly true for alcohol or substance abuse therapy, $X^2(9, N = 6,976) = 593.58$, $p < .001$ (see Figure 3.1), which children in Class 4 were more likely to have received than those in Classes 10 and 6, even though children in Classes 10 and 6 had much higher probabilities (19.3% and 7.1%, respectively) of alcohol or substance abuse problems than those in Class 4 (4.7%).

There are multiple interpretations for these findings. For example, children in Class 4 may have had some problems of which caregivers were unaware. Diagnostic information indicated that children in Class 4 were the second most likely to have adjustment disorders, following children in Class 7. When analyzing youth self-report of delinquent behaviors and substance use, it was found that for several of the problems, children in Class 4 were not the least likely to have them. However, children in Class 4 actually had a higher probability of having some problems than children in most of the other classes. Specifically, children in Class 4 were the fourth most likely to report alcohol drinking and marijuana use in the 6 months prior to entry into systems of care, after children in Classes 2, 3, and 7. The same was true for selling drugs or helping others sell drugs: Children in Class 4 were the fourth most likely to report having done that at least once in the past 6 months. A second possible interpretation is that the service needs of children in Classes 10 and 6 were not fully met in that few children in those two classes were receiving alcohol

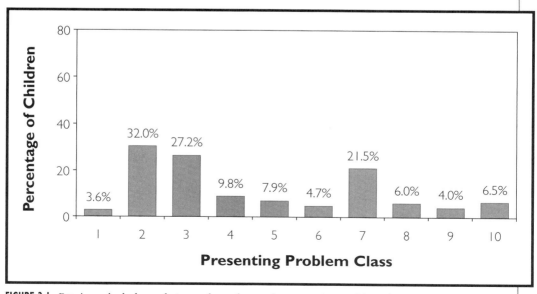

FIGURE 3.1. Previous alcohol or substance abuse therapy by presenting problem class.

or substance abuse therapy; however, no data were available to further explore this possibility.

These findings suggest that children were referred to system-of-care programs for a variety of presenting problems, and many of them had co-occurring problems in both internalizing and externalizing domains. The fact that 10 classes, rather than a smaller number of classes, emerged from the LCA analysis suggests the complexity of presenting problem combinations. Although these children appeared to have received services that were designed to address some of these specific problems, prior to entering systems of care, some of these services may have been insufficient in fully addressing their needs. It is important for case managers and service providers working with these children and families to fully understand the nature and patterns of these problems so that appropriate decisions can be made on the services provided to these children. In addition, understanding the patterns of problems across children referred into systems of care provides valuable information to program managers in their efforts to make decisions regarding changes in the available service array and programmatic resource allocation.

DIFFERENCES IN CLINICAL AND FUNCTIONAL OUTCOMES BY PROGRAM FOCUS (1997–2000)

Analyses in the previous sections focused on differences and similarities in demographic and psychosocial characteristics. In some communities, these variations may be due to the differences in program focus. Although the Guide for Applicants (GFA) provides general target population guidelines around child age, diagnosis, disability, multi-agency involvement, and duration and level of intensity of functional challenges, each grant community has the flexibility to choose its own program focus for serving that target population. For example, some grant communities may focus on serving minority children, while others may serve older children who have had troubles with the law prior to entry into the programs. Program focus may help to explain differences and similarities in demographic characteritics, functioning, and emotional and behavioral problems among children served.

This section focuses on the comparison of clinical and functional outcomes for children served in communities with two different foci: juvenile justice and school-based programs. There were three grant communities funded between 1997 and 2000 with a programmatic focus to serve youth returning to the community from juvenile detention or corrections and four that had school-based programs that out-stationed staff from the mental health agency to the local schools. Across these communities, there were 779 children in the juvenile justice programs and 1,147 children in the school-based programs with at least one piece of outcome information.

Clinical and functional outcomes were measured at entry into system-of-care services using the following three instruments: the *Behavioral and*

Emotional Rating Scale (BERS; Epstein & Sharma, 1998), the *Child Behavior Checklist* (CBCL; Achenbach, 1991), and the *Child and Adolescent Functional Assessment Scale* (CAFAS; Hodges, 1990). The BERS identifies the emotional and behavioral strengths of children. Whereas most existing assessment measures focus on deficits and problems, the BERS focuses on areas of strength and resiliency. The principal uses of the BERS include identifying children with limited strengths, targeting goals for an individual treatment plan, identifying strengths and weaknesses for intervention, documenting progress in a strength area as a consequence of specialized services, and measuring strengths in research and evaluation projects. The CBCL is designed to provide a standardized measure of symptoms and behavioral and emotional problems among children aged 4 through 18 years. The CBCL has been widely used in children's mental health services research and for clinical purposes to assess social competence, behaviors, and feelings. The CBCL elicits a rich and detailed description of behaviors and symptoms that provides different information than diagnosis alone would be able to provide. The CAFAS is a widely used measure of child functioning. It assesses the degree to which a youth's mental health or substance abuse disorder is disruptive to his or her functioning in everyday life in each of eight psychosocial domains: the community, the school, the home, substance use, moods and emotions, self-harming behavior, behavior toward others, and thinking. The CAFAS is designed to assess the *impact* of the child's challenges and behaviors on his or her ability to function successfully in various life domains.

The following analyses were conducted on a sample of children with information on their clinical and functional status upon entry into systems of care. To examine the differences and similarities in clinical and functional status at intake among children served in programs with a juvenile justice, as compared to a school-based, focus, three independent sample *t* tests were conducted separately for the following three areas: (a) overall behavioral and emotional strengths (total BERS strength quotient), (b) overall functional impairment (total CAFAS score), and (c) overall behavioral and emotional problems (total CBCL score). No significant differences were found for the overall behavioral and emotional strengths and problems between children served in the two programs. However, there was a significant difference in the level of overall functional impairment, with children served in the juvenile justice programs having a significantly higher average level of functional impairment than that of those served in school-based programs ($M = 120.95$ vs. $M = 102.21$), $t(756) = 5.74$, $p < .001$.

Analyses of the subscales for each of these three measures were then conducted. No significant differences were found for the BERS subscales, with the exception of school functioning. Not surprisingly, children referred into the school-based programs had lower strengths related to school functioning ($M = 6.77$ vs. $M = 7.27$) than did children referred into the programs focusing on youth with juvenile justice involvement, $t(606) = 2.05$, $p = .041$.

Analysis of the eight CAFAS subscales indicated that children served in programs with a juvenile justice focus had more severe impairment across all the domains of functioning, including the school role and home role (see

Figure 3.2), although the differences in the domains of moods/emotions and self-harmful behavior were not significant. This may suggest that children who have had contact with juvenile justice authorities also have problems in other areas of functioning, such as school and social functioning. However, children with problems or challenges at schools did not necessarily have high levels of impairment in other areas. This is most apparent in the Community Role subscale, where only 9.4% of the children from school-based programs were reported to have a severe impairment, as compared to 33.9% of those in the juvenile justice programs.

It is worth noting that although both the BERS and the CAFAS have a school subscale, the foci of the two subscales are different. The School Strength subscale on the BERS focuses only on strengths related to academic perfor- mance (e.g., completing homework on time), whereas the School Role Per- formance subscale on the CAFAS has a broader focus and includes discipli- nary actions (e.g., expulsion), as well as school performance. This may explain the apparent discrepancies in findings on these two subscales, such as those seen for children served in juvenile justice programs.

Analyses of the CBCL subscales indicated significant differences be- tween the program focus groups in internalizing behaviors, somatic com- plaints, social problems, and delinquent behaviors (see Table 3.6). Children enrolled in school-based programs had more problems with internalizing

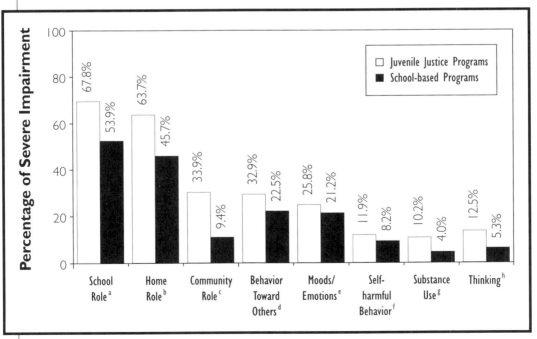

FIGURE 3.2. Percentage of children with severe functional impairment by program focus.
[a]$\chi^2(3, N = 744) = 17.30, p < .01.$ [b]$\chi^2(3, N = 744) = 23.94, p < .001.$ [c]$\chi^2(3, N = 744) = 81.23, p < .001.$ [d]$\chi^2(3, N = 744) = 14.79, p < .01.$ [e]$\chi^2(3, N = 744) = 6.04, p = ns.$ [f]$\chi^2(3, N = 744) = 4.63, p = ns.$ [g]$\chi^2(3, N = 744) = 17.16, p < .01.$ [h]$\chi^2(3, N = 744) = 17.68, p < .01.$

TABLE 3.6

Mean Scores (and Standard Deviations) in Behavioral
and Emotional Problem Scores by Program Focus

Problem	Juvenile Justice Programs	School-Based Programs	Statistical Test and Significance
Internalizing behaviors	63.4 (12.1)	65.1 (11.2)	$t\,(773) = -2.06, p < .05$
Somatic complaints	59.1 (9.6)	61.7 (10.1)	$t\,(773) = -3.65, p < .001$
Social problems	64.4 (11.6)	67.2 (11.1)	$t\,(773) = -3.36, p < .01$
Delinquent behaviors	70.4 (10.2)	67.2 (8.9)	$t\,(773) = 4.61, p < .001$

Note. Only subscales with significant differences included.

behaviors, somatic complaints, and social problems than did those in programs with a juvenile justice focus, while children in the latter programs had more severe problems in delinquent behaviors than did those in school-based programs. These findings suggest that children in school-based programs were more likely to have internalizing problems while children in juvenile justice programs were more likely to have externalizing problems.

These findings indicate that the most significant differences in program focus for child clinical and functional characteristics occurred in functional impairment (i.e., CAFAS scores). This may be due to the fact that many communities use the CAFAS score as one of the criteria to determine eligibility for receiving services in system-of-care programs or may indicate that programs with differing foci are serving children with varied levels of need or needs in different domain areas (e.g., schools vs. communities). Previous studies have indicated that these baseline differences may be related to sector of entry into services (e.g., schools vs. juvenile justice agencies). For example, in an analysis using data from the Great Smoky Mountains Study, it was found that baseline problem severity was one of the factors related to portal of entry into services and sequences of services received (Farmer, Burns, Phillips, Angold, & Costello, 2003).

Regardless, practitioners must take into account baseline differences in the level of functional impairment and in the areas of behavioral and emotional problems when planning services for children and must recognize the importance of environments, other than traditional mental health environments, for the organization and delivery of services. As Leaf and colleagues (1996) noted in their analysis of the MECA study data, the schools serve as an important point of resource mobilization and early detection for youth with serious emotional disturbance.

CONCLUSIONS

When interpreting these findings, one must consider their limitations. First, children with serious emotional disturbance referred into system-of-care services may in some way differ from other children with similar problems receiving services in traditional service environments, and from children receiving mental health services but not having serious emotional disturbance. In addition, these data were collected from an array of funded communities, each potentially with its own unique target population, referral process, and program design. Finally, as with any large-scale community-based data collection effort, patterns of missing data and how they may or may not be related to the characteristics of the children must be considered.

Regardless of these limitations, over the last decade tens of thousands of children with serious emotional disturbance have been referred into system-of-care services across the United States and its territories. These children, who differ in age, race, and ethnicity, enter services for a variety of reasons and with a variety of diagnoses. They bring with them diverse personal, family, and service histories and are accompanied by differing levels of strengths, problems, and functional challenges. As we continue to investigate the similarities and differences among these children at the time of their referral into service—whether the investigation focuses on differences as a function of demographic characteristics, program foci, or in clusters of children with common indicators—we are continually reminded of the complexity of these children's lives, experiences, and challenges.

There are similarities and differences between and among groups of children entering services. For example, there may be differences in lifetime risk exposure, educational indicators, and diagnoses as a function of age, race, and gender; differences in behavior and functioning as they relate to the focus of the system-of-care program; or differences in prior service use among groups of children classified by the number and type(s) of their presenting problems.

The complex clinical and psychosocial characteristics of these children at intake into services highlight their varied and unique service needs. Understanding and accepting the complexity and diversity further informs our efforts to appropriately expand service arrays, triage children into specialized services, and develop and implement individualized service plans.

REFERENCES

Achenbach, T. M. (1991). *Manual for the Child Behavior Checklist/4–18 and 1991 Profile.* Burlington: University of Vermont, Department of Psychiatry.

Costello, E. J., Messer, S. C., Bird, H. R., Cohen, P., & Reinherz, H. Z. (1998). The prevalence of serious emotional disturbance: A re-analysis of community studies. *Journal of Child and Family Studies, 7*(4), 411–432.

Epstein, M. H., & Sharma, J. (1998). *Behavioral and Emotional Rating Scale: A Strength-Based Approach to Assessment.* Austin, TX: PRO-ED.

Farmer, E. M. Z., Burns, B. J., Phillips, S. D., Angold, A., & Costello, E. J. (2003). Pathways into and through mental health services for children and adolescents. *Psychiatric Services, 54*(1), 60–66.

Hodges, K. (1990). *Child and Adolescent Functional Assessment Scale* (CAFAS). Ypsilanti: Eastern Michigan University, Department of Psychology.

Landrum, T. J., Singh, N. N., Nemil, M. S., Ellis, C. R., & Best, A. M. (1995). Characteristics of children and adolescents with serious emotional disturbance in systems of care: Part II. Community-based services. *Journal of Emotional and Behavioral Disorders, 3,* 141–149.

Leaf, P. J., Alegria, M., Cohen, P., Goodman, S. H., Horowitz, S. M., Hoven, C. W., et al. (1996). Mental health service use in the community and schools: Results from the four-community MECA Study. *Journal of the Academy of Child and Adolescent Psychiatry, 35*(7), 889–887.

Liao, Q., Mantueffel, B., Paulic, C., & Sondheimer, D. L. (2001). Describing the population of adolescents served in systems of care. *Journal of Emotional and Behavioral Disorders, 9,* 13–29.

Reid, R., Riccio, C. A., Kessler, R. H., DuPaul, G. J., Power, T. J., Anastopoulos, A. D., et al. (2000). Gender and ethnic differences in ADHD as assessed by behavior ratings. *Journal of Emotional and Behavioral Disorders, 8,* 42–54.

Rosenblatt, J., Robertson, M. B., Wood, M., Furlong, M. J., & Sosna, T. (1998). Troubled or troubling? Characteristics of youth referred to a system of care without system-level referral constraints. *Journal of Emotional and Behavioral Disorders, 6,* 38–48.

Stroul, B. A., & Friedman, R. M. (1986). *A system of care for children and youth with severe emotional disturbances.* Washington, DC: Georgetown University Child Development Center.

U.S. Department of Health and Human Services. (1999). *Mental health: A report of the Surgeon General.* Rockville, MD: Author.

Walrath, C., dosReis, S., Miech, R., Liao, Q., Holden, E. W., De Carolis, G., et al. (2001). Referral source differences in functional impairment levels for children served in the Comprehensive Community Mental Health Services for Children and Their Families Program. *Journal of Child and Family Studies, 10*(3), 405–417.

Assessment, Methodology, and Evaluation Models

Research Designs for Children's Mental Health Services Research

CHAPTER 4

Stephanie Reich and Leonard Bickman

Research in children's mental health services is focused on determining what treatments and methods for delivering services work best for children with mental health needs. To answer these questions, researchers often employ experiments and quasi-experiments in an attempt to identify a causal relationship between variables (e.g., Does this treatment result in better outcomes for children?). There are many different ways to study a causal relationship, and each method has potential problems associated with it. This chapter describes the criteria needed to determine causality and the key features of experimentation and quasi-experimental designs, and then enumerates the many issues that threaten the validity of a study and potential interpretations of the study results.

DETERMINING CAUSALITY

To determine that a causal relationship exists, several criteria must be met. First, the temporal order must be that the cause precedes the effect. Second, there should be temporal contiguity between the cause and effect; that is, the cause and the effect appear relatively close in time. Third, there should be a level of common variation, known as covariation, between the cause and the effect. When the cause is present, the effect is present, and when the cause is absent, the effect is absent. Fourth, there should be congruity between both. Typically, a small cause should result in a small effect, whereas a large cause should result in a large effect. When there is a mismatch (e.g., small cause produces big effect), more evidence is usually needed to explain this discrepancy (Cordray, 2000). Finally, plausible rival explanations of the observed effect should be improbable. Ruling out other explanations supports the proposed causal relationship. This is accomplished best by addressing the threats to validity described later in the chapter.

COUNTERFACTUAL CONDITION

The ideal way to test a causal relationship is to study a person or situation with an intervention and without it. This enables a research investigation to determine the effect of the cause by comparing what happened with the intervention to what would have happened without it. The "what would have happened" condition is called the *counterfactual condition* (Corrin & Cook, 1998; Holland, 1989) and is based on the assumption that everything else is the same except for the presence of the intervention (Shadish, Cook, & Campbell, 2002). In the real world, testing the counterfactual condition is not possible. Often the intervention has a lasting effect that would influence a later studied no-treatment condition. Participants who experience an educational intervention could not easily "unlearn" the program in order to be measured again in a no-treatment condition. Even if the intervention effects could be removed, there are many other characteristics that would be altered. The time period would be different and the participants would be more experienced with the study. This is why using each person as his or her own control is fraught with problems. Typically, the closest a researcher can come to the counterfactual condition is to use a comparison group.

A comparison group is a group of people who do not receive the "cause" (i.e., treatment or intervention) and who are compared to the group that does (treatment group). The difference between these groups, if everything else is the same, is the effect of the intervention. The more similar the comparison group is to the treatment group, the greater the confidence in the causal relationship or that the effect was produced by the cause.

EXPERIMENTS AND QUASI-EXPERIMENTS

Two ways researchers can investigate a causal relationship is through a randomized experiment or a quasi-experiment. In a randomized experiment, the researcher randomly assigns participants into groups, levels, or conditions such that each participant has an equal chance (i.e., independent, nonzero probability) of being assigned to any of the experimental groups, levels, or conditions (Keppel, 1991). In quasi-experimental designs, participants are not randomly assigned to conditions.

Random assignment reduces the possibility of systematic bias from characteristics of the participants appearing more often in one group than the other (Hill, Rubin, & Thomas, 2000). Participants may vary in many ways, and some of these characteristics may affect the behavior (effect) being studied. Without random assignment, these differences may be associated with how a person is placed in a group. When random assignment is carried out successfully, there is greater confidence that the treatment and control groups were equivalent on both measured and unmeasured variables before the treatment was initiated.

Imagine we believe that caregivers of children with severe emotional disturbance (SED) feel additional stress by having chaotic schedules in which they have to juggle their own agenda with their children's school schedules and mental health appointments. In response, we create a program that is designed to help people better manage their time. We decide to conduct an experiment in which half of the caregivers receive the program and the other half do not receive assistance with scheduling. We ask all 40 parents to come to the study facility at one specific time and we assign them to groups on a first-come basis. The first 20 parents to arrive are placed in the treatment group and the next 20 are assigned to the no-treatment group. At the end of the program we find that our treatment group members, who arrived earlier, are much more organized with their time than the other group. Is the difference observed at the end of the study because of the program or some other factor? Perhaps the caregivers who are punctual are already better at scheduling their time than the late-arriving ones are. Another explanation accounting for the difference could be that more of the people who arrived on time have cars, which provide more flexibility in scheduling, whereas people who arrived later rely on the bus and have less freedom in scheduling. If we had randomly assigned caregivers to groups, it would be more likely that the early- and late-arriving people would be equally distributed among the groups. Instead, we may have introduced systematic bias into our study.

Randomization works best when applied to large groups of participants. For example, if you flip a coin once, you have a $\frac{1}{2}$ chance of getting a head. If you flip it five times, you have a $(\frac{1}{2})(\frac{1}{2})(\frac{1}{2})(\frac{1}{2})(\frac{1}{2}) = \frac{1}{32}$ chance of getting all heads. The more people in the study, the less likely similar characteristics will disproportionately appear in one group more than the other. A researcher must be sure that the random assignment process is truly random and not simply haphazard. In an evaluation of a treatment, it is often better if the researcher, rather than the people delivering the services, conducts the random assignment. This helps ensure that the randomization process is not corrupted, for example, by assigning more "needy" cases to the treatment group.

A key factor in maintaining the credibility of a study design is that others consider it to be as unbiased as possible. When feasible, it is best to collect baseline (pretest) data prior to randomly assigning participants to groups. This helps ensure that the groups are equivalent because early dropouts (persons who do not complete the baseline data collection) will have dropped out before random assignment and thus will not contribute to differences between the groups. The data collected can also provide information on persons who drop out early. Moreover, if there is a key variable that the researcher wants to have randomly distributed, baseline data will allow for pairing participants on that variable and then randomly assign each member of a pair. Random assignment does not guarantee equivalent groups; it just increases the probability that influential variables will be equally distributed between groups rather than disproportionately clustering in one. In the next section, we describe a randomized study of children's mental health services to illustrate these points.

All research, including the examples cited in this chapter, requires ethical considerations in its design and implementation. Research procedures should be designed to protect the privacy and safety of participants. Each of the examples of children's mental health services research in this chapter was reviewed and approved by a university institutional review board (IRB), which has the express purpose of protecting the rights of children and their families. For more information on ethical conduct for research with human participants, please see Appendix 4.A.

The Stark County Study: Example of a Randomized Experiment

The Stark County study was an evaluation of a comprehensive system-of-care model using a randomized design (Bickman, Summerfelt, & Noser, 1997). The term *system of care* is a concept of integrated comprehensive care for children and was developed in response to problems concerning the availability and delivery of mental health services for children; this framework is discussed elsewhere in this volume. To recruit participants for the study, names and contact information from families seeking services were obtained from either the Department of Human Services or the local community mental health center. The center intake worker followed the clinic's usual guidelines to determine eligibility for services. Children were excluded from the evaluation if they were too young (less than 5 years old), did not have an SED, had too low an IQ (less than 85), or if the admitting center personnel considered the child to be in need of emergency services. The clinic intake staff, based on their usual procedures, made the determination of SED and also asked for permission for the Vanderbilt University evaluators to contact the parent. When contacted by the evaluation staff, 85% of the parents agreed to participate in the study and be interviewed.

Only after the interview data were collected did a computer program randomly assign the family to either the system of care (treatment group) or usual care from the community (comparison group). In this latter group, caregivers were told that they had to arrange services for their children on their own and were given a list of community providers.

The evaluation staff carried out the random assignment process after baseline data had been collected, reducing the potential threats to validity caused by differential attrition (e.g., families drop out at different rates from the treatment and comparison groups). The primary advantage of random assignment in this study was the increased probability of initially equivalent groups. However there were also potential problems associated with such a design; for example, critics of the evaluation claimed that the comparison group children were deprived of better services. The sole purpose of the study was to determine if a system-of-care model was more effective than treatment as usual. This model of care had not been tested and whether it was better was unknown. Therefore, it could have been argued that it was more unethical to continue to provide untested services to children and families than it was to withhold experimental services of unknown effectiveness.

Another potential problem with this experimental design was that although random assignment was used, it was not employed for all possible participants. Certain children were excluded from the study because they were in need of immediate care. Random assignment for such cases was not possible because collecting pretest data before assignment would have delayed treatment. As will be discussed later, the exclusion of this group limits the generalizability of the findings to nonemergency cases but does not affect the researcher's ability to make a conclusion about causality. Although randomization is often preferable, there are times when it is inconvenient, impractical, or unethical (Lipsey & Cordray, 2000).

At times, randomizing participants is burdensome and expensive. In such instances, relying on naturally occurring groups is more practical. School-based programs often utilize comparisons of students between schools rather than trying to randomly assign children to schools. At other times, randomization is simply not possible. If a program has full coverage, in which every member of the population receives the treatment, then it is not possible to randomly assign people to a treatment or no-treatment comparison group. This is often the case when entitlement policies are studied or if the study deals with a natural disaster (Hendrick, Bickman, & Rog, 1993). For example, if federal law entitles a certain class of people to services, it would be illegal to deny services to anyone in that group. Randomization is also impossible if a condition occurs in only a subset of the population. For example, a researcher cannot assign people to have major depression or to be female rather than male. It is difficult to imagine assigning someone to the conditions of poverty, incarceration, or homelessness. Finally, at times randomization may be possible but unethical. A researcher comparing two different effective types of services in order to determine which is more effective could not add a no-treatment control condition because an effective treatment exists. However, if there is no effective treatment, random assignment to a no-treatment control condition is acceptable. In practice, there is no ethical way to control whether people obtain services outside of the study. Thus, the comparison group is often labeled a treatment as usual group (TAU) rather than a no-treatment control group. More information about the use of randomized designs can be found in Boruch (1997).

When random assignment is not possible due to expense, practicality, or ethics, a researcher must rely on quasi-experimental designs. Although there are several types of quasi-experimental research designs, the three most relevant to mental health services are the (a) nonequivalent comparison group design, (b) the interrupted time series design, and (c) the regression discontinuity design.

Nonequivalent Comparison Group Design

When randomization is not possible, a researcher can use a nonequivalent comparison group design in which groups are identified by some naturally occurring criteria. This design is the most common quasi-experimental design used in the behavioral sciences (Rosenthal & Rosnow, 1991). Nonequivalent group designs can compare the treatment group to a deliberately chosen group, normed data from another group/sample, or secondary data collected from other studies (Shadish et al., 2002). Deliberately selecting a comparison group that is most similar to the treatment group is often the best method for making causal inferences.

Technically, the nonequivalent group design could include measurement as a pretest (before the intervention) and posttest (after the intervention) or only as a posttest (Reichardt & Mark, 1998). Because the groups were determined on some criteria other than randomization, using only posttest data renders causal explanations fraught with problems. Without measuring baseline status, it is difficult to conclude that differences between the groups were due to the intervention rather than to another factor that existed before the intervention.

The Fort Bragg Evaluation: A Nonequivalent Comparison Group Quasi-Experiment

The largest nonequivalent comparison group study evaluating child and adolescent mental health services was the Fort Bragg Demonstration Project and Evaluation (Bickman, 1996a, 1996b; Bickman et al., 1995). The Fort Bragg study was designed as an independent evaluation of the Fort Bragg Child and Adolescent Mental Health Demonstration to test the efficacy of providing a full continuum of community-based services. The goal was to determine if this continuum of services resulted in improved treatment outcomes while decreasing the cost of care when compared to treatment as usual.

The evaluation results revealed that the demonstration successfully implemented a continuum of care and that it dramatically increased access to mental health services. However, children at both the demonstration and comparison sites improved on measures of mental health outcomes. Children in the demonstration showed no greater improvement than did children at the comparison site, and the costs of services at the demonstration site were higher than at the comparison site. Instead of confirming strongly held beliefs, the evaluation reported that the continuum was less cost-effective than the fragmented treatment found in the comparison site.

The initial intent was to use a randomized design for the Fort Bragg evaluation. However this was not possible because the system-of-care intervention was a full-coverage program affecting all children in Fort Bragg, North Carolina. Every family in the area had access to the demonstration; therefore, none of the families could be assigned to a comparison group. Because the project was unable to use random assignment of participants to different models of care, families and children from other military bases served as comparison participants to facilitate examination of the effectiveness of the demonstration. Army officials designated two comparison sites that were approximately the size of Fort Bragg: Fort Campbell, Kentucky, and Fort Stewart, Georgia. Both bases provided children with traditional mental health services.

One of the major challenges with quasi-experimental designs is ensuring that the treatment and comparison groups are equivalent at the start of the study. Although modern statistical techniques make potential lack of equivalency less of a problem than in the past, differences at the start of the study clearly complicate interpretation of causal relationships. The study therefore needed to assess whether the families and the service settings were similar before the introduction of the demonstration.

The Fort Bragg evaluation was fortunate to have military posts as the sites of both the treatment and comparison conditions, because separate posts tend to be quite similar. In contrast to families in different cities or different parts of a city, military families and posts are very comparable regardless of where they are located.

However, these similarities did not guarantee that the families and children from each site would be the same on important mental health variables. Therefore, the evaluation staff compared the children and families on 103 mental health variables at baseline. This large number of variables was selected because the investigators wanted the comparisons to be exhaustive and include all subscales of the instruments. The sites differed statistically on 14 variables, with the comparison site children appearing more impaired on 9 variables and the demonstration children seeming more impaired on 5 other variables. These differences in groups were very small, and the researchers concluded that it was unlikely that they would account for differential outcomes in the posttest. Because this was not a randomized experiment, the researchers could not be sure that the groups did not differ on some important variable that they did not measure. It was believed, however, that this was unlikely given the number and importance of the variables tested.

Thus, although a randomized experiment could not be conducted, the quasi-experiment had the advantage of being able to include all families, even families in crisis, in contrast to the randomized Stark County study, discussed earlier, which eliminated this group of families. Another advantage of this design was the lack of delay in treatment because children were recruited as soon as they entered services. In a randomized experiment, there may be a delay in the receipt of services if the researcher wants to collect pretest data before the child is assigned to either the treatment or the comparison group. As noted earlier, children who are in need of immediate services could not participate in a randomized study (such as Stark County) but could be part of the quasi-experiment. In such cases where there is a choice of designs, a researcher will have to compare the benefits of randomized versus nonequivalent comparison group designs. These trade-offs address issues of internal and external validity of designs and will be discussed in greater depth later in the chapter.

Interrupted Time Series Design

When there are many data collection periods before and after an intervention, the quasi-experimental design is known as an interrupted time series design, which may or may not include a nonequivalent comparison group. A time series design is the repeated measure of a variable over time. An interrupted time series design is the repeated measurement of a variable before and after the introduction of a new variable, such as a treatment or intervention. The more often the variable is measured over time, the more sensitive the study will be to changes caused by the introduction of the treatment. By determining the typical trend of the variable before and after the intervention, researchers can identify the degree of impact, or effect, of the intervention. Typically, estimating the effect can be determined by calculating the slope or rate of change before and after the intervention. Data collection may look like this:

$$O_1 \qquad O_2 \qquad O_3 \qquad O_4 \qquad X \qquad O_5 \qquad O_6 \qquad O_7 \qquad O_8$$

Os indicate the measurement periods and X indicates the introduction of the intervention.

The change in the data may look like a large level shift, a slow increase or decrease, a temporary change, a delayed change, or an abrupt change that decays (Reichardt & Mark, 1998). Figure 4.1 demonstrates some of these changes. Interrupted time series designs allow the treatment group to serve as

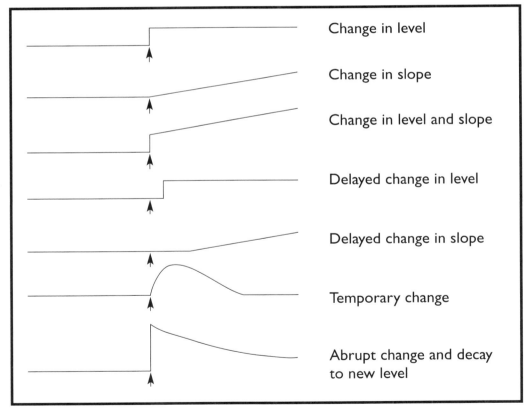

Change in level

Change in slope

Change in level and slope

Delayed change in level

Delayed change in slope

Temporary change

Abrupt change and decay to new level

FIGURE 4.1. Possible patterns that a treatment effect could follow over time. *From* "Quasi Experimentation," by C. Reichardt and M. Mark, in *Handbook of Applied Social Research Methods* (pp. 193–227) by L. Bickman and D. Rog (Eds.), 1998, Thousand Oaks, CA: Sage. Copyright 1998 by Sage. Reprinted with permission. This figure was originally adapted from "Estimating Effects of Community Prevention Trials: Alternative Design and Methods," by C. Reichardt, in *Community Prevention Trials for Alcohol Problems: Methodological Issues* (pp. 137–158) by H. D. Holder and J. M. Howard (Eds.), 1992, Westport, CT: Praeger. Copyright 1992 by Greenwood Publishing Group, Inc. Adapted with permission.

its own comparison group. Multiple measurement points before and after the intervention allow researchers to compare how the measured variables were changing over time without the intervention and how they changed after the intervention. Interrupted time series designs can use a nonequivalent comparison group as well. In such situations, both the treatment group and the comparison groups are measured at multiple times before and after the intervention is introduced to the treatment group. Such a design would look like the following:

Treatment group: O_1 O_2 O_3 O_4 X O_5 O_6 O_7 O_8

Comparison group: O_1 O_2 O_3 O_4 O_5 O_6 O_7 O_8

Wraparound Services: An Interrupted Time Series Example

In 1996 Congress mandated that the Department of Defense (DoD) develop, implement, and evaluate a demonstration project that utilized a "wraparound" service system for child and adolescent military dependents. Congress defined "wraparound" as a community-based program developed with a focus on individual needs to support normalized and inclusive options for child and adolescent mental health patients and their families. The evaluation addressed child and family outcomes and costs. A randomized experiment was not acceptable to DoD, so a nonequivalent comparison group design was used (Bickman, Smith, Lambert, & Andrade, 2003). The treatment group contained the children and families who entered the wraparound program. However, a comparison group was not easily established. The evaluators chose to recruit families who had been referred to the demonstration but did not participate in it. The logic was that the groups should start out equivalent because the children were referred by the same sources. However, it was possible that the demonstration's eligibility criteria and the self-selection of the families into the demonstration could produce two very different groups of children. Therefore, a comparison of the baseline data of those who agreed to participate in the evaluation and those who did not was conducted; this showed only 5 statistically significant differences out of 90 variables (which would be expected by chance alone).

Although the clinical outcomes for this study were evaluated in a nonequivalent group design, the cost analysis used a form of the interrupted time series design with a nonequivalent comparison group. This design is very useful for studying variables like service use or cost, which are usually collected frequently.

For service utilization and the cost analysis of the wraparound program, data from the Health Care Services Record (HCSR) were used. HCSR data report the volume and type of services children received and the dollar amount providers billed for those services. Summaries of these data were supplied for the services children received over the 3 years preceding the start of the wraparound demonstration and ended 1 month before any child received the last wraparound service. A summary was done per child for each month of care. On average, the HCSR data contained 48 months of service utilization and mental health expenditures per child.

When analyzing monthly HCSR information, we used a nonlinear longitudinal hierarchical model known as a piecewise linear model (PWLM). The main advantage of using a PWLM is that it allows measurement of changes in expenditures between groups across different time segments (Lambert, Wahler, Andrade, & Bickman, 2001; Snijders & Bosker, 1999). The results indicated that both groups had equivalent cost histories for the 30 months before the wraparound demonstration. In the 6 months preceding the demonstration, both groups experienced an equivalent dramatic rise in costs. However, in the 6 months following the start of the demonstration, costs dropped more dramatically for the comparison group than for the wraparound demonstration group, resulting in significantly lower costs for the comparison group. As in the two studies discussed above, child and family outcomes were equivalent but costs were higher in the experimental condition.

Regression Discontinuity Design

One of the risks of not randomly assigning participants to groups is that unmeasured characteristics may bias the effects. However, if we attempt to understand the criteria for how people are assigned to groups, we can attempt to control for their influence. Regression discontinuity designs determine a priori the criteria for how people are assigned to groups. Therefore, the selection process, as with random assignment, is known perfectly, at least in theory (Cook & Campbell, 1979).

In a regression discontinuity design, a researcher creates or identifies an assignment variable, which can be any measure taken at baseline. Once a measure is identified, the researcher determines a critical cutoff point. Participants with scores above this point are assigned to one group, and those below are assigned to the other. The cutoff point should be precise so that variations around this point are not mistaken for effects (Cook & Campbell, 1979). In a regression discontinuity design, the method for assignment can be perfectly measured and implemented (Shadish et al., 2002). Figure 4.2 illustrates the implementation of a regression discontinuity design. This design would be very useful if a service used objective measures and consistent cutoff points to assign different levels of care. However, this type of decision making is rare in mental health services, and this design is not frequently used.

THREATS TO VALIDITY

All experimental designs, including quasi-experiments and randomized experiments, are susceptible to external variables that can threaten the conclusions of a study. Inferences (e.g., conclusions and generalizations) about the findings are vulnerable to the threats in four categories of validity: (a) statisti-

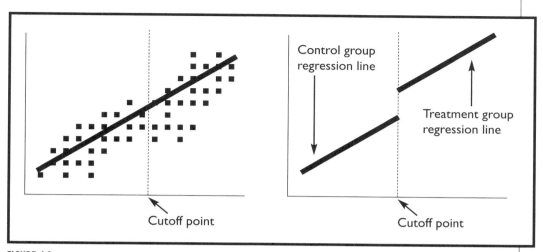

FIGURE 4.2. Assigning a treatment and control group in a regression discontinuity design.

cal conclusion validity, (b) internal validity, (c) construct validity, and (d) external validity (see Table 4.1). Internal validity deals directly with the causal relationship: Did A cause B? Statistical conclusion validity determines if there is quantitative evidence of a covariation between A and B. Construct validity deals with inferences made from findings: Are A and B conceptually what the researcher believes them to be, or has the relationship been mislabeled? External validity describes what applications of the causal relationship can be made. Specifically, can finding that A causes B be applied to other people, places, or times than this study? Understanding how these threats operate is critical to designing good studies. Because the goal of the good designer is to eliminate as many of these threats as possible, they are described in some detail in this chapter.

These four threats to validity apply to randomized experiments and noncausal relationships (e.g., correlations), but quasi-experimental designs are often more vulnerable to their effects. Therefore, this section will focus on how threats to statistical conclusion, internal, construct, and external validity can threaten the interpretations of causal relationships in quasi-experimental designs.

Statistical Conclusion Validity

If a study has statistical conclusion validity, then "conclusions about covariation are made on the basis of statistical evidence" (Cook & Campbell, 1979, p. 37). In quasi-experimentation, these conclusions are drawn about the cause and effects on the basis of proper statistical methods applied appropriately to reliable information (Wortman, 1994). Basically, statistical procedures can demonstrate that the cause is related to a change in the effect. To assess the statistical conclusion validity of a study, one must determine if (a) the study design is sensitive enough to detect covariation between two variables (i.e.,

TABLE 4.1
Threats to the Four Types of Validity

Statistical conclusion validity
  Low statistical power
  Fishing and error rate
  Unreliability of measures
  Unreliability of treatment implementation
  Random irrelevancies in the setting
  Random heterogeneity of respondents
  Violation of statistical tests

Internal validity
  History
  Maturation
  Testing
  Instrumentation
  Statistical regression
  Selection
  Attrition (mortality)
  Demoralization
  Contamination
  Compensation
  Interactions with selection
  Ambiguity about the direction of the causal inference

Construct validity
  Inadequate preoperational explication of the constructs
  Mono-operational bias
  Mono-method bias
  Hypothesis guessing
  Evaluation apprehension
  Experimenter expectancies
  Confounding of constructs
  Interaction of different treatments
  Interaction of testing and treatment
  Restricted generalization across related constructs

External validity
  Interaction of selection and treatment
  Interaction of setting and treatment
  Interaction of history and treatment

cause and effect), and (b) if so, what the evidence of the covariation is, and (c) given the evidence, how strong the covariation is (Rosenthal & Rosnow, 1991).

There are seven major threats to statistical conclusion validity that make drawing conclusions about covariation difficult. These are (a) low statistical power, (b) fishing and error rate, (c) unreliability of measures, (d) unreliability of treatment implementation, (e) random irrelevancies in the setting, (f) random heterogeneity of respondents, and (g) violation of statistical tests (Cook, Campbell, & Peracchio, 1990).

Statistical Power

Experimentation is based on supporting or rejecting the null hypothesis. The null hypothesis is the hypothesis that would be true if the experimental one is false. The null hypothesis is assumed to be true in generating the sampling distribution used in the study (Hays, 1994). For example, if a study hypothesizes that A causes B, the null hypothesis would state that there is no causal relationship between A and B. Thus, if the study fails to reject the hypothesis, then it cannot conclude that there was an effect (B) produced by a cause (A). On the other hand, if the study is able to reject the null hypothesis, it has demonstrated that there appears to be a relationship between the two variables.

In testing causal relationships, there are four possible findings: (a) that a relationship between the cause and effect exists and the study statistically identifies it, (b) that no such relationship exists and the study incorrectly concludes that there is one (false positive), (c) that no relationship exists and the study indicates no relationship, and (d) there is a relationship and the study falsely concludes that there is none (false negative). A Type I error occurs when covariation is found to be statistically significant but in actuality there is no relationship. The Greek letter α (alpha) represents the probability of such a false positive. When there is covariation and the researcher does not identify it (i.e., false negative), this is known as a Type II error. The Greek letter β (beta) represents the probability of making this error. *Statistical power* is the probability of identifying the covariation between the cause and effect when it is does, indeed, exist. This probability is $1 - \beta$. Several factors affect the statistical power of a study. These are the sample size (number of people in each condition of the study), alpha level (the probability of a false positive), the type of statistical test applied, and the effect size (the difference between the means of the treatment and comparison groups divided by their standard deviation; Lipsey, 1998).

Low statistical power is a threat to statistical conclusion validity because it increases the likelihood of falsely concluding that there is no relationship between the cause and the effect. Low statistical power is similar to saying a study is not very sensitive. To guard against this, the researcher should increase sample sizes, raise the alpha level, use more powerful statistics, or assess larger effect sizes. It is absolutely critical that statistical power be calculated during the design of the study. If the power is not sufficient to detect the expected effect size, it may not be wise to conduct the study.

Fishing and Error Rate

The alpha level is the probability of making a false positive. In the behavioral sciences this is typically set at $p < .05$. This means that out of every 100 studies conducted, 5 will be found significant by chance alone. Fishing occurs when multiple analyses of the data are conducted without adjusting the significance level. The more statistical comparisons that are conducted in a single study, the greater likelihood chance will bias the results. This threat can be decreased by reducing the number of analyses conducted, making statistical adjustments (corrections that lower the significance level, such as the Bonferroni procedure) when performing multiple analyses, and using multivariate techniques when testing relationships among many variables (Cook et al., 1990).

Reliability of Measures and Restriction of Range

The reliability of measures poses a particular threat to statistical conclusion validity. Reliable measures consistently measure a construct (Shadish et al., 2002). If a measure is unreliable, unintended variation is added to the research design. Unreliability may lead to nonsignificant findings when there was actually an effect produced. Therefore, unreliable measures threaten validity in either direction (i.e., false negative or false positive; Rogosa, 1980). Additionally, measures that restrict the range of data will not be sensitive to changes in participants. This is likely to occur when a large proportion of participants have extremely low or extremely high scores. They either cluster near the lowest possible score (floor effect) or at the highest possible score (ceiling effect). In either case, it is difficult to measure change because scores are already at the range limits and can be neither lower nor higher (Shadish et al., 2002).

Reliability of Treatment Implementation

To test whether the cause (e.g., treatment) produces an effect, it is important that the cause be implemented consistently. This reliability in implementation allows for greater causal inferences. For example, conclusions about the effects of a system-of-care model for children's mental health would be difficult to draw if some sites did not apply the model or only did so sporadically. Low treatment reliability or fidelity could also occur if one site used the system-of-care model for some families and not others within the same study.

Extraneous Variance in Setting

Variations in the setting in which the treatment occurs may have an influence on the effect. These influences can be any type of environmental factor (e.g., time of day, temperature, noise) that varies at different time points or between the comparison and intervention groups. This added variance makes it more difficult to identify which effects were produced by the intervention rather than the setting. Studies conducted within laboratory settings use a much smaller sample of participants to detect smaller effects than "real-world" field-based studies because the researcher or investigator can control and reduce the effects of setting variation. The ability to control the setting is almost absent in studies of treatment or services that take place in the real world.

Random Heterogeneity of Respondents (Units)

If the participants in a study are very different from one another, they may produce findings with a great deal of variation that is not due to the treatment. This extra variance may obscure covariation between the cause and effect, either by exacerbating or minimizing it. For example, laboratory studies of psychotherapy usually reduce variability by severely limiting the participants to a single diagnosis, a luxury that is not available in a community-based mental health center or clinic.

Violation of Statistical Test

Statistical conclusion validity is based on the statistical evidence of covariation between two variables. This evidence is obtained through statistical analysis. Each statistical test has certain assumptions that must be met for it to be valid. These assumptions should be known before the researcher applies them to data. False conclusions may be drawn if an inappropriate test is used to assess covariation. For example, analysis of variance (ANOVA) is intended for normally distributed data. If the data are highly skewed or bimodal, transformation may need to be conducted first or perhaps a different analytic procedure applied.

Statistical conclusion validity, although very important for assessing covariation and drawing causal inferences in quasi-experimental and experimental designs, has been written about the least in the research methodology literature. However, there is growing concern over this lack of awareness (Lipsey, 2000). Specifically, a lack of statistical power is an especially large threat to statistical conclusion validity. In 1962, Cohen found that social research had enough power to detect expected effects only half the time (Cohen, 1962). Twenty-seven years later, Sedlmeier and Gigerenzer (1989) found little improvement in the social sciences. Overall, most social science is underpowered, meaning that it is not sensitive enough to detect important smaller effect sizes. Clearly, there is no point in conducting well thought out and designed studies if they are not powerful enough to identify covariation when it is present. To avoid this, all planning for experimentation (including quasi-experimentation) should include a power analysis. Otherwise, treatments may be labeled as ineffective when, in actuality, they may be of benefit. Consumers of research should be aware of issues of power when reading studies that conclude no effect. Readers should be cognizant of sample sizes, alpha levels, the types of statistical tests conducted, and the effect sizes anticipated by the researchers. (For more information on statistical power, see Cohen & Cohen, 1983; Lipsey, 1990.)

Internal Validity

Internal validity refers to the truthfulness "with which statements can be made about whether there is a causal relationship from one variable to another" (Cook & Campbell, 1979, p. 38). Many factors can threaten the internal validity of a design. These include history, maturation, testing, instrumentation, statistical regression, selection, attrition (mortality), demoralization, contamination, compensation, interactions with selection, and ambiguity about the direction of the causal inference. Each of these will be briefly discussed.

History

Events other than the treatment that have an influence on participants' behavior can threaten internal validity (Shaughnessy & Zechmeister, 1994). These events typically occur after the pretest and before the posttest so that changes or lack of changes could be due to the intervention or some other event. A historical event may exaggerate or cloud findings (McCleary, 2000). Imagine the implementation of a school-based program to identify signs of depression and suicidal risk in teens. At the same time the program is being implemented, the city begins to air public service announcements detailing the warning signs of suicide and providing information on services. The posttest of the school-based program shows that there is an increase in staff and students' identification of depressive and suicidal behaviors. With these findings, it is difficult to conclude whether the program worked, the changes were due to the commercials appearing nightly, or the changes were due to a combination of the program and the announcements. Historical events thus make causal inferences difficult. Historical threats can apply to randomized designs if one group is exposed to some influencing event that the other group is not.

Maturation

Studies that occur over time are susceptible to the influence of historical changes as well as changes within participants that were not intended by the treatment. These changes could include growing older, stronger, wiser, more fatigued, or bored. If the changes affect the intended outcome, inferences about the effects of the treatment are difficult. This threat to internal validity is a common concern when researchers are working with young children. Because children grow and change quickly, it is often more difficult to separate changes due to natural maturation from effects of the intervention. For example, in a program to treat hyperactive and inattentive behaviors in young children, significant findings may be attributable to either the program or to the fact that the children have matured and display more age-appropriate self-regulation. This is a serious concern for research in the field of child and adolescent mental health services.

Testing

Testing participants multiple times also may affect the answers they give. This is called *reactivity*. Reactivity to testing can occur in several ways. Sometimes participants want to be consistent with previous answers, thus minimizing changes over time. The test may pique participants' curiosity about something on the pretest and provoke them to look up the answers or at least think more about the topic. Both thinking more and obtaining information may improve participants' performance on the subsequent testing. In such cases, their improvements are not due to the intervention but to their own studying. These reactive testing effects are sometimes referred to as *practice effects*.

There are several ways to assess the impact of testing effects. Item response theory (IRT) enables researchers to calibrate participants' performance through the use of multiple measures (Lord, 1980). Additionally, research designs can detect the influence of testing effects by providing comparisons between groups with and without pretest measures. The Solomon four-group design is the best example of this (Hendrick et al., 1993; Solomon, 1949). This design utilizes four groups: two intervention groups and two comparison groups. One of the intervention groups and one of the comparison groups are given a pretest, and all four groups are given a posttest. This allows inferences about the reactivity of testing.

Instrumentation

In addition to participants changing from pretest to posttest, the data collection process may change. This change could be due to an alteration in the person or method for collecting data. This threat is especially salient when the data are collected through observational methods and the observer is replaced during the course of the study (Shaughnessy & Zechmeister, 1994). The new person assigned to observe may be less experienced than the previous observer or use slightly different criteria for judging and categorizing observations.

Changes in the method of collecting data may also alter the data obtained. For example, a researcher studying insurance use for psychiatric services relies on data collected by the insurance company. If the company changes to a new system with different coding structures, the data given to the researcher may be very different from the data obtained earlier. In this situation, findings of changes in service use may be due to actual changes or to alterations in the coding process. This is a common problem in using administrative data and requires a vigilant investigator. Instrumentation changes are also common in the study of young children. For tests to be age appropriate, the method for collecting data is often different. Measuring behaviors in an infant would be different from measuring behaviors in a 10-year-old child.

Statistical Regression to the Mean

If respondents are assigned to treatment or comparison groups on the basis of an extreme and unreliable pretest score, the study is at risk for the artifact of statistical regression to the mean. Statistical regression to the mean occurs when scores are inflated or deflated due to error in measurement. Because the pretest score may be abnormally high or low, subsequent testing will most likely yield scores closer to the population mean (Cook & Campbell, 1979). A pretest that measures depressive symptoms may question a woman who had very little sleep and was feeling a bit overwhelmed. Her depressive symptoms may appear quite high at that time. However, retesting after she has had a good night's sleep and a productive day at work may show very little depressive symptomology. Her pretest score was unexpectedly high, but later testing will be much closer to the average population score of symptoms. Regression to the mean is especially a problem when a group is selected or self-selects based on a high and unreliable score. Thus, selecting the sickest children for treatment will almost always result in improvement regardless of the treatment.

Statistical regression to the mean is associated with random measurement error, which is often due to unreliability of measures. Although the use of more reliable measures will not eliminate this problem, it can minimize the influence of statistical regression to the mean (Shadish et al., 2002).

Selection

How participants are selected can be a threat to validity when the average person in one of the groups differs from the average person in the other groups. This nonequivalence confounds treatment effects with participant characteristics, making causal inferences difficult. This threat is greatest in quasi-experimental research because random assignment is not employed. As described at the start of the chapter, the Fort Bragg evaluation has been the largest nonequivalent comparison group study in children's mental health services. Because random assignment was not used, the threat of selection bias is present. Several statistical techniques can be used to ameliorate selection factors (e.g., propensity analysis), but it is better, when feasible, to avoid selection factors through the use of a well-planned and implemented research design.

Attrition (Mortality)

Attrition, also known as mortality, has an effect on internal validity similar to that caused by selection. Attrition occurs when people drop out of a study and do not complete posttests. If the people who drop out of one group are different from those that remain in another group, individual participant characteristics can influence the outcomes. In such cases, causal inferences are difficult because one cannot determine if differences are due to the treatment or participant characteristics. Imagine a therapy targeted at reducing depression. What if some people in the treatment group begin to feel much better after therapy, decide they no longer need it, and stop attending sessions? This results in the treatment group containing only people who have not felt a large improvement. Comparisons of the therapy to no-treatment groups may show no or even negative effects, when the treatment may have been quite effective. Almost every mental health study has attrition. It is important that the investigator attempt to retain participants, record in detail the extent of attrition (Cordray & Pion, 1993), and conduct an attrition analysis to determine if there are biases (Foster & Bickman, 1996).

Demoralization and Compensatory Rivalry

In addition to participants being different from the way they were at the start of the study, they can also behave differently during the study. Participants who somehow learn that they are in the comparison group may feel disappointed about not being in the treatment group and simply give up. This demoralization will tend to inflate the differences between the groups because the comparison group will perform more poorly than a typical comparison group. Conversely, rather than give up, the comparison group may work harder to overcome differences from the group that receives treatment. This compensatory rivalry by the comparison group will reduce the difference between the groups, thus reducing the treatment effect. Whether participants know their group assignment is dependent on the research design and consent procedures of the study.

Contamination and Diffusion

Elements of the treatment may unintentionally be provided to the comparison group in two ways. First, participants in the comparison group may accidentally receive some of the treatment through communication with the treatment group. This is known as *diffusion of treatment.* Also, participants may accidentally get aspects of the treatment from program personnel. This is known as *contamination of the comparison group.* For example, in a program that provides hot meals to children in the treatment group, extra food may be given to the comparison group children as well. Both diffusion of treatment and contamination of the comparison group will minimize the difference between the two groups because to some degree they are both getting the treatment.

Interactions: Selection Maturation, Selection History, Selection Instrumentation

Although the threats to validity are described individually, they seldom work in isolation. Of the threats to internal validity, several are more likely to work in conjunction. These are (a) selection maturation, (b) selection history, and (c) selection instrumentation. Selection maturation is the additive effect of nonequivalence groups that are also maturing at differential rates. Selection history refers to nonequivalent groups that experience different influential historical events. Selection instrumentation occurs when nonequivalent groups are tested using different measurements. Measurement differences could include a change in measures, time intervals of measurement, or the presence of ceiling or floor effects in the data.

Ambiguity About the Direction of Causal Inference

As mentioned earlier, the cause must precede the effect in order for the researcher to determine causality. If measurement is cross-sectional, meaning it occurs only at one point in time, then it is difficult to claim that A causes B and B did not cause A, or perhaps that some other variable, such as C, caused A and B. When both A and B are measured at the same time, then the study is correlational because temporal order is unknown and no inferences about causality can be made.

Importance of Internal Validity

Traditionally, internal validity has been written about as the most important type of validity. It is the only type of validity that directly examines a causal relationship. As Campbell and Stanley (1963) claimed, "Internal validity is the basic minimum without which any experiment is uninterpretable" (p. 5). Often, the more complicated the study question, the more frequently it will encounter potential threats to validity (Mark, 2000).

In addition to identifying threats to interpreting causal relationships, the researcher is interested in specifying the contingencies of such relationships. Examples of these contingencies include: "Under what conditions and to whom does the causal relationship apply?" Contingency questions are addressed through construct and external validity.

Construct Validity

Construct validity is focused on whether the study is measuring what it intends to measure. To make causal inferences, it is necessary to ensure that the study is assessing the intended cause and effect and has not mislabeled or confounded them with other variables during operationalization. The measurement of the cause and effect variables should have convergent and discriminant validity, meaning that it is similar to other measures of the same construct and unlike measures of different constructs. For example, a measure of major depression should be similar to some measures of bipolar disorder but different from measures of schizophrenia. In mental health services research, the construct validity of the cause (i.e., services or treatment) is usually very weak. There are no clear operational definitions of what is meant by such "treatments" as outpatient care or hospitalization. These can be seen as simply locations of treatment and not as describing treatment. Similar problems exist in the introduction of new treatments or services such as wraparound. A clear and precise definition is required to enhance the construct validity of the service or treatment being delivered (i.e., cause). Additionally, a method for monitoring the fidelity of implementation of services or treatments is needed to ensure that the construct is actually delivered as planned and promised. Variability in implementation can also affect statistical conclusion validity. In children's mental health, we have less of a problem with the construct of effect because usually a great deal of effort is expended to determine the psychometric qualities of the outcome measures. However, even if these concerns are dealt with, there are still threats that the investigator must be vigilant about.

There are 10 potential threats to construct validity. Each of these threats can occur at the same time and greatly influence any interpretation that may be drawn from the data.

Inadequate Preoperational Explication of the Constructs
Prior to implementing a study, researchers must clearly articulate the constructs they intend to measure. They must clearly state what the cause and the effect are. Mislabeling them may lead to incorrect causal inferences.

Mono-Operational Bias

Most studies use only one measure of a construct. However, the use of only one measure will tend to inadequately represent the construct and may include irrelevancies and other constructs (Shadish et al., 2002). It is often not much of an added cost to include more measures of a construct.

Mono-Method Bias

In addition to using multiple measures of a construct, using different methods of data collection is preferable. This is due to the risk that the method of data collection will influence the data obtained. For example, if all the measures for self-efficacy are given as written surveys and some participants are uncomfortable reading, they may feel less efficacious while completing the form and report lower levels of self-efficacy. However, an interview with the same questions may yield different, more favorable, responses.

Hypothesis Guessing

Another threat to construct validity is that participants will be able to guess the hypothesis of the study and alter their behavior as a result. The best way to avoid this threat is to make the hypotheses difficult to identify, decrease the level of reactivity of the study, and, if possible, give different hypotheses to different participants (Cook & Campbell, 1979).

Evaluation Apprehension

Many people are apprehensive about being evaluated and may alter their behaviors to appear in a more positive light (Campbell & Russo, 1999). This evaluation apprehension typically results in people attempting to portray themselves as competent and psychologically healthy (Cook & Campbell, 1979). Such behaviors may magnify or obscure treatment effects.

Experimenter Expectancies

In addition to the participants having expectations about the purpose of the study, researchers might have expectations that could bias data. If the researcher believes in a treatment and is aware of who obtains the treatment there is an opportunity for conscious or unconscious bias. This problem can be avoided through the use of masking, in which the researcher is unaware of either the research hypothesis or the group membership of each participant. However, it is usually not possible to mask the person delivering the treatment. In psychotherapy research, this may lead to the allegiance effect. This effects occurs in the situation where positive results are only associated with the investigator who developed the therapy being tested.

Confounding of Constructs

Confounding of constructs occurs when the cause and effect vary at different levels such that A at one level causes B but at a different level has no effect on B. This is most common when continuous constructs are measured discretely or when only one level of a construct is measured. For example, a medication at 1 mg will reduce seizures, but at less than .8 mg or above 1.4 mg it will have no effect. A design that only measures 2 mg would be insensitive to the dose response and would erroneously indicate that the medication had no effect on seizures.

Interaction of Different Treatments

Studies that provide more than one treatment to the same participants may yield an effect from the interaction of the two treatments. Although this is more common in laboratory studies than field settings, there is a risk to testing more than one treatment at a time. To avoid this threat, researchers should test each treatment separately or provide several treatment groups, one for each treatment and one for each interaction. However, in services research it is often not feasible to isolate the critical elements of an intervention.

Interaction of Testing and Treatment

The treatment and testing process can potentially interact, reducing the generalizations that can be made about the effects of the treatment. For example, would a study that used three pretests have found the same effects if it had one pretest? The interaction of the treatment with the method and time interval of testing may have an effect on the conclusions that are drawn.

Restricted Generalization Across Related Constructs

If a causal relationship is established, it is necessary to determine the breadth of effects that may be influenced by the cause. For example, a program to reduce hyperactive behavior in children may show success in increasing overall attention but have little influence on other constructs, such as school performance and compliance with adult demands. How findings can generalize to other constructs is an important question for social interventions.

Overall, construct validity is important for applications of findings from studies. If a causal relationship is identified, it is necessary to determine that the constructs underlying the relationship are valid. For example, a researcher could conduct a study to improve mathematic ability through an intensive program that uses word problems. As a consequence of going over word problems, the participants improve their reading ability. At the conclusion of the study, the children perform better on mathematical word problems. Although a causal relationship was demonstrated, the cause was mislabeled. The improvement in the testing was not due to improved mathematical skill but increased reading ability. Inferences and applications from this study may be invalid while the causal relationship may have been internally valid.

External Validity

Social research is often focused on identifying causal relationships to determine how best to help people. The process of generalizing findings from a study to other people, settings, or times is referred to as *external validity* and is based on a correspondence between target populations, study populations, and the achieved sample. The more representative of the target population the people in the study are, the higher the external validity. Like the other forms of validity, external validity has threats as well. These are (a) an interaction of selection and treatment, (b) interaction of setting and treatment, and (c) interaction of history and treatment.

Interaction of Selection and Treatment

Selection bias affects not only causal inferences but also generalizations about findings. Perhaps the people who volunteer for a study are systematically different from those who do not. In such cases, selection is not a threat to internal validity because volunteers would be present in both the treatment and comparison groups; however, the interaction of selection and treatment could threaten external validity such that the findings of the study may not apply to other (nonvoluntary) people.

Research on the characteristics of people who volunteer for studies has shown them to be more motivated to comply (West & Sagarin, 2002), better educated, have higher incomes, and be of nonminority group status (Rosnow & Rosenthal, 1976) compared to the typical members of the population. If participants who volunteer for research are different from those who do not volunteer, the strength of generalizations of findings to other groups is weak.

Interaction of Setting and Treatment

The setting in which the treatment is implemented may also influence the generalizability of findings. For example, a program that is very effective in an in-service psychiatric hospital may be less effective when provided as an after-school program. Perhaps the intensive setting of a residential facility is more engaging for participants, whereas seeking services at school is perceived as stigmatizing. In this example, both the treatment and the setting interact with each other, influencing the application of causal relationships. The same program may be effective in one setting but not another. Of greater concern is the possibility that results obtained from a demonstration project cannot be replicated when applied in more typical settings.

Interaction of History and Treatment

The effects of treatment are influenced by the historical context in which they occur. A treatment may be very effective at one point in time but not very effective at another. In the area of mental health, attitudes and public awareness about mental illness have been changing. A program to identify children with mental health problems may have experienced less success in the 1950s than it would today, when seeking services is more socially accepted. The program may be exactly the same in 1954 and 2004 but be successful only in the present day due to children and families' being more willing to seek services and comply with treatment.

RANDOMIZED EXPERIMENTS VERSUS QUASI-EXPERIMENTAL DESIGNS: TRADE-OFFS

Experimental and quasi-experimental designs are susceptible to threats to validity. Some designs are more vulnerable to certain threats than others; however, none are immune. Additionally, all four types of validity are interrelated. As noted by Cook and Campbell (1979), "increasing one kind of validity will probably decrease another kind" (p. 82).

Although randomized experiments greatly reduce the threat of selection bias and therefore increase internal validity, they may create a nontypical environment and therefore reduce external validity. For example, an experimental study may be able to randomly assign participants, but few programs have the resources or flexibility to implement such a procedure. Experimental studies may strengthen statistical conclusion validity through increasing participant numbers and number of measurement points, but this may be more burdensome to participants and result in greater attrition and more unreliability in measurement, thus reducing statistical and internal validity. Using multiple measures to improve construct validity may increase cost, resulting in lower numbers of participants, and may be more burdensome, leading to greater attrition. In this case, both internal validity and statistical conclusion validity will be lower.

All research designs involve trade-offs among the different types of validity. Therefore, researchers need to determine, a priori, which types of validity are most important. For instance, is the researcher predominately interested in determining the causal relationship between two variables or in the generalizability of the effects of a program to other groups? An explicit statement of the goals of the research will help determine which threats will be most severe and what design steps are needed to control for them.

Although random assignment helps protect against the threat of selection bias, randomized experiments are not free from its effects. If attrition is high or differential, the protective effects of randomization may be lost. Additionally, quasi-experimental designs that lack randomization can still control for its effects. Regression discontinuity designs enable researchers to determine the assignment criteria and control for it in subsequent analyses. Also statistical procedures such as the use of propensity scores in nonequivalent comparison group designs allow researchers, through the use of logistic regression, to predict group membership based on scores on other relevant factors (Rosenbaum & Rubin, 1985; Rubin & Thomas, 2000).

Although randomized experiments are viewed as the gold standard for research, quasi-experimental designs, when designed well, can support the same causal inferences while increasing external validity. This chapter placed a great deal of emphasis on the types of and threats to the validity of a study. Armed with an understanding of these threats, researchers will be able to design better studies and consumers of research will be able to judge the quality and veracity of conclusions.

APPENDIX 4.A

Ethical Considerations for Research in Children's Mental Health Services

Awareness of the rights of people participating in research is relatively recent, with most legislative changes occurring since the 1960s. When considering the historical lack of protection of human participants, most people recall the atrocious medical experimentation conducted by the Nazis during World War II. However, even the United States has a very checkered past of infringing on the rights of its citizens when conducting medical research. The most common of our unprotected participants have been veterans, children, inmates, psychiatric patients, impoverished minorities, and persons with developmental disabilities.

As a result of public attention, especially regarding the Tuskegee Syphilis Study, the National Research Act of 1974 was passed. This act created the National Commission for the Protection of Human Subjects of Biomedical and Behavioral Research, which eventually published the Belmont report in 1979. The Belmont report identified three essential areas for ethical research: (a) respect for persons such that each person enters into research voluntarily and well informed; (b) beneficence as a rule so that research does not harm participants, maximizes their benefit, and minimizes harm to them; and (c) justice so that every participant is treated fairly and not exploited.

Additionally, the U.S. Department of Health and Human Services (DHHS) regulations for the protection of human participants (Title 45 *Code of Federal Regulations* Part 46) offer special protections for children and adolescents. In addition to consent from parents, researchers must explain the study to children and obtain their assent to participate. This requirement can be even more challenging for research on children's mental health services, in which the function and comprehension of some children, adolescents, and families may be lower than those of typically developing peers. Additionally, confidentiality is of utmost importance because of potential stigmatization and discrimination.

To ensure that the recommendations of the Belmont report and regulations of DHHS were used, many universities and research institutions created IRBs. These committees, typically composed of researchers, community members, and religious leaders, review proposed research projects and ensure that they meet federal and institutional criteria for ethical research. IRBs also conduct training for investigators and periodically audit research projects to ensure compliance with proposed protocol. Last, participants may contact the IRB if they suspect their rights as participants are not being protected. At all research institutions, the IRB has the ability to halt research.

All research, especially research with children, should address participants' rights, protection, benefit, and potential risk. Ideally, an external body, such as an IRB, will oversee empirical works to promote ethical behavior. Because children, especially children with special needs, are considered a vulnerable population, researchers must design consenting and assenting procedures that best inform them of their rights and ensure their confidentiality. Ethical research does not entail a static, rule-following process, but rather an iterative process of balancing research questions with the best interest of children, their families, and society. Although there may be an added challenge for research with children with mental disorders, ethics are a paramount concern in design and execution. For more information on ethical research in children's mental health, we highly recommend Hoagwood, Jensen, and Fisher (1996), *Ethical Issues in Mental Health Research with Children and Adolescents.* The protection of human participants applies equally to quasi-experimental and experimental designs. Both warrant the same level of ethical considerations and scrutiny in recruitment, implementation, and execution.

REFERENCES

Bickman, L. (1996a). A continuum of care: More is not always better. *American Psychologist, 51*(7), 689–701.

Bickman, L. (Ed.). (1996b). Special issue: The Fort Bragg experiment. *Journal of Mental Health Administration, 23*(1).

Bickman, L., Gutherie, P. R., Foster, E. M., Lambert, E. W., Summerfelt, W. T., Breda, C. S., et al. (1995). *Evaluating managed mental health services: The Fort Bragg experiment.* New York: Plenum Press.

Bickman, L., Smith, C. M., Lambert, E. W., & Andrade, A. R. (2003). Evaluation of a congressionally mandated wraparound demonstration. *Journal of Child and Family Studies, 12*(2), 135–156.

Bickman, L., Summerfelt, W. T., & Noser, K. (1997). Comparative outcomes of emotionally disturbed children and adolescents in a system of services and unusual care. *Psychiatric Services, 48*(12), 1543–1548.

Boruch, B. F. (1997). *Randomized experiments for planning and evaluation.* Thousand Oaks, CA: Sage.

Campbell, D. T., & Russo, M. J. (1999). *Social experimentation.* Thousand Oaks, CA: Sage.

Campbell, D. T., & Stanley, J. C. (1963). *Experimental and quasi-experimental designs for research.* Boston: Houghton Mifflin.

Cohen, J. (1962). The statistical power of abnormal–social psychological research: A review. *Journal of Abnormal and Social Psychology, 65,* 145–153.

Cohen, J. (1992). A power primer. *Psychological Bulletin, 112*(1), 155–159.

Cohen, J., & Cohen, P. (1983). *Applied regression/correlation analysis for the behavioral sciences.* Hillsdale, NJ: Erlbaum.

Cook, T. D., & Campbell, D. T. (1979). *Quasi-experimentation.* Boston: Houghton Mifflin.

Cook, T. D., Campbell, D. T., & Peracchio, L. (1990). Quasi experimentation. In M. D. Dunnette & L. M. Hough (Eds.), *Handbook of industrial and organizational psychology* (Vol. 1, pp. 491–576). Palo Alto, CA: Consulting Psychologists Press.

Cordray, D. (2000). Enhancing the scope of experimental inquiry in intervention studies. *Crime and Delinquency, 46*(3), 401–424.

Cordray, D., & Pion, G. (1993). Psychosocial rehabilitation assessment: A broader perspective. In R. L. Glueckauf, L. B. Sechrest, G. R. Bond, & E. C. McDonel (Eds.), *Improving assessment in rehabilitation and health* (pp. 215–240). Newbury Park, CA: Sage.

Corrin, W., & Cook, T. (1998). Design elements of quasi-experiments. *Advances in Educational Productivity, 7,* 35–57.

Foster, M., & Bickman, L. (1996). An evaluator's guide to detecting attrition problems. *Evaluation Review, 20*(6), 695–723.

Hays, W. (1994). *Statistics.* Fort Worth, TX: Harcourt Brace College Publishers.

Hendrick, T. B., Bickman, L., & Rog, D. J. (1993). *Applied research design: A practical guide.* Thousand Oaks, CA: Sage.

Hill, J., Rubin, D., & Thomas, M. (2000). The design of the New York school choice scholarship program evaluation. In L. Bickman (Ed.), *Research design* (pp. 155–180). Thousand Oaks, CA: Sage.

Hoagwood, K., Jensen, P., & Fisher, C. (1996). *Ethical issues in mental health research with children and adolescents.* Mahwah, NJ: Erlbaum.

Holland, P. (1989). Comment: It's very clear. *Journal of the American Statistical Association, 84,* 875–877.

Keppel, G. (1991). *Design and analysis: A researcher's handbook.* Upper Saddle River, NJ: Prentice Hall.

Lambert, E. W., Wahler, R. G., Andrade, A. R., & Bickman, L. (2001). Looking for the disorder in conduct disorder. *Journal of Abnormal Psychology, 110*(1), 110–123.

Lipsey, M. (1990). *Design sensitivity: Statistical power for experimental research.* Thousand Oaks, CA: Sage.

Lipsey, M. (1998). Design sensitivity: Statistical power for applied experimental research. In L. Bickman & D. Rog (Eds.), *Handbook of applied social research methods.* Thousand Oaks, CA: Sage.

Lipsey, M. (2000). Statistical conclusion validity for intervention research: A significant ($p < .05$) problem. In L. Bickman (Ed.), *Validity and social experimentation* (pp. 101–120). Thousand Oaks, CA: Sage.

Lipsey, M., & Cordray, D. (2000). Evaluation methods for social intervention. *Annual Review of Psychology, 51,* 345–375.

Lord, F. (1980). *Applications of item response theory to practical testing problems.* Hillsdale, NJ: Erlbaum.

Mark, M. (2000). Realism, validity, and the experimenting society. In L. Bickman (Ed.), *Validity and social experimentation* (pp. 141–168). Thousand Oaks, CA: Sage.

McCleary, R. (2000). Evolution of the time series experiment. In L. Bickman (Ed.), *Research design* (pp. 215–234). Thousand Oaks, CA: Sage.

National Commission for the Protection of Human Subjects of Biomedical and Behavioral Research. (1979). *The Belmont report: Ethical principles and guidelines for the protection of human subjects of research.* Washington, DC: Belmont Conference Center at the Smithsonian Institution.

Reichardt, C. (1992). Estimating effects of community prevention trials: Alternative designs and methods. In H. D. Holder & J. M. Howard (Eds.), *Community prevention trials for alcohol problems: Methodological issues* (pp. 137–158). Westport, CT: Praeger.

Reichardt, C., & Mark, M. (1998). Quasi-experimentation. In L. Bickman & D. Rog (Eds.), *Handbook of applied social research methods* (pp. 193–228). Thousand Oaks, CA: Sage.

Rogosa, D. (1980). A critique of cross-lagged correlation. *Psychological Bulletin, 88,* 245–258.

Rosenbaum, P., & Rubin, D. (1985). Constructing a control group using multivariate matched sampling incorporating the propensity score. *American Statistician, 39,* 33–36.

Rosenthal, R., & Rosnow, R. (1991). *Essentials of behavioral research: Methods and data analysis.* Boston: McGraw-Hill.

Rosnow, R. L., & Rosenthal, R. (1976). The volunteer subject revisited. *Australian Journal of Psychology, 28*(2), 97–108.

Rubin, D., & Thomas, N. (2000). Combining propensity score matching with additional adjustments for prognostic covariates. *Journal of the American Statistical Association, 95,* 573–585.

Sedlmeier, P., & Gigerenzer, G. (1989). Do studies of statistical power have an effect on the power of studies? *Psychological Bulletin, 105,* 309–316.

Shadish, W., Cook, T., & Campbell, D. (2002). *Experimental and quasi-experimental designs for generalized causal inference.* New York: Houghton Mifflin.

Shaughnessy, J., & Zechmeister, E. (1994). *Research methods in psychology.* New York: McGraw-Hill.

Snijders, T., & Bosker, R. (1999). *Multilevel analysis: An introduction to basic and advanced multilevel modeling.* Thousand Oaks, CA: Sage.

Solomon, R. (1949). An extension of control group design. *Psychological Bulletin, 46,* 137–150.

West, S., & Sagarin, B. (2002). Participant selection and loss in randomized experiments. In L. Bickman (Ed.), *Contributions to research design: Donald Campbell's legacy* (pp. 117–154). Thousand Oaks, CA: Sage.

Wortman, P. (1994). Judging research quality. In H. Cooper & L. Hedges (Eds.), *The handbook of research synthesis* (pp. 97–110). New York: Russell Sage Foundation.

Multiple Perspectives on Family Outcomes in Children's Mental Health

CHAPTER 5

Barbara J. Friesen, Michael Pullmann, Nancy M. Koroloff, and Theresa Rea

onsider the following hypothetical research priorities:

- Examine the impact of caregiver support on the progression of Alzheimer's disease.
- Study how changes in caregivers' coping affect the cognitive functioning of their children with developmental disabilities.

These examples are, of course, far-fetched. In Alzheimer's disease and developmental disabilities, the clear focus of family support research is on how to preserve and support families who are faced with extraordinary challenges and caregiving demands as a result of the disability of their adult or child family members (Friesen, 1989; Grant et al., 2002; Harahan, 2001). Family support intervention is not expected to change the course of the primary condition.

Children's mental health differs from many other disability fields in the degree to which it is expected that services to families should result in changes in the child's clinical and functional status. Within the children's mental health field, goals such as reducing caregiver stress and improving family quality of life through support for caregivers and other family members are not yet universally accepted as worthwhile endeavors unless they are linked to other outcomes such as changes in the functioning of the child or reductions in out-of-home placement. Certainly, family members see the need for such support, and a national family support and advocacy organization, the Federation of Families for Children's Mental Health, explicitly addresses this issue in a statement on family support (Federation of Families for Children's Mental Health, 2002). Referring to respite care, the statement reads, "Family support services include … in-home and out-of-home respite care, with an emphasis on neighborhood and community participation for the child, and conceptualized *not as a clinical service but as a support for the whole family*" (p. 1).

Attention to family needs characterizes both research and service provision across many fields of human services and rehabilitation. There is an extensive literature focusing on understanding and addressing the responses of caregivers for persons with Alzheimer's disease. Studies address such concerns as loss, depression, social isolation, and burnout, with the central focus being on promoting the well-being of the caregiving partner (Grant et al., 2002; Ho, Weitzman, Cui, & Levkoff, 2000). In the field of developmental disabilities, studies address the reactions of parents to the circumstance of having a child with a cognitive disability, with major purposes of this research being to understand and help parents cope with negative feelings (grief, loss, frustration) and to provide an intervention to help them improve their family circumstances (Bowman, 2001; Dunn, Burbine, Bowers, & Tantleff-Dunn, 2001). Considerable research has also been conducted in the areas of childhood disability and chronic illness, again with a central focus on providing support and assistance to families who are caring for a child with special needs (Macias, Clifford, Saylor, & Kreh, 2001; Svavarsdottir, McCubbin, & Kane, 2000).

Significant advances have been made in the availability of services for families whose children have emotional, behavioral, or mental disorders since the Child and Adolescent Service System Program was authorized by Congress in 1984 with the goal of improving services for children with mental health problems and their families (Stroul, 1996). At that time there were very few services and supports for parents, siblings, and other family members except for therapeutic services designed to address the mental health issues of other family members, or of entire families, thought to cause or prolong the problems of the identified child. Services such as individual psychotherapy for caregivers, couples' counseling, or family therapy were usually offered in conjunction with mental health services for children. Services such as respite care, sibling support groups, and other family support services were, with rare exceptions, not seen as a part of children's mental health services (Friesen, 1993).

Over the last two decades, advocates have asserted that the field of children's mental health should move from a child-centered to a family-centered perspective (Friesen, 1993; Friesen & Koroloff, 1990), acknowledging and addressing the needs of the entire family, including the child with a serious emotional disorder. The rationale for this position is that it is both humane and socially responsible to be concerned with the well-being of all family members, acknowledging that change or disturbance in any part of the family system affects all members (e.g., that a child's acting-out behavior increases parental concern and stress, which may, in turn, reduce parenting effectiveness in the form of appropriate structure and discipline).

Early studies of the circumstances and needs of families (Friesen, 1989; Greenley & Robitschek, 1991; Tarico, Low, Trupin, & Forsyth-Stephens, 1989) revealed that many families felt blamed and disrespected by service providers, were frustrated by the lack of appropriate services and by access barriers, and experienced difficulty coping effectively with the needs and behaviors of their children. This research formed a foundation upon which to envision systems of care that were more family friendly, promoted family–professional collaboration, and provided services that were responsive to the support needs of families (Federation of Families for Children's Mental Health, 2002; Friesen & Koroloff, 1990).

In this chapter we assert that the somewhat fragmented research about family issues in children's mental health reflects the confusion and conflict that surround the topic, and that both greater clarity and consensus about the intended outcomes of services to families are necessary to develop and advance a coherent research agenda for the field. We also examine some of the approaches that researchers have used for defining and studying family outcomes in children's mental health. We address six general perspectives about these outcomes (see Figure 5.1):

1. the effect of family (mostly caregiver) characteristics and circumstances on the child's mental health;
2. the effect of the child's mental health problems and difficulty in obtaining services on the caregiver and family;
3. the mutual effects of child on family and family on child;
4. caregiver characteristics and responses conceptualized as mediating variables, with the outcomes of interest being variables relevant to the child's well-being;
5. studies that focus on the well-being of caregivers and the family as a whole, regardless of the outcomes for the target child; and
6. studies that examine the implications of family outcomes for communities and society as a whole, the focus being on the population of families whose children have mental disorders within a given community or society.

In the following discussion we have not undertaken to review and synthesize all of the research literature relevant to each perspective, but rather to present examples of studies that exemplify each viewpoint. The amount of research that is directly relevant to children's mental health varies greatly across perspectives. For some, such as Perspective 1, there are many studies, but for others, such as Perspective 6, it has been necessary to rely on literature from other fields because of the paucity of relevant research. We conclude the chapter with recommendations about research that is needed to fill in gaps in our current knowledge.

PERSPECTIVE 1: PARENTAL INFLUENCE ON CHILDREN'S MENTAL HEALTH

Perspective 1 focuses on the powerful influence that parents have on the cognitive, emotional, and behavioral development of their children. Both research and practical experience have produced a detailed literature about the norms of childhood, provided descriptions of the anticipated age-appropriate progressions through those norms, and emphasized the importance of the parent as a principal influence on determining a child's developmental trajectory. Research detailing normative development provides a foundation for understanding development that is delayed, abnormal, or absent. The primary goal of research concerned with deviations from the norm has been to be able to predict, prevent, or treat children's mental, emotional, and behavioral challenges and to understand parental impact on them.

The Surgeon General's Report on Mental Health (U.S. Department of Health and Human Services, 1999) stated that the "science of mental health in

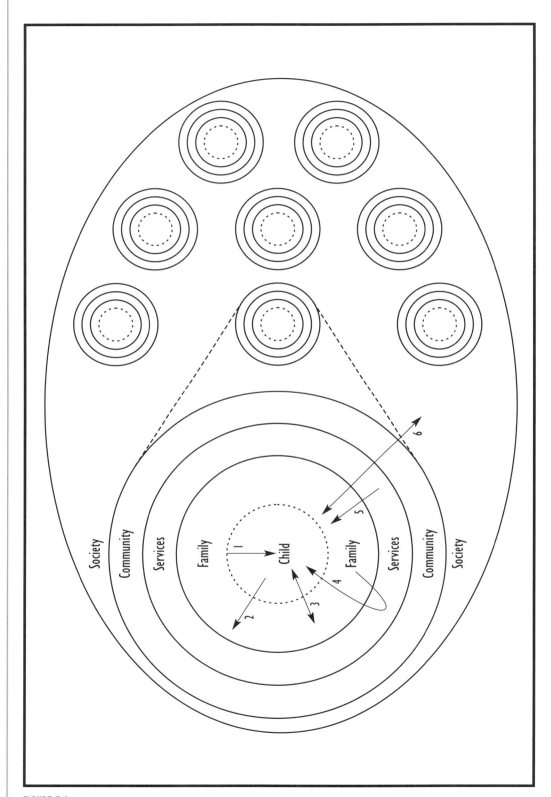

FIGURE 5.1. Perspectives on family outcomes.

childhood and adolescence is a complex mix of the study of development and the study of discrete mental or addictive disorders, combined conditions, or disorders" (p. 124). Within this framework, family variables are said to contribute in a significant way to children's mental health problems.

Research involving children and families has placed high value on parents as the primary contributors to child development. Emphasis on the parent or caretaker as the most influential person in a child's development dates back to the early work of pioneers such as Sigmund Freud, Jean Piaget, and Erik Erikson. These theorists contributed to the understanding of cognitive, emotional, and personality development from an organismic and intrapersonal perspective by defining the stages in childhood that may determine adult characteristics. They believed that if a person's internal cognitive and emotional processes were known, it was possible to not only predict that person's behavior but also to link the behavior back to some childhood event. In all cases, the parent played an integral role in facilitating the negotiation of these childhood stages and was believed to be the primary conductor of development. These early theorists of child development were followed by the advent of behaviorism and the work of B. F. Skinner, who introduced learning theory. Social learning theorists such as Albert Bandura subsequently built upon learning theory and added the cognitive components of memory and attention. This was a pivotal contribution because it widened our knowledge of behavior to include not only how children learn behavior but also how attitudes, values, and ideas pass from person to person.

Behavioral and social learning proponents argue that children, to a large degree, are taught behavior, have behavior modeled for them, and are reinforced for their own behavior. Many current prominent researchers and professionals in children's mental health believe that if a child is struggling with mental health problems in the form of emotional or behavioral disturbances, the parent is the primary reinforcer of those issues. Evidence exists about the negative repercussions on child emotional and behavioral development due to coercive parenting practices (Capaldi & Patterson, 1991; Stoolmiller, Patterson, & Snyder, 1997). Within a social learning framework, angry, aggressive, and coercive behaviors exhibited by parents are adopted and integrated into children's behavioral repertoires. Harsh and inconsistent discipline, inadequate supervision, and parental rejection are high on the list of critical predictors of such problems as antisocial behaviors, conduct disorder, and difficult-to-control behaviors (Arnold, O'Leary, Wolff, & Acker, 1993; Dix, 1991; Lindahl, 1998; Shaw & Bell, 1993).

In an attempt to understand why some parents apparently choose to parent in ways that are coercive and potentially damaging to their children, researchers began asking the question, "When and how does this type of parenting occur?" It became apparent that such parental behavior often happened in conjunction with tremendous stresses in the parent or caretaker's life. Conditions such as poverty, domestic violence, and drug abuse acted as barriers to the parents' ability to function in their parenting roles. What often emerged were parenting practices that exacerbated any emotional or behavioral challenges that the children of that family faced (Barkley, 2000). Coupled with ineffective parenting, the children were often believed not to have the level of resilience necessary to thrive in such adverse conditions.

Over time it became apparent that not only were there unfavorable environmental circumstances that stood to pose a threat to the developing children, in some cases the parents or caretakers suffered from mental health problems, such as depression or other serious and persistent mental illness (Oyserman, Mowbray, Meares, & Firminger, 2000), that left them vulnerable to parenting stresses. There is considerable evidence linking a mother's affective dysfunction, how she relates and responds to her child, and the negative influence that her behavior has on the emotional and behavioral development of the child (Katsurada & Sugawara, 2000; Larson & Almeida, 1999).

Although there can be no dispute about the important influence that parents have on their children's development, increasingly researchers have also examined the many other influences that work in concert with parents to shape children's emotional and behavioral development. For example, Bronfenbrenner (1979) introduced the biopsychosocial perspective, which recognized the importance of the interactions between the biological makeup of the child and experiences within the family and other environments. Thus, two children who share the attribute of being highly reactive to noise and social stimuli may fare very differently, depending on whether they are provided with support, structure, and a simplified environment at home, at school, and in recreational settings. Recognition of the influence of the environment and other social partners on the developing child reveals the limitations of the older literature, with its exclusive focus on the relationship between parental characteristics and children's mental health problems. Another widely recognized limitation of much early research within Perspective 1 is the use of correlational data to assert causation from parental characteristics to child outcomes. These limitations are gradually being overcome as the complexities of the etiology, course, and treatment of children's mental health problems are incorporated into research and evaluation designs.

PERSPECTIVE 2: CHILD'S INFLUENCE ON THE CAREGIVER

Perspective 2 reverses the causal lens used in the previous view and examines the impact on caregivers and other family members of living with and caring for a child with a serious mental disorder. Although most of the research in this category has its roots in the "caregiver burden" concept found in the adult mental health and gerontology literature, a few researchers have included the possibility that living with or caring for a child with mental health needs may have a positive effect on other family members (Friesen, 1989; McDonald, Poertner, & Pierpont, 1999; Yatchmenoff, Koren, Friesen, Gordon, & Kinney, 1998). Some researchers have also broadened this view, referred to as the "effects of the situation" (Yatchmenoff et al., 1998) to include the impact of an inadequate service system, financial demands, and other ecological variables on the family. Studies investigating the effects of living with and caring for a child with mental health challenges have shown consistent findings related to parenting stress. The most significant predictors of parental stress are child symptomatology, the severity of the child's disorder (Richardson & Heflinger, 2002; Yatchmenoff et al., 1998), child functioning (Floyd & Gallagher, 1997; Smith, Oliver, & Innocenti, 2001), and externalizing behaviors (Brannan & Heflinger, 2001).

There is ample agreement across researchers about the construct of "parental stress." Parental stress includes three areas: stress related to the child, to the parents' view of themselves, and to life events in general. Stress related to the child has included personal and social development; parent–child interactions (Smith et al., 2001); externalizing behaviors (Brannan & Heflinger, 2001); conflicts with family members, neighbors, peers, or police; or need for hospitalization. This sphere of influence targets the strain created by the direct behaviors and actions of the child. Children with mental health challenges often exhibit externalizing behaviors and lack sufficient social skills, making it difficult for them to appropriately interact with adults and peers. Depending on the age of the child, these behaviors may include tantrums, defiance, ignorance of or refusal to follow directions, displays of verbal or physical aggression, destruction of property, infliction of injury on themselves or others, antisocial behavior, delinquency, and drug abuse. Directly dealing with these types of difficult behaviors on a daily basis creates a heightened level of stress and challenge for these parents.

Stress that reflects the parents' view of themselves is a broad domain that generally covers the emotional and cognitive strain that is experienced by parents when confronted with problematic child situations. These are often referred to as guilt, shame, stigma, anger, worry, and attributions for their child's challenges. Brannan and Heflinger (2001) have described this dimension as "subjective caregiver strain." Additionally, an important piece of the subjective stress that parents feel, but that has not received much attention, is blame. A study that investigated the amount of blame that professionals placed on parents whose children had emotional and behavioral disorders indicated that 57% of the respondents agreed that parental dysfunction is the primary cause of serious mental illness in children (Rubin, Cardenas, Warren, Pike, & Wombach, 1998). Brannan and Heflinger (2001) have also discussed "objective caregiver strain," defined as "observable negative occurrences and constraints resulting directly from the relative's problems" (p. 406). These include the secondary effects of the child's behavior on the parents, which can be difficulties with neighbors and police, disrupted family relationships (between spouses, between parents and other children, or between siblings), struggles working with teachers and professionals, missed time from work, difficulty getting needed mental health services, no respite, and little social support from friends and relatives.

The last category of parental stress includes life events that can be very stressful in and of themselves. However, when these events are coupled with a child with mental health challenges, they can be particularly overwhelming. Life events can consist of remarriage, divorce, birth or death in the family, moving, financial issues, health-related matters, and unemployment or job change.

Critiques of this perspective are similar to those of Perspective 1. Most of the studies are correlational in nature, and although causality is assumed, it cannot be accepted without question. There is substantial evidence to support caregiver burden hypotheses, and researchers have shown that the greatest single predictor of parent quality of life (after controlling for socioeconomic disadvantage, parent stress and psychopathology, interpersonal relations, and social support) is child psychological functioning (Crowley & Kazdin, 1998). Many questions remain, however, about whether the stress parents and families feel is related to the child with mental illness or to other stressors that are erroneously attributed to the child.

PERSPECTIVE 3: MUTUAL EFFECTS OF PARENT ON CHILD AND CHILD ON PARENT

Perspective 3 examines the outcomes of the interaction between the child's needs and behaviors (Perspective 2) and those of other family members (Perspective 1). A preponderance of this literature examines the relationships between target children and their caregivers, although some recent studies have assessed the transactions between the affected child and his or her siblings. Studies conducted from this perspective often use conceptual frameworks similar to those that Farmer and Farmer (2001) have described as a *developmental science perspective* wherein "the individual functions as an integrated organism and development arises from the dynamic interrelations among systems existing within and beyond the person" (p. 172). In a review of the role of the family in relation to childhood disorders, Wamboldt and Wamboldt (2000) have presented an interactive view as part of their findings, concluding that "families can cause problems, but many times the problem families have are in response to a child's problems" (p. 1212).

Assessing possible mutual effects of parent on child and child on parent requires measurement of parent and child behavior or functioning or other variables on at least two points in time. Studies that specifically attend to possible mutual effects of parent and child are, unfortunately, scarce. However, an exception is a study by Early, Gregoire, and McDonald (2002), who examined the relationships between child functioning and caregiver well-being at two points in time (12–18 months apart) in a sample of the caregivers of 164 children receiving mental health services. These researchers examined the impact of caregiver well-being at Time 1 on child functioning at Time 2 and child functioning (at Time 1) on caregiver well-being at the second measurement point. These researchers concluded that "child functioning and caregiver well-being mutually affect each other and measures of both child functioning and caregiver well-being are fairly stable over time" (p. 385), and "when controlling for the mutual effects of Time 1 and those effects on caregiver well-being, child functioning continues to significantly affect caregiver well-being at Time 2" (p. 387). Early et al. (2002) suggested that their analysis should be considered exploratory, with additional research needed to untangle the mutual effects of child and caregiver over time.

Stoolmiller (2001) examined the mutual effects of children's behavior and parents' behavior, focusing on the relationship between manageability problems in boys and parental disciplinary practices. He described these effects as "synergistic" and was most concerned with predicting future increases in externalizing behavior. Stoolmiller used a social learning framework, coercion theory, which has at its core a negative reinforcement mechanism. The cycle described by Stoolmiller includes the caregiver's attempt to intervene in the child's behavior, followed by the child's resisting the intrusion, perhaps through a tantrum. The caregiver then backs down and withdraws the demand for change, and then the child ceases the aversive resistance. According to this framework, the child learns that such aversive behavior is very effective for controlling the behavior of others. This cycle is thought to undermine parental discipline and to put the child at risk for continued antisocial behavior.

A similar phenomenon is described by Bailey, Barton, and Vignola (1999) but viewed through a different lens. They compared the coping styles of a group of mothers whose children had attention-deficit/hyperactivity disorder (ADHD) with a control group of mothers whose children did not have ADHD or any other disability or illness. They found that mothers of children with ADHD used significantly more indirect coping, which the authors called a "wise strategy" (p. 46), devised to avoid direct confrontation with their difficult children. This is in contrast to the coercive theory perspective explicated by Stoolmiller (2001), which posits that these mothers may be inadvertently teaching their children that aggressive behavior is effective.

Another somewhat specialized area in which research has been conducted from a transactive perspective is in the examination of family outcomes when parents have a severe and persistent mental illness. The dual focus includes the effect of the children's behavior and the parenting role on persons with mental illness, as well as the influence of the parents' behavior on child outcomes. Although early studies in this area were primarily concerned with the needs and responses of the adult parent with mental illness (both positive and negative), recently, researchers in this area have proposed a "family model" (Falkov, 1998) that takes into account the needs for treatment and support of parents with psychiatric illness along with a concern for the healthy development of children in these families.

PERSPECTIVE 4: CAREGIVER CHARACTERISTICS AS MEDIATORS

In Perspective 4, caregiver variables are treated as mediators and outcome variables are service system variables or the child's functioning. The service system variables include likelihood of receiving mental health services, type or amount of mental health services received, recidivism, and out-of-home placements. Child functioning has generally been operationalized using standardized clinical or functional measures, such as the *Child Behavior Checklist* (CBCL; Achenbach & Rescorla, 2001) and the *Child and Adolescent Functional Assessment Scale* (CAFAS; Hodges, Doucette-Gates, & Liao, 1999), service usage (e.g., hospitalization or arrests), and behavioral indicators (e.g., suicide attempts). Additionally, research in this perspective often includes an intervention with the caregiver based on the assumption that changes in the caregiver's behaviors will have an effect on the child. Commonly used interventions are parent training or psychoeducation, sibling workshops, and respite care.

As with any of the perspectives, research in this perspective can be explicit (in this case, directly testing caregiver variables as possible mediators) or implicit (completing descriptive or bivariate analyses as support for a theoretical mediating relationship). Regardless, within this perspective a major justification for studying caregiver variable(s) is their theoretical mediating relationship with an aspect of the child's functioning or experience with the service system.

Child's Experience with the Service System as Outcome

Research on caregiver strain and burden provides a good example of research focusing on the mediating influence of caregiver variables between child functioning and aspects of the child's experience with the service system. Angold et al. (1998) examined caregiving burden "as a factor in propelling parents to seek help for their children's disorders" (p. 75). The researchers found that the best predictors of any burden, and the best predictors of level of burden, were the child's symptoms and functioning (measured by the total *DSM–III–R* symptom score and the total functional impairment score from the *Child and Adolescent Psychiatric Assessment*). The caregiver's history of mental health problems was also a predictor of burden, among other variables. Demonstrating the mediating effect of caregiver variables, the strongest predictor of entry into and use of child specialist mental health services was parental burden. Similarly, Brannan, Heflinger, Schweitzer, and Orten (2001) found that caregiver strain was predictive of the amount of overall service use and type of service use (e.g., support, intermediate outpatient, and residential/inpatient services).

McKay, Pennington, Lynne, and McCadam (2001) found that the level of child mental health need and demographic factors such as gender and age of the child were not significantly related to initial attendance at a mental health service or to the number of sessions attended. Again, the best predictors of the use of mental health services were caregiver factors, in this case, parental beliefs about mental health and parental discipline; children of parents who reported skepticism about mental health treatment and parents who reported problems with discipline were less likely to receive services. As in previous studies, the researchers found that the number of mental health sessions was explained by family stress, as well as by the presence of another adult in the home and parental discipline efficacy. These findings are startling in that child functioning did not predict service use; only parental factors were predictive. As in the Angold et al. (1998) study, a mediating relationship was implicit but not directly tested.

The common theme throughout these studies is the emphasis on a stated or implied causal link between caregiver factors and children's experience with the service system. In each case, the ultimate outcome of interest is service use. The justification for examining caregiver factors is not necessarily an inherent interest in the quality of life of the caregiver or the entire family; rather, studying caregiver factors is considered essential to understanding child-related service issues. Other studies discussed later examine how caregivers' behaviors and beliefs mediate the effects of family interventions on the outcome of child functioning.

Child's Functioning as Outcome

Parent Training

Possibly the most widespread research exemplifying Perspective 4 is parent training. For this discussion we are including a broad range of interventions intended to educate parents about their child's disability or train them to manage typical problems, often in combination with social support or group education. These interventions have been conducted in a wide variety of locations (e.g., hospitals, residential programs, support groups) by a variety of people (e.g., psychiatrists, caseworkers, paraprofessionals, peer mental health consumers) in a variety of ways (e.g., individual meetings, group meetings, family groups, handouts, books, board games) about a variety of topics (e.g., education on medication, behavior management, course and prognosis of illness, recovery, consumer rights) for a variety of problems (e.g., bipolar disorder, schizophrenia, developmental disabilities, depression; Bisbee, 2000; McFarlane, Dushay, Stastny, Deakins, & Link, 1996; Reinares, Colom, Martinez-Aran, Benabarre, & Vieta, 2002). Not surprisingly, research in this area has produced a variety of findings, including significant and positive changes in caregiver knowledge, beliefs, and attitudes (Matthews & Hudson, 2001); decreased caregiver stress, increased caregiver self-efficacy, and improved family quality of life (Feldman & Werner, 2002); decreased symptoms and rehospitalization rates (McFarlane et al., 1996; Reinares et al., 2002); and decreased adolescent suicidal ideation and improved child behavior (Kazdin, 1997).

The fundamental logic in these studies is the belief that intervention will change aspects of the caregiver's knowledge and behavior, which in turn will change the child's behavior. What places these studies into Perspective 4 is that caregiver variables are mediators between the intervention and the child's behavior. The intervention is a tool to affect the caregiver and achieve the ultimate goal—improving the child's functioning. Some research focuses on this goal to the near exclusion of possible impacts on the caregiver or family. For example, Kazdin (1997), in a review of research on parent management training (PMT), described the technique as focusing on the specific behaviors of caregivers and children, with sparse research available on other outcomes such as marital satisfaction and family cohesion. A few researchers have assessed outcomes beyond caregiver behavior change, but they consider these outcomes secondary to improvement in child functioning. For example, Feldman and Werner (2002) stated that they were interested in "positive side-effects of Behavioral Parent Training on the parents and families" (Feldman & Werner, 2002). In this case, the impact on the caregiver is described as "collateral effects" and "positive side-effects" (p. 75) of training rather than an intended target of the intervention. Importantly, these researchers found reduced caregiver stress, increased family quality of life, and increased caregiver self-efficacy to be outcomes of parent training.

Although training intended to modify parent behavior is one of the most studied interventions in this perspective, researchers have also examined caregiver and family interventions intended to modify other caregiver variables. The next section discusses studies of progressive interventions such as services designed to increase caregiver empowerment (e.g., parent partners) and services designed to reduce caregiver strain or burden (e.g., respite care).

Other Interventions

Taub, Tighe, and Burchard (2001) examined the relationship between changes in caregiver empowerment as measured by the *Family Empowerment Scale* (FES; Koren, DeChillo, & Friesen, 1992) and changes in child mental health as measured by the *Child Behavior Checklist* (CBCL) and the *Youth-Self Report* (YSR; Achenbach & Rescorla, 2001). In their study, Taub et al. argued that families enrolled in the statewide system of care participated in services designed to promote family empowerment, among myriad other goals. Findings about the relationships between child functioning and empowerment were mixed; empowerment was not related to the YSR, but an increase in family empowerment over time was predictive of an improvement in child functioning as measured by the CBCL Total Problems and Externalizing scores. As with other examples, this article is not confined to Perspective 4. Although part of the analysis focused on the relationship between empowerment and child outcomes, in the literature review, these researchers also discussed the inherent value of caregiver empowerment independent of child outcomes.

Respite care is another intervention that is targeted at the caregiver but thought to affect the entire family. Supporters of respite care have long argued that it can benefit the whole family, but there has been little research into this matter in the field of children's mental health. Generally, researchers have reported a positive impact on caregiving burden but little or no effect on child outcomes. A wide range of possible outcomes of respite care, including improvements in child and family functioning, lessening of caregiver strain, and better service usage, were examined in a study by Bruns and Burchard (2000). Only one statistically significant relationship was found with regard to child functioning: Families who received respite care reported that their children had fewer community externalizing behaviors (police contact, truancy, suicide attempts, or alcohol/drug use), and because of the low incidence of these behaviors, even this relationship was suspect. Regardless, the researchers framed this piece of analysis in Perspective 4, postulating that an intervention targeting the caregiver would have positive and measurable effects on the child.

In the following sections, Perspectives 5 and 6 shift the focus from the target child to the well-being of all members of the family and to the good of society as a whole.

PERSPECTIVE 5: FAMILY OUTCOMES AS PRIMARY GOALS

The most salient feature of Perspective 5 is that positive outcomes within the family system are valued whether there is any change in the child's symptoms, behavior, living situation, educational progress, or legal status. For this perspective, the condition of the child with a mental, emotional, or behavioral disorder can remain static or decline without affecting the value of the family outcomes. What is important is that the family, while maintaining the child in the home and community, can effectively work and thrive as any other family would.

Perspective 5 examines the outcomes associated with an intervention that targets change in family members other than the child with the mental, behavioral, or emotional disorder. These outcomes may include internal aspects of family members (such as feelings or attitudes), be related to the impact of the intervention on the family members' behaviors, or address how family members are able to carry out their multiple roles. Sometimes more than one type of outcome is included in a study. For example, respite care is an intervention that is offered to families with the expectation that it will allow them to take a break from caregiving, thus reducing the families' stress levels. In Perspective 4, this reduced stress level would be important because of its influence on the family's ability to maintain the child in their home or its influence on the child's behavior. In Perspective 5, however, reduced family stress may be valued because we believe that all families function more effectively if the stress in their lives is lowered periodically. Or, we may believe that if a mother's stress is lowered, her ability to participate in treatment planning for her child or to parent her other children will increase. Both are examples of outcomes that focus on the well-being and internal functioning of the family itself.

Perhaps the most common outcome associated with Perspective 5 is the psychological health of family members, specifically, the mental health of mothers. Maternal anxiety, maternal depression, and the mother's psychological status are all examples of outcomes that are primarily important from the family's point of view. Examples of this focus are found in a series of studies on families of children with chronic illness by Ireys and colleagues (Ireys, Chernoff, Stein, DeVet, & Silver, 2001). These authors summarized the results of three randomized clinical trials of community-based support programs for parents of children with chronic physical illnesses. Variables such as depression, anxiety, anger, and psychiatric symptoms were used as outcomes in preventive efforts designed to support caregivers. Ireys et al. reported that maternal anxiety was significantly lowered for mothers in the intervention condition across all three studies.

Another study led by Ireys (Ireys & Blue, 2002) examined the impact of a similar parent-to-parent support intervention on families with children with emotional, mental, or behavioral disabilities. In this study, the outcomes included both the impact on the mothers' mental health and stress levels and the impact of the intervention on the children's mental health status.

It appears that mental health researchers are more likely than their health or disability colleagues to expect that family support interventions should have an impact on the child's mental health symptoms, no matter what the target. By contrast, in their review of parent-related research in the field of early childhood education, Brooks-Gunn, Berlin, and Fuligni (2000) reported a series of studies on the effects of programs such as home visiting and parent education paired with classroom supports for the child. For all of these programs, they examined the impact on maternal mental and physical health. The outcomes they focused on included maternal depressive symptoms, life satisfaction, and child-rearing attitudes.

Other examples of outcomes consistent with Perspective 5 are the family's satisfaction with services and the family's quality of life. Both of these variables suffer from imprecise definitions and measurement challenges, but both also represent outcomes that are important to the families individually yet may not be a high priority to the larger social system unless connected to a socially valued outcome, such as decreased use of government subsidies or increased ability to participate in the workforce. A final example, important because it comes from the field of mental health, is a study of respite care by Bruns and Burchard (2000), which was also discussed in relation to Perspective 4. This was a controlled longitudinal study of the short-term impact of respite care on families of children with mental and emotional disorders. The outcomes measured included a variety of family-related variables (perceived need for future out-of-home placement and crisis intervention, family functioning, caregiving stress, and parent's general stress). They also included measures of service use (actual use of out-of-home placement, crisis intervention), as well as child behavior. Families who had received respite care services were significantly less likely to need out-of-home placement for their child and reported less personal strain of caregiving than did families who did not receive respite care.

PERSPECTIVE 6: COMMUNITY AND SOCIETAL BENEFITS OF CAREGIVER AND FAMILY WELL-BEING

Perspective 6 focuses on positive outcomes that accrue to the community or to society as a result of providing services to families caring for children with disabilities. In this regard, positive outcomes are posited as occurring for both the family itself and for the community and society within which they live. In Perspective 6, the emphasis is on community or societal outcomes; thus, although the community may care in an altruistic way about the mother's mental health, it is the impact of her poor mental health—her inability to parent or work—that has a noticeable effect on the community.

Increased self-sufficiency is an obvious example of a Perspective 6 outcome because of the focus on returning mothers from welfare to the workforce. Lee, Sills, and Oh (2002) have documented the work participation rate of mothers on welfare who have a child with a disability. Their work participation rate is slightly lower than that of mothers of children without disabilities and higher than that of mothers who themselves have a disability. In their study of families on welfare, Meyers, Brady, and Seto (2000) found that mothers with at least one child with a severe disability were 20% to 30% less likely to have worked in the previous month. The ability of the caregiver to work outside of the home is a positive outcome that would result in improved community and societal conditions.

Other examples of outcomes at the societal level are the ability to pay taxes and support oneself without government subsidies, the ability to return to or continue with an education or training, and the ability to do volunteer work, help another family member, or contribute to church and community. Leonard, Brust, and Sapienza (1992) also noted that the long-term caregiving provided by families, especially for children with disabilities, is an important resource for society. In the Meyers et al. (2000) study of families on welfare, the researchers found that 45% of the families were absorbing the direct costs of their child's disability for such things as specialized child care, transportation, or medicine.

Although examples of research that have incorporated outcomes consistent with this perspective are rare in the field of mental health, a few can be found in related fields. In their meta-analysis, Brooks-Gunn et al. (2000) examined the impact of several types of early childhood programs on maternal employment and education. Of the 17 programs reviewed, each had at least some impact on education, employment, and self-sufficiency, with the most comprehensive, a home-visiting approach based on the work of Olds et al. (1999), having the most impact. From the field of aging, Mittelman, Ferris, Shulman, Steinberg, and Levin (1996) conducted a randomized clinical trial to examine the impact of a family support program for families of persons with Alzheimer's disease who were living at home. Those families receiving the support services were two-thirds less likely to place their family member in a nursing home. For family members who were placed, the length of stay was reduced by approximately 1 year and 1 month, representing a large cost saving for society. Similarly, Heller, Factor, Hsieh, and Hahn (1998) found that families caring for adults with developmental disabilities were less likely to place their adult family member out of the home if they were provided with family support services. They also found that the adults with developmental disabilities whose families received support services earned higher wages and were more integrated into the community than those in the control group. These examples provide a reason to believe that families who receive support can contribute in concrete ways to their community and society, whereas families without support will consume community resources.

SUMMARY AND DISCUSSION

In this chapter we have identified six research perspectives addressing family issues and outcomes in children's mental health. There are many research examples of Perspective 1, probably reflecting the long tradition of studying mother–child relationships in an attempt to explain emotional, behavioral, and mental disorders in children. Interest in the possible impact of a child's mental health needs on the caregiver, siblings, or the entire family is relatively new, which may explain the few studies that reflect Perspective 2. A more transactive view of parent–child relationships and influences is found in Perspective 3. Much more research is needed to understand the mutual effects of child and caregiver over time. A considerable amount of research is available to illustrate Perspective 4, which includes both the consequences of the caregiver's response to the child's problems and intervention research designed to influence caregiver attributes that may affect the child's clinical symptoms or functioning. This latter area of intervention research is particularly in need of better conceptual frameworks and program theory. Perspectives 5 and 6 consider caregiver and family outcomes as important goals for families and communities. These two perspectives do not require that the child's outcomes necessarily change as a result of changes in family circumstances.

This review of research on outcomes related to family/caregiver topics in children's mental health raises a number of issues for discussion. First, it is clear that the term *family outcomes* is in large part a misnomer; most of the research that we reviewed addresses a single caregiver, most often the mother, although more recent studies have also included fathers (Almeida, Wethington, & Chandler, 1999; Brody & Ge, 2001; Crawford & Manassis, 2001) and siblings (Bullock & Dishion, 2002; Wamboldt & Wamboldt, 2000). Attention to the outcomes for all family members individually and of the family unit will provide a deeper understanding of the complex family issues related to children who have serious mental health problems.

The second issue concerns the scope of the research addressing family outcomes in children's mental health. Much of the research focuses on some aspect of the relationship between child and caregiver characteristics or outcomes and does not take into account the ecological context within which the child and family live. Increasingly, researchers are urged to consider the impact of poverty and other factors on the health, productivity, physical environment, and emotional well-being of families (Earls & Carlson, 2001; Park, Turnbull, & Turnbull, 2002; U.S. Department of Health and Human Services, 1999). This approach is exemplified by studies that examine parental stress in relation to both child functioning and broader ecological variables. For example, in a study of parents of children with serious emotional disorders, McDonald et al. (1999) found that the child's behavior was a very important predictor of parental stress, along with other issues such as employment, more social and formal support, relationship to the child (mothers reported more stress), and race (whites had more stress). In contrast, in a sample of families whose children had developmental disabilities, Smith et al. (2001) reported that factors such as income, time available for interaction with the child, and social support predicted parenting stress better than child functioning. Despite the somewhat conflicting results of these two studies, they represent a beginning step in considering the child and family in an ecological context, and they emphasize the need for further study.

A final area of discussion has to do with the need for a more planful approach to both program development and research about family issues within children's mental health. Three important areas for development are (a) better program theory and logic models that map anticipated links between the independent variables and expected outcomes, (b) more sophisticated research designs and analysis methods that take into account complex family circumstances and relationships, and (c) an inclusive process for identifying and prioritizing research topics related to family outcomes in children's mental health that include the concerns of affected youth and families.

Better program theory and logic models could assist both program developers and researchers to specify intended connections among independent variables such as family needs and responses, interventions, and expected outcomes. Interventions could be more carefully focused and implemented, and studies would then be better able to address questions such as, "Why should respite care for overstressed caregivers necessarily result in changes in child symptoms or functioning?" "What specific changes in parent behavior do we expect to result from parent training?" And, "Why should these changes make a difference?"

Research that takes into account complex family circumstances and relationships requires large sample sizes and designs that account for the "nested arrangement of family, school, neighborhood, and community contexts in which children grow up" (Earls & Carlson, 2001, p. 143). The work of Felton Earls and colleagues constitutes an example of this work in the area of child health. Parallel work in children's mental health that includes the development and testing of interventions is needed.

The process of identifying and prioritizing research topics related to family outcomes in children's mental health should not be left exclusively to researchers or government representatives. The process should involve families, researchers, program developers, funders, and policymakers, all of whom have a stake in these issues. Although the final list of topics should be left to these stakeholders, some areas that have had little or no attention in children's mental health include

- intervention studies that examine a wide range of possible outcomes of family support services;
- attention to the implications for society of the collective experiences of individual caretakers and families;
- research regarding the effects of caregiving on the health and ability of caregivers to function effectively in adult roles; and
- examination of the financial impact, both direct and indirect, of caregiving for children and youth with serious emotional disorders, along with the implications for society of various choices about the provision of services and supports.

In recommending strategies and topics for future research, it is important to acknowledge that the choices made by researchers about what to study are influenced by previous research, including the conceptual frameworks and availability of measures, societal attitudes, and the availability of support for particular research directions. Fortunately, there is now a small body of research on the outcomes of family support (Perspectives 4, 5, and 6) on which to build a research agenda. In addition, society's interest in promoting the well-being of caregivers in less stigmatized populations, such as those with other childhood disabilities or Alzheimer's disease, offers a rationale and some support for the study of parallel topics in children's mental health. For example, a recent federal research initiative addressing informal caregiving for chronic conditions (National Institutes of Health, 2002) covered caregiving for persons with mental illness, including children. Such a focus on the well-being of caregivers across disability groups should help (a) to build a knowledge base that can be used to improve the lives of families whose children have emotional, behavioral, or mental disorders and (b) to highlight the importance of their circumstances for the communities in which they live.

AUTHORS' NOTE

Preparation of this chapter was partially supported by Grant H133B40021, National Institute on Disability and Rehabilitation Research, U.S. Department of Education, and Center for Mental Health Services, Substance Abuse, and Mental Health Services Administration. The views expressed in this chapter are not necessarily those of the funders.

REFERENCES

Achenbach, T. M., & Rescorla, L. A. (2001). *Manual for the ASEBA school-age forms and profiles.* Burlington, VT: ASEBA.

Almeida, D. M., Wethington, E., & Chandler, A. L. (1999). Daily transmission of tensions between marital dyads and parent–child dyads. *Journal of Marriage and the Family, 61*(1), 49–61.

Angold, A., Messer, S. C., Stangl, D., Farmer, E. M. Z., Costello, E. J., & Burns, B. J. (1998). Perceived parental burden and service use for child and adolescent psychiatric disorders. *American Journal of Public Health, 88*(1), 75–80.

Arnold, D. S., O'Leary, S. G., Wolff, L. S., & Acker, M. M. (1993). The parenting scale: A measure of dysfunctional parenting in discipline situations. *Psychological Assessment, 5,* 137–144.

Bailey, J., Barton, B., & Vignola, A. (1999). Coping with children with ADHD: Coping styles of mothers with children with ADHD or challenging behaviours. *Early Child Development and Care, 148,* 35–50.

Barkley, R. A. (2000). *Taking charge of ADHD: The complete, authoritative guide for parents.* New York: Guilford Press.

Bisbee, C. C. (2000). Psychiatric patient education. *Psychiatric Times, 17*(4). Retrieved July 10, 2002, from www.psychiatrictimes.com/p000476.html

Bowman, R. (2001). *Quality of life assessment for young children with developmental disabilities and their families: Development of a quality of life questionnaire.* Unpublished doctoral dissertation, West Virginia University, Morgantown.

Brannan, A. M., & Heflinger, C. A. (2001). Distinguishing caregiver strain from psychological distress: Modeling the relationships among child, family, and caregiver variables. *Journal of Child and Family Studies, 10*(4), 405–418.

Brannan, A. M., Heflinger, C. A., Schweitzer, T. B., & Orten, P. (2001). Child and family predictors of service use in two service systems: Role of caregiver strain. In C. Newman, C. J. Libertori, K. Kutash, & R. M. Friedman (Eds.), *14th annual research proceedings, a system of care for children's mental health: Expanding the research base* (pp. 267–270). Tampa: University of South Florida, Louis de la Parte Florida Mental Health Institute, Research and Training Center for Children's Mental Health.

Brody, G. H., & Ge, X. (2001). Linking parenting processes and self-regulation to psychological functioning and alcohol use during early adolescence. *Journal of Family Psychology, 15*(1), 82–94.

Bronfenbrenner, U. (1979). *The ecology of human development.* Cambridge, MA: Harvard University Press.

Brooks-Gunn, J., Berlin, L. J., & Fuligni, A. S. (2000). Early childhood intervention programs: What about the family? In J. P. Shonkoff & S. J. Meisels (Eds.), *Handbook of early childhood intervention* (2nd ed., pp. 549–588). Cambridge, England: Cambridge University Press.

Bruns, E. J., & Burchard, J. D. (2000). Impact of respite care services for families with children experiencing emotional and behavioral problems. *Children's Services: Social Policy, Research, and Practice, 3*(1), 39–61.

Bullock, B. M., & Dishion, T. J. (2002). Sibling collusion and problem behavior in early adolescence: Toward a process model for family mutuality. *Journal of Abnormal Child Psychology, 30*(2), 143–153.

Capaldi, D. M., & Patterson, G. R. (1991). Relation of parental transitions to boys' adjustment problems: I. A linear hypothesis. II. Mothers at risk for transitions and unskilled parenting. *Developmental Psychology, 27*(3), 489–584.

Crawford, A. M., & Manassis, K. (2001). Familial predictors of treatment outcome in childhood anxiety disorders. *Journal of the American Academy of Child and Adolescent Psychiatry, 40*(10), 1182–1189.

Crowley, M. J., & Kazdin, A. E. (1998). Child psychosocial functioning and parent quality of life among clinically referred children. *Journal of Child and Family Studies, 7*(2), 233–251.

Dix, T. (1991). The affective organization of parenting: Adaptive and maladaptive processes. *Psychological Bulletin, 110,* 3–25.

Dunn, M. E., Burbine, T., Bowers, C. A., & Tantleff-Dunn, S. (2001). Moderators of stress in parents of children with autism. *Community Mental Health Journal, 37*(1), 39–52.

Earls, F., & Carlson, M. (2001). The social ecology of child health and well-being. *Annual Review of Public Health, 22,* 143–166.

Early, T. J., Gregoire, T. K., & McDonald, T. P. (2002). Child functioning and caregiver well-being in families of children with emotional disorders: A longitudinal analysis. *Journal of Family Issues, 23*(3), 374–391.

Falkov, A. (1998). *Crossing bridges: Working with mentally ill parents and their children.* Southampton, England: Pavilion Press.

Farmer, T. W., & Farmer, E. M. Z. (2001). Developmental science, systems of care, and prevention of emotional and behavioral problems in youth. *American Journal of Orthopsychiatry, 71*(2), 171–181.

Federation of Families for Children's Mental Health. (2002). *Federation of families web page: Who we are.* Retrieved September 5, 2002, from http://www.ffcmh .org/Eng_one.htm#WhatIsNew

Feldman, M. A., & Werner, S. E. (2002). Collateral effects of behavioral parent training on families of children with developmental disabilities and behavior disorders. *Behavioral Interventions, 17*(2), 75–83.

Floyd, F. J., & Gallagher, E. M. (1997). Parental stress, care demands, and use of support services for school-age children with disabilities and behavior problems. *Family Relations: Interdisciplinary Journal of Applied Family Studies, 46*(4), 359–372.

Friesen, B. J. (1989). *National study of parents whose children have serious emotional disorders.* Paper presented at conference: Children's Mental Health Services and Policy: Building a Research Base, Tampa.

Friesen, B. J. (1993). Family support in child and adult mental health. In G. H. S. Singer, L. E. Powers, & A. L. Olson (Eds.), *Redefining family support: Innovations in public–private partnerships* (pp. 260–289). Baltimore: Brookes.

Friesen, B. J., & Koroloff, N. M. (1990). Family-centered services: Implications for mental health administration and research. *Journal of Mental Health Administration, 17,* 13–25.

Grant, I., Adler, K. A., Patterson, T., Dimsdale, J. E., Ziegler, M. G., & Irwin, M. R. (2002). Health consequences of Alzheimer's caregiving transitions: Effects of placement and bereavement. *Psychosomatic Medicine, 64*(3), 477–486.

Greenley, J. R., & Robitschek, C. G. (1991). Evaluation of a comprehensive program for youth with severe emotional disorders: An analysis of family experiences and satisfaction. *American Journal of Orthopsychiatry, 61*(2), 291–297.

Harahan, M. F. (2001). New paradigms for guiding research, interventions and policies for family caregivers. *Aging and Mental Health, 5(Supp. 11),* S52–S55.

Heller, T., Factor, A. R., Hsieh, K., & Hahn, J. E. (1998). The impact of age and transitions out of nursing homes for adults with developmental disabilities. *American Journal on Mental Retardation, 103,* 236–248.

Ho, C. J., Weitzman, P. F., Cui, X., & Levkoff, S. E. (2000). Stress and service use among minority caregivers to elders and dementia. *Journal of Gerontological Social Work, 33*(1), 67–88.

Hodges, K., Doucette-Gates, A., & Liao, Q. (1999). The relationship between the Child and Adolescent Functional Assessment Scale (CAFAS) and indicators of functioning. *Journal of Child and Family Studies, 8*(1), 109–122.

Ireys, H. T., & Blue, R. (2002). *Developing, implementing, evaluating, and replicating a successful family-to-family support and education program.* Paper presented at conference: Building on Family Strengths, Portland, OR.

Ireys, H. T., Chernoff, R., Stein, R. E. K., DeVet, K. A., & Silver, E. J. (2001). Outcomes of community-based family-to-family support: Lessons learned from a decade of randomized trials. *Children's Services: Social Policy, Research, and Practice, 4*(4), 203–216.

Katsurada, E., & Sugawara, A. I. (2000). Moderating effects of mothers' attribution on the relationships between their affect and parenting behaviors and children's aggressive behaviors. *Journal of Child and Family Studies, 9*(1), 39–50.

Kazdin, A. E. (1997). Parent management training: Evidence, outcomes and issues. *Journal of the American Academy of Child and Adolescent Psychiatry, 36*(10), 1349–1357.

Koren, P. E., DeChillo, N., & Friesen, B. J. (1992). Measuring empowerment in families whose children have emotional disabilities: A brief questionnaire. *Rehabilitation Psychology, 37*(4), 305–321.

Larson, R. W., & Almeida, D. M. (1999). Emotional transmission in the daily lives of families: A new paradigm for studying family process. *Journal of Marriage and the Family, 61*(1), 5–20.

Lee, S., Sills, M., & Oh, G.-T. (2002, June 20). *Disabilities among children and mothers in low-income families.* Institute for Women's Policy Research. Retrieved August 20, 2002, from http://www.ipr.org

Leonard, B., Brust, J., & Sapienza, J. (1992). Financial and time costs to parents of severely disabled children. *Public Health Reports, 107*(3), 302–311.

Lindahl, K. M. (1998). Family process variables and children's disruptive behavior problems. *Journal of Family Psychology, 69*(1), 100–109.

Macias, M. M., Clifford, S. C., Saylor, C. F., & Kreh, S. M. (2001). Predictors of parenting stress in families of children with spina bifida. *Children's Health Care, 30*(1), 57–65.

Matthews, J. M., & Hudson, A. M. (2001). Guidelines for evaluating parent training programs. *Family Relations: Interdisciplinary Journal of Applied Family Studies, 50*(1), 77–86.

McDonald, T. P., Poertner, J., & Pierpont, J. (1999). Predicting caregiver stress: An ecological perspective. *American Journal of Orthopsychiatry, 69*(1), 100–109.

McFarlane, W. R., Dushay, R. A., Stastny, P., Deakins, S. M., & Link, B. (1996). A comparison of two levels of family-aided assertive community treatment. *Psychiatric Services, 47*(7), 744–750.

McKay, M. M., Pennington, J., Lynne, C. J., & McCadam, K. (2001). Understanding urban child mental health service use: Two studies of child, family, and environmental correlates. *Journal of Behavioral Health Services and Research, 28*(4), 475–484.

Meyers, M. K., Brady, H. E., & Seto, E. Y. (2000). *Expensive children in poor families: Intersection of childhood disabilities and welfare.* San Francisco: Public Policy Institute of California. Retrieved August 29, 2002, from the http://www.ppic.org

Mittelman, M. S., Ferris, S. H., Shulman, E., Steinberg, G., & Levin, B. (1996). A family intervention to delay nursing home placement of patients with Alzheimer disease. A randomized controlled trial. *Journal of the American Medical Association, 276*(21), 1725–1731.

National Institutes of Health. (2002). *NIH guide: Informal caregiving research for chronic conditions* [Web page]. Retrieved September 8, 2002, from http://grants1.nih.gov/grants/guide/pa-files/PA-02-155.html

Olds, D. L., Henderson, C. R., Kitzman, H. J., Eckenrolde, J. J., Cole, R. E., & Tatelbaum, R. C. (1999). Prenatal and infancy home visitation by nurses: Recent findings. *The Future of Children, 9,* 44–65.

Oyserman, D., Mowbray, C. T., Meares, P. A., & Firminger, K. B. (2000). Parenting among mothers with a serious mental illness. *American Journal of Orthopsychiatry, 70*(3), 296–315.

Park, J., Turnbull, A. P., & Turnbull, H. R. (2002). Impacts of poverty on quality of life in families of children with disabilities. *Exceptional Children, 68*(2), 151–170.

Reinares, M., Colom, F., Martinez-Aran, A., Benabarre, A., & Vieta, E. (2002). Therapeutic interventions focused on the family of bipolar patients. *Psychotherapy and Psychosomatics, 71*(1), 2–10.

Richardson, K. D., & Heflinger, C. A. (2002). *Caregiver strain in families of children with serious emotional disorders: Does relationship to child make a difference?* Paper presented at conference: A System of Care for Children's Mental Health: Expanding the Research Base, Tampa.

Rubin, A., Cardenas, J., Warren, K., Pike, C. K., & Wombach, K. (1998). Outdated practitioner views about family culpability and severe mental disorders. *Social Work, 43,* 435–445.

Shaw, D. S., & Bell, R. Q. (1993). Developmental theories of parental contributors to antisocial behavior. *Journal of Abnormal Child Psychology, 21*(5), 493–518.

Smith, T. B., Oliver, M. N. I., & Innocenti, M. S. (2001). Parenting stress in families of children with disabilities. *American Journal of Orthopsychiatry, 71*(2), 257–261.

Stoolmiller, M. (2001). Synergistic interaction of child manageability problems and parent-discipline tactics in predicting future growth in externalizing behavior for boys. *Developmental Psychology, 37*(6), 814–825.

Stoolmiller, M., Patterson, G. R., & Snyder, J. (1997). Parental discipline and child antisocial behavior: A contingency-based theory and some methodological refinements. *Psychological Inquiry, 8*(3), 223–229.

Stroul, B. A. (1996). Introduction: Progress in children's mental health. In B. A. Stroul (Ed.), *Children's mental health: Creating systems of care in a changing society* (pp. xxi–xxxii). Baltimore: Brookes.

Svavarsdottir, E. K., McCubbin, M. A., & Kane, J. H. (2000). Well-being of parents of young children with asthma. *Research in Nursing and Health, 23*(5), 346–358.

Tarico, V. S., Low, B. P., Trupin, E., & Forsyth-Stephens, A. (1989). Children's mental health services: A parent perspective. *Community Mental Health Journal, 25*(4), 313–326.

Taub, J., Tighe, T. A., & Burchard, J. (2001). The effects of parent empowerment on adjustment for children receiving comprehensive mental health services. *Children's Services: Social Policy, Research, and Practice, 4*(3), 103–122.

U.S. Department of Health and Human Services. (1999). *Mental health: A report of the Surgeon General.* Rockville, MD: U.S. Department of Health and Human Services, Substance Abuse and Mental Health Services Administration, Center for Mental Health Services, National Institutes of Health, National Institute of Mental Health.

Wamboldt, M. Z., & Wamboldt, F. S. (2000). Role of the family in the onset and outcome of childhood disorders: Selected research findings. *Journal of the American Academy of Child and Adolescent Psychiatry, 39*(10), 1212–1219.

Yatchmenoff, D. K., Koren, P. E., Friesen, B. J., Gordon, L. J., & Kinney, R. F. (1998). Enrichment and stress in families caring for a child with a serious emotional disorder. *Journal of Child and Family Studies, 7*(2), 129–145.

Strength-Based Assessment in Children's Mental Health

CHAPTER 6

Mark K. Harniss and Michael H. Epstein

In recent years, individuals who work in fields that address the needs of children and youth at risk for emotional and behavioral disorders have seen the development of assessment and treatment approaches that focus on the strengths and assets of these children in addition to their deficits or weaknesses. Some would call this emphasis on strengths a fundamental shift in thinking, while others perceive it more as a necessary reminder to caregivers and mental health workers to more systematically do something they have always done. Regardless, the emphasis on looking at the whole child (strengths as well as deficits) and using all this information in treatment planning has received increasing attention in many fields, including juvenile justice (Clark, 1996; Marquoit & Dobbins, 1995), child welfare (Saleeby, 1992), social work (Early, 2001; Graybeal, 2001), mental health (Lourie, Katz-Leavy, & Stroul, 1994), family services (Dunst, Trivette, & Deal, 1994), and education (Nelson & Pearson, 1991). In addition, a number of established treatment models and education and mental health initiatives have focused attention on the need for strength-based assessment. These initiatives and models include the U.S. Department of Education's *National Agenda for Achieving Better Results for Children and Youth with Serious Emotional Disturbance* (1994), the wraparound approach (VanDenberg & Grealish, 1996), multisystemic therapy (Henggeler, Schoenwald, Borduin, Rowland, & Cunningham, 1998), and systems of care (Stroul & Friedman, 1994). The increased emphasis on holistic, strength-based approaches in the social science fields mirrors developments in other areas, such as health. The *International Classification of Functioning, Disability, and Health (ICD–10;* World Health Organization, 2001) is an example where the emphasis has changed from a focus on impairments and disease states to a focus on overall health states in which disease or impairment is one part of the information collected.

Strength-based approaches are growing in large part due to a sense that focusing solely on deficits and weaknesses limits service providers' ability to think broadly about treatment opportunities. As Clark (1996) noted regarding the juvenile justice field, the problem-focused approach "drives our workers to assess primarily what offenders cannot do or have failed to do. We are then consumed by work to 'fix the failure.' This focus is so pervasive and entrenched we are often left blind to any alternatives" (p. 33). More importantly, focusing on strengths may result in more positive treatment plans. As Rockwell (1998) noted, "Armed with knowledge of characteristics exhibited by resilient youth, educators can actively search for and find ways to enhance those factors in the students they teach. They can emphasize what is healthy, strong, and potentially resilient about youth, rather than concentrating on repairing what is wrong" (p. 15).

In this chapter, we discuss strength-based assessment as a component of a comprehensive model of assessment and evaluation. Strength-based assessment has been defined as "the measurement of those emotional and behavioral skills, competencies, and characteristics that create a sense of personal accomplishment; contribute to satisfying relationships with family members, peers, and adults; enhance one's ability to deal with adversity and stress; and promote one's personal, social, and academic development" (Epstein & Sharma, 1998, p. 3). We begin with a brief overview of strength-based assessment, discuss informal and formal assessment techniques, and end with applied examples of strength-based assessment.

OVERVIEW OF STRENGTH-BASED ASSESSMENT

Strength-based assessment is premised upon the following set of beliefs:

1. All children have strengths.
2. Assessing a child's strengths in addition to his or her deficits may result in enhanced motivation and improved performance from the child.
3. Deficits should be viewed as opportunities to learn rather than as fixed or stable.
4. Families and children are more likely to positively engage in treatment when service plans include a focus on strengths.

All Children Have Strengths

Many formal assessment instruments in the field of emotional and behavioral disorders possess strong psychometric properties and provide useful information to practitioners and researchers. These include the *Behavior Rating Profile* (Brown & Hammill, 1990), the *Revised Behavior Problem Checklist* (Quay & Peterson, 1987), and the *Child Behavior Checklist* (Achenbach, 1991). In general, these instruments have been used to identify deficits or problems in an individual's or a group's performance for the purpose of screening, diagnosis, identification, or remediation. However, the focus on deficits may unnecessarily limit the information collected about children's behavior by restricting the field of vision of those who gather the data, and as a result, professionals may fail to collect additional information that could be relevant to developing, implementing, and monitoring comprehensive service plans.

Salvia and Ysseldyke (1998) defined assessment at its most general level as a process for gathering data to inform decisions about a group or an individual.

Thus, it seems obvious that the field of assessment is not limited merely to the identification of problems and weaknesses. Rather, from this broader standpoint, information about strengths should be equally as important as information about weaknesses. Strength-based assessment, then, fits within a model in which each child is viewed holistically as an individual possessing both strengths *and* weaknesses. This approach to assessment is a change from an emphasis on "patching up" those parts of a child that are broken or poorly developed to an emphasis on identifying, building, and strengthening a child's assets. It is important to note that "the identification of strengths is not the antithesis of the identification of problems. Instead it is a large part of the solution" (Graybeal, 2001, p. 234). If professionals focus on the identification and development of strengths, they may be able to help children develop a stronger foundation upon which to face personal challenges.

Every child and family has personal and unique individual strengths. Although we typically do not acknowledge that children with emotional and behavioral disorders possess personal strengths, recent research has indicated that these children demonstrate sufficient strengths in important areas. For example, Walrath, Mandell, Holden, and Santiago (2004) assessed the strengths of 1,838 children who entered community-based mental health programs. Along with assessing for functional impairments, the researchers also measured the emotional and behavioral strengths of children. They noted that the children, even those with severe functional impairments, demonstrated levels of average personal strengths similar to their peers without disabilities. More important, they noted that strengths and impairments were not opposite ends of the same continuum but rather were separate constructs.

Focus on Strengths

When professionals focus on a child's deficits, they may inadvertently respond to the child more negatively and with less enthusiasm. According to Kral (1989), "If we ask people to look for deficits, they will usually find them, and their view of the situation will be colored by this. If we ask people to look for successes, they will usually find it, and their view of the situation will be colored by this" (p. 32). A child or caregiver may read this negativity as "giving up" or a lack of interest, which may lead to less motivation to change or grow. Rockwell (1998) noted that professionals are susceptible to four myths about children that are reinforced by a solely deficit-based approach to assessment: the *myth of irreparable damage,* in which professionals posit that the abuse and emotional damage created early in a child's life can never be fixed or improved; the *myth of predetermination,* in which professionals believe that a child's circumstances, genetics, or upbringing predetermine him or her to be unsuccessful; the *myth of identity,* in which professionals believe that children are their label (e.g., abused, behavior disordered, emotionally disturbed) and that the label defines their identity; and finally, the *myth that ultimately "it doesn't matter,"* in which burnout and stress lead providers to believe that for all the efforts they put into working with a challenging child, nothing positive will come of their effort. Rockwell noted that in reality providers must learn that they cannot give up on children based upon current status or functioning. Instead, providers must inform children that they are in control of their own lives regardless of current circumstance. According to Rockwell, "Even when these children throw the worst they have to give in our directions, we must reflect back to them the best that they can be and reassure them that nothing is predetermined. They can make their own decisions." (p. 17). In addition, providers who work with these youth should be constantly "engaged in a talent search, defining the identities of those youth in terms of their strengths" (p. 17). And finally, providers need to find ways to see that what they do matters, even if they do not see the immediate positive outcomes of their efforts. Strength-based assessment offers service providers a more concrete view of positive outcome and helps them focus on the areas where improvement is most likely to occur.

Opportunity To Learn: Focusing on Positive Interventions

When children have problems learning or applying information, we tend to focus on solutions that involve teaching and instruction. We often are more willing to assume that academic problems are a "cannot" problem rather than a "will not" problem. That is, we assume that if we adapt our instruction, students will learn a skill they did not know before and the problem will be solved. With behavioral problems, however, we tend to assume that students have the skills in their repertoire and that for some reason they are choosing to not use them. For example, we might assume that a student who is physically aggressive in class (e.g., hitting, pinching other students) knows that what she is doing is not appropriate and thus we focus on reducing the behavior. In fact, the child may know that the approach is not the most appropriate action but might not have any other behaviors in her repertoire that achieve the same outcome (e.g., the reduction of task requirements).

Strength-based assessment can aid in the selection of replacement behaviors by highlighting those areas where a child does in fact excel. In the previous example, if the child was highly verbal, it might make sense to teach her to request a "quiet time." As Graybeal (2001) noted, "The fundamental premise is that individuals will do better in the long run when they are helped to identify, recognize, and use the strengths and resources available in themselves and their environments" (p. 234). Strength-based assessment aids providers in developing interventions that accomplish this goal.

Service Plans

Service plans that begin with a focus on strengths are more likely to be acceptable to children, families, and service providers as they provide a foundation of competence upon which to improve rather than a focus on incompetence and failure (Saleeby, 1992). Collecting a range of assessment data that represents both strengths and weaknesses may be very useful in communicating with parents and caregivers who are interested not only in what is "wrong" with their child but also in knowing what is "right" and in building upon the skills and competencies they see in their child. Moreover, such an orientation to families may lead to a positive parent–professional relationship characterized by mutual trust, supportiveness, and clarity of goals.

Strength-based practices are also increasingly being written into federal legislation. The reauthorization of the Individuals with Disabilities Education Act (IDEA) in 1997 stated that the Individualized Education Program (IEP) team shall consider "the strengths of the child and the concerns of the parents for enhancing the education of their child" (34 C.F.R. 300.346). This added strength-based component of IDEA has the potential to change the IEP process from a focus solely on a child's problems to a broader focus on the child's presenting strengths in combination with her or his areas for improvement. With this information, the IEP team could develop an assessment inventory that highlights a child's current strengths and resources, identifies critical needs across all life domains, includes parental goals, and provides the services and supports that will be used to build upon the child's strengths.

INFORMAL STRENGTH-BASED ASSESSMENT

In informal approaches to strength-based assessment, a professional usually engages in a "strength chat" with the child, family, and informal supports (e.g., relatives, friends, pastors). During this "chat," the professional asks questions about the resources, strengths, goals, and vision for the future for the child and family. This information is used to identify the needs of the child and family. The questions, data collection, and format of this chat vary from professional to professional. Questions that might appear in an informal interview include the following: "What do you see yourself doing in 3 years?" "If you were in trouble, whom would you ask for help?" and "What are your favorite hobbies or activities?" Counselors and diagnosticians have frequently practiced informal strength-based assessment (VanDenBerg & Grealish, 1996, 1998). However, there is no single model of informal strength-based assessment that applies to all situations. The chief benefit of informal approaches to strength-based assessment is in their clinical utility for service planning. In the following section, a brief case study is presented that illustrates how an informal strength-based assessment could be used to identify goals and establish a treatment plan.

Applied Example

Jim is a fourth grader at Covey Green Elementary. Jim's immediate family is composed of his older brother, Greg (sixth grade); his younger sister, Laura (second grade); his dad, Jake; and his dad's live-in girlfriend, Rachel. His dad is a salesman for a pharmaceutical company and travels frequently, leaving the children in Rachel's care. Jim's biological parents have been divorced for 2 years. In the first year following their divorce, he and his siblings lived with his mother, Sara. However, Sara has rapid cycling bipolar disorder, and her wide mood swings and difficulty in staying on a treatment plan affected the safety of the children. For this reason, Jake was awarded custody of the children. Sara is currently participating in a court-ordered mental health program in order to regain visitation rights to the children.

Jim has been missing a lot of school, ostensibly due to illness. When he is in class, teachers have noted that he is not engaged and has become increasingly withdrawn. Sometimes he lays his head on the desk and will not work on projects even if the teacher gives him a direct request. His grades are suffering due to his lack of work completion. At recess he begs to stay inside with the excuse that he is not feeling well. He has also been increasingly requesting to visit the school nurse, and the teacher has noted that this usually happens when the class is engaged in collaborative activities. The second-grade teacher has noted similar but less severe withdrawal by Laura, his younger sister. In contrast, Greg, his older brother, has been sent to the principal's office multiple times for noncompliance and recently was picked up by the truant officer after he ran away from school.

Jim's teacher suggested to Jake that the family get involved in a statewide project called Healthy Families, Healthy Communities. During intake to the program, Jake met with Janice, the family service worker, to participate in an informal strength-based assessment. The purpose of the assessment was to gain more information about the family's strengths, interest, experiences, goals, values, and traditions. The questions and Jake's answers are presented in Figure 6.1.

The information gathered from the interview was useful for Janice in planning an approach to intervention. It seemed clear that the family had things they liked to do together (e.g., hiking, playing with the dog, watching movies). There were people in their extended family and community who cared about them, were trusted, and were available to help. Jake very much wanted the children in his life and was willing to make changes to ensure that they were happy. In particular, he wanted to be home more and was considering changing jobs. And Rachel, even though she had only been in their lives a brief time, also cared about and was invested in the children, who related well to her and treated her like an aunt or older sister.

This information, combined with the data collected at the school, was used by a family planning team consisting of Jake, Rachel, Jake's dad, the school counselor, and Janice. In their first meeting, they worked through a solution-oriented interview process (e.g., Clark, 1996) in which Jake identified goals that he had for the family and then linked those goals to strategies that might move the family toward achievement of those objectives. The goals were categorized into three categories (a) counseling support for the children, (b) development of extracurricular activities and friends for the children, and (c) a job change for Jake.

Name of family: Anderson
Parent/guardian interviewed: Jake (father)

1. **The things I like most about my child(ren) are:**
   They take good care of each other. They are caring and gentle.

2. **My life would really be better 6 months from now if:**
   I could be at home more. If I were traveling less.

3. **My child's/children's life would be really better 6 months from now if:**
   If they had more friends and activities to keep them busy. If they could visit their mother when she was stable and know that she is all right.

4. **The most important thing I have ever done is:**
   Regain custody of my children.

5. **I am happiest when:**
   My family is happy. When I feel like I've done something good as a father.

6. **The best times we have as a family are:**
   Saturday morning at the park, playing Frisbee with the dog, and throwing rocks in the river. Backpacking once a year.

7. **My best qualities as a parent are:**
   I take care of them. I make enough money to support them and give them what they need.

8. **Name some special rules that your family has:**
   We don't criticize. We respect each other's privacy.

9. **Who are persons you call when you need help and want to talk? Who have you turned to in the past for support?**
   College friend (Rick); Sara's parents; my dad.

10. **What activities does your family enjoy?**
    Like to read, watch movies, eat out for breakfast on Saturday, hike in the mountains.

11. **What are your family traditions? In which cultural events does your family participate?**
    My grandparents are Norwegian and they have always taken the kids to the local Scandinavian festival. At Christmas, they eat lutefisk and decorate the tree with Christmas baskets.

12. **Are there any special values or beliefs that were taught to you by your parents or others who are important to you?**
    Be honest, be kind, help others when they need it.

13. **Does your family belong to any part of the faith community? In what way?**
    The kids go to a local Methodist church with Rachel. They attend summer vacation Bible school. Jake is agnostic.

FIGURE 6.1. Example of an informal strength-based assessment.

Janice noted that there was a project at the local college that was providing counseling groups for children whose parents had recently divorced. She suggested that the two younger children, Laura and Jim, might benefit especially from talking to children their own age who lived in similar family situations. The school counselor mentioned that she had recently heard of a program funded by the state department of community health that worked with children who had a parent with mental illness. She thought the children might benefit from learning more about their mother's illness. The principal suggested that the older sibling, Greg, might benefit from having a Big Brother to do things with who could get him involved in extracurricular activities. In addition, the whole team thought that the children would enjoy being involved in the Brownies, Cub Scouts, or Scouts (depending upon age), as they enjoyed camping and the outdoors. Jake's dad, who is retired, agreed to help out with afterschool activities by transporting the children where they needed to go. Finally, they suggested that Jake work with a local employment counselor to identify other jobs he might perform that wouldn't require the extensive travel of his current position. All of these solutions take advantage of individual and family strengths and are linked to personal goals and to assets in the community.

FORMAL STRENGTH-BASED ASSESSMENT

Although informal strength-based assessment can be a powerful tool, as demonstrated in the previous section, it is difficult to be certain that these measures reliably assess the variables of interest. Informal strength-based measures also lack normative data that would allow practitioners to identify an individual's strengths relative to other individuals from a specific population. Recently, strength-based assessment has begun to receive the same rigorous psychometric consideration as deficit-oriented approaches. Specifically, proponents of strength-based assessment are beginning to investigate the reliability, validity, and fidelity of implementation of strength-oriented measures.

Several standardized strength-based measures have been developed, field-tested, and published in recent years (Early, 2001). Some of these measures are targeted toward families (e.g., *The Family Resource Scale;* Dunst & Leet, 1987), while others are targeted toward children (e.g., *The Reasons for Living Inventory for Adolescents;* Osman et al., 1998). In the following section, we review a few of the most commonly used instruments and discuss their psychometric qualities. Specifically, we briefly review the *Child and Adolescent Strengths Assessment Scale* (CASA; Lyons, Kisiel, & West, 1997; Lyons, Uziel-Miller, Reyes, & Sokol, 2000), the *Strengths and Difficulties Questionnaire* (SDQ; Goodman, 1997), and *Profiles of Student Life: Attitudes and Behaviors* (PSL-AB; Benson, Leffert, Scales, & Blyth, 1998; Leffert et al., 1998). Finally, we review in detail the *Behavioral and Emotional Rating Scale* (BERS; Epstein

& Sharma, 1998) and describe how formal strength-based data can be used for treatment planning and program evaluation purposes.

Child and Adolescent Strengths Assessment Scale

The CASA is a strength-based tool designed to be included as part of an overall mental health evaluation. A child's caregiver or therapist administers the CASA, which is a 30-item scale divided into six domains. These domains are as follows:

1. morality/spirituality (e.g., has developed values/morals; 4 items),
2. peer strengths (e.g., has close friend[s]; 3 items),
3. psychological strengths (e.g., has the ability to adapt to stressful life circumstances; 5 items),
4. school/vocational strengths (e.g., excels in at least one subject; 8 items),
5. family strengths (e.g., has strong positive relationship with at least one parent; 6 items), and
6. extracurricular strengths (e.g., has a hobby or hobbies; 4 items).

The rater evaluates the child on a 3-point scale for each item (1 = *no evidence*, 2 = *interest/potential*, 3 = *yes, definitely*). Each point on the scale is linked to an anchor that provides a foundation for the rating. For example, when rating the item "Has a strong positive relationship with a parent," a professional would see that the anchor for the third point on the scale reads as follows:

> *Yes, definitely* would be used to rate an individual for whom there is a warm, loving relationship with a parent or caregiver. This relationship would be characterized by reciprocal attachment and strong communication. If the caregiver is not a parent, then the relationship must be at least 3 months in duration before using this level. (Lyons et al., 2000, p. 178)

When finished, the rater can identify the presence of strength in each domain and the potential for development of that strength. The scale appears to possess adequate content and concurrent validity as well as internal reliability (Lyons et al., 2000).

Strength and Difficulties Questionnaire

The SDQ is a brief (one-page) screening instrument with 25 positive and negative items. A widely accepted measure, the SDQ is used in basic and applied research and as a screening tool in educational and mental health environments. It is available online in more than 40 languages. The measure is divided into five domains, each of which is represented by 5 items:

1. prosocial behavior (e.g., considerate of other people's feelings),
2. peer problems (e.g., has at least one good friend),
3. emotional symptoms (e.g., many worries, often seems worried),
4. inattention/hyperactivity (e.g., easily distracted, concentration wanders), and
5. conduct problems (e.g., often has temper tantrums).

Parents, teachers, or mental health professionals complete the primary version of the SDQ; youth (ages 11–16) can complete a self-report version themselves. The measure has been validated in a large-scale ($N = 10,000$) study (Goodman, 2001) and possesses adequate concurrent and predictive validity as well as test–retest reliability (Goodman, 1997; Goodman & Scott, 1999).

Profiles of Student Life: Attitudes and Behaviors

The Developmental Asset Framework (a set of benchmarks for positive development of children and adolescents) and the Asset-Building Community (a model for developing communities with more positive supports for youth) were developed by the Search Institute, a nonprofit social science research organization that seeks to promote positive youth development (Benson et al., 1998; Leffert et al., 1998). The institute focuses on community-based programs that address the strengths and assets of families and individuals.

The Developmental Asset Framework is operationalized in the Search Institute's revised PSL–AB, which is a self-report survey designed to measure developmental assets. Developmental assets are defined as "a set of 'building blocks' that when present or promoted appear to enhance significant developmental outcomes among youth" (Benson et al., 1998, p. 142). The 156-item survey measures 40 developmental assets as well as other constructs (e.g., developmental deficits, thriving indicators, high-risk behaviors). The developmental assets are grouped into categories that represent external (i.e., environmental) and internal (i.e., values) assets. In the PSL–AB, these broad categories are divided into eight additional external or internal subcategories. External developmental assets are (a) support, (b) empowerment, (c) boundaries and expectations, and (d) constructive use of time. Internal developmental assets are (a) commitment to learning, (b) positive values, (c) social competencies, and (d) positive identity. The PSL–AB possesses reasonable internal consistency and strong content validity (Leffert et al., 1998). It has been used in a large-scale study ($N = 99,462$) to evaluate the developmental assets of communities in the United States and to investigate relationships between developmental assets and risk behavior (Benson et al., 1998).

Behavioral and Emotional Rating Scale

The BERS is a 52-item strength-based assessment tool. Each item is rated on a scale from 0 to 3 (0 = *not at all like the child;* 1 = *not much like the child;* 2 = *like the child;* 3 = *very much like the child*). Five subscales of emotional and behavioral strengths and an overall strength quotient were derived from the BERS using factor analysis (Epstein, Ryser, & Pearson, 2002). A confirmatory factor analysis study with a sample of 1,799 children with serious emotional disturbance indicated that the original five-factor structure of the BERS was well established (Liao, Holden, & Epstein, 2002). Those five factors are as follows:

1. Factor 1, Interpersonal Strengths (14 items) measures a child's ability to control his or her emotions or behaviors in social situations (e.g., accepts criticism).
2. Factor 2, Family Involvement (10 items) measures a child's participation and relationship with his or her family (e.g., interacts positively with parents).
3. Factor 3, Intrapersonal Strengths (11 items) assesses a child's outlook on his or her competence and accomplishments (e.g., is self-confident).
4. Factor 4, School Functioning (9 items) focuses on a child's competence on school and classroom tasks (e.g., completes school tasks on time).
5. Factor 5, Affective Strengths (7 items) assesses a child's ability to accept affect from others and express feelings toward others (e.g., acknowledges painful feelings).

The initial items used in the BERS were developed through rigorous content validity procedures (Epstein, 1999). The BERS was also normed using national samples of children with ($N = 861$) and without ($N = 2,176$) emotional disturbance (Epstein et al., 2002; Epstein & Sharma, 1998). It also has demonstrated convergent and discriminant validity with students with emotional disturbance and without disabilities (Epstein, Nordness, Nelson, & Hertzog, 2001; Harniss, Epstein, Ryser, & Pearson, 1999; Reid, Epstein, Pastor, & Ryser, 2000; Trout, Ryan, LaVigne, & Epstein, 2003) and has shown short-term (10 days) and long-term (7 months) test–retest and interrater reliability (Epstein, Harniss, Pearson, & Ryser, 1998; Epstein, Hertzog, & Reid, 2001; Friedman, Leone, & Friedman, 1999). These studies suggest that the BERS is a psychometrically sound, norm-referenced assessment tool possessing acceptable content validity, strong internal consistency, moderate to high convergent and discriminant validity, high interrater and test–retest reliability, and stability over time. The BERS is recommended for the following uses: (a) documenting children's emotional and behavioral strengths, (b) identifying children with limited emotional and behavioral strengths, (c) setting goals for an individual education program, and (d) documenting progress in strength areas as a result of intervention.

APPLIED EXAMPLES OF STRENGTH-BASED ASSESSMENT

In this section, we provide two examples of the use of the BERS in evaluating two national programs for children with or at risk of behavior disorders. In the first example, the BERS was used as an outcome measure in a national study on children's mental health. In the second example, the BERS was used to monitor the outcomes of the Families and Schools Together program, a national school-based program to prevent violence, dropout, and substance abuse for at-risk children.

Comprehensive Community Mental Health Services Program

The Comprehensive Community Mental Health Services for Children and Their Families program was funded in 1992. The program was initiated to increase the availability of systems of care for children with serious emotional disturbance and their families. The program was based on system-of-care principles (Stroul & Friedman, 1994), including (a) the creation of partnerships between parents and professionals; (b) the delivery of services in an individualized, strength-based, and culturally competent manner; and (c) the facilitation of collaboration among mental health, education, child welfare, juvenile justice, and related sectors (Holden, Friedman, & Santiago, 2001). By 2003, the program had funded more than 60 communities, services had been provided to more than 40,000 children and families, and more than $400 million in federal funds had been used to support the program.

A national comprehensive evaluation of the program was mandated by the federal legislation authorizing the program. The evaluation focused on six questions: Who are the children and families served by the program? How do systems of care develop over time? To what extent do children's clinical and functional outcomes improve over time? What are the service utilization patterns of children and families in systems of care and what are the associated costs? Are improvements greater in a system-of-care approach compared to a traditional service delivery approach? To what extent are children's, families', and providers' experiences consistent with the system-of-care philosophy? (Holden et al., 2001). The design of the national evaluation was based on these questions, and in effect, each question led to a specific study, such as the child and clinical outcome study.

The outcome study was designed to assess how a system of care affects a child's clinical and functional status, family functioning, and satisfaction with services. Data were collected on the children and families who entered the system-of-care communities at intake and at 6-month intervals. The dependent measures included a number of standardized psychometrically sound instruments, as well as some instruments designed specifically for the national evaluation. The BERS is one of the measures used to assess the child outcomes and has been included as part of the national evaluation since 1998. Parents or caregivers complete the BERS on the children receiving services at intake and at 6-month intervals.

Intake BERS data have been collected on almost 2,200 children. The average standard score for each of the five subscales of the BERS appears in Figure 6.2. The data indicate that even upon entrance to a community-based system of care, children with serious emotional disturbance demonstrated important strengths in their functioning. The highest area of strength was in the affective domain ($M = 9.4$), whereas the area of lowest strength was in the school functioning domain ($M = 7$). These areas of strength can be used by caregivers and service providers to design individualized service plans. At 6 months, the data indicated significant improvement in the children. Specifically, for the 1,069 children assessed at intake and then at 6 months, 47% demonstrated improvement in their total BERS score, 28% were stable, and 25% had deteriorated. These results demonstrated that this national program was achieving its goal of improving the mental health status of children with emotional disturbance.

Families and Schools Together

The Families and Schools Together (FAST) program is a collaborative prevention and parent involvement program designed to reduce factors related to alcohol and drug abuse, violence and delinquency, and school dropout (Epstein et al., 2003). FAST is a 2-year program focused on strengthening the entire family unit. The program invites families with children ages 4 to 9 who

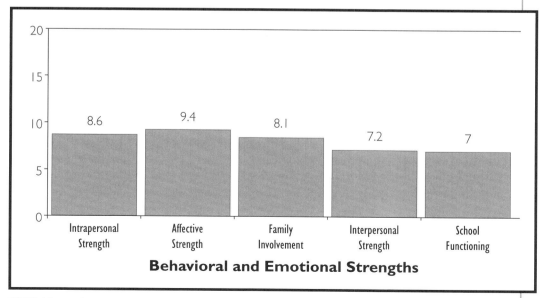

FIGURE 6.2. Intake *Behavioral and Emotional Rating Scale* (BERS; Epstein & Sharma, 1998) scores for children entering a system of care.

display behavior problems at school or at home, low self-esteem, short attention span, or hyperactivity to participate in 8 or 10 weekly multifamily meetings at their child's school. During the sessions, families participate in activities that are designed to build on the natural strength of the family unit. The FAST curriculum works toward four general goals: (a) enhancing family functioning, (b) promoting child success in school, (c) preventing substance abuse by the child and the family, and (d) reducing the stress that parents and children experience from daily life situations.

A collaborative team composed of four community members—a parent partner, a school partner, a community-based mental health partner, and a community-based substance abuse partner—facilitates FAST weekly sessions. These four core team members operate as a team of coaches supporting the parents in strengthening their own family units, building a social support network of their design, and modeling the power of a respectful and supportive team approach to problem solving. Furthermore, the team facilitates communication among program administrators, collaborative community partners, and parents.

Each of the weekly sessions includes six key components: (a) a meal shared as a family unit, (b) several communication games played at the family table, (c) time for adults to talk one-on-one with another adult, (d) a parent self-help group, (e) one-to-one quality play, and (f) a door prize that each family wins once. The six components are designed to strengthen the bonds within and between families and their community. Following the weekly sessions, the families graduate into FASTWORKS, a 2-year follow-up program that meets monthly to continue building on the bonds created during FAST.

In a recent evaluation, FAST was found to reduce factors related to alcohol and drug abuse, violence and delinquency, and school dropout (Epstein et al., 2003). Outcomes reported in child behavior, family functioning, and parent involvement indicate positive changes at the home, school, and community levels. In addition, the results showed statistically significant parent and teacher changes over time (6% and 12%, respectively, on the overall behavioral and emotional strength score of the BERS). Epstein et al. also reported statistically significant increases on each of the five subscales: a 10% increase in Interpersonal Strength, a 7% increase in Family Involvement, a 7% increase in Intrapersonal Strength, a 7% increase in School Functioning, and a 5% increase in Affective Strength. After the program, teachers' ratings revealed statistically significant increases on each of the three measured subscales, including a 12% increase in Interpersonal Strength, a 13% increase in Intrapersonal Strength, and an 11% increase in School Functioning.

CONCLUSION

Direct service providers can gain several advantages by adding a strength-based assessment to their battery of assessments. In particular, strength-based assessment is useful both for planning for individual child interventions and for evaluating program outcomes.

Strength-based assessment is useful for planning purposes because it allows service providers to write and implement treatment plans related to a child's strengths. These plans can involve family members and others in working toward positive outcomes. Because strength-based assessment serves to minimize the frustration of parents and practitioners by emphasizing solutions as opposed to problems, it can engage the child and family in a positive way in receiving specialized services. Assessment that focuses on strengths can foster positive parent–professional relationships by encouraging open communication, mutual trust, cooperation, and supportiveness. Because strength-based assessment helps to identify what is going well in the life of a child and what skills and competencies can be developed, it can empower the family and, in some cases, the child to assume responsibility for decisions and actions.

Strength-based assessment is also useful as an outcome measure. When professionals are trained and supported so that they regularly gather and use strength-based information, such information can be highly useful in monitoring the extent to which service plans and treatments result in positive changes in their clients. In addition, agencies can use such information to monitor the effectiveness of their organization and their models of service, and finally, at both state and national levels, individuals can use such information to identify the extent to which initiatives result in improved outcomes for all children. The addition of a positive strength-based component to the existing needs-based assessment infrastructure has the potential to amplify and enhance the information-gathering function of social services and may result in more targeted, appropriate interventions that take a holistic perspective of a child that includes not only weaknesses but also strengths.

REFERENCES

Achenbach, T. M. (1991). *Manual for the Child Behavior Checklist/4–18 and 1991 profile.* Burlington: University of Vermont, Department of Psychiatry.

Benson, P. L., Leffert, N., Scales, P. C., & Blyth, D. A. (1998). Beyond the "village" rhetoric: Creating healthy communities for children and adolescents. *Applied Developmental Science, 2*(3), 138–159.

Brown, L. L., & Hammill, D. D. (1990). *Behavior Rating Profile: An Ecological Approach to Behavioral Assessment.* Austin, TX: PRO-ED.

Clark, M. D. (1996). Solution-focused interviewing: A strength-based method for juvenile justice. *Journal for Juvenile Justice and Detention Services, 11*(1), 33–39.

Dunst, C. J., & Leet, H. E. (1987). Measuring the adequacy of resources in households with young children. *Child Care Health and Development, 13*(2), 111–125.

Dunst, C. J., Trivette, C. M., & Deal, A. G. (Eds.). (1994). *Supporting and strengthening families: Methods, strategies, and practice* (Vol. 1). Cambridge, MA: Brookline.

Early, T. J. (2001). Measures for practice with families from a strengths perspective. *Families in Society: The Journal of Contemporary Human Services, 82*(2), 225–232.

Epstein, M. H. (1999). Development and validation of a scale to assess the emotional and behavioral strengths of children and adolescents. *Remedial and Special Education, 20,* 258–262.

Epstein, M. H., Harniss, M. K., Pearson, N., & Ryser, G. (1998). The Behavioral and Emotional Rating Scale: Test–retest and inter-rater reliability. *Journal of Child and Family Studies, 8,* 319–327.

Epstein, M. H., Harniss, M. K., Robbins, V., Wheeler, L., Cyrulik, S., Kriz, M., et al. (2003). Strength-based approaches to assessment in schools. In M. Weist, S. Evans, N. Lever, & M. D. Conefry (Eds.), *Handbook of school mental health* (pp. 285–299). New York: Kluwer/Plenum.

Epstein, M. H., Hertzog, M. A., & Reid, R. (2001). The Behavioral and Emotional Rating Scale: Long-term test–retest reliability. *Behavioral Disorders, 26,* 314–320.

Epstein, M. H., Nordness, P. D., Nelson, J. R., & Hertzog, M. (2002). Convergent validity of the Behavioral and Emotional Rating Scale with primary grade-level students. *Topics in Early Childhood Special Education, 2*(2), 114–121.

Epstein, M. H., Ryser, G., & Pearson, N. (2002). Standardization of the Behavioral and Emotional Rating Scale: Factor structure, reliability, and criterion validity. *Journal of Behavioral Health Services and Research, 29,* 208–216.

Epstein, M. H., & Sharma, J. (1998). *Behavioral and Emotional Rating Scale: A Strength-Based Approach to Assessment.* Austin, TX: PRO-ED.

Friedman, K. A., Leone, P. E., & Friedman, P. (1999). Strengths-based assessment of children with SED: Consistency of reporting by teachers and parents. *Journal of Child and Family Studies, 8*(2), 169–180.

Goodman, R. (1997). The Strengths and Difficulties Questionnaire: A research note. *Journal of Child Psychology and Psychiatry, 38,* 581–586.

Goodman, R. (2001). Psychometric properties of the Strengths and Difficulties Questionnaire. *Journal of the American Academy of Child and Adolescent Psychiatry, 40*(11), 1337–1345.

Goodman, R., & Scott, S. (1999). Comparing the Strengths and Difficulties Questionnaire and the Child Behavior Checklist: Is small beautiful? *Journal of Abnormal Child Psychology, 27,* 17–24.

Graybeal, C. (2001). Strengths-based social work assessment: Transforming the dominant paradigm. *Families in Society: The Journal of Contemporary Human Services, 82*(3), 233–242.

Harniss, M. K., Epstein, M. H., Ryser, G., & Pearson, N. (1999). The Behavioral and Emotional Rating Scale: Convergent validity. *Journal of Psychoeducational Assessment, 17*(1), 4–14.

Henggeler, S. W., Schoenwald, S. K., Borduin, C. M., Rowland, M. D., & Cunningham, P. B. (1998). *Multisystemic treatment of antisocial behavior in children and adolescents.* New York: Guilford.

Holden, E. W., Friedman, R. M., & Santiago, R. L. (2001). Overview of the national evaluation of the Comprehensive Community Mental Health Services for Children and Their Families Program. *Journal of Emotional and Behavioral Disorders, 9,* 4–12.

Kral, R. (1989). *Strategies that work: Techniques for solutions in the schools.* Milwaukee: Brieg Family Therapy Center.

Leffert, N., Benson, P. L., Scales, P. C., Sharma, A. R., Drake, D. R., & Blyth, D. A. (1998). Developmental assets: Measurement and prediction of risk behaviors among adolescents. *Applied Developmental Science, 2*(4), 209–230.

Liao, Q., Holden, E. W., & Epstein, M. H. (2002). *Confirmatory factor analysis of the Behavioral and Emotional Rating Scale.* Paper presented at the Research and Training Center's Florida Mental Health Institute's Fifth Annual Conference, Tampa.

Lourie, I. S., Katz-Leavy, J., & Stroul, B. A. (1994). Individualized services in a system of care. In B. A. Stroul (Ed.), *Children's mental health: Creating systems of care in a changing society* (pp. 429–452). Baltimore: Brookes.

Lyons, J. S., Kisiel, C., & West, C. (1997). Child and Adolescent Strengths Assessment: A pilot study. *Family Matters, 3,* 30–33.

Lyons, J. S., Uziel-Miller, N. D., Reyes, F., & Sokol, P. T. (2000). Strengths of children and adolescents in residential settings: Prevalence and associations with psychopathology and discharge placement. *Journal of the American Academy of Child and Adolescent Psychiatry, 39*(2), 176–181.

Marquoit, J. W., & Dobbins, M. (1995). Do juvenile sex offenders have strengths? *Reclaiming Children and Youth, 7*(1), 31–33.

Nelson, C. M., & Pearson, C. A. (1991). *Integrating services for children and youth with behavioral disorders.* Reston, VA: Council for Exceptional Children.

Osman, A., Downs, W. R., Kopper, B. A., Barrios, F. X., Baker, M. T., Osman, J. R., et al. (1998). The Reasons for Living Inventory for Adolescents (RFL–A): Development and psychometric properties. *Journal of Clinical Psychology, 54*(8), 1063–1078.

Quay, H. C., & Peterson, D. (1987). *Revised Behavior Problem Checklist.* Coral Gables, FL: University of Miami, Department of Psychology.

Reid, R., Epstein, M. H., Pastor, D. A., & Ryser, G. (2000). Strengths-based assessment differences across students with LD and EBD. *Remedial and Special Education, 21*(6), 346–355.

Rockwell, S. (1998). Overcoming four myths that prevent fostering resilience. *Reaching Today's Youth, The Community Circle of Caring Journal, 2*(3), 14–17.

Saleeby, D. (Ed.). (1992). *The strengths perspective in social work practice.* New York: Longman.

Salvia, J., & Ysseldyke, J. (1998). *Assessment* (7th ed.). Boston: Houghton Mifflin.

Stroul, B. A., & Friedman, R. M. (1994). *A system of care for children and youth with severe emotional disturbances.* Washington, DC: Georgetown University, CASSP Technical Assistance Center.

Sugai, G., & Horner, R. H. (1999). Discipline and behavioral support: Practices, pitfalls, and promises. *Effective School Practices, 17*(4), 10–22.

Trout, A. L., Ryan, J. B., LaVigne, S. B., & Epstein, M. H. (2003). Behavioral and Emotional Rating Scale: Two studies of convergent validity. *Journal of Child and Family Studies, 12*(4), 399–410.

U.S. Department of Education. (1994). *National agenda for achieving better results for children and youth with serious emotional disturbance.* Washington, DC: Author.

VanDenBerg, J. E., & Grealish, E. M. (1996). Individualized services and supports through the wraparound process: Philosophy and procedures. *Journal of Child and Family Studies, 5,* 7–22.

VanDenBerg, J. E., & Grealish, E. M. (1998). *The wrap-around process: Training manual.* Pittsburgh: Community Partnership Group.

Walrath, C. M., Mandell, D. S., Holden, E. W., & Santiago, R. L. (2004). Assessing the strengths of children referred for community-based mental health services. *Mental Health Services Research, 6*(1), 1–8.

World Health Organization. (2001). *International classification of functioning, disability, and health* (10th ed.). Geneva, Switzerland: Author.

Assessing the Child and Family Outcomes of Systems of Care for Youth with Serious Emotional Disturbance

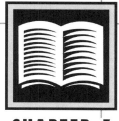

CHAPTER 7

Abram Rosenblatt

As chronicled throughout this book, innovative care systems and service interventions designed to address and remedy the plight of children and adolescents with serious emotional disturbance (SED) have spread exponentially in the last decade, through both local and federal initiatives. There is considerable excitement, enthusiasm, and hope regarding the potential of these innovations to provide better care for children and their families. Nonetheless, there is also considerable dread, doubt, and worry about the future of reform efforts. Federal, state, and local human services budgets are facing the closest scrutiny in years as resources become increasingly scarce. New models of health-care delivery generally subsumed under the rubric of managed care are creating uncertainty regarding the future of reform efforts in children's services (Stroul, 1996).

It is just this trepidation about the future that is feeding a groundswell of interest in whether systems of care are an effective and efficient model of service delivery that can survive in a rapidly changing human service delivery environment. Although a number of research programs deriving from investments in child services research capacity over the last several years are beginning to yield results, the research findings remain limited. Few of the research results have been published (Burns & Friedman, 1990; Stroul, 1993), making an evaluation of the quality of the findings difficult. Consequently, in spite of a number of notable local and state attempts to reform service systems, critically needed information regarding effective treatment and service system strategies was either unavailable or incomplete during the recent federal health-care reform process of 1993–1994 (McGuire, Frank, & Goldman, 1992; National Advisory Mental Health Council, 1993; Scallet, 1994).

In part, the lack of information on systems of care for youth with SED derives from the difficulty in conducting outcome studies of these multi-layered systems. In this chapter, the outcomes of system-of-care research are reviewed in the context of the central challenges to assessing the effectiveness of these reform efforts. These challenges are grouped into three core questions pertaining to outcomes research: (a) What is the independent variable (in this case, a system of care)? (b) What is an outcome? and (c) How are the independent variable and the outcomes linked, and what is the methodology? The chapter concludes with an overview of the strengths and weaknesses of the knowledge base regarding child and family outcomes of systems of care for children with SED. Implications for the future are also discussed.

THE PROBLEM OF THE INDEPENDENT VARIABLE: WHAT IS A SYSTEM OF CARE?

By any definition, a system of care is a complex intervention, and this chapter does not attempt to comprehensively define system of care (see instead National Institute of Mental Health [NIMH], 1983; Stroul & Friedman, 1986). Nonetheless, an understanding of the levels of a system of care is essential to assessing the outcomes of it. Although human service systems can be analyzed from a wide range of perspectives, current research on systems of care tends to focus on three levels of analysis: the systems level, the programmatic level, and the clinical level.

The Systems Level: Structure, Organization, and Financing

System-level reforms initially coming out of the mental health sector in the last decade have been dominated by two emergent concepts: the systems-of-care approach described initially by Stroul and Friedman (1986) and the wraparound approach (Burchard & Clark, 1990) associated with pioneering work by Dennis, VanDenBerg, Burchard, Tannen, Lourie, and others, and most frequently exemplified by the Kaleidescope program in Chicago, the Alaska Youth Initiative, and Project Wraparound in Vermont.

The systems-of-care approach, spearheaded through the NIMH and Center for Mental Health Services (CMHS) Child and Adolescent Service System Program (CASSP), was designed to provide assistance to states and communities in the development of comprehensive, coordinated systems of care for children and adolescents (Day & Roberts, 1991; National Institute of Mental Health, 1983). Local examples of programs firmly rooted in this tradition include ones created in Ventura County, California (Jordan & Hernandez, 1990), and North Carolina (Behar, 1985, 1992).

Systems of care place a special emphasis on linkages among child-serving agencies such as mental health, juvenile justice, social welfare, and education; on community-based care in lieu of restrictive placements; on developing a continuum of services; and, in some cases, on measuring the costs and outcomes of care. All of these elements are also essential to the wraparound process (VanDenBerg & Grealish, 1996). Analogously, although wraparound efforts are historically known for their emphasis on individualized services, on the unconditional provision of care, and on flexible funding, many locales following the systems-of-care approach incorporate these ideals and services into their service arrays. Both systems of care and the wrap-around process fully share the principle of involving parents in all aspects of service delivery. They also emphasize providing culturally competent, community-based, integrated care. Results from research on reform efforts that are most firmly rooted in the system-of-care approach to service delivery will be presented in this chapter.

The Program Level: Components of a System of Care

A system of care is composed of programmatic components that may include traditional clinical services, such as outpatient and inpatient care, or more innovative, blended services, such as therapeutic foster care, case management, and individualized care. In theory, a system of care should have component services that are themselves effective. However, the overall effectiveness of any of these individual components has not been well documented (Kutash & Rivera, 1996). Although some findings are promising, on the whole the evidence is nonexistent, sparse, or not encouraging regarding the positive effectiveness of most individual program components. It is still important to note that the general lack of encouraging findings regarding the components of a system of care does not necessarily preclude discovering more encouraging results for an entire system of care. The whole may be greater than the sum of its parts. Different components may interact with each other to produce effective change.

The Clinical Level: Caseworker Behaviors, Skills, and Tools

Regardless of the level of innovation at the program or system levels, the ultimate success of any care is dependent on what occurs at the clinical level. This level refers to the ways in which a caseworker (or a team of caseworkers) interacts directly with children, their families, and their support systems. Clinical interventions in a system of care may include a range of office-based psychotherapeutic approaches, such as cognitive-behavioral therapy, family therapy, and play therapy. In a system of care, however, interventions at the clinical level also encompass the interactions of line-level staff with children and families across a continuum of settings and interventions. These settings may include the home, the school, the juvenile courts, and the foster care system. The interventions used in these settings are often loosely articulated and consist of the capacity of line staff to collaborate successfully with probation officers, teachers, and foster parents in providing services to the child and family.

Given the range of skills required to work in the natural environments in which children and families live, it is not surprising that the voluminous and relatively sophisticated literature on the outcomes of psychotherapy does not adequately inform the development of a system of care, because of a lack of external validity (Weisz, Donenberg, Han, & Kauneckis, 1995). Research on mental health services to children and adolescents at the clinical level has focused on the efficacy of various treatment interventions for a variety of specific disorders. Based on a meta-analysis of outcome studies of psychotherapy for children ages 4 to 18, Weisz, Weiss, Alicke, and Klotz (1987) concluded that the average treated individual was better adjusted after treatment than 79% of those not treated. This cumulative finding may provide support for the efficacy of outpatient psychotherapy interventions provided to children presenting with specific mental health problems and behavioral disorders. In fact, when results from clinic-based trials are examined, the findings are less positive than those conducted in university-based laboratories (Weisz et al., 1995).

Historically, clinical interventions were designed to reside in only one programmatic component of a system of care: outpatient therapy. A similar body of knowledge does not exist regarding more novel treatment approaches, such as therapeutically enhanced foster care or individualized service programs. Remarkably little is empirically known about what clinicians actually do when they provide many of the services within more novel care modalities. An exception to this tradition is the work conducted by Henggeler and colleagues on developing multisystemic therapy (MST; Henggeler & Borduin, 1990; Henggeler, Melton, & Smith, 1992). This treatment approach is consonant with the principles of a system of care and focuses on interventions that are tied to the multiple environments or systems in which a child lives.

Assessing the Intervention: The Strength, Integrity, and Ecology of a System of Care

Given the multilayered nature of systems of care, assessing whether a system can or should be called a system of care is a difficult task. Concepts deriving from program evaluation, such as the strength and integrity of an intervention, can be applied to help understand the dimensions that need to be assessed to determine whether a system of care follows the intent of the model. In addition, complex social interventions such as systems of care evolve and change over time, requiring an ecological approach to understanding their evolution.

Strength and Integrity

In order for a program to be effective, it must be implemented with sufficient strength and integrity (e.g., Sechrest & Rosenblatt, 1987; Sechrest, West, Phillips, Redner, & Yeaton, 1977). The most straightforward analogy is to medicine: Penicillin may cure an infection, but if it is administered in an insufficient dose (strength) or on an irregular schedule (integrity), it will not be effective. Similarly, systems of care may constitute a completely correct theory of service delivery. Nonetheless, if the intensity of services that are provided in a given community is insufficient, if interagency coordination is not complete, if staff commitment is lacking, and if programs within a continuum of care are ineffective, the system of care may not be strong enough to affect the children and families served. Likewise, if treatment teams are not composed of the people necessary to create change for a child and family, if treatment plans are poorly conceived, if children and families irregularly receive needed services, if target populations are not clearly specified, and if interagency coordination does not exist, the program as implemented may not have sufficient integrity to achieve results.

The lack of strength and integrity in the implementation of a program can lead to erroneous conclusions regarding whether a program can be effective. As one example, less than a decade ago, the general conclusion was that community-based diversion programs for juvenile delinquency did not work (Quay, 1987); that is, it was concluded that they were no more effective in preventing rearrests than jail or no treatment. At that point, we examined the literature and found that little attention had been paid to the strength and integrity of the so-called ineffective treatments. In one instance, children and families rarely attended the group therapy sessions that were at the core of a diversion program (Sechrest & Rosenblatt, 1987). As a result, we concluded that the hypothesis of whether community-based treatments could reduce rates of relapse into the juvenile justice system had not been tested and that little could really be concluded about the effectiveness of community care with this population.

Evaluation and the Ecology of Systems of Care

Ensuring that a system of care has sufficient strength and integrity to create outcomes requires ongoing evaluation of which elements of the care system are effective. Historically, studies that evaluated the implementation of a program were called process (after Cronbach, 1964), or formative (Scriven, 1967), evaluations. These kinds of evaluations stood in contrast to outcome (Cronbach, 1964), or summative (Scriven, 1967), evaluations. Close to two decades ago, however, Tharp and Gallimore (1979) broke down the distinction between these two types of evaluations by applying the language of ecology to social programs. Although these concepts were designed to describe the development of programs, they are perhaps even more applicable to the development of systems. Tharp and Gallimore argued that social programs evolve over time through a series of relatively transitory stages until they reach a stable condition. This stable condition was described as "an association of program elements, organized for and producing a defined social benefit, which will continue to exist, and in which there will not be a replacement by other element types, so long as social values, goals and supporting resources remain constant" (Tharp & Gallimore, 1979, p. 43). They further described four conditions required for a program to reach this stable state: (a) longevity (stability requires time), (b) stability of values and goals (the program must meet a stable value), (c) stability of funding (a program must remain consistently funded in order to survive), and (d) power of the evaluator (the influence of an evaluator must be maintained to influence the integrity of program research and development).

Taken seriously, the implications for outcomes research of considering the evaluation of systems of care from this ecological framework are profound. Most systems of care are relatively new, and few could meet the aforementioned four conditions for program stability. In particular, few systems of care have an integrated evaluation process that influences system development. Conducting "outcome" evaluations of such programs is liable to produce premature and erroneous results. Put another way, systems that are not in a stable condition are unlikely to have sufficient strength and integrity to achieve results.

THE DEPENDENT VARIABLE: MEASURING OUTCOME

A system of care is obviously a complex intervention that attempts to achieve positive change in children and families across a range of behaviors, settings, and contexts. Consequently, the goals of a system of care are highly varied. Ideally, the outcomes of a system of care ought to derive directly from the goals of the care system. Because care systems do not have a single goal, a single outcome cannot capture the desired effects of the care system. Just as several authors have pointed out the need for multiple measures and approaches to measuring outcomes both for persons suffering from the most severe disorders (Attkisson et al., 1992; Hargreaves & Shumway, 1989; NIMH, 1991) and for persons suffering from a range of mental disorders (Ciarlo, Brown, Edwards, Kiresuk, & Newman, 1986), so, too, do outcomes need to be considered from a multidimension framework with respect to children with SED.

The potential list of outcome indicators for children with SED could easily number in the hundreds. It is therefore helpful to have a mechanism for grouping measures on some set of criteria. A model that can be used to stratify the various kinds of measurement that may be undertaken in outcome research on systems of care is summarized in this section. This model consists of four treatment outcome domains (what is measured), five respondent types (who participates as a respondent), and four behavioral contexts of measurement (where the measured phenomena occur). The model is presented more fully elsewhere (Rosenblatt & Attkisson, 1993).

Systematic Domains of Service Outcome

The first question concerns the content areas or outcome domains that are included in the conceptual framework. We derive four domains of treatment outcome. In Table 7.1, each of these domains, along with examples of measures or indicators of that domain, is presented. The first is called the clinical status domain. This domain encompasses the dual concepts of mental and physical health and includes measurement and indices of psychopathology and symptomatology encompassing both classification and severity. The domain thereby focuses on impairments in both psychological and physical status. Measures of clinical status are defined as processes that document and assess the physical, emotional, cognitive, and behavioral signs and symptoms related to disorder. Common measures of clinical status in children include the problem domains of the *Child Behavior Checklist* (CBCL; Achenbach & Edelbrock, 1993), the *Child Depression Inventory* (Kovacs, 1991), and the *Diagnostic Interview Schedule for Children* (DISC–2.1; Shaffer, Fisher, Piacentini, Schwab-Stone, & Wicks, 1989).

The second domain, called functional status, captures the ability to effectively fulfill social and role-related functions. This area includes measures of ability to function in a variety of life settings. These functions include the maintenance of interpersonal and familial relationships and the development of school, employment, and vocational capacities. Examples of functional adaptation include the ability to work, attend school, learn, remain in home or maintain independent living, and maintain positive and enhancing social relationships. Common measures or indicators of functional status include the competency domains of the CBCL, the role performance scales of the *Child and Adolescent Functional Assessment Scale* (CAFAS; Hodges, 1994), and functional indicators such as rearrest rates and educational attainment.

The third dimension is called life satisfaction and fulfillment. Contained within this dimension is an attempt to capture the human struggle to achieve some level of personal fulfillment during the course of a life. This domain, in many ways the most conceptually intricate, relies on prior work that defines the meaning of concepts such as well-being, life satisfaction, objective quality

TABLE 7.1
Examples of Measures and Indicators of Outcome Domains

Clinical Status	Functional Status	Life Satisfaction and Fulfillment	Safety and Welfare
• satisfaction scales	CBL/YSR Problem • Presence of scales	• CBCL/YSR Competency with services	• Child and parent abuse or neglect
• *Child Depression Inventory*	• CAFAS Role Performance scales	• *Family Empowerment Scale*	• Presence of criminal victimization
• CAFAS Moods and Emotions scale	• Educational attendance and achievement	• Satisfaction with living situation	• Presence of communicable disease
• *Diagnostic Interview Schedule for Children* (DISC–2.1)	• Juvenile justice arrest rates	• Satisfaction with school or work	• Drug or alcohol abuse
		• Self-esteem and happiness	

Note. CBCL = *Child Behavior Checklist* (Achenbach & Edelbrock, 1993); YSR = *Youth Self-Report;* CAFAS = *Child and Adolescent Functional Assessment Scale* (Hodges, 1994); DISC–2.1 = *Diagnostic Interview Schedule for Children* (Shaffer, Fisher, Piacentini, Schwab-Stone, & Wicks, 1989).

of life, subjective quality of life, and happiness. The life satisfaction and fulfillment domain focuses on the subjective appraisal of well-being. This is distinguished from subjective quality of life in that subjective quality of life is usually understood to encompass both subjective appraisal of well-being and also positive and negative affect. Affective and mood states are included as part of the clinical status domain within our model and do not need to be included again in this domain. In our model, quality of life and well-being measures will often span the two domains of functional status and life satisfaction. Importantly, life satisfaction may include satisfaction with services, as measured by instruments such as the *Client Satisfaction Questionnaire* (Attkisson & Greenfield, 1995). Life satisfaction may also include a family's sense of empowerment, as measured by instruments such as the *Family Empowerment Survey* (Koren, DeChillo, & Friesen, 1992).

The final domain, welfare and safety, encompasses the safety and welfare problems posed by SED to the individual, the family, their social network, and the community in which they live. Such problems include self-injurious behaviors and acts such as suicide, substance abuse, and lack of basic sanitation; infectious diseases such as AIDS, other sexually transmitted diseases, and tuberculosis; abuse, neglect, or other forms of violence suffered by the youth; and violent and illegal acts committed by the youth.

Type of Respondent

Measures of outcome must reflect a range of social perspectives. The range of respondent types in the outcome frame can include (a) the client, (b) family members, (c) members of the social network, (d) clinical practitioners, and (e) scientists. These can be operationalized as varying sources of outcome information. The perception of psychopathology, for instance, may vary depending on the source of the information. The method of data collection may also vary within and between respondent types. Self-reports, interviews, behavioral observations, and other types of assessments can all be used to collect data from different respondent types. The scales developed by Achenbach and colleagues (Achenbach & Edelbrock, 1993), for example, collect a range of perspectives on the functioning of the child, including those of the teacher, parent or caregiver, researcher or independent rater, and the child.

Social Contexts in the Measurement of Outcomes

The cost-outcome model stipulates four social contexts of measurement: (a) the individual/self, (b) the family, (c) the work setting or school, and (d) the community. The levels move from the individual unit to the broader scope of individual life contexts.

Measures taken within the individual/self context focus on the characteristics, symptoms, and adaptational responses of the youth. Examples of this context would include presence or absence of physical disease in the individual, presence or absence of a clinical diagnosis for the individual, and level of symptomatology for an individual. However, most human abilities and characteristics vary across social contexts. Some children function well at school but not at home, for example. Others function well in the presence of their family but are unable to function socially in the broader community. Measures within the family context focus on the child in the context of family life. Importantly, *family life* is broadly defined to include a range of persons with whom the child may live and may be considered part of a "family" social structure or environment. Measures within the school or work context focus on the youth in the work or educational setting. Measures at the level of the community context focus on youth in the context of the broader community in which they live. One example, the CAFAS, measures role performance (functioning domain) at the school, community, and family (termed *home* on the CAFAS) contexts.

Integration of Cost, Service Use, and Outcome Data

Outcome information, regardless of its quality, is an insufficient basis for sound public policy in mental health. Cost data are equally essential for public mental health policy—as well as for managing and marketing systems of care in mental health. Research and evaluation efforts that integrate cost, service use, and outcome data are those that are most likely to have an impact on practice, administration, and policy (Phillips & Rosenblatt, 1992). Costs and outcomes are usually combined in two separate types of analyses: cost-effectiveness analysis (CEA) and cost–benefit analysis (CBA).

Cost-effectiveness analysis traditionally combines cost measures with measures of effectiveness or outcome (Sorensen & Grove, 1978). For example, one program may cost less than another but demonstrate roughly equivalent reductions in symptomatology. In such a case, one program may be considered more cost-effective than another. In CBA, dollar values are assigned to the cost of delivering services in the same manner as in CEA. In CBA, however, dollar values are also assigned to outcomes or benefits. Total dollar costs are subtracted from total benefits costs to provide the net benefit of a program. In these analyses, one program, for example, may have a net benefit of $100 for each person served when compared to another program. Such studies have typically assigned dollar values (such as lost earnings) to mortality and morbidity. Assigning dollar values to other types of outcomes, such as happiness or well-being, is extremely difficult.

In both types of studies, the measurement can be classified within the framework according to the measure of "effectiveness" or "benefit." Thus, studies that combine assessment of costs with the measurement of psycho-pathology might fall into the clinical status domain. Similarly, if benefits are measured in terms of dollar values associated with decreased job productivity, the outcome measure would fall into the functional adaptation domain in the work/school context. Better classification and understanding of which dimensions are being measured is critical in cost studies. This is especially the case when attempts are made to synthesize the results from several cost-effectiveness, cost–benefit, or other cost studies.

There are, however, practical difficulties in applying these methods to children enrolled in systems of care. These problems revolve largely around the capacity to collect detailed utilization data regarding a specific time span or episode of treatment. Many of the children enrolled in systems of care receive services from multiple child-serving sectors (e.g., mental health, juvenile justice, social welfare). Each of these sectors may contain within them a wide range of programs. A significant and clinically important proportion of these children will likely have complex treatment histories that span a number of different care sectors. Existing automated records do not typically track children across these multiple-care systems, either making a labor-intensive review of charts necessary for constructing treatment history careers or requiring complex and often difficult linkages across care sector data systems.

Selecting Outcome Measures

As our conceptual model illustrates, there is a wide range of outcome measures from which to choose in determining the results of a system of care. Resources rarely exist to collect all possible kinds of outcome data, and even when resources do exist, it may not be desirable to do so. Difficult decisions must be made about which measures need to be included in an outcome study. A number of strategies, or perhaps more accurately, approaches, can be described for selecting measures, including (a) selecting all possible measures (the "kitchen sink" approach), (b) selecting measures by what is available, (c) selecting measures that best match the goals of a program, (d) selecting measures according to their desired impacts or purpose, and (e) selecting measures by some combination of the above strategies. Each of these strategies is discussed next.

The Kitchen Sink Approach

It is tempting to measure virtually all possible domains with all possible youth when conducting outcome research on systems of care. This approach appears the most certain way to find some kind of significant change on at least one of the measures. The potential does exist for capitalizing on chance (e.g., if 20 measures are administered, the odds are that 1 of the measures will be significant at the .05 probability level just by chance). It is usually, however, neither possible nor wise to select all possible measures. If, for example, 6 critical outcomes are significantly positive out of the 20 that were measured, conclusions regarding the effectiveness of the program may be confusing. Multiple measures can distract from more central indicators of effectiveness.

This dilemma for program evaluators is magnified in the case of evaluating a system of care. Historically, programs designed to focus on a single problem (e.g., teen pregnancy) are relatively more focused in their intended outcomes when compared to many systems of care. Both statistical and methodological strategies exist for determining whether an intervention "succeeds" based on a range of potentially contradictory outcomes, although these strategies require skill to properly apply them. There is considerable ongoing debate, for example, about a portion of findings from a major recent study of a continuum of care in which 3 of 12 tests were found to be significant (Friedman & Burns, 1996; Lambert & Guthrie, 1996). One set of authors considered this to be somewhat discouraging, whereas others considered the findings to be somewhat encouraging. Of course, selecting too few measures can give the appearance of measuring too few domains.

Availability

Systems of care are a relatively new approach to serving youth with SED. Many of the key aspects of these systems deviate from more traditional modes of treatment. Most well-validated measures were developed to assess the kinds of domains and perspectives found in more traditional treatment approaches (e.g., the clinical or scientific perspective on clinical status, such as depression inventories developed to assess changes in level of depression among adolescents). For example, a range of long-standing service models focus on the alleviation of psychopathology and the reduction of symptoms. Consequently, many measures exist for measuring psychopathology and symptoms. Systems of care, however, are often based on building strengths as opposed to alleviating weaknesses, and they may focus more directly on improving social and academic functioning. Few strength-based measures exist, however, and measures of social and even academic functioning are not always included in studies of systems of care.

The present situation places the researcher in a considerable quandary regarding the selection of measurement tools: Should selection focus on more psychometrically sound measures that do not directly match the goals of the care system, or should selection focus on less psychometrically sound measures that more directly match the goals of the care system? Relying on unproven measures is clearly risky for any large-scale evaluation. Any results are subject to extensive reinvestigation regarding the reliability and validity of the measure. Many measures of functional status and of safety and welfare can be collected as concrete indicators with limited "measurement" error (Rosenblatt, 1993). Youth either are arrested or they are not, they live either in the community or in a hospital, they are in school or they are not, they are the victim of a crime or not. Although considerable subtlety and effort is required to collect this type of information, doing so is not necessarily dependent on the creation of psychometric tools.

Matching of Goals

Measures that fail to match the goals of a system of care may be inappropriate for assessing the outcomes of that system. In the field of services to adults with severe mental illness, for example, vocational programs may improve the level of employment of individuals enrolled in the program without reducing psychiatric symptomatology. A service system designed to promote keeping youth in the most homelike environment may improve the stability of a youth's residential location without significantly improving levels of depression or anxiety. Although most systems of care have wide-ranging goals for the youth they serve, and many measures and domains are intercorrelated, priorities often need to be established regarding which of these goals are going to be the subject of ongoing evaluation.

Desired Impact

We have presented a model of outcome assessment that delineates five domains of outcome measurement: clinical status, functional status, service satisfaction, life satisfaction and fulfillment, and safety and welfare. Different domains of outcome measurement will likely have different kinds of impacts or will be targeted toward varying audiences. Ultimately, the utilization of outcome results rests on the matching of outcome domains with the desired arenas of impact. Data collected in the clinical status domain are most likely to appeal to clinical practice or the research community. Many clinicians are conversant with the language of test scores and clinical assessment devices. Clinicians often must work at the symptom level, attempting to reduce the occurrence of more harmful thoughts and behaviors and increase the occurrence of more beneficial ways of acting in the world. Clinical status measures may have some utility to program administrators if the data are quickly scored and analyzed. Clinical status measures, taken alone, will likely have relatively less impact on organization, financing, and policy. Such measures are less likely to reflect the more concrete and practical considerations faced by those who work in the political and regulatory arenas (Rosenblatt, 1993).

Data collected in the functional status domain will appeal to a number of audiences. Clinicians, especially those working within a strength-based model, are likely to be especially concerned about the ability of their clients to remain in school, to stay out of trouble, or to continue living at home. Administrators are also likely to find functional status data valuable. For example, information on work and school performance can point to vocational or academic programs that need to be integrated with the care system. Similarly, the public, and hence politicians and legislators, are often concerned that all members of society engage in productive roles.

One of the more subtle areas of data collection pertains to life satisfaction and fulfillment. This domain can potentially affect a wide range of audiences. Job or educational satisfaction, service satisfaction, satisfaction with the home environment, and the like have obvious value to administrators and clinicians who provide a range of services. Satisfaction or dissatisfaction with services can, when voiced by consumers and consumer advocates, be a powerful agent for political change (Attkisson & Greenfield, 1994, 1995).

Finally, measures of safety and welfare are especially germane to the policy arena. Public perceptions of safety and public health undeniably drive part of the mental health policy debate. Interventions that are able to reduce public fears will likely be more easily embraced by policymakers from the "grass roots" to the elected level. As a result, interventions designed to affect policy must consider measuring variables such as arrest rates, suicide rates, and rates of comorbid conditions such as drug use.

Mixing Strategies

In reality, the ultimate choice of which outcome measures to select will rest on some combination of the goals of the service system, the desired impacts, the availability of measures, and the available resources. However, the success of outcome studies relies on the congruence among goals, desired impacts, and the availability of quality measures or indicators. As care systems evolve, so too must measurement strategies. For example, system reform may begin by focusing on creating interagency teams and placement screening processes. The goal of these new interventions may be to reduce placements in restrictive levels of care. Consequently, the ability of youth in the care systems to remain at home becomes a critical measure of system outcome, given these new interventions. Although it may be desirable to measure other outcome domains, reductions in rates of placements may not translate into reductions in symptomatology. As the care system evolves, however, and begins interventions at the level of the child and family that are designed to reduce problematic behaviors in youth so that they can be maintained in their homes, measures of symptoms may become important outcomes.

Table 7.2 draws from our experiences to illustrate how the goals, programs or services, target populations, outcomes, and audiences or stakeholders may interrelate (Rosenblatt, 1993). The table demonstrates that it is important to achieve consistency among the goals, the target populations, and the outcomes of a care system. Choices regarding the selection of any of these individual components affect other components. For example, if a care system is attempting to keep youth in school, there ought to be programs targeted specifically toward helping a defined group of children reach that goal. Furthermore, measures need to be incorporated into an ongoing evaluation

TABLE 7.2
Examples of Matching Goals, Populations, Measures, and Impacts

Goal	Target Population	Program	Measure	Desired Audience
In home	Youth at risk of out-of-home placement	Interagency placement screening team	Placement and expenditures in restricted levels of care	Program managers, board members, and state policy
In school	Youth enrolled in special education programs	Special day schools	School attendance and school achievement	County supervisors and board of education
Out of trouble	Wards of the court	Juvenile hall support	Rearrest rates	State policy, county supervisors, and judges
Healthy	Younger youth with multiple risk factors	Outpatient therapy	*Child Behavior Checklist* (Achenbach & Edelbrock, 1993)	Clinical line staff and program managers

of the care system to ensure that the goal is met and that relevant audiences can be convinced of the utility of the program. In the case of keeping youth in school, such audiences might naturally include board of education members. Of course, although not illustrated in the table for purposes of simplicity, many measures may be suitable across a range of target populations and may have multiple impacts beyond those specified in the table.

System-of-Care Outcomes by Domain

There is a paucity of published, peer-reviewed research on the outcomes of systems of care for children and youth with serious emotional disturbance. A majority of the work in this area is available only as technical reports or as brief professional conference proceedings. Fortunately, Stroul (1993) undertook the task of summarizing the outcomes of systems of care to that point in time. This review relies on Stroul's (1993) work, along with newly published documents and reports obtained by the author, to overview the current status of system-of-care outcomes research. Because some documents could not be obtained and because unpublished reports often do not provide sufficient information regarding study design and methods, a review of this material can be neither critical nor comprehensive. Rather, the review demonstrates the focus of systems-of-care research to this point. Finally, this review does not examine the outcomes of various components within a system of care (for a complete review of system-of-care component outcomes, see Kutash & Rivera, 1996).

The results of the outcomes of 20 community-based systems of care by outcome domain are summarized in Table 7.3. The knowledge base is expected to grow further in the future as results from new systems of care become available. This is especially the case given the awarding, through the Center for Mental Health Services, of 22 grants across the nation designed to implement systems of care for youth with SED (McCormick, 1994).

As illustrated in Table 7.3, a range of studies have demonstrated reductions in either the cost of care or utilization of restrictive levels of care as measured

TABLE 7.3
Outcomes of Community-Based Systems of Care

Study (Primary Reference)	Clinical Status	Functional Status	Life Satisfaction and Fulfillment	Safety and Welfare	Cost or Utilization
New Directions, VT (Vermont DMHMR, 1993)	Improved	Improved	"Extremely satisifed"		Reduced
Ventura, CA (Jordan & Hernandez, 1990)		Improved		Reduced arrests	Reduced
Children's Initiative, NC (Behar, 1992)	Improved	Improved	"Very satisfied"	Reduced arrests	Reduced
Stark, OH (Stroul, 1992)					Reduced
Bennington, VT (Stroul, 1993)	Improved	Improved			Reduced
Dubuque, IA (Iowa DHS, 1992)					Reduced
Mountain State Network, WV (Rugs, 1992)				Reduced arrests	Reduced
Impact, KY (Illback, 1993)	Improved	Improved	Increased	Improved	Reduced
Fort Bragg, NC (Bickman, 1995)	Same as comparison	Same as comparison	Higher in demonstration		Higher in demonstration
Demonstration Projects, VA (Virginia DMHMRSA, 1992a)			"Excellent or good"		Reduced
AB377 Counties, GA (Rosenblatt et al., 1992)					Reduced
Northumberland, PA (Lourie, 1992)					Reduced
Augusta, GA (Georgia DMHMRSA, 1992)					Reduced
FMP, CA (Martinez & Smith, 1993)		Improved		Reduced detention	Reduced
Lucas, OH (Keros, cited in Stroul, 1993)					Reduced
AIMS, TN (Glisson, 1992)	Improved	Improved			Reduced
LIS Projects, VA (Virginia DMHMRSA, 1992b)	Improved	Improved			
Connections, OH (Hanna-Williams, cited in Stroul, 1993)	Improved	Improved			
North Idaho (Lubrecht, cited in Stroul, 1993)	Improved	Improved	"Good or very good"		
Franklin, OH (McCoard, 1993)					Reduced

through hospital admissions, inpatient lengths of stay, state hospital expenditures, and residential treatment center placements (e.g., Behar, 1992; Burchard & Clarke, 1990; Goldman, 1992; Illback, 1993; Jordan & Hernandez, 1990; Lourie, 1992; Rosenblatt & Attkisson, 1992; Stroul, 1992, 1993). Researchers have also shown improvements in clinical and functional status. For example, results from the Kentucky IMPACT project indicated reductions in internalizing and externalizing problem behaviors (Illback, 1993), as measured by the CBCL. Using the same instrument, evaluators in Tennessee found improved functioning of children involved in the AIMS project after 1 year (Glisson, 1992). Improvements in the safety and welfare domain have also been demonstrated. A range of studies demonstrated reduced juvenile justice recidivism, reduced incarceration rates, or improved school achievement and attendance (e.g., Jordan & Hernandez, 1990; Rosenblatt & Attkisson, 1997; Rugs, 1992). Investigators in North Carolina reported moderate to substantial improvements in functioning, as demonstrated by scores on the CAFAS after 1 year (Behar, 1992). A component of life satisfaction and fulfillment, satisfaction with services was also assessed in a half dozen of the studies, with generally high levels of satisfaction being reported.

However, a major recent and important study reported less positive results. The Department of Defense CHAMPUS program funded the creation of a continuum of care in Fort Bragg, North Carolina. Through this demonstration, military families in Fort Bragg were allowed to receive virtually any type of mental health service rather than more traditional inpatient, outpatient, and residential care (Behar, Macbeth, & Holland, 1993). An evaluation was conducted that compared the costs and outcomes of care for children and families who received services in Fort Bragg to the costs and outcomes of care for children and families who received a limited range of outpatient and inpatient care at a comparison site. Evaluators from the Fort Bragg project found no differences between the intervention and no-intervention groups in terms of child adaptive functioning, child psychopathology, or degree of family burden (Bickman et al., 1995). Differences were found in the Fort Bragg study for levels of family satisfaction in favor of the intervention group. This study, the most comprehensive child services research effort to date, is the subject of ongoing scientific discussion and debate (e.g., Bickman, 1996b, 1996c; Friedman & Burns, 1996).

A number of trends in system-of-care research to date emerge from the studies described in Table 7.3. The majority of the research has focused on demonstrating reductions in cost or utilization of restrictive service options, with all but five studies presenting findings in this domain. In some cases, these reductions were translated into dollar amounts. Fewer than half of the studies presented results on clinical or functional status, as typically measured on the CBCL, the CAFAS, or other scales. Direct indicators of safety and welfare, such as educational status and law enforcement status, were each assessed by fewer than 20% of the studies. Aside from client satisfaction, only a few of the investigators attempted to measure other indicators of satisfaction and fulfillment, such as family participation in services, amount of abuse or neglect inflicted upon the child, spousal and other family violence, and family burden.

LINKING THE INDEPENDENT AND DEPENDENT VARIABLES: THE QUALITY OF THE RESEARCH DESIGN

The results from system-of-care research illustrate that youth and families enrolled in systems of care do show improvements in a range of outcome domains. Making the causal link, however, between the implementation of these complex interventions and the outcomes achieved can be difficult. The capacity to draw these conclusions is at least in part a function of the research design of each study. The current attention focused on the Fort Bragg study is due largely to the inclusion of outcome measures that covered the range of domains typically considered relevant for assessing the effectiveness of systems of care along with the use of a comparison group. In this study, the results would have appeared completely positive if it were not for the inclusion of the comparison group. Youth in the demonstration site did show improvement, but youth in the comparison site showed similar levels of improvement on most measures (Bickman et al., 1995; Lambert & Guthrie, 1996).

Importantly, a distinction exists between making a causal link and making a plausible link between an intervention and an independent variable. Inferring causality (i.e., Did the intervention cause the outcome?) is largely a function of the internal validity (i.e., the strength of the design and the measures) of the research (Campbell & Stanley, 1966). The plausibility of a research finding to various audiences, such as scientists, program administrators, legislators, and clinicians, is a more complex matter that involves an interplay between the internal and external validity of the design (i.e., generalizability to other populations and interventions), along with how findings are presented. Weiss and Bucuvales (1980), for example, found that methodological rigor was only one of several factors (e.g., a perceived lack of bias in the conclusions) related to the judged utility of research findings. Similarly, Holland (1984) found that mental health providers did not distinguish between the "truthfulness" and the "usefulness" of research results.

It is possible to have a well-conducted research project that demonstrates a causal, but implausible, link between an intervention and an outcome. The most simple examples are internally valid studies that have little external applicability. An intervention may "cause" situationally depressed college students to feel better, but clinicians or program administrators would be unlikely to implement the intervention with persons who have a major affective disorder. More subtle examples exist. Considerable debate exists regarding why clinicians tend not to use the results of psychotherapy outcomes research in their practice. Weisz et al. (1995) offered a likely solution by noting that even though an extensive and sophisticated literature exists on psychotherapy outcomes with children in controlled settings, the literature on the "real-world" outcomes of psychotherapy is sparse. Most psychotherapists practice outside of the university-based clinics where most psychotherapy research is conducted, making many of the results from the psychotherapy outcomes literature remote, not relevant, unconvincing, or implausible compared to their own clinical experiences.

Inferring causality without randomized experiments is problematic (Sechrest, 1984), and even when randomized experiments are conducted, inferring causality may still not be possible. Randomized studies are rarely perfectly conducted, and deviations from treatment or intervention protocols, combined with inevitable disruptions in the random assignment process, can wreak havoc on sophisticated research designs conducted in applied settings. Although a randomized design was implemented in one study of a system of care in Ohio (Bickman, 1996a), results from that study are not yet available. It is highly unlikely that many further randomized trials will be implemented anytime in the near future. A system of care is an extensive intervention, usually aimed at counties, catchment areas, or communities. In all cases, it is unlikely that alternate care systems can be implemented within such geographical or regional boundaries. Although alternate systems may exist in neighboring communities, it is certainly not feasible, or ethical, to randomly request youth and families to move to a different county just so they can participate in a research study.

Consequently, the barriers to implementing a randomized design of a system of care are extensive, at least equal to those found in other social interventions (Weiss, 1972). Randomized designs of components of a system of care are feasible, have been conducted, and are yielding results (Kutash & Rivera, 1996). These studies can compare two different treatment options within a care system and randomly assign youth to two potentially equally attractive treatment options. Opportunities may exist in the future to conduct randomized designs of contrasting system models if multiple providers begin to move into communities and compete for public funds. The dawning of managed mental health care in both the private and public sectors may create scenarios where multiple providers exist in communities, each providing full arrays of services under different models. In such instances, random assignment, or a close variant of random assignment, may be feasible.

Nonetheless, research on systems of care has relied on quasi-experimental designs and will most likely continue to rely on more refined variants of these designs in the future. The wide range of potential research designs still used by most of the evaluation research world has changed little since the seminal work by Campbell and Stanley (1966) and Cook and Campbell (1979). Although innovations in research designs appear periodically, most quantitative evaluation work still draws on refinements of designs that originated more than a decade ago. The major nonexperimental research designs pertinent to systems of care are described in the following section.

Pre–Post Designs

Pre–post designs contain no comparison to a nontreatment group. In these designs, measurements are taken before and after an intervention. In some cases, these designs create relatively weak arguments for the link between an intervention and a set of outcome findings. However, these designs can have importance in relatively young fields, such as children's mental health services. Pre–post designs can be the blocks upon which more sophisticated research builds. They can demonstrate the possibility of change for populations where change is not a given, such as in the case of children with SED. In doing so, these designs can change the research and policy agenda from questions of whether youth can improve to questions of which factors or interventions lead to improvement. Furthermore, these designs may become the basis of policy formulation. For example, as illustrated earlier in this chapter, the majority of research on systems of care has focused on whether youth can be maintained in homelike environments. One research and policy question that derives from these studies is whether the youth who are either removed or diverted from residential care suffer poor outcomes as a result of controls on utilization. Pre–post designs can make plausible arguments that youth are faring well even when utilization of restrictive levels of care is controlled. These designs also have some value in the policy arena because of the relative simplicity and intelligibility of the results that derive from these studies.

Nonequivalent Comparison Group Designs

Nonequivalent comparison group designs (NECGDs) are likely to become the mainstay of research on systems of care as the field builds upon simple pre–post designs. These designs use a nonrandomly assigned comparison group to compare to a group receiving an intervention. The quality of these designs rests largely on the capacity to find or create two or more comparison groups that are as similar as possible. A range of techniques exists for equating the two groups either statistically (e.g., analysis of covariance, forced entry regression) or as design features (e.g., matching strategies).

Time Series and Multiple Time Series Designs

Interrupted time series designs can, if properly conducted, provide highly defensible conclusions regarding the effects of an intervention (Judd & Kenney, 1981). These designs require ongoing measurement of the variable of interest both before and after a specified intervention. They are distinguished from repeated measures designs in that they require a relatively large number of pre- and postmeasurement intervals. Consequently, these designs are often used to analyze data such as cost, utilization, and community indicators (e.g., crime rates) that are collected repeatedly over extended periods of time. Time series designs may be used to compare multiple series, such as crime rates in one community versus another. The statistical treatment of these designs is well established (McCleary & Hays, 1980) and can help create relatively powerful and plausible arguments regarding an intervention. The major limitation of these designs is the relatively large number of observations required over time to permit successful analyses.

Regression Discontinuity Designs

Regression discontinuity designs can be a fairly powerful design option (Trochim, 1984) that has not been used to date in system-of-care research. These designs require that youth be assigned to conditions on the basis of some cut point or cutting score. For example, if youth with a reading score below 80 are assigned to a remedial class whereas youth with a score of 81 or above remain in a regular class, it is possible to assess the relative effectiveness of each treatment option. These designs can also be used when youth are assigned to a treatment condition on the basis of age. For example, youth under 17 may be eligible for children's services, whereas youth 18 and over may be eligible only for adult services. Natural cut points may also occur on the basis of service utilization. It is common, for example, in managed care to allocate a set number of sessions (e.g., eight outpatient sessions) to anyone who requests care but to also require utilization reviews for persons who wish to receive more than the allowed number of sessions (e.g., nine or more). Although regression discontinuity designs can be difficult to implement and analyze (the cutting score often may not be exact or precise), the design is nonetheless a potentially rigorous option whenever youth are assigned to services on the basis of some type of cutting score.

Mixing Designs

In many cases, research on systems of care may be composed of a series of substudies that may feature varying design strategies. A randomized design of case management strategies may be nested as a separate, more intensive study contained within a broader, nonequivalent comparison group study of the system as a whole. Alternately, time series techniques may be used to compare cost data across systems, while pre–post designs are used to evaluate the effectiveness of specific programs within a system.

Review of Systems of Care and Research Designs

A summary of the research designs used to achieve the results given earlier in this chapter is presented in Table 7.4. At this writing, results from randomized research designs of systems of care are not available, and only one such

TABLE 7.4

Research Designs of Community-Based System-of-Care Studies

Study (Primary Reference)	Clinical Status	Functional Status	Life Satisfaction and Fulfillment	Safety and Welfare	Cost or Utilization
New Directions, VT	Pre–post	Pre–post	Post		Pre–post
Ventura, CA	Pre–post	Pre–post		Pre–post	Post/time series
Children's Initiative, NC	Pre–post	Pre–post	Post	Pre–post	Pre–post/NECGD
Stark, OH	Post	Post			Time series
Bennington County, VT	Post	Post			Time series
Dubuque, IA					Time series
Mountain State Network, WV				NECGD	NECGD
Impact, KY	Pre–post	Pre–post	Pre–post		Pre–post/time series
Fort Bragg, NC	NECGD	NECGD	NECGD	NECGD	NECGD
Demonstration Projects, VA			Post		NECGD/Pre–post
AB377 Counties, CA					Mult. time series
Northumberland, PA					Repeated measures
Augusta, GA		Post			Time series/NECGD
FMP, CA				Pre–post	Pre–post
Lucas, OH					Pre–post
AIMS Project, TN	NECGD	NECGD			NECGD
LIS Projects, VA	Pre–post	Pre–post			
Connections, OH	Post	Post			
North Idaho	Pre–post	Pre–post	Post		
Franklin, OH					Pre–post

Note. NECGD = Nonequivalent comparison group design.

design is being implemented (Bickman, 1996a). The most frequent research design used across these studies was a pre–post design. Time series designs of varying quality are also frequently used in assessing service use outcomes. Three studies used nonequivalent group comparison designs to measure child and family outcomes.

Research designs vary considerably by the type of outcome variable analyzed. Several of the studies applied a range of time series methods to cost and utilization data, and some types of external comparisons were utilized with these types of outcome indicators more frequently than with other outcomes. Cost and utilization data are frequently found in a variety of management and billing information systems and have been collected and stored over time in a wide range of locales, making the application of time series and multiple time series designs feasible. Client outcome data are not as readily available as certain types of cost and utilization data and, consequently, often require more time, effort, and resources to collect. As a result, time series designs are not typically used with these types of variables.

When considered in the context of the research designs, the positive findings for systems of care presented in Table 7.3 offer a far less consistent picture. The findings are universally positive, with the critical exception of the Fort Bragg study, which included a comparison group. In terms of scientific and political significance, the reality that the results from the Fort Bragg study may overshadow the results from 19 other research efforts is largely a testimony to the power of more sophisticated research designs. Clearly, more studies that find ways to use some types of comparisons to communities implementing systems of care are needed.

CONCLUSIONS

Changes in child and adolescent mental health care are occurring in the context of dramatic shifts in the organization and financing of public mental health services, including (a) shifts toward managed care, resource capping, and capitation models (Hoge et al., 1994; Mechanic & Aiken, 1989); (b) increasing movement toward local control and responsibility for public mental health programs and systems; and (c) movement toward the privatization of what previously were public mental health services. All of these changes are occurring in the context of greatly diminished public resources and with the imperative to do more with less.

In such an environment, documenting the outcomes of care systems may determine whether models and systems continue to survive. Given the sociopolitical context in which the systems-of-care movement now exists, there is a strong tendency for a rush to judgment. As argued elsewhere (Rosenblatt, 1996), quick and easy answers to whether systems of care or other complex social programs are working do not provide the basis for sound policy development.

Nonetheless, the first decade of research on the outcomes of systems of care for youth with SED did yield a knowledge base that researchers can build upon. This base includes the following broad conclusions:

- Across a range of outcome domains, youth with SED who are enrolled within innovative systems show improvement.
- The Fort Bragg study (Bickman et al., 1995) raises the question of whether these improvements are due to being enrolled in a system of care, are simply the result of obtaining any kind of services, or constitute the natural course of SED (youth would get better without any intervention). Given the severity of the problems faced by children and families who receive these services, as well as numerous reports citing the unfortunate plight of children and families, the latter conclusion is highly implausible.
- With the exception of the Fort Bragg study, the research has demonstrated that systems of care can manage costly out-of-home placements. The research methods for these studies were consistently more convincing than the methods for assessing child and family outcomes, with a number of studies having used time series methods or comparisons of some type. Consequently, there is substantial evidence that communities implementing systems of care can control residential placements (either lower or reduce the rate of increase). This finding is consistent with the concept of utilization and cost as indicators of change at the system level.

Still, as would be expected given the relative newness of the field, the existing literature has its share of weaknesses:

- The existing research on systems of care is extremely difficult to evaluate critically. Most studies are not published in scientific journals and thus are not subject to peer review; descriptions of methodology are generally inadequate; and statistical analyses are often either inappropriate or incomplete.
- The research methods used in evaluating the child and family outcomes of systems of care vary considerably but are all quasi-experimental. Pre–post designs are the norm. There is a need for more sophisticated research designs.
- Measure selection for evaluating systems of care is difficult both because of the range of outcomes that systems are designed to influence and because of limitations in measurement. Few measures exist that are designed specifically on the basis of the values and goals of the system-of-care approach.
- Care systems are complex interventions occurring at many levels. Relatively little is empirically known regarding how different levels of a system of care may interact to produce change across a range of potential outcome domains.

- Given the complexity of multilayered systems, it is not entirely surprising that the term *system of care* is often used loosely and is not objectively defined. This makes it difficult to determine whether the care systems studied in the literature truly embody the concepts or theory behind the system-of-care movement.

Linking Systems of Care and Outcomes

As this chapter has emphasized, research on the outcomes of systems of care rests on making plausible links between a multilayered social intervention and a multidimensional set of potential outcomes. The relationships between these two multidimensional constructs are likely to be neither direct nor linear. Rather, the ultimate effectiveness of a system of care relies on the independent and interactive effectiveness of systemic, programmatic, and clinical reforms. Changes at different levels of the systems may correspond to changes in different types of outcomes. The quality of clinical interventions, for example, may be most directly related to changes in symptomatology, whereas the quality of system organization may be most directly related to improvements in the efficiency of service delivery. It is tempting to view any outcome of a system of care as a function of system change alone, which can be expressed as

$$Oi = f(S) \tag{1}$$

where Oi is the outcome for an individual, i, and S represents some kind of system-level reform. A great deal of the current research essentially relies on this level of model; for example, whether systems of care can reduce utilization of out-of-home placements or improve clinical status. A slightly more complex version of this line of thought may be expressed as follows:

$$Oitdcp = f(S) \tag{2}$$

where $Oitdcp$ is the outcome for an individual at time t, for clinical domain d, in context c, and by perspective p. This model acknowledges that changes may occur in a range of different types of outcomes and may vary by the outcome domain, the perspective on outcome measurement, and the context in which outcomes are assessed, as well as by the time interval during which change in an outcome is assessed. A few researchers of systems of care followed this type of model by studying a range of outcomes of system-level reform efforts without explicitly or clearly attending to reform at programmatic and clinical levels. This model therefore is overly simplistic, given the multiple levels found within a system of care. The more inclusive, and more appropriate, way of envisioning the relationships between levels of care and outcome expands on this and may be expressed as

$$Oitdcp = f(S, P, C) \tag{3}$$

where *P* reflects some constellation of programmatic reforms and *C* some constellation of clinical reforms. Systemic, programmatic, and clinical changes may interact with one another within this framework to produce different types of outcomes. This perspective also allows for the exploration of how specific types of outcomes may relate only to specific combinations of system, program, and clinical interventions. The research on systems of care reviewed in this chapter does not fully embrace this last perspective, no doubt in part because of the difficulty of conducting such research.

The direct implications of this model for analyzing the outcomes of a system of care are threefold: (a) Systems of care need to be created, understood, studied, and described, and their strength and integrity assessed, at multiple levels; (b) outcomes within a system of care need to be thought of as multidimensional and multidetermined; and (c) the relationships between levels of intervention delivered within a system of care and the multiple outcomes of the system of care can be interactive as well as additive.

Even this final model is oversimplified. Many factors can mediate the relationship between multiple levels of a system of care and multiple outcome domains. The characteristics of the children, their families, and the communities in which they live are bound to mediate the relationships between systems and outcomes. Similarly, different research designs may yield different levels of confidence in the strength of the linkages between system change and child and family outcomes. The quality of the data-analytic strategies are yet another factor in understanding outcomes that are not discussed in this chapter.

Although models like the one presented here may lead to applied research problems that rapidly approach a level of incomprehensible complexity, they are important to keep in mind in evaluating and discussing the current state of systems-of-care outcomes research. Even the most sophisticated existing studies relevant to systems of care focus almost exclusively on the system, the program, or the clinical level. Most system-of-care studies do not measure outcomes across a range of measurement domains, perspectives, and contexts. Too often, results are presented as though system change can be expected to lead directly to changes in individual-level outcomes. The strength and integrity of a system of care needs to be better elucidated and ensured. Finally, relatively new systems are often expected to produce a range of outcomes before they have reached a sufficient level of maturity. Additional multidimensional models need to be developed that acknowledge the complexities inherent in the relationships between systems and outcomes, and these kinds of models need to be kept in mind in interpreting the existing literature.

Although the challenges are clearly great, the future of research on systems of care for youths with SED can be bright. Already, researchers involved at the systemic, programmatic, and clinical levels of a care system are exchanging ideas regarding how research at different levels may be more coherently conducted. As an example, attention is now being focused on how clinical efficacy research can bridge the gap into effectiveness research (Hoagwood, Hibbs, Brent, & Jensen, 1995; Weisz et al., 1995). A model of clinical intervention that is based on the multisystemic needs of youth is being implemented in a range of systems of care and may provide bridges among the clinical, programmatic, and systemic levels of care systems (Henggeler & Borduin, 1990; Henggeler et al., 1992). The components of systems of care are receiving increasing levels of attention, and individualized service approaches are being integrated into systems of care (VanDenBerg & Grealish, 1996).

The first generation of research on the outcomes of systems of care for youth with SED did yield the beginnings of a knowledge base. This research also, however, yielded something else: an evolutionary revolution in how research can be conducted on human service systems and how researchers can cross their own disciplinary and topical boundaries to produce more integrative, holistic, and, it is hoped, ultimately meaningful research. It is appropriate that a service reform movement based on principles of collaboration and integration should encourage collaboration and integration among researchers working in often disparate traditions.

Finally, from a broader perspective, systems of care for youth with SED are one of a number of efforts to better integrate services for children and families. Although a range of attempts at service integration date to the 1970s, there remains precious little information on the costs and effects of these efforts (Kagan & Neville, 1993). The current wave of interest in service integration provides an opportunity to begin to answer a host of questions about its ultimate success. Without these answers, the social and political pendulums will certainly swing as dictated by the fashions and forces of the times. Without these answers, it will be impossible to know whether the pendulums are swinging in a benign and beneficial direction, or whether they are headed on a collision course with positive outcomes for families and children.

AUTHOR'S NOTE

Preparation of this chapter was supported in part by evaluation research contracts from the Center for Mental Health Services and the California State Department of Mental Health (89-70225, 90-70195, 91-71106, 92-72090, 92-72347, 93-73346, 94-74252, 94-74285, and 95-75217) and a center grant from the National Institute of Mental Health (P50MH43694).

REFERENCES

Achenbach, T. M., & Edelbrock, C. S. (1993). *Manual for the Child Behavior Checklist and Revised Child Behavior Profile.* Burlington: University of Vermont, Department of Psychiatry.

Attkisson, C. C., Cook, J., Karno, M., Lehman, A., McGlashan, T. H., Meltzer, H. Y., O'Connor, M., et al. (1992). Clinical services research. *Schizophrenia Bulletin, 18*(4), 561–626.

Attkisson, C. C., & Greenfield, T. K. (1994). *Client Satisfaction Questionnaire-8* and *Service Satisfaction Scale-30*. In M. E. Maruish (Ed.), *The use of psychological testing for treatment planning and outcome assessment.* Hillsdale, NJ: Erlbaum.

Attkisson, C. C., & Greenfield, T. K. (1995). The Client Satisfaction Questionnaire (CSQ) Scales. In L. L. Sederer & B. Dickey (Eds.), *Outcome assessment in clinical practice.* Baltimore: Williams & Wilkins.

Behar, L. (1985). Changing patterns of state responsibility: A case study of North Carolina. *Journal of Clinical Child Psychology, 14,* 188–195.

Behar, L. (1992). *The children's initiative, North Carolina mental health services program for youth.* Raleigh: North Carolina Division of Mental Health, Developmental Disabilities, and Substance Abuse Services, Child and Family Services Branch.

Behar, L. B., Macbeth, G., & Holland, J. M. (1993). Distribution and costs of mental health services within a system of care for children and adolescents. *Administration and Policy in Mental Health, 20,* 283–295.

Bickman, L. (1996a). *Preliminary findings from a randomized trial in Stark County, Ohio.* Paper presented at an NIMH-sponsored workshop, "Moving from Efficacy to Effectiveness in Children's Research," Washington, DC.

Bickman, L. (1996b). The evaluation of a children's mental health managed care demonstration. *Journal of Mental Health Administration, 23,* 7–15.

Bickman, L. (1996c). Reinterpreting the Fort Bragg evaluation findings: The message does not change. *Journal of Mental Health Administration, 23,* 137–145.

Bickman, L., Guthrie, P., Foster, E. M., Lambert, E. W., Summerfelt, W. T., Breda, C., et al. (1995). *Managed care in mental health: The Fort Bragg experiment.* New York: Plenum.

Burchard, J. D., & Clarke, R. T. (1990). The role of individualized care in a service delivery system for children and adolescents with severely maladjusted behavior. *Journal of Mental Health Administration, 17,* 48–98.

Burns, B. J., & Friedman, R. M. (1990). Examining the research base for child mental health services and policy. *Journal of Mental Health Administration, 17,* 87–98.

Campbell, D. T., & Stanley, J. C. (1966). *Experimental and quasi-experimental designs for research.* Skokie, IL: Rand McNally.

Ciarlo, J. A., Brown, T. R., Edwards, D. W., Kiresuk, T. J., & Newman, F. L. (1986). *Assessing mental health treatment outcome measurement techniques* (National Institute of Mental Health Series FN No. 9, DHHS Publication No. ADM 86-1301). Washington, DC: Superintendent of Documents, U.S. Government Printing Office.

Cook, T. D., & Campbell, D. T. (1979). *Quasi-experimentation design: Design and analysis in field settings.* Skokie, IL: Rand McNally.

Cronbach, L. J. (1964). Evaluation for course improvement. In R. W. Heath (Ed.), *New curricula* (pp. 231–248). New York: Harper & Row.

Day, C., & Roberts, M. C. (1991). Activities of the Child and Adolescent Service System Program for improving mental health services for children and families. *Journal of Clinical Child Psychology, 20,* 340–350.

Friedman, R. M., & Burns, B. J. (1996). The evaluation of the Fort Bragg demonstration project: An alternative interpretation of the findings. *Journal of Mental Health Administration, 53,* 128–136.

Georgia Division of Mental Health, Mental Retardation, and Substance Abuse (DMHMRSA). (1992). *A report on the August SED project.* Athens: Author.

Glisson, C. (1992). *The adjudication, placement, and psychosocial functioning of children in state custody.* Knoxville: University of Tennessee, College of Social Work.

Goldman, S. (1992). Ventura County, California. In B. Stroul, S. Goldman, I. Lourie, J. Katz-Leavy, & C. Zeigler-Dendy (Eds.), *Profiles of local systems of care for children and adolescents with severe emotional disturbances* (pp. 287–337). Washington, DC: Georgetown University, CASSP Technical Assistance Center.

Hargreaves, W. A., & Shumway, M. (1989). Effectiveness of mental health services for the severely mentally ill. In C. A. Taube, D. Mechanic, & A. Hohmann (Eds.), *The future of mental health services research* (DHHS Publication No. ADM 89-1600, pp. 253–284). Washington, DC: U.S. Government Printing Office.

Henggeler, S. W., & Borduin, C. M. (1990). *Family therapy and beyond: A multisystemic approach to treating the behavior problems of children and adolescents.* Pacific Grove, CA: Brooks/Cole.

Henggeler, S. W., Melton, G. B., & Smith, L. A. (1992). Multisystemic treatment of serious juvenile offenders: An effective alternative to incarceration. *Journal of Consulting and Clinical Psychology, 60,* 953–961.

Hoagwood, K., Hibbs, E., Brent, D., & Jensen, P. (1995). Introduction to the special section: Efficacy and effectiveness in studies of child and adolescent psychotherapy. *Journal of Consulting and Clinical Psychology, 63*(5), 683–687.

Hodges, K. (1994). *The Child and Adolescent Functional Assessment Scale.* (Available from Kay Hodges, Eastern Michigan University, Psychology Department, Ypsalanti, MI 48197)

Hoge, M. A., Davids, L., Griffith, E. E., Sledge, W. H., et al. (1994). Defining managed care in public sector psychiatry. *Hospital and Community Psychiatry, 45,* 1085–1089.

Holland, R. S. (1984). *Perceived truthfulness and perceived usefulness of program evaluations by direct services staff.* Unpublished doctoral dissertation, University of Michigan.

Illback, R. (1993). *Evaluation of the Kentucky Impact program for children and youth with severe emotional disabilities, Year 2.* Frankfort, KY: Division of Mental Health, Children and Youth Services Branch.

Iowa Department of Human Services (DHS). (1992). *Dubuque County progress report.* Dubuque: Iowa Department of Human Services, Dubuque Area Office.

Jordan, D. D., & Hernandez, M. (1990). The Ventura Planning Model: A proposal for mental health reform. *Journal of Mental Health Administration, 17,* 26–47.

Judd, C. M., & Kenney, D. A. (1981). *Estimating the effects of social interventions.* New York: Cambridge University Press.

Kagan, S. L., & Neville, P. R. (1993). *Integrating services for children and families: Understanding the past to shape the future.* New Haven, CT: Yale University Press.

Koren, P. E., DeChillo, N., & Friesen, B. J. (1992). Measuring empowerment in families whose children have emotional disabilities: A brief questionnaire. *Rehabilitation Psychology, 37,* 305–321.

Kovacs, M. (1991). *The Children's Depression Inventory.* North Tonawanda, NY: Multi-Health Systems.

Kutash, K., & Rivera, V. R. (1996). *What works in children's mental health services? Uncovering answers to critical questions.* Baltimore: Brookes.

Lambert, W. E., & Guthrie, P. R. (1996). Clinical outcomes of a children's mental health managed care demonstration. *Journal of Mental Health Administration, 53,* 51–68.

Lourie, I. (1992). Northumberland County, Pennsylvania. In B. Stroul, S. Goldman, I. Lourie, J. Katz-Leavy, & C. Zeigler-Dendy (Eds.), *Profiles of local systems of care for children and adolescents with severe emotional disturbances* (pp. 87–149). Washington, DC: Georgetown University Child Development Center, CASSP Technical Assistance Center.

Martinez, M., & Smith, L. (1993). *The Family Mosaic Project.* Report submitted to the Washington Business Group on Health. San Francisco: Family Mosaic Project.

McCleary, R., & Hays, R. A., Jr. (1980). *Applied time series analysis for the social sciences.* Beverly Hills, CA: Sage.

McCoard, D. (1993). *10 KIDS: An interprofessional managed care approach to returning SED youth placed out-of-county using nontraditional cross-system collaborative strategies.* Paper presented at the sixth annual research conference, A System of Care for Children's Mental Health: Expanding the Research Base, Tampa.

McCormick. (1994). *Measuring outcomes of systems of care.* Paper presented at 1994 CASSP Biennial Training Institutes, Traverse City, MI.

McGuire, T. G., Frank, R. G., & Goldman, H. H. (1992). Designing a benefit plan for child and adolescent mental health services. *Administration and Policy in Mental Health, 19,* 151–157.

Mechanic, D., & Aiken, L. H. (1989). Capitation in mental health: Potentials and cautions. *New Directions for Mental Health Services, 43,* 5–18.

National Advisory Mental Health Council. (1993). Health care reform for Americans with severe mental illness: Report of the National Advisory Mental Health Council. *American Journal of Psychiatry, 150*(10), 1447–1465.

National Institute of Mental Health. (1983). *Program announcement: Child and Adolescent Service System Program.* Rockville, MD: Author.

National Institute of Mental Health. (1991). *Caring for people with severe mental disorders: A national plan of research to improve services* (DHHS Publication No. ADM 91-1762). Washington, DC: Superintendent of Documents, U.S. Government Printing Office.

Phillips, K. A., & Rosenblatt, A. (1992). Speaking in tongues: Integrating psychology and economics into health and mental health services outcomes research. *Medical Care Review, 49*(2), 191–230.

Quay, H. C. (1987). *Handbook of juvenile delinquency.* New York: Wiley.

Rosenblatt, A. (1993). In home, in school, and out of trouble. *Journal of Child and Family Studies, 2*(4), 275–282.

Rosenblatt, A. (1996). Bows and ribbons, tape and twine: Wrapping the wraparound process for children with multi-system needs. *Journal of Child and Family Studies, 5,* 101–116.

Rosenblatt, A., & Attkisson, C. C. (1992). Integrating systems of care in California for youth with severe emotional disturbance: I. A descriptive overview of the California AB377 Evaluation Project. *Journal of Child and Family Studies, 1,* 93–113.

Rosenblatt, A., & Attkisson, C. C. (1993). Assessing outcomes for sufferers of severe mental disorder: A review and conceptual framework. *Evaluation and Program Planning, 16,* 347–363.

Rosenblatt, A., & Attkisson, C. C. (1997). Integrating systems of care with severe emotional disturbance: IV. Educational attendance and achievement. *Journal of Child and Family Studies, 6*(1), 113–129.

Rosenblatt, A., Attkisson, C., & Mills, N. (1992). *The California AB377 evaluation, 3-year summary report.* San Francisco: University of California.

Rugs, D. (1992). *Mountain state network project* (Unpublished report). Tampa: Florida Mental Health Institute, Department of Child and Family Studies.

Scallet, L. J. (1994). The unintended consequences of health care reform for children's mental health services. *Behavioral Healthcare Tomorrow, 3*(2), 68–69.

Scriven, M. (1967). The methodology of evaluation. In R. W. Tyler, R. M. Gagne, & M. Scriven (Eds.), *Perspectives on curriculum evaluation.* Chicago: Rand McNally.

Sechrest, L. (1984). *Evaluating health care.* Unpublished manuscript, University of Arizona.

Sechrest, L., & Rosenblatt, A. (1987). Research methods. In H. C. Quay (Ed.), *Handbook of juvenile delinquency* (pp. 81–101). New York: Wiley.

Sechrest, L., West, S. G., Phillips, M. A., Redner, R., & Yeaton, W. (1977). Some neglected problems in evaluation research: Strength and integrity of treatments. In L. Sechrest, S. G. West, M. A. Phillips, R. Redner, & W. Yeaton (Eds.), *Evaluation studies review annual* (Vol. 4, pp. 15–35). Beverly Hills, CA: Sage.

Shaffer, D., Fisher, P., Piacentini, J., Schwab-Stone, M., & Wicks, J. (1989). *Diagnostic Interview Schedule for Children (DISC–2.1).* New York: New York State Psychiatric Institute.

Sorensen, J. E., & Grove, H. D. (1978). Using cost-outcome and cost-effectiveness analyses for improved program management and accountability. In C. C. Attkisson, Q. A. Hargreaves, M. J. Horowitz, & J. E. Sorensen (Eds.), *Evaluation of human service programs* (pp. 371–408). New York: Academic Press.

Stroul, B. A. (1992). Stark County, Ohio. In B. Stroul, S. Goldman, I. Lourie, J. Katz-Leavy, & C. Zeigler-Dendy (Eds.), *Profiles of local systems of care for children and adolescents with severe emotional disturbances* (pp. 211–286). Washington, DC: Georgetown University Child Development Center, CASSP Technical Assistance Center.

Stroul, B. A. (1993). *Systems of care for children and adolescents with severe emotional disturbances: What are the results?* Washington, DC: Georgetown University Child Development Center, CASSP Technical Assistance Center.

Stroul, B. A. (1996). *Managed care and children's mental health: Summary of the May 1995 state managed care meeting.* Washington, DC: Georgetown University Child Development Center, National Technical Assistance Center for Children's Mental Health.

Stroul, B. A., & Friedman, R. M. (1986). *A system of care for seriously emotionally disturbed children and youth.* Washington DC: Georgetown University Child Development Center, CASSP Technical Assistance Center.

Tharp, R. G., & Gallimore, R. (1979). The ecology of program research and evaluation: A model of evaluation succession. In L. Sechrest, S. G. West, M. A. Phillips, R. Redner, & W. Yeaton (Eds.), *Evaluation studies review annual* (Vol. 4, pp. 39–60). Beverly Hills, CA: Sage.

Trochim, W. M. K. (1984). *Research design for program evaluation: The regression discontinuity approach.* Beverly Hills, CA: Sage.

Trupin, E. W., Forsyth-Stephens, A., & Low, B. P. (1991). Service needs of severely disturbed children. *American Journal of Public Health, 81,* 975–980.

VanDenBerg, J. E., & Grealish, E. M. (1996). Individualized services and supports through the wraparound process: Philosophy and procedures. *Journal of Child and Family Studies, 5,* 7–22.

Vermont Department of Mental Health and Mental Retardation. (1993). *Vermont new directions evaluation of children and adolescent services.* Waterbury: Division of Mental Health.

Virginia Department of Mental Health, Mental Retardation, and Substance Abuse Services (DMHMRSA). (1992a). *Demonstration project interim evaluation results.* Richmond: Office of Research and Evaluation.

Virginia Department of Mental Health, Mental Retardation, and Substance Abuse Services (DMHMRSA). (1992b). *Local interagency service projects initiative.* Richmond: Office of Research and Evaluation.

Weiss, C. H. (1972). *Evaluation research: Methods of assessing program effectiveness.* Englewood Cliffs, NJ: Prentice Hall.

Weiss, C. H., & Bucuvales, M. J. (1980). Truth tests and utility tests: Decision makers' frames of reference for social science research. *American Sociological Review, 45,* 302–313.

Weisz, J. R., Donenberg, G. R., Han, S. S., & Kauneckis, D. (1995). Child and adolescent psychotherapy outcomes in experiments versus clinics: Why the disparity? *Journal of Abnormal Child Psychology, 23*(1), 83–106.

Weisz, J. R., Weiss, B., Alicke, M. D., & Klotz, M. L. (1987). Effectiveness of psychotherapy with children and adolescents: A meta-analysis for clinicians. *Journal of Consulting and Clinical Psychology, 55*(4), 542–549.

Measuring Fidelity Within Community Treatments for Children and Families

CHAPTER 8

Challenges and Strategies

Eric J. Bruns, John D. Burchard, Jesse C. Suter, and Michelle D. Force

Over the past decade and a half, the mental health field has made great advances in the design of community systems to combat serious emotional and behavioral problems in childhood. There is now nationwide consensus that services for these children and young people should be individualized, family centered, community based, culturally competent, and provided in the least restrictive setting possible (Stroul & Friedman, 1986). At the same time, the science of studying the efficacy of mechanisms to address mental health problems of children and adolescents has advanced considerably. Whereas once there was a near absence of such a research base, now agency heads, clinicians, and parent advocates alike are all clamoring for the latest information on evidence-based practices.

Nonetheless, we continue to be deflated by research findings that show service systems' failure to affect child outcomes (Bickman, Summerfelt, & Noser, 1997), as well as the inability of promising interventions to be effective in "real-world" settings (Kazdin & Weisz, 1998). Standing in our way have been both systemic and scientific barriers. Systemically, we continue to allocate the majority of our mental health resources to restrictive care settings, which have the poorest research base on effectiveness (Burns, Hoagwood, & Maultsby, 1998). Meanwhile, even though the research base on both diagnosis-specific and multimodal community-based treatments for children and families is advancing, major gaps in our knowledge base persist. For many of the comprehensive multimodal community interventions, the specification of service delivery approaches is emergent and not well understood, resulting in providers who are uncertain how to effectively implement services. In addition, although much of the extant research base is encouraging, outcome studies featuring adequate methodologies remain scarce. Those studies that do exist often neglect to adequately describe the intervention and specify its "ingredients." Finally, even when an intervention is well described, studies often overlook the importance of assessing whether it was implemented as intended, leading to confusion about interpretation.

To improve outcomes for families with children with emotional and behavioral disturbance (EBD), we first must move away from the vague descriptions of services that are prevalent in the literature and more clearly define our terms (Hoagwood, 1997). Although it is a critical step, specifying program models is often ignored in mental health services research (Bickman, 1987; McGrew, Bond, Dietzen, & Salyers, 1994). Lack of specification leaves interventions difficult to replicate, vulnerable to "program drift" (Bond, 1991, p. 74) and susceptible to dilution and alteration in response to local conditions.

Once an intervention has been fully described and operationalized, and adequate training and supervision are in place to ensure that the treatment protocol is implemented as intended, advancing the science of measuring service processes within the intervention becomes critical. A key concept within this science is treatment fidelity. Although the dynamics of defining, maintaining, and assessing fidelity to community treatments for youth are complex, psychometrically sound fidelity measurement holds promise for advancing both research and practice within children's mental health. The current chapter will discuss the importance of treatment fidelity and the many applications of and approaches to its measurement. The chapter will then describe specific approaches to measuring fidelity within children's mental health, paying particular attention to the wraparound process as a salient example with which to illustrate the development of treatment fidelity approaches for a community-based treatment for youth.

TREATMENT FIDELITY

Treatment fidelity refers to how well a specific program conforms to its defined program model, protocol, or standards (Bond, Evans, Salyers, Williams, & Hea-Won, 2000). Thus, fidelity measures assess the adequacy of program implementation. The implicit assumption is that better adherence to the specified model will result in better outcomes for the program's participants. Such measures have their origins in the 1950s with Eysenck's (1952) well-publicized critiques of psychotherapy models, as well as the 1960s, when the emerging community mental health movement led to demands for better treatment specification to allow for replication of treatment methods (Moncher & Prinz, 1991). Assessing treatment fidelity serves both practice purposes and several research purposes.

Practical Uses of Fidelity Assessment

Chief among the practical uses of fidelity measures is their utility in facilitating service delivery. At the outset, when an intervention is introduced to a program site, fidelity measures can offer a template for providers to understand the required practice guidelines (Bond et al., 2000). During the course of providing services, fidelity scores from rating scales, checklists, logs, or clinical records can be continuously fed back to providers and supervisors to inform areas in which service delivery is not adequately conforming to the program model. Finally, summary fidelity scores for an entire program or system can be analyzed to assess areas in which more comprehensive training, technical assistance, or tangible resources is required.

Developers and proponents of well-established interventions have promoted the clinical use of fidelity measures because of their concern with ensuring strict adherence to their models. In the adult psychiatric rehabilitation field, for example, concerns about improper dissemination led to development of standards and checklists for the Fountain House clubhouse model (Beard, Propst, & Malamud, 1982; Propst, 1992), even though the program originally had been designed nearly 50 years earlier (Bond et al., 2000). Fidelity assessment can also inform service delivery that is not intended to be implemented via a single specific model. Within the medical field, for example, *practice guidelines* are prominent mechanisms for recommending types and levels of treatment for a certain population. Within mental health, such guidelines were originally developed for adult populations, such as persons with schizophrenia (see Lehman, Steinwachs, & PORT Co-Investigators, 1998). Within children's mental health, such guidelines now exist for disorders such as attention-deficit disorder, anxiety disorder, conduct disorder, and mental retardation (Burns, 2002). Measures of adherence to system-of-care principles—to be discussed later in this chapter—provide another example of measuring fidelity to guidelines or principles.

Research Uses of Fidelity Assessment

Fidelity assessment is an essential, yet underemployed, component of evaluation research. Perhaps most critically, in research designs that feature intervention and control groups, fidelity measures are necessary to examine the extent of treatment differentiation between groups. Without such information, interpretation of between-group differences may be difficult or impossible. For example, in a multisite study of assertive community treatment (ACT; Stein & Santos, 1998) for adults with schizophrenia, fidelity tools were instrumental in documenting that some control programs that were supposed to be delivering standard case management services scored quite high on ACT fidelity scales (Teague, Drake, & Ackerson, 1995). In children's mental health, conclusions from the Fort Bragg Demonstration Project (Bickman, 1996) that a system-of-care site fared no better than a comparison site were challenged because of the lack of an extensive implementation study (Vinson, Brannan, Baughman, Wilce, & Gawron, 2001). Indeed, post hoc studies of the "systemness" of the comparison site suggested that the comparison site fared at least as well as the system-of-care site on certain variables (Hoagwood, 1997).

In addition to documenting whether the systematic variance between groups is adequate, fidelity tools are also useful in research that aims to identify critical ingredients of program models, regardless of whether treatment and control groups are used in the design. To accomplish this purpose, fidelity tools tend to be constructed to include subscales that correspond to different "ingredients" of the intervention. Scores on such subscales are then correlated with a criterion, such as client outcomes (Bond et al., 2000). For example, McGrew et al. (1994) found that of 17 fidelity items on a measure of fidelity to ACT, reduction in hospital use was predicted by 5: shared caseloads, total contacts, presence of a nurse on the team, daily team meetings, and 24-hour availability. Variants of fidelity can often illuminate the relationship between service processes and outcomes. For example, in an outcome study of respite care services for children with EBD, greater intensity of respite care services and parent satisfaction with scheduling flexibility were associated with outcomes (Bruns & Burchard, 2000).

Finally, consistent fidelity assessment can help synthesize a body of research (Bond et al., 2000). Using identical fidelity tools across evaluations of similar programs would allow one to determine whether the program being studied in each evaluation met the criteria for inclusion in a review. Ideally, meta-analyses attempting to determine the effectiveness of a treatment could also use fidelity score as an independent variable. Also, evaluations of generic interventions (e.g., residential treatment or case management) that are implemented differentially in various sites could be better interpreted if consistent fidelity measures were employed, allowing a reviewer to discern the variations in the independent variable. However, as pointed out by Moncher & Prinz (1991), achieving such an ideal would require that treatment fidelity be consistently measured and reported in outcome studies.

Approaches to Measuring Treatment Fidelity

The full constellation of potential data sources available to researchers and program administrators examining treatment fidelity includes manuals and program descriptions, staffing and budget data, management information systems data on procedure or reimbursement codes, and observations of service processes (McGrew et al., 1994). In assessing fidelity to medication regimens—which would more accurately be referred to as treatment compliance—this universe could be expanded to include pill counts, blood or urine drug levels, and microelectronic monitoring of medication containers (Hack & Chow, 2001). However, within mental health and social services, most fidelity assessments rely primarily on reviews of available clinical records, logs of staff contact, observations, and checklists or surveys completed by staff and clients.

Because the range of treatments to which fidelity measures can be applied varies so greatly, there is no way to determine the relative superiority of different data collection methods. However, the complexity of an intervention may inform the selection of specific data sources for fidelity assessment. For example, in measuring medication compliance—where the prescribed treatment is well defined—the relative cost-efficiencies of the various methods will likely be the most salient factor in the decision: monitoring blood or urine drug levels or microelectronic monitoring will be less commonly used because of the expenses incurred, whereas face-to-face interviewing of the client or monitoring of prescription use through calls to pharmacies will likely be more commonly used (Hack & Chow, 2001).

Similarly, within mental health interventions, psychotherapy models that focus on a specific behavior or diagnosis and that use sequential intervention steps (e.g., parent–child behavior training or manualized cognitive-behavioral therapy) will also be relatively less complex to measure. For example, the *Cognitive Therapy Scale* (Dobson, Shaw, & Vallis, 1985), comprising a relatively brief set of items completed by expert raters based on reviews of therapy session audiotapes, has been found to be adequately sensitive to detect deviations from protocol within cognitive-behavioral therapy for depression (Schoenwald, Henggeler, Brondino, & Rowland, 2000). However, more complex and multifaceted interventions may require more complex fidelity measurement. For example, in a study of the effectiveness of ACT for adults with dual diagnoses, McHugo, Drake, Teague, and Xie (1999) conducted intensive longitudinal data collection, including interviews with clinical and administrative staff, activity logs collected by case managers, clinical records, and direct observations. Although the intensity of this process resulted in fidelity ratings that predicted several outcomes and guided formation of recommendations for future policy, more cost-efficient mechanisms for collecting fidelity data will generally be demanded if fidelity assessment is to become commonplace[1] (Manderscheid, 1998).

MEASURING FIDELITY TO COMMUNITY TREATMENTS FOR YOUTH

As suggested by the preceding sections, there are two interrelated challenges in measuring fidelity to complex mental health interventions for children and families. The first is the lack of treatment specification. This is a particular challenge within more generic—but often very prevalent—mental health intervention models for children and families, such as intensive case management, residential treatment, and psychiatric hospitalization, which have generally been poorly specified (Schoenwald et al., 2000). In addition, the system-of-care framework that undergirds many communities' service delivery to families presents challenges to treatment specification. With respect to both system-of-care principles and complex mental health services models, even when critical ingredients or practice guidelines have been identified, operational definitions of how these principles are actually implemented in service delivery often are lacking, hampering both service delivery and fidelity measurement.

The second challenge to measuring fidelity is the complexity and individualized nature of mental health service models for children and families.

---

[1] Indeed, within research on ACT, other fidelity tools, such as the *Index of Fidelity to Assertive Community Treatment* (McGrew et al., 1994), have been developed that can be completed following a review of program materials and interview with a program administrator.

Measuring fidelity within psychotherapy primarily requires attention to the therapist's behaviors. In community-based interventions, however, comprehensive fidelity assessments require attention to provider behaviors as well as multiple structural and administrative characteristics of both the program and overall system of care. Some of these potential organizational and system-level characteristics are listed in Table 8.1. The primary point to be made here, however, is that the complexity of children's mental health interventions makes them more difficult to specify in a treatment manual, which in turn makes fidelity assessment more complicated and challenging. As summarized by Bond et al. (2000) in describing the adult psychiatric rehabilitation field, community-based interventions "are inherently more difficult ... because the interventions occur in multiple settings, with multiple providers and recipients, and involve diverse activities that go far beyond a counseling setting" (p. 78).

TABLE 8.1

Structural and Administrative Characteristics
Amenable to Fidelity Assessment in Community Interventions

Organizational-Level Characteristics	System-Level Characteristics
Hiring practices	System partners' support of intervention core values
Staff education and qualifications	System partners' ability to collaborate
Staff salaries	Autonomy granted to provider organizations to develop services and supports
Training, supervision, and support provided	Documentation requirements
Caseload sizes	Reimbursement structures
Location of services	Blended funding mechanisms/degree of "categorization" of services
Availability and accessibility of services	Infrastructure for information sharing across agencies and organizations (e.g., services and costs data)
Referral and eligibility determination process	Characteristics of system governance structure (including representation of family voices)
Organization's support of intervention core values	
Organization's support of staff members' full participation in intervention	
Working conditions that enable quality service provision	
Policies on access to flexible funds	
Infrastructure for collecting monitoring and cost data	
Characteristics of organization governance structure (including representation of family voices)	

Specific Approaches to Measuring Fidelity

Despite the challenges of model specification and model complexity, the heightened recognition of the importance of fidelity measurement in children's mental health has led to a relative explosion in the development of fidelity measures. In an almost paradoxical development, the need to devise such measurement approaches has also contributed to better model specification within children's mental health. As summarized by Burns (2002), adherence measures are one of a set of approaches to improving the consistency and quality of care that also includes clinical protocols and manuals, practice guidelines, quality monitoring, and regulations. Among the major community-based interventions for children and youth with EBD, three have "reasonably well-developed" (Burns, 2002, p. 11) methods for assessing fidelity: multisystemic therapy (MST; Henggeler, Schoenwald, Borduin, Rowland, & Cunningham, 1998), treatment foster care (TFC), and the wraparound process. The rest of this section will briefly describe fidelity measurement approaches for the first two of these interventions, as well as describe approaches to measuring fidelity to system-of-care principles. The chapter will conclude with an in-depth description of approaches to measuring fidelity to the wraparound process.

System-of-Care Principles

Although the system of care model was initially articulated in the mid-1980s (Stroul & Friedman, 1986), published assessments of communities' system development did not emerge until a decade later. These initial studies tended to narrowly focus on how agencies develop linkages, primarily using techniques such as network analysis (e.g., Morrissey, Johnsen, & Calloway, 1997). Results of attempts to comprehensively measure fidelity to the tenets of the system-of-care model—including previously unassessed principles such as family involvement and cultural competence—have recently surfaced as part of the evaluation of the federal Comprehensive Community Mental Health Services for Children and their Families (CCMHS) program (Manteuffel, Stephens, & Santiago, 2002).

Evaluators of the CCMHS program have devised a system-level assessment (SLA) that results in both qualitative descriptions of grantee sites' approaches to developing systems of care, and quantitative ratings that describe how well each principle was achieved. Based on systems-of-care theory, SLAs are structured to assess eight components within two primary domains. The *infrastructure* domain consists of governance, management, service array, and quality-monitoring components, whereas the *service delivery* domain contains entry, service planning, service provision, and case-monitoring components. For each domain component, researchers attempted to create a measurable indicator of how well each of the eight system-of-care principles (e.g., family focused, accessible) was being achieved. For example, at the intersection of the service planning component and the accessible principle, indicators included "service planning occurs at flexible times to maximize the convenience for the child and family" and "the service plan is fully accessible to families." Ratings for indicators were then generated from information gleaned via semistructured interviews of individuals such as administrators, family members, and providers at each funded site.

Results of these SLAs demonstrated that over 5 years, sites made significant progress in achieving certain system-of-care principles, whereas other principles (e.g., family involvement in system governance, interagency collaboration in funding) have been more difficult to achieve (Vinson et al., 2001). Results of SLAs in funded versus comparison sites showed that progress toward achieving system-of-care principles was better in funded sites than matched comparison sites, but that infrastructural improvements in funded sites were more likely to be achieved than were service delivery improvements (Brannan, Baughman, Reed, & Katz-Leavy, 2002). Overall, the profiles of challenges and successes described by the quantitative and qualitative results of the SLAs were instrumental in generating recommendations on how best to build a local system of care. In addition, such system implementation data also aided interpretation of between-group results from the comparison study. Finally, researchers' experiences in developing the SLAs generated myriad examples of the challenges that must be addressed when creating fidelity measures in this field. Primary among these challenges are the need to develop items that are pinned to well-defined and observable behavioral events wherever possible (as opposed to abstract constructs) and the importance of training raters to criteria for interrater reliability (Vinson et al., 2001).

Multisystemic Therapy

In children's mental health, MST has emerged as the comprehensive treatment with the most stringent program specifications. Not coincidentally, it also has demonstrated the best empirical support, with positive child outcomes determined through several randomized trials. Evidence that fortifying adherence to the MST's model is associated with better child outcomes has resulted in fidelity measures for both therapists and supervisors that are encouraged in national replications of the model. To measure therapist adherence, the MST adherence scale is administered to the therapist, caregiver, and youth at regular intervals during treatment. The adherence scale contains 26 Likert-scale items (e.g., "the therapist tried to change the ways some family members interact with one another," "not much was accomplished during therapy sessions") across six empirically derived factors. In ideal MST implementation, scores from the adherence scale are made immediately available to clinical supervisors to allow for ongoing feedback and better fidelity to the model (Schoenwald et al., 2000). Recent studies examining the transportability of MST also have employed a measure of supervisor fidelity that parallels the MST supervision manual (Schoenwald et al., 2000). Use of this measure encourages implementation according to the MST model while also allowing examination of associations among supervision practices, therapist adherence, and child outcomes (Schoenwald & Rowland, 2002).

Additional procedures—including an adherence questionnaire completed by a MST expert after review of audiotaped therapy sessions—have also been added to fortify adherence to MST. Use of such intensive fidelity measures has been found to improve ratings on the MST adherence forms, while information from both methods has been instrumental in determining pathways among MST processes, instrumental outcomes, and ultimate child and family outcomes (Schoenwald et al., 2000).

Treatment Foster Care

First introduced in the mid-1970s, TFC provides treatment to children with behavioral and mental health problems within private homes of trained families (Chamberlain, 2002) and is now considered the most widely used alternative to restrictive care settings for this population (Kutash & Rivera, 1996). Like many complex community-based treatments, the model features specific core practice elements for which implementation guidelines are adequately flexible to be tailored to the needs of a specific child and family. Fidelity assessment in the TFC program run by colleagues at the Oregon Social Learning Center takes several forms. Daily phone calls to TFC parents by case managers function both as a fidelity assessment and as an essential supervision practice. Case managers also complete weekly checklists rating adherence to key program activities by TFC parents (e.g., use of contingencies, providing alternatives to delinquent peer association). These checklists provide a more formal and consistent assessment of fidelity.

In addition, formal TFC program standards were recently published (Foster Family-Based Treatment Association, 1995), providing the foundation for construction of a fidelity measure titled the *Standards Review Instrument* (SRI; Farmer, Burns, Dubs, & Thompson, 2002). The SRI is a 55-item instrument administered by a trained interviewer assessing administrative-level conformity to the model across three constructs: (a) Conformity of Program Standards; (b) Conformity of Treatment Parent Standards; and (c) Conformity on Children, Youth, and their Family Standards. Results from Farmer and colleagues' study using the SRI to assess TFC fidelity across 45 programs in North Carolina indicated that implementation of the standards for TFC showed considerable variability across sites, with total scores ranging from 45 to 85 out of a possible 110. This suggests that real-world implementation of TFC is likely to deviate significantly from the stringent standards adhered to in, for example, the research-oriented Oregon TFC programs.

MEASURING TREATMENT FIDELITY TO THE WRAPAROUND PROCESS

Along with MST, TFC, and intensive case management, wraparound is generally cited among the promising community-based interventions for children with EBD and their families (Burns, 2002; Burns et al., 1998). Summarized briefly, it uses a definable, team-based planning process that results in a unique set of community services and natural supports that are individualized for a child and family to achieve a set of positive outcomes. The wraparound process has been described in several monographs (Burchard, Burchard, Sewell, & VanDenBerg, 1993; Burns & Goldman, 1999; Kendziora, Bruns, Osher, Pacchiano, & Mejia, 2001), in chapters in books on community-based interventions for children (e.g., Burchard, Bruns, & Burchard, 2002), and in manuals for trainers (e.g., Grealish, 2000; VanDenBerg & Grealish, 1998). Like MST and TFC, the wraparound process is guided by a set of elements and practice principles but is administered in an individualized manner, depending on the needs of the child and family.

However, unlike MST and TFC, the wraparound elements and practice principles were defined only recently, there are no nationally recognized standards, and there is no definitive blueprint or "manual" to guide service delivery activities. As a result, many of wraparound's philosophical principles have not been well operationalized into specific provider behaviors. Put simply, there is confusion about what the term *wraparound* means. To some, it simply connotes a community-based service, such as mentoring or respite. To others, a wraparound service suggests anything purchased with noncategorical care dollars. To others, wraparound is not a team-based, stepwise process, as is described in some resources (e.g., Kendziora et al., 2001), but a system organization philosophy.

The confusion about wraparound can largely be traced to the intervention's individualized, multimodal approach, which focuses on system improvements as well as specific activities. Such characteristics make wraparound a signature example of the challenges facing these types of interventions for families that are neither "macro level" enough to be defined by mere practice guidelines or administrative prerequisites nor adequately "micro level" to be prescribed by a strict treatment manual. As such, the wraparound process provides an excellent example with which to illustrate the development of treatment fidelity approaches in children's mental health.

Early Fidelity Assessment

Early attempts to measure fidelity to the wraparound process primarily rested within programs' quality assurance procedures (Bruns, 1999). For example, supervisors trained in the wraparound approach met regularly with wraparound care managers (sometimes called resource facilitators or care coordinators) to assess the fidelity of their performance vis-á-vis the wraparound principles and to problem-solve difficulties. Supervisors also conducted open-ended interviews with providers, youth, and families to determine whether services delivered were truly drawing upon child and family strengths; were utilizing nonprofessional services and supports in the community; and were responsive to family's opinions, preferences, and stated needs. Later, rating-scale surveys became the norm, wherein families were queried about their satisfaction with services and specific providers. Eventually, surveys incorporated questions that asked parents and youth whether services adhered to certain wraparound principles, such as whether they felt providers listened to them or whether they perceived that their services would be provided "no matter what" (Rosen, Heckman, Carro, & Burchard, 1994).

Another traditional approach that remains a crucial mainstay in fidelity assessment and quality monitoring is record reviews. Within wraparound programs, random sampling of families' case files can be used to investigate whether providers are following practice principles for a specific family. Examples of wraparound principles that can be investigated via case file review are listed in Table 8.2.

Observational Approaches

Team-based individualized service planning is a central component of the wraparound process, and the team process should reflect the principles of wraparound in specific and observable ways. As such, the child and family team process that occurs within wraparound is highly amenable to observational approaches to assessing fidelity.

The first such approach was developed by Singh and colleagues (1997), whose 42-item *Family Assessment and Planning Team Observation Form* (FAPT) was specifically designed to assess the family centeredness of professionals at team meetings. More recently, Epstein and colleagues (1998) developed the *Wraparound Observation Form* (WOF), the most current version of which—the WOF–2—evolved from FAPT items that were most reflective of the core wraparound principles. The WOF–2 includes 48 close-ended items arranged into eight dimensions. Some of the dimensions are specific to the wraparound principles (e.g., Individualized Services, Measurable Outcomes), whereas others are more specific to the team process (e.g., Management of Team Meetings). Examples of items within these three dimensions include, respectively, "Strengths of the family members are identified and discussed at the meeting," "The plan of care goals are discussed in objective, measurable terms," and "Plan of care is agreed on by all present at the meeting." For each WOF–2 item, the rater is asked to select one of three responses: yes, no, and not applicable. A detailed manual instructs on-site observers how to assign ratings based on operational definitions of team members' behaviors and team processes. The first version of the WOF demonstrated adequate overall reliability, including 95% overall interrater agreement and 70% to 100% agreement for specific items (Epstein et al., 1998).

Results from the WOF–2 demonstrate the potential utility of the instrument in assessing patterns of adherence to the wraparound approach for individual teams, programs, and entire service systems (Epstein et al., 2002). However, as its authors acknowledged, the approach has limitations. First, its scope is restricted to the team planning process, and as such the WOF cannot assess how well a planned intervention is actually carried out. Second, the WOF's reliance on ratings of occurrence versus nonoccurrence for each of its items does not allow for a finer level assessment of how fully an observed

TABLE 8.2

Principles of the Wraparound Approach and
Potential Case File Data Sources To Use in Assessing Fidelity

Wraparound Principle	Case File Data Sources and Indicators
Individualized services and supports	The case file includes an updated plan of care.
	The family's plan of care is unique to the child and family and does not resemble those of other families served by the same program.
	There is a list of a full range of potential interventions and informal service and support options for the family from which the plan of care was crafted.
	There is a specific and unique safety or crisis plan with specific responsibilities for each team member listed.
Community based	The family's plan of care includes a goal to achieve the least restrictive placements possible.
	If there is a goal to move to a less restrictive setting, specific steps are listed in the plan of care to do so.
Team-driven process	File includes full roster of participating team members.
	Frequency and recency of team meetings is documented.
	Attendance of team members is documented.
	Plan of care lists specific responsibilities for each team member in wraparound plan.
Family centered	Plan of care specifies clear roles and responsibilities for family members.
	Family members' attendance and full participation (including parents, siblings, and extended family) are documented.
	File contents include evidence that family members participated in planning process.
	File contents include evidence that family members received copies of service plan.
Flexible service delivery/ funding	The case file includes evidence of an individualized budget for the family.
	Budget or expenditure reports show evidence for availability of flexible funds to meet plan-of-care goals.
Formal and informal services and supports	The plan of care includes services and supports provided by informal resources.
	There is documentation that friends and advocates of the child and family, as well as community members, are represented at team meetings.
Collaborative interagency services and supports	There is documentation that all agencies and organizations who provide services to the family are in attendance at team meetings.
	A community collaborative structure has reviewed and signed off on the plan of care.
Strength based	An updated strengths inventory is included in the file, along with a service plan that clearly corresponds to child, family, and community strengths.

(continues)

TABLE 8.2 *Continued.*
Principles of the Wraparound Approach and
Potential Case File Data Sources To Use in Assessing Fidelity

Wraparound Principle	Case File Data Sources and Indicators
Culturally competent	Team planning process and general meeting minutes reflect that family members are given opportunities to describe their family's specific beliefs, traditions, and rituals.
	The plan of care reflects the family's specific traditions and rituals.
	Team membership reflects the characteristics of the family's specific support network.
Outcomes based	The plan of care includes goals with measurable indicators of success for each goal.
	There is evidence of formal satisfaction assessment.
	There is documentation of the child's progress in specific outcome domains, such as school attendance, school achievement, and behavioral functioning.

event may have been implemented. Third, although one of the strengths of the WOF is that it relies on expert observations rather than respondents' potentially subjective ratings, wraparound principles such as cultural competence, which are difficult to reliably observe in a team meeting, are not assessed via the WOF.

The Wraparound Fidelity Index

Like many other fidelity tools, the *Wraparound Fidelity Index* (WFI) was developed out of concerns about the misapplication of the term *wraparound* by providers who did not have adequate understanding of the full set of required service strategies or did not possess the resources to implement them. Aimed initially at generating interpretable feedback to providers to aid training and supervision, the WFI was intended to be a user-friendly and cost-efficient method for a program, service system, or research team to assess wraparound fidelity via the triangulation of ratings derived from interviews with a set of key informants. The process of operationalizing survey items for the WFI also served a key role in defining observable behaviors that should occur within the wraparound process, setting the stage for better definition of specific practices and provider behaviors within the intervention.

Development of WFI 1.0

The first iteration of the WFI (WFI 1.0) was created by (a) choosing items from an existing measure, the *Service Process Inventory for Families and Youth* (SPIFY; Bramley & Tighe, 1999), that corresponded well with the wraparound elements and principles; (b) incorporating other items identified by a small group of experts; and (c) arranging these items into three different forms—one each for parents/caregivers, resource facilitators/case managers, and youth. In WFI 1.0, the Resource Facilitator Form included items that assessed 8 of the 10 elements of wraparound, whereas the parent and youth versions each assessed 4 elements. For each respondent form, 4 items were included for each element, yielding a 32-item scale for the Resource Facilitator Form and a 16-item scale for the Caregiver and Youth Forms. Respondents answered each item on a 3-point scale, where 2 = *yes,* 1 = *sometimes or somewhat,* and 0 = *no.* Combining scores from across informants, a full profile of adherence to the 10 elements could be constructed for individual families, which could then be aggregated within a site or program to create an overall fidelity score, as well as a profile of element scores for the site.

Pilot Test of WFI 1.0

Preliminary pilot studies (Bruns, Ermold, & Burchard, 2001) were intended to assess the WFI's face validity and ease of administration and to establish properties and psychometrics. WFI 1.0 was piloted with 60 families at four sites nationally. To assess the construct validity of the WFI 1.0, a national expert on wraparound visited three of the sites. Following a protocol that included record reviews and intensive interviews with family members and providers, the expert assigned fidelity scores for each element included on the WFI for each family. WFI scores were then correlated with the expert's ratings across the elements for each family. At the fourth site, the WFI was administered on two occasions 2 weeks apart to assess test–retest reliability.

A major finding of this series of preliminary pilot studies was that summed element scores for the WFI 1.0 were very high (range = 5.88–7.50 out of a possible score of 8.0), such that variability was limited and a ceiling effect was observed. Internal consistency was found to be adequate for total fidelity scores; however, for individual elements, alphas were low. (This was not surprising, given that individual element scores comprised only 4 items, whereas total fidelity scores comprised 32). Test–retest results revealed that percentage of total agreement between administrations (all items) was acceptable for the Caregiver and Resource Facilitator Forms but poorer for the Youth Form.

With respect to construct validity, results from the pilot study indicated that correlations between the expert's overall ratings and WFI total fidelity scores were significant. However, for 3 of the 10 individual element scores, the WFI was not significantly associated with the expert's rating. These results were interpreted to be due to two major shortcomings in the scale. First, as described above, the WFI 1.0 exhibited a lack of sensitivity that was largely due to items that were not operationalized well. Second, the WFI relied on a single informant for scores on 6 of the elements, reducing the opportunity for multi-informant triangulation of information on fidelity. The WFI's failure to query parents across all wraparound elements was also critiqued by parents and parent advocates.

Revision of WFI 1.0

Despite the challenges that emerged, the results of the initial study were encouraging, especially with respect to the ability of WFI 1.0 to assess the overall adherence to the wraparound elements for a family in a way that correlated with external criteria. To make the WFI more psychometrically sound and better able to distinguish fully versus partially implemented wraparound, a number of changes were initiated:

1. One element of wraparound, "services will be individualized and strengths-based," was split into two elements, to reflect the independence of the constructs "individualized" and "strengths-based." This resulted in 11 elements to be assessed via WFI 2.0.
2. WFI 2.0 assessed each informant (parent/caregiver, youth, and resource facilitator) for each element. This was intended to increase the variability in scores, increase the social validity of the tool for family members, and increase the construct validity across elements and for total fidelity scores.
3. For all respondent forms, WFI 2.0 items were better operationalized and made more stringent with respect to the element being assessed. This was intended to increase variability of scores and reduce the ceiling effect observed in WFI 1.0. Examples of items that were better operationalized from the Caregiver Form include the following:
   - "As the primary caregiver, are you given highest priority when making major decisions?" (Element 1: Voice and Choice)
   - "Is there a friend or advocate of your family or child who is an active participant on the team?" (Element 2: Youth and Family Team)
   - "Are more than half of the participants on the team professionals?" (Element 7: Natural Supports)
4. WFI 2.0 included reverse-scored items to vary the response pattern for respondents and thus contribute to greater variability in scores. An example of a reverse-scored item from the Youth Form is the following: "If you were to get into big trouble, do you think the team would give up on you and not be there to help you out?" (Element 8: Continuation of Care)
5. A WFI 2.0 user's manual that includes scoring criteria for each item within each element was completed. Many items now do not require a respondent to simply respond "yes," "sometimes," or "no." Instead, the interviewer must be able to assign a rating of 2, 1, or 0 based on the respondent's description.

Results Using WFI 2.0

Because of the improvement in its face validity, WFI 2.0 was made available to wraparound program providers nationally who agreed to provide data to the WFI research team. Results compiled for more than 250 families in 12 sites nationally revealed that items on WFI 2.0 demonstrated substantially more variance, less skewness, and a far less pronounced ceiling effect than the WFI 1.0 items (Bruns, Burchard, Suter, Leverentz-Brady, & Force, 2004). In addition, internal consistency for WFI 2.0 was greatly improved over that of WFI 1.0, increasing from .72 to .90 for the Caregiver Form, from .74 to .78 for the Resource Facilitator Form, and from .63 to .90 for the Youth Form. However, internal consistency for several individual elements remained inadequate for between-group comparisons, meaning that overall fidelity scores remain the primary research metric. Nonetheless, element scores continued to be calculated and graphed in profiles for sites' use in quality improvement activities.

The improvements in properties of the WFI after its revision were extremely encouraging. Although evidence from the pilot test of WFI 1.0 suggested the tool's construct validity and test–retest reliability, the improved variance for WFI 2.0 suggested improved utility in quality improvement activities. In addition, despite the addition of items, mean administration times remained under 15 minutes for all three WFI 2.0 forms. Providers also reported that standardized profiles of wraparound adherence across elements were useful and easily interpretable. Figure 8.1 provides an example of an adherence profile for one service delivery site, in which scores for each respondent are presented together for each element. As shown, adherence for the site was generally high; however, scores were lower for certain aspects of service delivery, including the use of natural supports (especially from the perspective of the resource facilitators and caregivers). Closer examination of specific items within the Natural Supports element are provided in a second adherence profile in Figure 8.2. Here, one can observe that 8 of 10 resource facilitators and 7 of 10 parents assessed via the WFI reported that their team relied "mostly on professional services," contributing significantly to the low score for the Natural Supports element. Feedback of WFI data such as these should prompt administrators at this site to initiate policies that reward less reliance on formal professional services in child and family plans, as well as training and supervision that help resource facilitators design more creative service plans that capitalize on families' natural supports.

Association of WFI 2.0 with Outcomes

The improved psychometrics of WFI 2.0 suggested the measure would be adequate for use in research studies, such as those aiming to determine whether service characteristics predict outcomes. Pursuant to this goal, an initial exploration of the association between wraparound fidelity and child and family outcomes was conducted (Bruns, Suter, & Burchard, 2002). The study correlated WFI scores for both resource facilitators and caregivers with outcome measures assessed both concurrently and 6 months post–WFI assessment. Outcome measures used included the *Child and Adolescent Functional Assessment Scale* (CAFAS; Hodges, 1999); the *Behavioral and Emotional Rating Scale* (BERS; Epstein & Sharma, 1998), a measure of behavioral strengths; a measure of residential restrictiveness; and two satisfaction questions asking the caregiver about satisfaction with services overall and the child's progress.

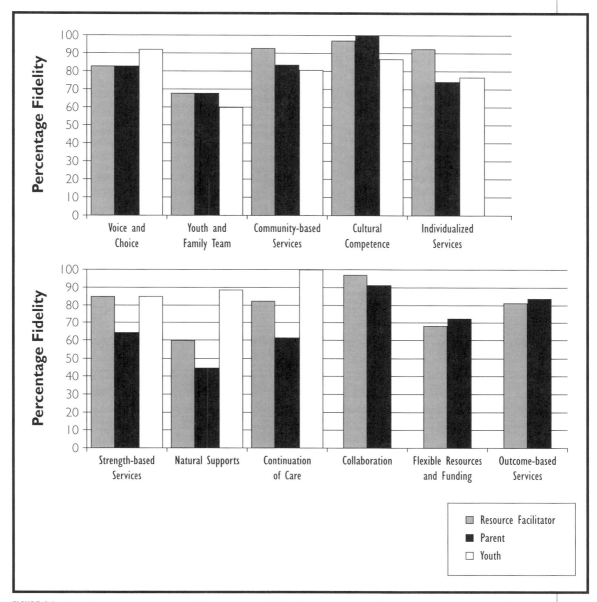

FIGURE 8.1. Graphic depiction of mean *Wraparound Fidelity Index* scores for all 11 elements and across all three respondent types (resource facilitators, caregivers, and youth) for 10 families in one service delivery site.

Participants in the final sample included 36 families with children experiencing emotional and behavioral disturbance in one federally funded system-of-care site.

Results demonstrated that WFI caregiver scores were significantly correlated with service satisfaction at Time 1, child behavioral strengths at Time 1, and satisfaction with the child's progress at Time 2. WFI resource facilitator scores were significantly associated with restrictiveness of living scores at both

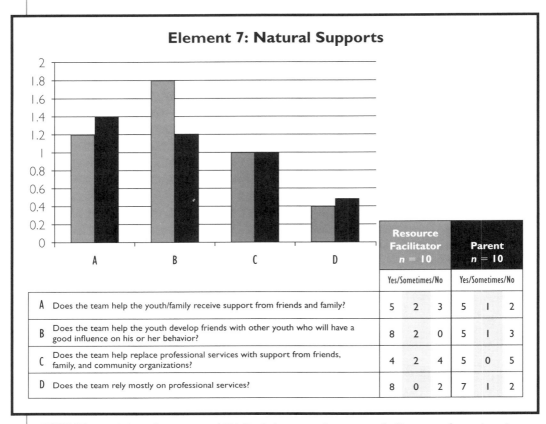

FIGURE 8.2. Depiction of *Wraparound Fidelity Index* scores for resource facilitators and caregivers in one service delivery site for the four items in the Natural Supports element.

Time 1 and Time 2, behavioral strengths at Time 1 and Time 2, and child functioning as measured by the CAFAS at Time 1. Overall, out of 16 correlations conducted, 15 coefficients were in the hypothesized direction, with 5 reaching statistical significance at $p < .05$ and an additional 3 correlations reaching marginal levels of significance at $p < .1$. No significant correlations opposite the hypothesized direction were found.

Thus, the weight of evidence in this exploratory study suggests that wraparound fidelity is associated with both concurrently assessed and future outcomes. With respect to the types of outcomes to which wraparound fidelity may be related, it is apparent that service outcomes, such as satisfaction and residential restrictiveness, are well associated with fidelity as assessed via the WFI. This is in keeping with other systems-of-care research showing that these types of outcomes may be most sensitive to the development of systems of care (see Bickman, 1999). However, the results of the current study also indicate that outcomes such as child behavior may be predicted by how well providers adhere to the core principles of wraparound, which is likely to be an even more important implication of the current results. Overall, although the sample sizes were small and the pattern of associations found was somewhat mixed, this preliminary study provided support for the importance of maintaining fidelity to the wraparound process, as well as to service delivery processes for children and families in general. The results also provided additional evidence for the construct validity of the WFI.

Future WFI Development

Because community treatments such as wraparound propose specific provider activities as well as program and systemic procedures and policies (Koroloff, Walker, & Schutte, 2002), a program administrator interview (WFI–PA) has been developed to assess the presence of the elements of wraparound from an infrastructural level. The WFI–PA is administered in an interview format to program administrators or local agency heads, with ratings based on operational criteria derived from model specifications, such as case manager caseload size, number of agencies participating on community teams, and flexibility of funds. Administered along with the other WFI forms, the WFI–PA will provide a more comprehensive fidelity or it can be administered by itself, across sites or over time. In addition to development of WFI–PA, WFI 2.0 has been revised again in response to the more extensive piloting of WFI 2.0. WFI 3.0 is identical in structure to WFI 2.0 except that it attempts to improve item variability and face validity in response to WFI 2.0 data and feedback from parents and providers.

CONCLUSION

In addition to providing examples of fidelity measurement approaches, this chapter has attempted to make several major points. First, treatment model specification is challenging in community treatments for children and youth, but it is a prerequisite for both quality service delivery and effective fidelity measurement. Second, even well-defined mental health interventions often suffer from inadequate fidelity measurement in outcome studies, which confuses interpretation of results and hinders our understanding of important service processes. Finally, there exists a vast array of potential data sources from which a fidelity measure can be derived, and selecting the most appropriate data source(s) and structure is a difficult task. As for many measurement issues, the balancing act between a cost-effective approach that can be completed consistently and a comprehensive approach with adequate psychometrics is a major challenge.

In attempting to determine the quality of a potential measure, Calsyn (2000) published a highly informative checklist that considers issues of validity, reliability, and generalizability from the perspective of fidelity assessment. Calsyn's criteria are stringent, and many tools discussed in the current chapter would not meet several basic prerequisites. For example, does the measure assess service dimensions that are unique to the intervention as well as those that are nonspecific to or prohibited by the intervention? Does it adequately assess the amount or dosage of the intervention components as well as their simple presence or absence? With respect to validity, has the measure been found to correlate with other measures of the same construct? Finally, has the measure been found to be associated with measures of program effectiveness, such as client outcomes?

Indeed, it is unlikely that fidelity measures meeting all the above criteria would be parsimonious or cost-efficient. Given the current primordial state of treatment specification and fidelity assessment in children's mental health, Calsyn's criteria should be carefully considered, but with simultaneous thought given to the most fundamental—and useful—fidelity constructs. Such fundamental constructs include ensuring that providers have a full understanding of the activities they should be undertaking with families, that supervisors have basic information about prescribed procedures and how well their providers are adhering to them, and that program administrators understand the system prerequisites for implementing an intervention and which prerequisites they do not meet. At this exciting but formative stage in developing community treatments for children and families, even incremental steps to providing answers to these questions hold the potential to greatly improve the quality of treatment delivered to children and families.

AUTHORS' NOTE

This work was supported in part by the U.S. Substance Abuse and Mental Health Services Administration Center for Mental Health Services, Child, Adolescent, and Family Branch through a subcontract with ORC Macro, Inc.

REFERENCES

Beard, J. H., Propst, R. N., & Malamud, T. J. (1982). The Fountain House model of rehabilitation. *Psychosocial Rehabilitation Journal, 5,* 47–53.

Bickman, L. (1987). The functions of program theory. In L. Bickman (Ed.), *Using program theory in evaluation* (pp. 5–18). San Francisco: Jossey-Bass.

Bickman, L. (1999). Practice makes perfect and other myths about mental health services. *American Psychologist, 54,* 966–978.

Bickman, L., Summerfelt, W. T., & Noser, K. (1997). Comparative outcomes of emotionally disturbed children and adolescents in a system of services and usual care. *Psychiatric Services, 48,* 1543–1548.

Bond, G. R. (1991). Variations in an assertive outreach model. *New Directions for Mental Health Services, 52,* 65–80.

Bond, G. R., Evans, L., Salyers, M., Williams, J., & Hea-Won, K. (2000). Measurement of fidelity in psychiatric rehabilitation. *Mental Health Services Research, 2,* 75–87.

Bramley, J., & Tighe, T. (1999). The *Service Process Inventory for Youth* (SPIFY). Poster presented at the 12th Annual System of Care Conference: Building the Research Base, Tampa, FL.

Brannan, A. M., Baughman, L. N., Reed, E. D., & Katz-Levy, J. (2002). System of care assessment: Cross-site comparison of findings. *Children's Services: Social Policy, Research, and Practice, 5,* 37–56.

Bruns, E. J. (1999). *National approaches to measuring and monitoring treatment fidelity.* Paper presented at the 12th Annual Research Conference: A System of Care for Children's Mental Health, Clearwater Beach, FL.

Bruns, E. J., & Burchard, J. D. (2000). Impact of respite care services for families with children experiencing emotional and behavioral problems and their families. *Children's Services: Public Policy, Research and Practice, 3,* 39–61.

Bruns, E. J., Burchard, J. D., Suter, J. C., Leverentz-Brady, K., & Force, M. D. (2004). Fidelity to the wraparound process and its association with child and family outcomes. *Journal of Emotional and Behavioral Disorders, 12,* 2.

Bruns, E. J., Ermold, J., & Burchard, J. D. (2001). The Wraparound Fidelity Index: Results from an initial pilot test. In C. Newman, C. Liberton, K. Kutash, & R. Friedman (Eds.), *A system of care for children's mental health: Expanding the research base. Proceedings of the 13th annual conference* (pp. 339–342). Tampa: Florida Mental Health Institute Research and Training Center for Children's Mental Health.

Bruns, E. J., Suter, J., & Burchard, J. D. (2002). Pilot test of the Wraparound Fidelity Index 2.0. In C. Newman, C. Liberton, K. Kutash, & R. Friedman (Eds.), *A system of care for children's mental health: Expanding the research base. Proceedings of the 14th annual conference* (pp. 235–238). Tampa: Florida Mental Health Institute Research and Training Center for Children's Mental Health.

Burchard, J. D., Bruns, E. J., & Burchard, S. N. (2002). The wraparound approach. In B. J. Burns, and K. Hoagwood (Eds.), *Community treatment for youth: Evidence-based treatment for severe emotional and behavioral disorders* (pp. 69–90). Oxford, England: Oxford University Press.

Burchard, J. D., Burchard, S. N., Sewell, R., & VanDenBerg, J. (1993). *One kid at a time: Evaluative case studies and descriptions of the Alaska Youth Initiative Demonstration Project.* Washington, DC: SAMHSA Center for Mental Health Services.

Burns, B. K. (2002). Reasons for hope for children and families: A perspective and overview. In B. J. Burns & K. Hoagwood (Eds.), *Community treatment for youth: Evidence-based treatment for severe emotional and behavioral disorders* (pp. 3–15). Oxford, England: Oxford University Press.

Burns, B. J., & Goldman, S. K. (1999). Promising practices in wraparound for children with serious emotional disturbance and their families. *Systems of care: Promising practices in children's mental health, 1998 series* (Vol. 4). Washington, DC: Center for Effective Collaboration and Practice, American Institutes for Research.

Burns, B. J., Hoagwood, K., & Maultsby, L. T. (1998). Improving outcomes for children and adolescents with serious emotional and behavioral disorders: Current and future directions. In M. H. Epstein, K. Kutash, & A. Duchnowski (Eds.), *Outcomes for children and youth with behavioral and emotional disorders and their families* (pp. 685–708). Austin, TX: PRO-ED.

Calsyn, R. J. (2000). A checklist for critiquing treatment fidelity studies. *Mental Health Services Research, 2,* 107–113.

Chamberlain, P. (2002). Treatment foster care. In B. J. Burns & K. Hoagwood (Eds.), *Community treatment for youth: Evidence-based treatment for severe emotional and behavioral disorders* (pp. 117–138). Oxford, England: Oxford University Press.

Dobson, K., Shaw, B. F., & Vallis, T. M. (1985). Reliability of a measure of the quality of cognitive therapy. *British Journal of Clinical Psychology, 24,* 295–300.

Epstein, M., Jayanthi, M., McKelvey, J., Frankenberry, E., Hary, R., Potter, K., et al. (1998). Reliability of the Wraparound Observation Form: An instrument to measure the wraparound process. *Journal of Child and Family Studies, 7,* 161–170.

Epstein, M. H., Nordness, P. D., Duchnowski, A., Kutash, K., Schrepf, S., & Benner, G. (2002). Assessing the wraparound process during family planning meetings. *Journal of Behavioral Health Services and Research, 29,* 208–216.

Epstein, M. H., & Sharma, J. M. (1998). *Behavioral and Emotional Rating Scale: A strength-based approach to assessment.* Austin, TX: PRO-ED.

Eysenck, H. (1952). The effects of psychotherapy, an evaluation. *Journal of Consulting Psychology, 16,* 319–324.

Farmer, E. M. Z., Burns, B. J., Dubs, M. S., & Thompson, S. (2002). Assessing conformity to standards for treatment foster care. *Journal of Emotional and Behavioral Disorders, 10,* 213–222.

Foster Family-Based Treatment Association. (1995). *Program standards for treatment foster care.* New York: Author.

Grealish, M. (2000). *The wraparound process curriculum.* McMurray, PA: Community Partners.

Hack, S., & Chow, B. (2001). Pediatric psychotropic medication compliance: A literature review and research-based suggestions for improving treatment compliance. *Journal of Child and Adolescent Psychopharmacology, 11,* 59–67.

Henggeler, S. W., Schoenwald, S. K., Borduin, C. M., Rowland, M. D., & Cunningham, P. B. (1998). *Multisystemic treatment for antisocial behavior in children and adolescents.* New York: Guilford Press.

Hoagwood, K. (1997). Interpreting nullity: The Fort Bragg experiment—A comparative success or failure. *American Psychologist, 52,* 546–550.

Hodges, K. (1999). Child and Adolescent Functional Assessment Scale (CAFAS). In M. E. Maruish (Ed.), *Use of psychological testing for treatment planning and outcome assessment* (2nd ed., pp. 631–664). Mahwah, NJ: Erlbaum.

Kazdin, A. E., & Weisz, J. R. (1998). Identifying and developing empirically supported child and adolescent treatments. *Journal of Consulting and Clinical Psychology, 66,* 19–36.

Kendziora, K., Bruns, E. J., Osher, D., Pacchiano, D., & Mejia, B. (2001). Wraparound: Stories from the field. *Systems of care: Promising practices in children's mental health, 2001 series* (Vol. 1). Washington, DC: Center for Effective Collaboration and Practice, American Institutes for Research.

Koroloff, N., Walker, J., & Schutte, K. (2002). *Implementing high-quality team-based individualized services planning: Necessary and sufficient conditions.* Portland, OR: Research and Training Center on Family Support and Children's Mental Health.

Kutash, K., & Rivera, V. R. (1996). *What works in children's mental health services? Uncovering answers to critical questions.* Baltimore: Brookes.

Lehman, A. F., Steinwachs, D. M., & PORT Co-Investigators. (1998). At issue: Translating research into practice: The Schizophrenia Patient Outcomes Research Team (PORT) treatment recommendations. *Schizophrenia Bulletin, 24,* 1–10.

Manderscheid, R. W. (1998). From many to one: Addressing the crisis of quality in managed behavioral health care at the millennium. *Journal of Behavioral Health Services and Research, 25,* 233–238.

Manteuffel, B., Stephens, R. L., & Santiago, R. (2002). Overview of the national evaluation of the Comprehensive Community Mental Health Services for Children and Their Families Program and summary of current findings. *Children's Services: Social Policy, Research, and Practice, 5,* 3–20.

McGrew, J. H., Bond, G. R., Dietzen, L. L., & Salyers, M. P. (1994). Measuring the fidelity of implementation of a mental health program model. *Journal of Consulting and Clinical Psychology, 62,* 670–678.

McHugo, G. J., Drake, R. E., Teague, G. B., & Xie, H. (1999). The relationship between model fidelity and client outcomes in the New Hampshire Dual Disorders Study. *Psychiatric Services, 50,* 818–824.

Moncher, F. J., & Prinz, R. J. (1991). Treatment fidelity in outcome studies. *Clinical Psychology Review, 11,* 247–266.

Morrissey J. P., Johnsen, M. C., & Calloway, M. O. (1997). Evaluating performance and change in mental health systems serving children and youth: An interorganizational network approach. *Journal of Mental Health Administration, 24,* 4–22.

Propst, R. (1992). Standards for clubhouse programs: Why and how they were developed. *Psychosocial Rehabilitation Journal, 16,* 25–30.

Rosen, L., Heckman, M., Carro, M., & Burchard, J. (1994). Satisfaction, involvement and unconditional care: The perceptions of children and adolescents receiving wraparound services. *Journal of Child and Family Studies, 3,* 55–67.

Schoenwald, S. K., Henggeler, S. W., Brondino, M. J., & Rowland, M. D. (2000). Multisystemic therapy: Monitoring treatment fidelity. *Family Process, 39,* 83–103.

Schoenwald, S. K. & Rowland, M. D. (2002). Multisystemic therapy. In B. J. Burns & K. Hoagwood (Eds.), *Community treatment for youth: Evidence-based treatment for severe emotional and behavioral disorders* (pp. 91–116). Oxford, England: Oxford University Press.

Singh N. N., Curtis W. J., Wechsler H. A., et al. (1997). Family friendliness of community-based services for children and adolescents with emotional and behavioral disorders and their families: An observational study. *Journal of Emotional and Behavioral Disorders, 5,* 82–92.

Stein, L. I., & Santos A. B. (1998). *Assertive community treatment of persons with severe mental illness.* New York: Norton.

Stroul, B. A., & Friedman, R. M. (1986). *A system of care for children and adolescents with severe emotional disturbance.* Washington, DC: Georgetown University Child Development Center, National Technical Assistance Center for Children's Mental Health.

Teague, G. B., Drake, R. E., & Ackerson, T. H. (1995). Evaluating use of continuous treatment teams for persons with mental illness and substance abuse. *Psychiatric Services, 46,* 689–695.

VanDenBerg, J. E., & Grealish, M. E. (1998). *The wraparound process training manual.* Pittsburgh: The Community Partnerships Group.

Vinson, N., Brannan, A. M., Baughman, L., Wilce, M., & Gawron, T. (2001). The system-of-care model: Implementation in 27 communities. *Journal of Emotional and Behavioral Disorders, 9,* 30–42.

Cross-Agency Data Integration Strategies for Evaluating Systems of Care

CHAPTER 9

Steven M. Banks, John A. Pandiani, Monica M. Simon, and Nancy J. Nagel

Over the past decade, increasing demands for program accountability and the requirements of fee-for-service reimbursement systems have led to the creation of client- and service-level data sets in human service agencies at the local, state, and national levels. Inexpensive data processing and storage currently make it possible for even small organizations to maintain comprehensive databases. The same technology, in conjunction with user-friendly analytical software, makes it possible for program evaluators, researchers, and administrators to access and analyze these comprehensive data sets.

Historically, the wealth of information contained in these data systems has had only limited utilization for program evaluation. The field has had only a few limited models to follow on how to use administrative data sets to answer questions about the availability, access, cost, and effectiveness of services. Traditional research methods that were taught to a generation of evaluation researchers focused on instrumentation, sampling, and data collection because they were developed in an age of information scarcity. These issues are not a primary concern in the analysis of comprehensive administrative data sets in the new age of data abundance. Issues of concern to analysts of administrative and operational data sets are more likely to focus on linking data sets, longitudinal analysis, and data aggregation.

This chapter will illustrate the utility of a virtual management information system (virtual MIS) approach to evaluating behavioral health-care programs and systems of care (Pandiani, 2000b). Traditional approaches to evaluation and research relied heavily on special purpose data collection efforts (e.g., consumer surveys, case manager reports). More recently these approaches have been augmented by attempts to build massive human services and health-care data sets based on unique person identifiers. A virtual MIS uses a different approach. It integrates extracts from existing administrative databases that are maintained by state agencies to address a specific research/evaluation question.

A number of treatment outcomes for children and adolescents have been measured using this approach. For example, rates of incarceration have been measured for young men served by children's mental health, social services, and special education programs (Pandiani, Schacht, & Banks, 2001). The virtual MIS comes into existence when data from these child-serving agencies are brought together with data maintained by the state correctional authority. Maternity rates for female clients of these same agencies were measured by bringing data from vital records databases together with data from the child-serving agencies. Numerous other aspects of system and program performance have been measured in similar ways.

There are three key elements to the virtual MIS. The first is to break free from the data collection reflex (the habit of approaching every research question as if it required new data collection) that is the legacy of research and evaluation paradigms developed in an era of information scarcity. In today's era of data abundance, most research and evaluation questions can be answered by bringing existing data sets together. The second key is the adoption of systems perspective to program evaluation. The virtual MIS tells you *how many* children and adolescents had specified outcomes; it does *not* tell you *who*. Program evaluators do not need to know who experienced the positive or negative outcomes under evaluation. They need to know how many. The virtual MIS does not support clinical and billing functions that require unique personal identifiers. It does, however, provide powerful measures of program and service system performance without additional data collection and without raising issues regarding the confidentiality of medical records. The third key is the statistical technology of probabilistic population estimation (Banks & Pandiani, 2001). This technology provides precise estimates of the number of people shared across data sets that do not share unique person identifiers. These estimates are based on a statistical comparison of the distribution of dates of birth observed in a data set with the distribution of dates of birth that is expected based on knowledge of the distribution of dates of birth in the general population. Probabilistic population estimation will be described in more detail later. Most questions about treatment outcomes are questions about caseload overlap—the number of people shared by data sets—and can be answered by applying this statistical technique to anonymous data sets.

The virtual MIS approach that will be used in the case studies in this chapter has a number of advantages over traditional approaches. First, because it does not rely on personally identifying information, the confidentiality of medical records is protected (Pandiani, Banks, & Schacht, 1998a). Second, because it relies on existing data resources, it is possible to compare past program performance to current performance. The impact of changes in systems of care, such as funding levels and treatment approaches, can be evaluated in a way that is impossible using special or single purpose data collection that begins about the time the change is being implemented. Third, because the existing databases used in these analyses are comprehensive, they provide measures of the indicator under examination for the general population as well as for the population of service recipients. The combination of general population measures with the same measures for service recipients allows for the determination of relative risk associated with mental health needs. Finally, because the virtual MIS relies on existing data resources, it produces measures of program performance much more quickly and economically than traditional approaches.

This approach to outcome measurement has two additional advantages over methodologies based on self-reports or clinician reports. First, issues of respondents' willingness or ability to provide valid information are avoided because authoritative records from official databases are used in the calculations. Second, critical events (e.g., hospitalization, incarceration, death) that occur after the termination of treatment can be measured; traditional MIS systems tend to collect information regarding only active clients. In every application described in this chapter, critical indicators of service system performance are produced without special purpose data collection and without threat to the personal privacy of individuals and the confidentiality of medical records.

MEASURES OF PROGRAM PERFORMANCE

Conceptually, measures of program performance can be divided into three categories: measures of access to care, measures of practice patterns, and measures of treatment outcomes. The distinction among these categories is more a matter of the relative time than of the content of the observation. Treatment outcomes can be conceptualized as things that occur after treatment, whereas measures of access to care tend to focus on things that come before treatment. Practice patterns are those things that are part of the treatment process.

Admission to a hospital, for example, in and of itself does not necessarily belong exclusively to any one of these domains. Rates of admission to a hospital *after community treatment* are measures of poor treatment outcomes. In this example, the hospitalization rate is calculated as a percentage of the people previously served by the community-based child-serving agency. Hospitalization rates can also provide an important measure of access to care when the focus is on episodes of hospitalization that occur before community treatment. Here access rates are calculated by dividing the number of people entering treatment after hospitalization by the total number of people discharged from inpatient care and expressing the results as a percentage of all people discharged during the earlier period. Finally, hospitalization during the same period of time as community-based care can be thought of as a measure of practice patterns. Here hospitalization is thought of as part of the treatment process and is usually expressed as a percentage of the total number of people receiving community treatment. In every case, the temporal relationship between events and the way the indicator is conceptualized are key to categorizing the indicator as a measure of access to care, practice patterns, or treatment outcome.

Access to Care

Mental health program administrators are increasingly called upon to provide information to both consumers and funding agencies on the level of access provided by their own programs and by their contracted organizations.

Boyle and Callahan (1995) identified access to care as one of the core ethical concerns regarding behavioral health care. Valid and reliable quantitative indicators of the level of access to care can provide a very powerful measure of the performance of child-serving agencies.

In this chapter, we describe an approach that overcomes two core problems in measuring access to care: the complexity of service delivery systems and the lack of common person identifiers across service sectors and providers. The lack of common identifiers is no longer a problem, and the complexity problem is greatly simplified when the statistical method of probabilistic population estimation is applied to existing data sets. The application of this technology to the measurement of access to care has been illustrated in a number of recent studies (Banks & Pandiani, 1998; Pandiani, Banks, Bramley, Pomeroy, & Simon, 2002; Pandiani, Banks, & Gauvin, 1997). The first case study in this chapter provides an example of a measure of access to children's services in a statewide system of care in Vermont.

Practice Patterns

Most services research focuses on issues regarding the treatment process. Such research may focus on the amount and type of service provided or received (e.g., out-of-home placement, medication, wraparound, multisystemic therapy), degree of adherence to clinical practice guidelines, and consumers' perceptions of the appropriateness and the effectiveness of services. This research tends to be clinical in nature and orientation.

A broader, systems-oriented approach to research on practice patterns in children's systems of care is provided by a study of the degree of caseload integration across child-serving agencies (Pandiani, Banks, & Schacht, 1999). This study measured the degree of shared responsibility for children and adolescents among three child-serving agencies (community mental health, child protection, and special education) over a 4-year period. The results indicate that there is a great deal of variation in caseload integration among regions in a statewide system of care. The amount of caseload integration varies with levels of funding of mental health programs. Variation in service system integration (a practice pattern) is related to a number of important treatment outcomes (e.g., rates of out-of-home placement, criminal justice involvement; Pandiani, Banks, & Schacht, 2001). The second case study in this chapter provides an example of the use of this measure of practice patterns in Colorado.

Treatment Outcomes

The past decade has seen increasing interest in the development of standardized measures of treatment outcomes that can be used to evaluate community mental health program performance (American College of Mental Health

Administration, 2001; Kramer, Daniels, & Mahesh, 1995; Mental Health Statistics Improvement Project, 1996; National Association of State Mental Health Program Directors, 1998). Prominent among the proposed measures of treatment outcomes are rates of hospitalization, incarceration, and mortality subsequent to treatment. More positive measures, such as high school graduation and employment rates for children and adolescents, are frequently mentioned as well.

We have used existing data resources to measure a wide range of treatment outcomes for recipients of mental health services. These studies indicated that adult recipients of mental health services are at an elevated risk of incarceration (Pandiani, Banks, Clements, & Schacht, 2000) and mortality (Pandiani, Banks, Bramley, & Moore, 2002). Risk of hospitalization for adults decreases when clients in community programs are treated in conformity to practice guidelines (Banks et al., 1998). Youthful recipients of community mental health services are at elevated risk of trouble with the law and maternity, but the relative risk decreases over time (Pandiani, Schacht, & Banks, 2001).

The third and fourth case studies in this chapter provide examples of outcome measures for children and adolescents. The third case study focuses on school performance in Vermont. The fourth case study focuses on youth involved in the legal system in the Tampa Bay area of Florida.

METHOD

There are three approaches to determining the number of people shared across different data sets. Direct record linkage, the most widely used approach, relies on unique person identifiers that are shared across data sets to determine the number of people in both data sets (i.e., caseload overlap). The second method uses constructed identifiers to approximate unique person identifiers by pooling semi-unique attributes of people. Finally, probabilistic population estimation measures caseload overlap, without personal identifiers, using calculations based on probability theory. Each approach is described in this section.

Direct Record Linkage

Direct record linkage relies on preexisting unique identifiers, such as Social Security number, Medicaid number, driver's license number, or any other person identifiers that are contained across multiple data sets. Caseload overlap is determined by linking records from two (or more) data sets that contain the same person and counting the number of identifiers that appear in both (or all) data sets.

Direct record linkage is considered by many to be the gold standard for measuring the number of people occurring in multiple data sets (i.e., caseload overlap). In addition to providing measures of the magnitude of caseload overlap, direct record linkage also identifies the individuals who appear in multiple data sets. Direct record linkage technology, however, assumes that no identifier is used by more than one person and no person has more than one identifier—one Social Security number per person, for example. In the real world, there are conditions under which these assumptions are violated. Direct record linkage also raises issues of personal privacy and the confidentiality of medical records. The U.S. General Accounting Office report on record linkage and privacy (U.S. GAO, 2001) provides an excellent overview of methods for reducing threats to privacy while using direct record linkage such as data masking, list inflation, and third-party vendors. Another major disadvantage of unique identifiers systems is the cost and time required to build these systems and the continuing cost and time required to ensure that all individuals are assigned one, and only one, unique identifier.

Constructed Identifiers

Constructed identifiers use combinations of personal attributes, such as name fragment, date of birth, race/ethnicity, and gender, to build pseudo-unique person identifiers. The unique identifier used by the State of Vermont for the federal substance abuse treatment episode data set (TEDS) uses a constructed identifier that includes the first three letters of the client's first name, the first three letters of the client's mother's maiden name, and the client's date of birth. Caseload overlap is determined by linking records from two (or more) person-level data sets and counting the number of identifiers that appear in both (or all) data sets based on the occurrence of identical constructed identifiers. This method has the advantage of being based on widely available data items that exist in multiple data sets.

There are two risks associated with using constructed identifiers for record linkage. Constructed identifiers can link records for different people (false positive) or can fail to link records for the same individual (false negative). The risk of each type of error changes with the number of data elements used in the constructed identifier. The frequency of the false positives can be understood based on the probability of coincidences (Diaconis & Mosteller, 1989). This mathematical observation shows that when two data sets include a large number of individuals, each of whom has a small probability of falsely matching, there is a high probability of false matches for the group as a whole. Constructed identifiers based on fewer data elements (e.g., date of birth and gender only) are likely to produce false positive matches in data sets with more than 40,000 people.

The frequency of false negatives can be understood using the volatility of name fragments as an example. Names frequently have a number of forms (Robert/Bob for instance) and may change over time (marriage, divorce, etc.). Constructed identifiers based on larger numbers of data elements (e.g., the previously mentioned TEDS identifier, which includes name fragments) fail to link records from two data sets that describe the same individuals at an uncertain rate. The utility of constructed identifiers is related to the relative benefits and detriments associated with the inclusion of different numbers and different types of data elements in the constructed identifier.

Probabilistic Population Estimation

Probabilistic population estimation is a statistical procedure for measuring the number of people represented in data sets that do not share unique person identifiers (Banks & Pandiani, 2001; Pandiani & Banks, 2002). Probabilistic population estimation reports how many people are represented in both databases but does not reveal who the people are. For this reason, probabilistic population estimation is not suitable for clinical and case management applications that require the identification of individuals.

Probabilistic population estimation has three important advantages. First, the personal privacy of individuals and the confidentiality of medical records are assured because probabilistic population estimation does not depend upon information that identifies specific individuals. Second, because the method relies on existing databases, it does not require the commitment of substantial amounts of staff time or financial resources to collect new data. Finally, probabilistic population estimation can support evaluation of changes in systems of care that have occurred in the past and provide longitudinal baseline data for evaluating current or anticipated changes in systems of care wherever basic client information resides in electronic databases.

The Mathematics of Probabilistic Population Estimation

Probabilistic population estimation allows researchers, policy analysts, and evaluators to answer two basic questions that have frequently remained unanswered because existing data sets lack unique person identifiers across organizations and service sectors: How many people have contact with a service system? and How many people are served by more than one organization, service sector, or service system? Probabilistic population estimation provides answers to these questions by combining information on the distribution of dates of birth in data sets with information on the distribution of dates of birth in the general population to produce valid and reliable estimates of the number of people represented. The ability of this statistic to provide probabilistic estimates (with known confidence intervals) of these basic parameters of service systems is particularly valuable where issues of confidentiality or organizational complexity limit the availability of unique identifiers or where the lack of adequate financial resources inhibits the development of comprehensive integrated data warehouses.

Probabilistic population estimation is derived from the solution to the classic mathematical "coupon collector" problem (Feller, 1957). The solution to the original coupon collector problem answers the question, How many baseball cards must a collector collect to obtain a complete set of cards, when the probability of every card being in a given bubble gum package is known? In the current application, the same logic is used to answer two questions: How many unique individuals are represented in a data set that does not include a unique person identifier? and How many unique individuals are shared by data sets that do not include common person identifiers?

Determining Population Size

The number of individuals represented in a data set that does not include unique person identifiers can be determined by

$$P_j(l_j) = \sum_{i=1}^{l} \frac{365}{365-i}$$

where j represents a distinct gender/year of birth cohort and i is the number of observed birth dates within that cohort.

For example, if 231 dates of birth were represented in a data set of mental health service recipients who were male children born in 1975, the procedures described in the previous equation would indicate that 367 unique individuals were represented in that data set. Similarly, if a data set containing information on incarceration for a subsequent year with information on all men born in the same year included 280 dates of birth, that data set would represent 533 unique individuals.

Table 9.1 provides an example of the accuracy and the precision of estimates of population size that are provided by probabilistic population estimation. This table shows the number of people who were served by each of the 10 regional community mental health children's services programs in the State of Vermont during fiscal years 1997 and 1998. These person counts are determined by counting the unique identification numbers that were assigned by the local agency to each person who was served. Table 9.1 also includes the probabilistic estimate (with 95% confidence intervals) of the number of people served by each of these programs during each of these years. In this example, the probabilistic estimate fell within $\pm1\%$ of the true value in 15 out of 20 cases. The 95% confidence interval of the estimate included the true value in 18 out of the 20 cases. In a large number of applications, the 95% confidence interval will include the true value in 19 out of 20 cases.

Determining Population Overlap

To determine the number of children and adolescents shared across data sets that do not include a common person identifier, the sizes of three populations are determined and the results are compared. First, the number of young people represented in each of the original data sets is determined. In this case, the original data sets are the set that describes all community mental health

TABLE 9.1

Actual Counts and Probabilistic Estimates of Population Size
for the Number of Children Served by Mental Health Programs
in Vermont During Fiscal Years 1997 and 1998

Region	People Served	Probabilistic Estimate	95% CI	Accuracy Difference	Accuracy Within 95%
1997					
Chittenden	1,030	1,035.6	(1,020.6–1,050.6)	+0.5%	Yes
Southeast	1,435	1,406.6	(1,386.7–1,426.6)	−2.0%	Yes
Northeast	867	876.9	(863.6–890.3)	+1.1%	Yes
Rutland	693	690.0	(680.6–699.5)	−0.4%	Yes
Washington	560	560.3	(553.3–567.3)	+0.1%	Yes
Franklin	520	517.7	(510.3–525.1)	−0.5%	Yes
Addison	683	682.6	(673.7–691.5)	−0.1%	Yes
Bennington	474	475.2	(468.2–482.2)	+0.3%	Yes
Orange	523	524.3	(517.0–531.5)	+0.2%	Yes
Lamoille	203	203.6	(200.4–206.7)	+0.3%	Yes
1998					
Chittenden	1,027	1,020.8	(1,006.0–1,035.7)	−0.6%	Yes
Southeast	1,360	1,352.5	(1,333.3–1,371.7)	−0.06%	Yes
Northeast	967	984.9	(970.4–999.5)	+1.9%	No
Rutland	618	618.9	(610.2–627.6)	+0.1%	Yes
Washington	516	502.8	(496.3–509.4)	−2.6%	No
Franklin	484	481.3	(474.3–488.3)	−0.6%	Yes
Addison	641	633.9	(625.4–642.4)	−1.1%	Yes
Bennington	455	455.7	(448.9–462.6)	+0.2%	Yes
Orange	542	542.5	(534.6–550.4)	+0.1%	Yes
Lamoille	224	223.9	(220.5–227.3)	0.0%	Yes

clients for the base period and the data set that describes all individuals in
correctional facilities during the follow-up period. Second, these two data sets
are combined, and the number of unique individuals represented in this third
population is determined.

The number of people shared by the two data sets is the number of former clients of children's services programs who were incarcerated during the
follow-up period. Mathematically, the number of people who are shared by the
two data sets is the difference between the sum of the numbers of people represented in the two original data sets and the number of people represented
in the combined data set. In terms of mathematical set theory (Whitehead &
Russell, 1927), the size of the intersection of two sets ($A \cap B$) is the difference

between the sum of the sizes of the two sets $(A + B)$ and the size of the union of the two sets $(A \cup B)$:

$$(A \cap B) = A + B - (A \cup B)$$

The size of the two original data sets and the size of the combined data set may be determined using the probabilistic population estimation as described previously.

In the hypothetical example introduced previously, there were 231 dates of birth (representing $367[\pm]$ young people) in the mental health data set and 280 dates of birth (representing $533[\pm]$ individuals) in the corrections data set. (In the interest of readability, all estimates of caseload size and overlap will be accompanied by the symbol $[\pm]$ to indicate the associated uncertainty. Precise 95% confidence intervals are provided in the tables.) When the two data sets were merged, the combined data set contained 324 unique dates of birth. Probabilistic population estimation indicates that 802 individuals are represented in this combined data set. The overlap is the difference between the sum of the numbers of people in the two original data sets (900) and the number of people in the combined data set (802). In this hypothetical example, $98(\pm)$ of the total $367(\pm)$ youth, or 27%, who had been served by the children's mental health programs were later incarcerated.

Table 9.2 provides an example of the accuracy and the precision of estimates of population overlap that are provided by probabilistic population estimation. This table provides the number of people who were served by each community children's mental health services programs in each of the 10 regions in the State of Vermont during FY 1997 and FY 1998. These counts are based on identification numbers that are assigned to each person served by

TABLE 9.2

Actual Counts and Probabilistic Estimates of Population Overlap for the Number of Children Served by Mental Health Programs in Vermont During Fiscal Years 1997 and 1998

Region	Number Served Both Years	Probabilistic Estimate	95% CI	Accuracy Difference	Accuracy Within 95%
Chittenden	483	474.1	(458.9–489.2)	+1.8%	Yes
Southeast	730	730.0	(710.5–749.5)	0.0%	Yes
Northeast	487	481.8	(468.8–494.9)	−1.1%	Yes
Rutland	316	316.9	(307.7–326.1)	+0.03%	Yes
Washington	293	290.8	(284.7–297.0)	−0.7%	Yes
Franklin	207	209.6	(202.2–217.1)	+1.3%	Yes
Addison	352	348.4	(340.5–356.2)	−1.0%	Yes
Bennington	225	224.1	(217.4–230.9)	−0.4%	Yes
Orange	289	284.3	(277.6–291.0)	−1.6%	Yes
Lamoille	104	104.0	(101.2–106.9)	0.0%	Yes

the local agency. The table also includes the probabilistic estimates (with 95% confidence intervals) of the number of people shared by the two annual data sets. In this case, the probabilistic estimate fell within ±2% of the true value in all 10 cases and the 95% confidence interval of the estimate included the true value in all 10 of the cases.

CASE STUDIES

Case studies of four projects that use data integration across child-serving agencies for the purpose of measuring access to care, practice patterns, and treatment outcomes are presented in this section. These case studies use multiple administrative data sets. Both probabilistic measurement of caseload overlap and record linkage based on unique identifiers are demonstrated. In each case, a research question and a rationale for the investigation are provided. The data sources are identified and the methodology is described. The results are summarized in narrative, graphical, and tabular formats, and a few illustrative directions for further research are identified. In each case, the impact of gender on the findings is examined.

 CASE STUDY I

ACCESS TO CARE IN CHILDREN'S MENTAL HEALTH PROGRAMS IN VERMONT

Research Questions
Two research questions are addressed in this case study: Do residents of different regions of the State of Vermont have equal access to mental health services for children and adolescents? and Do levels of access to care vary among demographic groups and special populations? This analysis was conducted in response to the recommendations of a multistakeholder advisory group (Pandiani, 2000a). For purposes of this case study, penetration/utilization rates are defined as the proportion of a target population who receive services. These rates provide an indicator of access to care (Pandiani, Banks, Bramley, Pomeroy, & Simon, 2002).

Data Sources
Data were obtained from published reports and from databases provided by five state agencies. Published population estimates from statistical reports yielded the number of residents in specified age and gender categories. The state Department of Education provided demographic and clinical information for young people who had an Individualized Educational Program (IEP) due to an emotional or behavioral disorder (EBD). The Health Department's hospital discharge data set provided demographic and clinical information for all young people hospitalized for behavioral health care. The state Department of Social and Rehabilitation Services (SRS), which functions as both the state child

protection and juvenile justice agencies, provided demographic and case information for all young people served. The state Mental Health Division's database
provided demographic and clinical information for all young people served by
mental health providers. Finally, an extract from the Medicaid "eligibles" data
set provided eligibility information for all individuals covered by Medicaid.
The proportion of young people who have a serious emotional disorder (SED)
in each service area was based on national- and state-level estimates obtained
from the *Federal Register*. The number of young people with SED in each region
of Vermont was based on the population and these state-level estimates.

Method

Penetration/utilization rates were calculated for the population as a whole,
for six demographic groups, and for five special populations. In every case,
penetration/utilization rates were derived by dividing the number of people in
the specified population who received services by the total number of people in
the specified population residing in the service area. For demographic categories, the number of service recipients in an age or gender category was
divided by the total number of young people in the same category who resided
in the service area. Similar procedures were used to determine penetration/
utilization rates for youth with SED.

Probabilistic population estimation was used to measure caseload overlap between the community mental health programs and the inpatient, special
education, and social services caseloads because these data sets did not share
unique person identifiers. Where the special population was defined by participation in another program that shared a unique person identifier (i.e., Medicaid), direct record linkage was used to determine caseload overlap.

Findings

Results indicate that there was substantial variation in access to care among
Vermont's 10 regional children's services programs (see Figure 9.1 and Table 9.3).
There were also substantial differences in access to care among demographic
groups and special populations. Overall, 5% of all youth in Vermont participated in a community-based children's mental health services program during
the year examined, and utilization rates for the child-serving agencies ranged
from 3% to 8%. Utilization was highest for youth in the 13- to 17-year age
group: 13% of all state residents in this group participated in the mental health
service system, with regional utilization rates for this age group ranging from
10% to 24%. Boys and girls participated in mental health programs at about
equal rates.

Utilization rates for identified special populations were substantially
higher. Almost half (46%) of the young people discharged from inpatient care
were served by a community mental health program. Forty percent of the
young people with an IEP for EBD were served by their local community mental health program. About one-third (32%) of the young people on the SRS
caseload and 15% of the estimated young people with SED were served by a
children's mental health services program (Pandiani & Simon, 2001; Pandiani,
Simon, & Bramley, 2001). Figure 9.1 illustrates a rating of more than average,

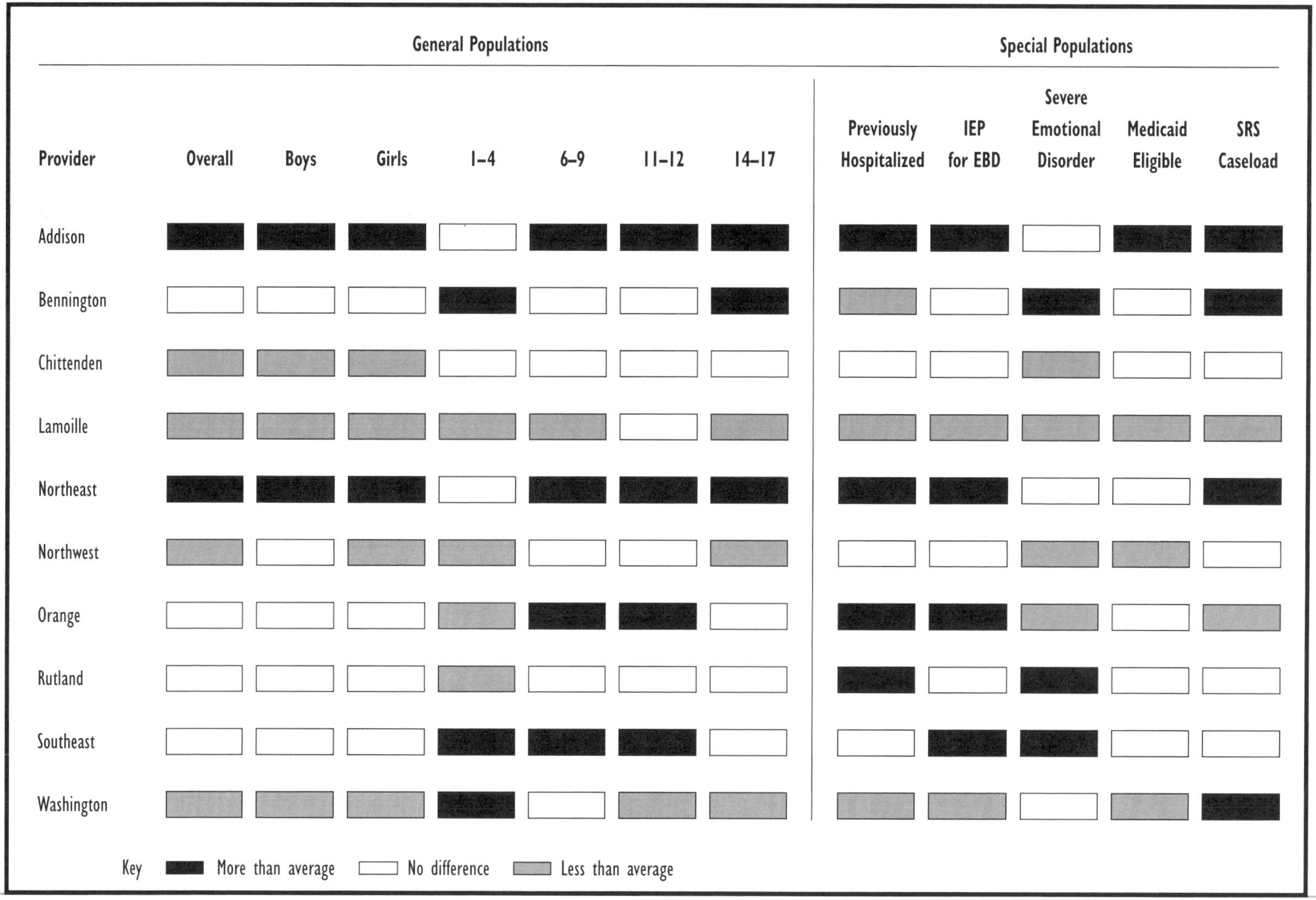

FIGURE 9.1. Access to child and adolescent mental health services by region, Vermont fiscal year 1999, compared to the statewide utilization rate for specific population. *Note.* Differences based on effect size as measured by statistical odds ratios where OR > 1.2 is considered greater than average and OR < .8 is considered less than average. EBD = emotional and behavioral disorders; SRS = Department of Social and Rehabilitative Services.

TABLE 9.3

Access to Care in Children and Adolescent Programs in Vermont During Fiscal Year 1999 (*Percentage Served*)

Provider	General Population							SRS Caseload	Severe Emotional Disorder	Special Populations		
	Overall	0–4 yrs.	5–9 yrs.	10–12 yrs.	13–17 yrs.	Boys	Girls			Hospitalized for Mental Health	IEP for EBD	Medicaid Eligible
Addison	8	1	6	5	24	9	7	50 ± 3	14	88 ± 6	62 ± 3	16
Bennington	5	1	3	3	16	6	5	39 ± 3	24	24 ± 9	35 ± 4	11
Chittenden	4	0	3	2	12	4	3	28 ± 2	10	43 ± 11	40 ± 3	11
Lamoille	3	0	2	2	9	3	2	22 ± 2	3	16 ± 7	15 ± 2	3
Northeast	6	1	5	5	16	7	6	47 ± 3	15	81 ± 6	55 ± 3	10
Northwest	4	0	3	3	10	5	3	30 ± 2	8	49 ± 14	35 ± 4	8
Orange	6	0	5	5	13	6	5	23 ± 3	11	67 ± 8	48 ± 3	12
Rutland	4	0	4	3	13	5	4	33 ± 3	18	51 ± 6	40 ± 3	9
Southeast	6	1	5	4	15	6	5	29 ± 3	20	43 ± 7	45 ± 4	11
Washington	4	1	3	3	9	4	3	49 ± 2	17	30 ± 2	32 ± 3	8
Statewide median	5	1	4	3	13	5	5	32	15	46	40	10

less than average, or no different from average for each of the specified populations in each of the community mental health providers. It is interesting to note that no community programs rated consistently higher than average or consistently lower than average in terms of access to care. No program provided equal access to all of the populations examined in this case study (Figure 9.1).

Next Questions

This case study examined levels of access to care during a single time period. As such, it can lead to important questions about change over time in levels of access to care. Repeated measures of access to care over time can provide a valuable assessment of the success of new initiatives, changes in eligibility criteria, and changes in funding levels. Fortunately, the data used in this analysis are available for several of the past years and will continue to be available in the future. As new high-risk special populations are identified for intervention, baseline measures of access to care can be provided and changes can be tracked on both the statewide and local levels as they occur. Information about relative access to care also provides a context within which variation in practice patterns and treatment outcomes may be understood and evaluated.

 ## CASE STUDY 2

PRACTICE PATTERNS FOR CASELOAD SEGREGATION/INTEGRATION IN COLORADO

Research Question

The research question addressed in this case study is, Does the degree to which child-serving agencies share responsibility for the children and adolescents vary among regions in a state and among age and gender groups? This question is based on the desire to determine the degree to which these regions have integrated service systems that follow the system-of-care philosophy (Stroul & Friedman, 1986).

Data Sources

Data were obtained from statewide databases maintained by four child-serving agencies in Colorado. These agencies are responsible for mental health, child welfare, youth corrections, and special education services for youth identified as having SEDs. Data sets containing the date of birth and gender of each child served, as well as the region of the state the children were served in, were obtained from each of these agencies. Data sets included information on all young people (less than 21 years of age) in Colorado who received services in one of the state's 16 service areas during FY 1999.

Method

For purposes of this study, the degree of cross-agency shared responsibility for children and adolescents in each region of Colorado was measured using the caseload segregation/integration ratio (CSIR; Pandiani et al., 1999). The CSIR is calculated using the following formula:

$$\text{CSIR} = \left[\left(\frac{D}{U} - 1\right) \div \left(\frac{D}{LU} - 1\right)\right] * 100$$

In this formula, D is the sum of the unduplicated counts of children and adolescents served by each sector. Children and adolescents served in more than one service sector are counted more than once in D. U is the unduplicated count of children and adolescents served by any of the four service sectors. LU is the unduplicated count of children and adolescents served by the largest service sector. Because none of the data sets used in this analysis share unique person identifiers, probabilistic population estimation was used to determine unduplicated counts of young people served across service sectors.

The quantity D/U is a raw segregation/integration ratio that is not suitable for comparison across service systems. To provide for comparison across local systems of care, this raw ratio was mathematically adjusted by determining the logically possible range of values for any given local service system and expressing the result on a scale that ranged from 0 to 100. A score of 0 would indicate that no child or adolescent was served by more than one agency. A score of 100 would indicate that all children and adolescents served by any agency are served by all agencies.

Findings

Results indicate that there was substantial variation in the degree of caseload integration among the regions of Colorado (see Figure 9.2). During FY 1999, levels of CSIR, our measure of service integration, ranged from 15 to 34. In every region, there was more caseload integration for girls than for boys, but the magnitude of the difference varied substantially. Caseload integration for girls was more than 50% greater than for boys in 5 of the state's 16 regions and less than 10% greater in 2 regions. There were also differences in the degree of caseload integration provided to young people in different age groups. Eighteen- to twenty-year-olds had the least caseload integration in every region of the state. The differences between 0- to 11-year-olds and 12- to 17-year-olds tended to be small (less than 10% in 8 of the 16 regions).

Next Questions

This case study examined levels of caseload integration in 16 regions in the state of Colorado. Research in Vermont has shown that caseload segregation/integration is related to a number of important treatment outcomes. Similar research in other states could provide external reference points in relation to which levels of service system integration in Colorado could be evaluated. Replication of this research in Colorado and other states could provide an important test of the generalizability of this finding. As the next two case studies will demonstrate, important treatment outcomes based on analysis of existing data sets can be easily measured using the approach described in this chapter.

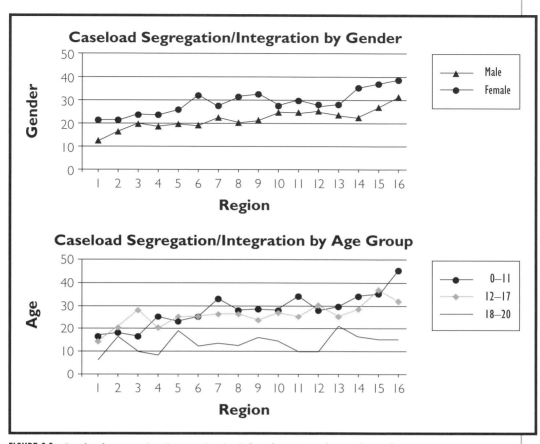

FIGURE 9.2. Caseload segregation/integration in Colorado FY 1999 by gender and age.

 CASE STUDY 3

TREATMENT OUTCOMES FOR EDUCATIONAL TEST SCORES IN VERMONT

Research Question

The research question for this case study is, How do the young people served by public sector human service agencies compare to other students in terms of school performance? This research question is based on growing concerns regarding educational outcomes for children and adolescents. Outcome measures for children frequently include "the ability to effectively fulfill social and role-related functions" (Rosenblatt, 1998, p. 336). It is important to point out that from the point of view of the National Association of State Mental Health Program Directors (NASMHPD), "school performance is not determined solely by the mental health services received" and "mental health service providers cannot be held responsible for school performance." Nevertheless, they concluded that school performance is a "critical objective of such services and mental health services should have some impact" (NASMHPD, 1998, p. 43).

Previous evaluations of mental health interventions and programs have measured school performance in a variety of ways. In much of this research, standardized tests were administered to service recipients to measure academic performance. These tests included the *Wide Range Achievement Test* (Duchnowski, Hall, Kutash, & Friedman, 1998), the *Stanford Achievement Test* (Rodick & Henggeler, 1980), and a number of other standardized test batteries (McConaughy, Kay, & Fitzgerald, 1999).

Data Sources

This analysis used data from four statewide databases. A statewide, standardized educational test score database provided a measure of school performance, and three state agency client databases provided information on recipients of children's services. This analysis used anonymous extracts from the Vermont Department of Education's *Mathematics Skills Assessment* for 4th-, 8th-, and 10th-grade students for 1998 through 2001 to measure school performance. The data from the statewide test score database included scores for all tests and the date of birth, gender, and school for each student who participated. The number of young people represented in these education data sets averaged 20,743 per year.

Anonymous data from the Vermont Mental Health Division's monthly service report database provided basic information on all young people who received community mental health services during the same time periods. The number of young people in the relevant age groups who were tested and represented in the community mental health data set averaged 889 per year. Anonymous extracts from statewide databases maintained by the Department of Social and Rehabilitation Services (SRS) provided basic demographic data for all young people in the caseload of the state's combined child protection and juvenile justice agencies. The number of young people in the relevant age groups who were tested and represented in the SRS data set averaged 312 per year. Anonymous extracts from statewide databases maintained by the Department of Education provided basic demographic data for all young people who were on an IEP due to an EBD at a point in time during the school year. The number of young people in the relevant age groups who were tested and represented in this data set averaged 260 per year.

Method

The relative school performance of recipients of children's mental health services were addressed by comparing the school performance of recipients of services from each of the three child-serving agencies with the performance of students who were not served by these agencies. The school performance of these three groups was compared for male and female students as well as for the total tested population. For purposes of this analysis, two data sets were constructed for the overall educational test data set. The first data set contained all individuals in specified age groups who completed the test. The second data set contained all individuals who met or exceeded the standard on the specified test.

School performance was measured using a three-step process. First, the overlap between the service sector data set and the data set of young people who scored at or above standard was determined. Second, the overlap between the same service sector and the data set of all students tested was determined. Finally, the percentage of service recipients who scored at or above the standard was determined by dividing the number scoring at or above by the total number tested. This procedure was repeated for each of the three service data sets and for the tested population as a whole. Because the education and the service data sets did not include unique person identifiers, probabilistic population estimation was used to determine caseload overlap between the data sets.

Findings

Young people in Vermont who received public sector human services during the period under examination were significantly less likely to perform at or above the standard set by the state for their grade level on the *Mathematics Skills Assessment* (see Figure 9.3). This difference was evident for both genders. There were no differences in school performance among young people served in the three service sectors. That is, youth served by community mental health centers, SRS, and individuals on an IEP performed similarly on the *Mathematics Skills Assessment.*

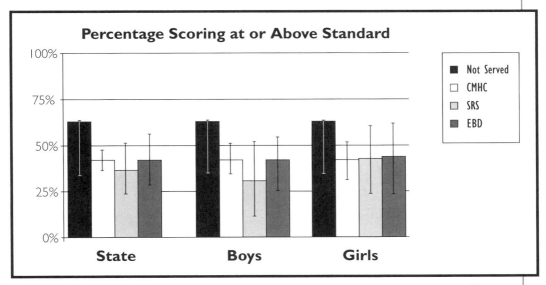

FIGURE 9.3. School performance on statewide mathematics skills assessment; young people served by child and adolescent programs in Vermont during 1998–1999 and other young people, by gender. *Note.* Child and adolescent programs include community mental health center (CMHC), child protection/juvenile justice (SRS), and special education programs for emotional and behavioral disorders (EBD). Analysis is based on data files provided by the departments of Developmental and Mental Health Services, Social and Rehabilitation Services, and Education. Analysis includes individuals who were tested on grade level or 1 year later. Because these data do not share unique person identifiers, probalistic population estimation was used to provide unduplicated counts of individuals shared across data sets (with 95% confidence intervals).

Next Questions

Three important questions are raised by these findings. First, does the school performance of service recipients (compared to other students) vary among regions of the state? This is an important question from a program evaluation perspective. Second, does school performance of service recipients improve over time at a rate that is greater than that of other students? These are important questions from a service system evaluation perspective. Finally, the question of the impact of any differences among regions in the characteristics of the youth (e.g., demographic, socioeconomic) should be addressed.

 CASE STUDY 4

TREATMENT OUTCOMES FOR ARREST RATES FOR CHILDREN'S SERVICES RECIPIENTS IN TAMPA

Research Question

The question addressed by this case study is, Does participation in community-based mental health services for adolescents have a favorable impact on levels of criminal justice involvement? This question is based on widespread recognition that criminal justice involvement is an important measure of community mental health program performance (Cocozza & Skowyra, 2000; Pandiani, Banks, & Schacht, 1998b; Rosenblatt, 1998). There is not, however, a single standard approach to measuring improvement in this area. Improvement might be inferred from evidence of low levels of criminal justice involvement after treatment. Decreased levels of criminal justice might also demonstrate improvement after treatment compared to before treatment.

Data Sources

Two data sets were used in this analysis. Anonymous data sets obtained from the Louis de la Parte Florida Mental Health Institute at the University of South Florida provided basic demographic information on all children and adolescents who received Medicaid-reimbursed child mental health services from 1995 through 1998 in the five-county Tampa Bay area. Anonymous data sets obtained from the Florida Department of Law Enforcement provided similar information on all people who were arrested in the same five counties during the study period.

Method

The proportion of young people receiving mental health services for 1995 through 1998 who were also arrested during each year was determined using probabilistic population estimation. These annual rates were averaged to provide an overview of levels of criminal justice involvement by youth receiving mental health services.

To provide a measure that focuses explicitly on treatment outcomes, the number of young people who had been arrested during the year before the treatment year was compared to the proportion of young people who were arrested during the year after the treatment year. For this analysis, the number of young people who appeared in both the 1996 mental health data set and the 1997 criminal justice data set, for instance, was determined. This result is the number of mental health service recipients who were subsequently arrested. The arrest rate for the Tampa Bay area was obtained by dividing the number arrested by the total number of mental health services recipients. Similar calculations using the 1995 criminal justice data set provided the arrest rate for the year prior to the treatment year.

Findings

The results of this analysis indicate that on average, almost one-third (30%) of all 14- to 16-year-old boys and almost one-fifth (18%) of all 14- to 16-year-old girls in Hillsborough County were arrested 1 year after receiving mental health care (see Figure 9.4). In surrounding counties, the arrest rates varied from more than one-fifth (22%) for 14- to 16-year-old boys to more than one-fourth (26%) for 17- to 19-year-old boys. Arrest rates for girls were lower. In Hillsborough County, 19% of 14- to 16-year-old girls and 11% of 17- to 19-year-old girls, on average, were arrested each year. In the surrounding counties, almost 1 in 10 (8%) of girls in both age groups, on average, were arrested each year. Comparison of arrest rates for the year before treatment with arrest rates for the year after treatment for 14- to 16-year-old boys indicate that arrest rates during the year after treatment were significantly higher than arrest rates prior to treatment in both regions.

Next Questions

A number of questions remain to be answered. First, and perhaps foremost, how do these arrest rates compare to arrest rates for other young people who live in the same regions? In Vermont, recipients of children's mental health services were found to have a much greater likelihood of getting into trouble with the law than other residents, but the degree of elevated risk decreased as these young people grew older (Pandiani, Schacht, & Banks, 2001).

Levels of criminal justice involvement prior to treatment provide a powerful measure of access to care for one of the groups of people who are most in need of services. From this perspective, programs that are serving more young people with a history of criminal justice involvement may be seen as doing a better job than programs that are not serving these high-risk young people.

Further research should also investigate the impact of race and ethnicity on access to mental health services and levels of criminal justice involvement for youthful recipients of mental health services. Types of criminal justice involvement should also be investigated. Finally, more attention to the treatment process could provide valuable information on the relationship between treatment approach and treatment outcomes. This information could help guide practice patterns with high-risk adolescents.

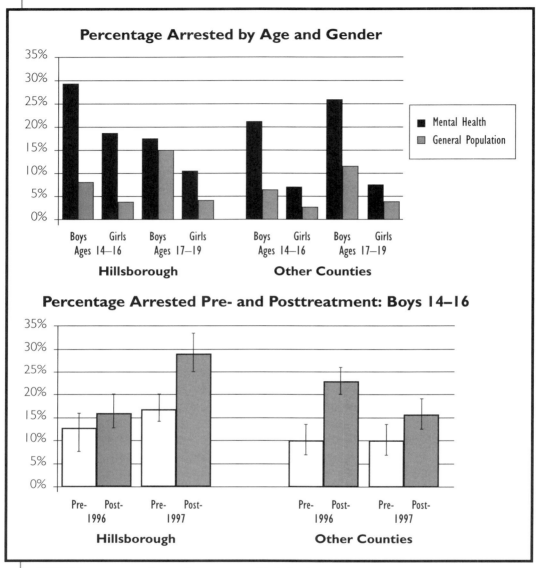

FIGURE 9.4. Arrest rates for youths receiving publicly funded mental health services, Hillsborough and other Tampa Bay, Florida, counties, fiscal years 1995–1998.

CONCLUSION

This chapter has demonstrated an incremental approach to children's services research and evaluation that relies heavily on existing data and emerging statistical technologies to answer questions whose results could guide further research. This incremental approach is designed to increase our understanding of patterns of access to care, practice patterns, and treatment outcomes in systems of care for children and adolescents.

This approach is most effective when it is complemented by widespread dissemination of incremental research results. Such dissemination should be designed to ensure that findings are interpreted from a variety of perspectives and that future analyses are guided by those interpretations. Electronic communications—such as e-mail or posting on a Web site—have made it easy to share findings with diverse and geographically dispersed communities of stakeholders. For example, the findings of the Vermont Performance Indicator Project are distributed to a wide audience and posted on the State of Vermont Web page on a weekly basis (Vermont Department of Developmental and Mental Health Services, 2002). The accumulated findings of these and similar projects can provide the basis for meta-analyses to identify patterns in findings much more quickly than has traditionally been the case.

The next questions that are raised during this incremental process tend to fall into three broad categories: time, space, and the imagination. We have found that explicitly referring to these categories helps to move the process of inquiry forward.

Attention to the dimension of time sensitizes both researchers and consumers of evaluation research to the need to consider the possibility that findings may change over time. Identification of the sources of potential changes over time in the phenomenon under examination can add a great deal to our understanding of the causal mechanisms involved. Attention to the dimension of time also sensitizes the reader to the temporal relationship between factors that are related in the analysis. As we pointed out at the outset, the difference between measures of access to care and treatment outcomes does not lie in the nature of the variable but in the temporal relationship between treatment and the other variable in the analysis.

Attention to the dimension of space sensitizes the reader to the need to consider the possibility that findings could vary among geographical areas or in different settings within the same geographical area. Identification of the sources of potential variation among settings and geographical regions can also add a great deal to our understanding of the causal mechanisms involved.

Finally, the most important dimension is the dimension of the imagination. What do we make of our empirical findings? What meaning do we attach to these findings? The dimension of imagination is also critical to the design of future research. What questions can we answer with the vast data resources and the powerful statistical tools that are currently available?

The approach to children's outcomes research that was described in this chapter also has important implications for the maintenance and use of electronic databases in human service programs. The case studies presented have demonstrated the utility of a wide range of existing databases, which extends well beyond their originally intended use. As statistical technology adjusts to the potential of our new age of data abundance, the utility of data archives will continue to increase. Historical databases will be able to support longitudinal research that will help policymakers and program administrators to better understand the long-term implications of their actions.

Administrative databases, of course, are better suited to addressing some research questions than others. Researchers are limited to the information that is routinely collected for these databases. Some information is collected more comprehensively than other information. Some information in administrative databases is more valid and reliable than other information. Information in administrative databases rarely, if ever, represents the perspective of the service recipients or significant others. The case studies presented tended to rely on data elements that had been comprehensively collected and were the most valid and reliable.

Electronic databases are a fragile resource from both technological and organizational perspectives. Technologically, electronic media tend to degrade. Also, upgrades of computer systems can render historical data unreadable. For many program administrators, the preservation of data archives has tended not to be a high priority. In many states, managers of information systems are expected to keep a close eye on emerging data processing technologies but are not expected to ensure the continued viability of data archives. This lack of attention to the preservation of an increasingly valuable data infrastructure, in conjunction with the Y2K crisis, has put large stores of archival data at risk. Policymakers and program administrators who invest in the preservation of their administrative and operational databases will be making an important contribution to the future knowledge and understanding of the functioning and outcomes of human services programs and systems of care.

REFERENCES

American College of Mental Health Administration. (2001). *A proposed consensus set of indicators for behavioral health.* Pittsburgh: Author.

Banks, S. M., & Pandiani, J. A. (1998). The use of state and general hospitals for inpatient psychiatric care. *American Journal of Public Health, 88,* 448–51.

Banks, S. M., & Pandiani, J. A. (2001). Probabilistic population estimation of the size and overlap of data sets based on date of birth. *Statistics in Medicine, 20,* 1421–1320.

Banks, S. M., Pandiani, J. A., Gauvin, L., Reardon, E., Schacht, L. M., & Zovistoski, A. (1998). Practice patterns and hospitalization rates. *Administration and Policy in Mental Health, 26*(1), 33–44.

Boyle, P. J., & Callahan, D. (1995). Managed care in mental health: The ethical issues. *Health Affairs, 14*(3), 7–22.

Children with Serious Emotional Disturbance Estimation Methodology for the Substance Abuse and Mental Health Services Administration, 63 Fed. Reg. 137, 38661–38665 (July 17, 1998).

Cocozza, J. J., & Skowyra, K. R. (2000). Youth with mental health disorders: Issues and emerging responses. *Juvenile Justice, 7*(1), 3–13.

Diaconis, P., & Mosteller, F. (1989). Methods of studying coincidences. *Journal of the American Statistical Association, 84,* 853–861.

Duchnowski, A., Hall, K. S., Kutash, K., & Friedman, R. (1998). The alternatives to residential treatment study. In M. H. Epstein, K. Kutash, & A. Duchnowski

(Eds.), *Outcomes for children and youth with severe emotional disorders and their families* (pp. 55–80). Austin, TX: PRO-ED.

Feller, W. (1957). *An introduction to probability theory and its applications* (2nd ed.). New York: Wiley.

Kramer, T., Daniels, A., & Mahesh, N. (1995). *Performance indicators in behavioral healthcare: Measures of access, appropriateness, quality, outcomes, and prevention* (Report). Portola Valley, CA: Institute for Behavioral Healthcare, National Leadership Council Task Force.

McConaughy, S. H., Kay, P. J., & Fitzgerald, M. (1999). The achieving, behaving, and caring project for preventing ED: Two year outcomes. *Journal of Emotional and Behavioral Disorders, 7,* 224–39.

Mental Health Statistics Improvement Project (MHSIP). (1996, April). *The final report of the MHSIP Task Force on a consumer-oriented mental health report card.* Waterford, NY: Author.

National Association of State Mental Health Programs Directors (NASMHPD). (1998). *Performance measures of mental health systems.* Arlington, VA: Author.

Pandiani, J. A. (2000a). *Vermont's mental health performance indicator project multi-stakeholder advisory group's recommendation.* Montpelier: Vermont Department of Developmental and Mental Health Services. Retrieved June 17, 2002, from http://www.state.vt.us/dmh/Data/PIPs/pipPerfIndRecs.pdf

Pandiani, J. A. (2000b). A virtual MIS for child and adolescent systems of care. *Data Matters: An Evaluation Newsletter, 1*(2), 2.

Pandiani, J. A., & Banks, S. M. (2002, April 9). *Probabilistic population estimation: The Bristol Observatory.* Retrieved May 12, 2002, from http://www.thebristol observatory.com/PPE1.htm

Pandiani J. A., Banks, S. M., Bramley, J. A., & Moore, R. (2002). Mortality of mental health service recipients in Vermont and Oklahoma. *Psychiatric Services, 53*(8), 1025–1027.

Pandiani, J. A., Banks, S. M., Bramley J. A., Pomeroy S. M., & Simon M. M. (2002). Measuring access to mental health care: A multi-indicator approach to program evaluation. *Program Planning and Evaluation, 25,* 271–285.

Pandiani, J. A., Banks, S. M., Clements, W., & Schacht, L. M. (2000). Elevated risk of being charged with a crime for people with a severe and persistent mental illness. *Justice Research and Policy, 2*(2), 9–26.

Pandiani, J. A., Banks, S. M., & Gauvin L. M. (1997). A global measure of access to mental health services for a managed care environment. *Journal of Mental Health Administration, 24*(3), 268–277.

Pandiani, J. A., Banks, S. M., & Schacht, L. M. (1998a). Personal privacy vs. public accountability: A technological solution to an ethical dilemma. *Journal of Behavioral Health Services and Research, 25*(4), 456–463.

Pandiani, J. A., Banks, S. M., & Schacht, L. M. (1998b). Using incarceration rates to measure mental health program performance. *Journal of Behavioral Health Services and Research, 25,* 300–311.

Pandiani, J. A., Banks, S. M., & Schacht, L. M. (1999). Caseload segregation/ integration: A measure of shared responsibility for children and adolescents. *Journal of Emotional and Behavioral Disorders, 7*(2), 66–71.

Pandiani, J. A., Banks, S. M. & Schacht, L. M. (2001). Caseload segregation/ integration and service delivery outcomes for children and adolescents. *Journal of Emotional and Behavioral Disorders, 9*(4), 232–238.

Pandiani, J. A., Schacht, L. M., & Banks, S. M. (2001). After children's services: A longitudinal study of significant life events. *Journal of Emotional and Behavioral Disorders, 9*(2), 131–138.

Pandiani, J. A., & Simon, M. M. (2001, February 2). *Access to child and adolescent mental health services by the population as a whole.* Montpelier: Vermont Department of Developmental and Mental Health Services. Retrieved June 17, 2002, from http://www.state.vt.us/dmh/Data/PIPs/2001/pip020201.pdf

Pandiani, J. A., Simon, M. M., & Bramley, J. A. (2001, February 9). *Access to child and adolescent mental health services: Specified target populations.* Montpelier: Vermont Department of Developmental and Mental Health Services. Retrieved June 17, 2002, from http://www.state.vt.us/dmh/Data/PIPs/2001/pip020901.pdf

Rodick, J., & Henggeler, S. (1980). The short-term and long-term amelioration of academic and motivational deficiencies among low-achieving inner-city adolescents. *Child Development, 51,* 1126–1132.

Rosenblatt, A. (1998). Assessing the child and family outcomes of systems of care for youth with serious emotional disturbance. In M. H. Epstein, K. Kutash, & A. Duchnowski (Eds.), *Outcomes for children and youth with severe emotional disorders and their families* (pp. 329–362). Austin, TX: PRO-ED.

Stroul, B. A., & Friedman, R. M. (1986). *A system of care for children and youth with severe emotional disturbances* (Rev. ed.). Washington DC: Georgetown University Child Development Center, CASSP Technical Assistance Center.

U.S. General Accounting Office (GAO). (2001, April). *Record linkage and privacy: Issues in creating new federal research and statistical information* (GAO-10-126SP). Washington, DC: Author.

Vermont Department of Developmental and Mental Health Services. (2002). Vermont Performance Indicator Project. Retrieved June 17, 2002, from http://www.state.vt.us/dmh/Data/PIPs/pips.htm

Whitehead, A. N., & Russell, B. (1927). *Principia mathematica* (Vol. 1, 2nd ed.). Cambridge, England: Cambridge University Press.

A Road Map for Cost Analyses of Systems of Care

CHAPTER 10

E. Michael Foster and Tim Connor

Systems of care offer a wealth of research topics and challenges to economists. Although many noneconomists associate economics with analyses of costs and cost-effectiveness, the range of possible research topics is far more extensive. For example, economists have a keen interest in how financial incentives shape the behavior of providers and consumers. A long stream of research has examined the impact of copayments, deductibles, and other forms of cost sharing on families' use of mental health services (e.g., Manning, Newhouse, Duan, Keeler, & Leibowitz, 1987). Additionally, the field of health economics has devoted considerable attention to the issue of how service delivery reflects the way care is financed (e.g., how does capitation affect service delivery?) (Mechanic, 1999). Given that systems of care span multiple child-serving sectors, questions about the way in which providers (and agencies) respond to financial incentives are magnified and multiplied. These issues are especially salient as managed care extends beyond mental health services to include child welfare (Courtney, 2000; Embry, Buddenhagen, & Bolles, 2000).

However, the interests of economists are not limited to matters of healthcare finance. A long tradition of research in economics has examined the determinants of children's health and its link to the "inputs" parents provide either directly (their time) or by purchasing them (food, clothing, and services). The theory of household production examines the way in which families combine these inputs to produce desirable child outcomes, such as emotional well-being. A key feature of this framework is that it recognizes that families make choices based on their children's "endowments" or time-invariant characteristics (Foster, 2002).

Systems of care raise a wealth of questions of interest to economists and noneconomists alike. For example, are school services and mental health services "substitutes" or "complements"? In other words, does using one type of services make others more (or less) effective? This question is particularly salient in thinking about the relationship between services and interventions and whether the latter might reduce the use of the former (Foster, Dodge, & Jones, 2003). In general, this framework shows great potential for thinking about the use of services and for understanding their impact (e.g., Davis & Foster, in press).

A key contribution of research in this area is that it highlights the difficulties with linking families' choices to children's outcomes. Policymakers and

225

researchers, for example, are currently quite interested in questions about dose response—the relationship between the amount of services received and child outcome (Angold, Costello, Burns, Erklani, & Farmer, 2000; Bickman, Andrade, & Lambert, 2002; Foster, 2000, 2003). The economic framework highlights the difficulties in addressing questions like these. When evaluated using the economists' framework for thinking about family's choices, it seems very likely that children receiving different doses differ systematically and in ways difficult to measure. As a result, simple (or even covariate-adjusted) comparisons of children receiving different treatments reflect more than the effect of services per se.

Although the avenues of potential research on systems of care by economists are many and broad, most researchers look to economists to first address questions about the costs of services. Indeed, the first question policymakers want answered is, "What will a system of care cost?" Given how little attention has been paid to the economics of systems of care, costs and expenditures represent a good starting point for research on the topic. Measures of costs provide the foundation for broader economic evaluation and inform critical policy decisions about systems of care. As discussed later, our hope is that research on the economics of systems of care will not end there.

Given that many systems of care are already in place, what information do policymakers and researchers need on the costs of systems of care? The former must determine whether to extend systems of care to new communities and, if so, how to set funding levels. Data on total and per-child expenditures represent a starting point, but policymakers need information on the variability of costs as well. This includes information on the distribution of expenditures across service types and across individuals. The former would be essential for gauging the adequacy of existing service capacity. Information on individual-level variability would be useful for creating reimbursement schemes (such as risk-adjusted capitation) and for determining which children to include in the system of care.

A full understanding of expenditures also requires an understanding of how a system of care affects other child-serving sectors, such as child welfare, juvenile justice, and special education. These sectors represent a potential source of funding for systems of care and, as discussed later, are quite likely to be affected by changes in the delivery of mental health services. These effects are either intentional or unintentional. Either way, a central theme of this chapter is that the true costs of a system of care cannot be judged solely by expenditures on mental health.

Finally, policymakers also need to understand how the impact of a system of care on mental health and broader measures of expenditures depends on community and other characteristics, such as the characteristics of a state's Medicaid program. Because systems of care are individualized and contextualized, this information is essential for understanding how prior research will apply to future implementations.

This chapter provides a road map, or research agenda, for thinking about the costs of systems of care and for providing a research base for policy making. First, we define what we mean by costs or expenditures and discuss how one might calculate them. The next section outlines three sets of questions. The first set involves questions regarding how the system of care affects expenditures on mental health services at both the system and individual levels. The former includes questions about the costs of establishing and sustaining systems of care. The second set of questions involves the impact of the system of care on other child-serving sectors, such as juvenile justice, child welfare, and education (especially special education). The third set involves community-level variations in the answers to the first two sets of questions.

The chapter's next section reviews existing evidence. The bottom line is that very little is known about the costs of systems of care. If we limit our review to studies comparing systems of care to a comparable community representing treatment as usual, we can identify only two studies (and, arguably, one of them does not involve a true system of care). The penultimate section examines the reasons so little is known and the barriers to developing better answers to the questions we identify. A discussion concludes the chapter.

WHAT DO WE MEAN BY THE COSTS OF SYSTEMS OF CARE?

Economists use the term *costs* to refer to the value of resources used in a given activity. The amount and value of resources depend on the perspective from which they are assessed. In general, the question "What do systems of care cost?" should really be reworded as "What do systems of care cost *to whom?*" Possible perspectives include that of the individuals treated or served or of payors, such as Medicaid or other government programs. The costs of an activity often vary according to the perspective chosen. The costs of a service to clients involve any payments they make; for poor families on Medicaid, these costs may be low or zero. When judged from the public or taxpayer perspectives, the costs of the same service may be much larger. For these reasons, the first step in thinking about costs is to define a perspective from which to measure them.

Our focus here is primarily on the perspective of government agencies—namely the state and local agencies primarily responsible for funding mental health services as well as the juvenile justice, education, and child welfare systems. *Costs* refer to the payments or expenditures made by these agencies to directly deliver and administer services, as well as those made to additional providers who deliver services. Per-unit costs generally can be calculated on cost per unit of service and multiplied by the number of units received by a given individual. As discussed later, the latter might be recorded in management information systems maintained by providers, obtained from inpatient records, or reported by clients in interviews. Per-unit costs could be derived from budgetary information or contracts. In some cases, billing records include both volume of services received and the relevant per-unit costs.[1]

It is important to note that supplemental information is often necessary to capture some expenditures. For example, additional budgetary data are often required to estimate administrative costs. Those expenses can be included in estimates of aggregate expenditures or assigned to specific children on a per capita or other basis. In addition, community agencies may contract for some services in terms of "slots," or positions. As a result, they may not record which individuals actually use those services. Payments for those services may be recorded in program budgets or contracts and can be included in estimates of the aggregate costs.

Economists generally favor a societal (or global) perspective that captures the impact of a given program or service on all members of society; when economists refer to costs, they almost always mean "societal costs." When gauged from a societal perspective, costs are best thought of not as payments but as *opportunity costs,* the value of alternatives to which resources used might have been devoted (Zerbe & Dively, 1994). In many instances, payments are a poor proxy for opportunity costs, and as a result, estimating social costs introduces a broad range of additional concerns. These issues are quite common in mental health and in health services more generally; payment levels are often determined through negotiation and only partially reflect the value of resources used (Hargreaves, Shumway, Hu, & Cuffel, 1998). Societal costs also include resources for which no out-of-pocket payments are made, such as donated space or time. From an economist's perspective, the time of volunteers has value in alternative uses and must be included in social costs. Placing a value on that time introduces an added range of technical issues (Gold, Russell, Siegel, & Weinstein, 1996; Zerbe & Dively, 1994).

In the discussion that follows, we recognize that the costs or expenditures we describe could be valued from any of several perspectives. Our goal is relatively modest; we focus on those payments made by public sources and avoid many of the issues involved in estimating social costs. For that reason, we use the terms *costs* and *expenditures* interchangeably, but the reader is reminded that the former really involves costs to public payors.

WHAT WE NEED TO KNOW ABOUT THE COSTS OF SYSTEMS OF CARE

In this section, we identify three sets of questions. The first involves the effect of the system of care on expenditures on mental health services. Included are

---

[1] Even when the focus of a study is limited to that of a public payor, there are many technical issues surrounding the calculation of per-unit costs. For example, the unit of service used to calculate per-unit costs must be the same as that used to record service use. These and other issues are discussed in detail in Wolff (1998a, 1998b), Wolff and Helminiak (1993), and Wolff, Helminiak, and Diamond (1995).

questions about how the system of care affects the variation of costs across treated individuals as well as system-level questions, such as the costs of establishing and sustaining systems of care. The second set of cost-related questions involves the impact of the system of care on other child-serving sectors, such as juvenile justice, child welfare, and education (especially special education). The third set of questions involves community-level variations in the answers to the first two sets of questions. The answers to these questions are essential to understanding the resource implications of existing systems of care and to making decisions about developing systems in new communities.

The Costs of Mental Health Services Under a System of Care

These questions include macro- or system-level questions, such as how a system of care affects aggregate expenditures on mental health services and the distribution of expenditures across types of services. These questions are critical for the program administrator or policymaker who is responsible for the overall mental health budget. The question on distribution might involve, for example, expenditures devoted to care in restrictive out-of-home placements versus that received in community-based settings.

Other relevant questions involve the system of care per se. These questions address the costs of implementing and administering such systems:

- What are the costs of establishing a system of care?
- How does the system of care affect the mix of expenditures devoted to administration versus direct patient care? How does this mix change over time?
- What level of expenditures are necessary to sustain the administrative structure of a system of care once it has been established?

The last two questions highlight the importance of the maturity of the system of care itself. A system of care takes time to develop. Administrative costs may change over time as relationships with other child-serving agencies and collaborative mechanisms evolve. Furthermore, different services may develop or become more widely available as the system builds or stimulates the services infrastructure. Other services may be eliminated as duplication of services is reduced.[2]

Other questions examine expenditures at the individual level:

- Does the system of care increase the concentration of expenditures on the most costly children, or does it spread resources across children more evenly?

---

[2] This question is particularly complex. The environment into which systems of care are introduced is not static. A wide range of changes are occurring, including the introduction, growth, and evolution of Medicaid-managed care. Distinguishing these changes from the maturation of the system of care is difficult.

- Does the system of care focus resources on the most needy? Does the system of care strengthen the relationship between mental health services and individual characteristics, such as symptomatology or functioning? Are the most costly children the most needy?
- How does the system of care affect the timing of expenditures? Does the system of care focus expenditures early in an episode of care? Does it lengthen treatment episodes and spread expenditures over time as a result?

The first of these questions addresses the fact that a small minority of treated children absorb the bulk of resources (Foster, Summerfelt, & Saunders, 1996). The last question highlights the point that both individuals and the system are maturing over time.

The Impact on Costs in Other Child-Serving Sectors

This first set of questions is critical, but a full understanding of systems of care involves its impact on expenditures by other child-serving sectors or agencies, such as child welfare, juvenile justice, and special education. Also included are expenditures on mental health services funded by other payors (e.g., facilities supported by block grants or inpatient stays financed directly by Medicaid). The impact on other child-serving sectors is particularly salient because the system-of-care philosophy presumes that many of the problems that bring children into contact with different systems are related to mental health. As a result, the system of care focuses on children with multi-agency needs and emphasizes interagency collaboration.

Research with adults has demonstrated that the costs of mental illness may be borne by a range of public programs, including criminal justice and various transfer programs (Weisbrod, Test, & Stein, 1980; Wolff et al., 1995; Wolff et al., 1997). Although available research is limited (as discussed later), the impact on other systems for children and adolescents is potentially large as well. Children using mental health services, for example, are substantially more likely to be arrested or otherwise involved in the juvenile justice system. In a study of Hillsborough County, Florida, boys between the ages of 14 to 16 years using mental health services were three times as likely to be arrested as their peers (see Chapter 9 in this book; Banks & Pandiani, 2002). Roughly 1 in 10 youth receiving services from the public mental health system in Colorado were detained by the juvenile justice system in the same year (Libby, Cuellar, Snowden, & Orton, 2002). Similar overlap exists between mental health and child welfare. Roughly 1 in 4 individuals using the public mental health system in Colorado, for example, had contact with the child welfare system during a given year (Libby et al., 2002).

Thus, if a system of care can provide effective mental health services, involvement with and expenditures by other child-serving agencies may fall. In fact, the potential cost savings in other child-serving sectors have the potential to be quite high; expenditures on those services often exceed those for mental health services themselves. Out of 450 children enrolled in a Center for Mental Health Services (CMHS) study in two counties in Ohio (to be discussed in detail later), 28% received services from juvenile justice, child welfare, or special education in the community over a 4-year period. For those youth, the costs of these other services ($22,735) dwarfed those for mental health per se ($9,180).

The potential effects of the system of care on other systems may take two forms: *cost shifting* or *cost offset.* Cost shifting occurs when the source of payment shifts from one agency to another but the type or content of services received does not change (Norton, Lindrooth, & Dickey, 1999).[3] Such shifting can be intentional. For example, the juvenile justice and mental health systems may work together to identify children with emotional and behavioral problems in the former and to offer treatment through the latter. In other instances, cost shifting may involve less coordinated but rational behavior on the part of public agencies. For example, the department of child welfare may recognize that the mental health system is better financed or otherwise equipped to offer care in group homes. This cost shifting may or may not be accompanied by appropriate transfers of funds from one agency to the other. Cost shifting might be driven by consumer choice as well. For example, families of children with attention-deficit/hyperactivity disorder (ADHD) may prefer medication monitoring by psychiatrists (financed through mental health budgets) rather than by pediatricians.

Changes in costs in other child-serving sectors also might involve so-called cost offset. This term is most often associated with medical expenditures (Marketing Department Practice Directorate, American Psychological Association, 2002). In this case, improvement in a child's mental health reduces the need for services in other sectors. Cost offset, for example, might occur if treating a child's anxiety reduces visits to the pediatrician for sleep problems. Cost offset, however, is not limited to the medical sector. Providing better mental health services (e.g., anger management classes), for example, might reduce the likelihood of involvement in juvenile justice.

Variability in the Impact of Systems of Care on Costs

Simply answering these first two sets of questions would provide an ambitious research agenda. However, to provide policymakers with the information they need, a third question must be addressed: How does the impact of

---

[3] To differentiate this concept from price discrimination, referred to as "cost shifting" in the economics literature (Morrisey, 1994), Libby et al. have referred to this concept as "cost substitution" (Libby, Cuellar, Snowden, & Orton, 2002).

care on mental health and other public expenditures vary across systems of care? This information is necessary because systems of care are individualized and contextualized. As a result, systems of care differ in terms of

- the target population,
- the level at which other child-serving sectors are integrated into the system of care,
- local service capacity,
- how mental health services are delivered or configured, and
- the broader policy context (such as characteristics of the Medicaid program).

Each of these may influence the impact of the system of care on expenditures.

Systems of care often differ in terms of the age and the nature and severity of mental health problems among children and youth served. For example, the CMHS-funded Vermont system of care targets preschool-age children (Center for Mental Health Services, 1999; Simpson, Jivanjee, Koroloff, Doerfler, & Garcia, 2001), whereas the Milwaukee system of care targets juvenile offenders. These variations can affect the types and volumes of services that are appropriate and the level and composition of expenditures as a result. Vermont's mental health services thus are more prevention oriented; Milwaukee's services focus more on treatment of conduct-related disorders. These variations are associated with differences in expenditures.

This variation highlights another factor—the level of integration between the mental health and other child-serving systems. Such integration has several dimensions—other agencies may serve as referral sources, they may coordinate services with the system of care, or they may contribute funding. For example, in Stark County, Ohio, child welfare is closely integrated with the mental health system. A mental health specialist participates in the screening administered to children entering child welfare. As previously discussed, such screening naturally has implications for the types of children entering mental health services. Child welfare agencies may refer a wide age range of children who may have disorders related to family dissolution, neglect, and abuse.

The level of integration also affects how services are delivered. Analyses of data from Stark County (described in this chapter) suggest that the use of group homes decreased in the child welfare system under the system of care. The coordination of services may reduce duplication as well. At the CMHS site in Nebraska, both the child welfare and mental health systems were providing case management prior to the system of care. Under the system of care, case management functions were combined in a single position (Center for Mental Health Services, 1999).

Integration also may involve various forms of financial cost sharing. The degree to which these payments reinforce and promote the other forms of integration is a critical research question in this area.

Local service capacity also may affect the impact of the system of care on costs. For example, counseling services may be widely available, but day treatment, partial hospitalization, and other so-called intermediate services may not. Population density in rural areas, for example, may be too low to support such services or may raise the costs of delivering services. As a result, the impact of the system of care may be greater in a community where such services are available and encouraged under that system.

The costs of a system of care may differ among communities even when the same broad categories of services are available in each. Such variation may reflect the fact that those services may be delivered in quite different ways. For example, the ratio of group to individual counseling may vary across communities: the more common group counseling is, the lower the expenditures on outpatient therapy. The configuration of services also may affect costs, depending on who delivers services (e.g., PhD psychologists versus master's-level therapists). Communities also may differ in the way different services are integrated or linked. For example, individuals discharged from inpatient facilities may be routinely referred for partial hospitalization or some other form of stepdown treatment. This linkage may create differences in expenditures even if the array of available services is the same for two communities.

State and federal policies may influence the impact of the system of care on expenditures as well. First and foremost is the influence of Medicaid policy. Medicaid is the largest payor for public children's mental health services, but Medicaid reimbursement rates and coverage vary by state and are heavily influenced by managed care. States also differ widely in their ability to draw upon alternative funding sources.

These factors highlight reasons for and manifestations of between-site differences in the system of care, and all potentially moderate the impact of a system of care on expenditures. As a result, decisions about whether to implement a system of care in a community cannot be made simply on the basis of a single study (no matter how well designed and thoughtful) of expenditures under such a system. A new community is not likely to match any existing system precisely across the whole range of factors that might moderate the impact of the system of care on expenditures. As a result, the experiences of a single community may be a poor guide for some communities. By looking across communities, however, one might gain an understanding of how a system of care will perform in a given community, with its own combination of child welfare, juvenile justice, and educational systems. Answering these three sets of cost-related questions would require an ambitious, multisite program of research.

WHAT LITTLE WE KNOW

Little evidence currently exists for answering the research questions posed previously. That paucity is especially striking if we restrict the scope of our review to studies with a plausible comparison group.[4] If we limit our review in this way, we are left with two studies: the Fort Bragg evaluation and the CMHS Comparison Pairs study. (The latter is part of the national evaluation of the Comprehensive Community Mental Health Services for Children and Their Families Program.) These studies have much in common (e.g., a quasi-experimental design), but differences between the studies illuminate the natural evolution of research in this area.

The Fort Bragg Evaluation

To evaluate the impact of improved mental health services on expenditures and outcomes, the U.S. Army offered dependents at Fort Bragg in North Carolina an expanded array of mental health services; the additional services included partial hospitalization, respite care, group homes, and other services unavailable through care as usual. The Fort Bragg Evaluation Project (FBEP) focused on the experiences of a sample of 984 children living at Fort Bragg and at two comparable military posts in Kentucky and Georgia. Beginning at study entry, participants and their families completed a series of interviews over several years. The first wave of data collection was treated as a pretest measure and used to assess initial (or preexisting) differences. Analyses of these data suggested that children at the treatment and comparison sites were comparable across a range of characteristics at study entry, including demographics and common measures of mental health status. Using data from interviews and administrative sources, the evaluation team described outcomes, service use, and expenditures for these children over time. Expenditures were evaluated from the perspective of the military's insurer (see Bickman et al., 1995).

The strengths and limitations of the FBEP have been discussed and debated extensively in the literature (e.g., Evans & Banks, 1996; Friedman, 1996; Kingdon & Ichinose, 1996; Weisz, Han, & Valeri, 1996). Two features of the study are especially relevant for understanding what it reveals about the costs of mental health services under the system of care. First, as noted, the demonstration lacked key features of the system of care. For that reason, the study provides limited information on the costs of implementing, administering, and sustaining a system of care. Second, administrative data were available only for care financed by the military, so little information was available on services obtained through other means (e.g., out of pocket). (Reports by families suggested that use of services financed in this manner was limited; Bickman et al., 1995.)

Even given its limitations, the Fort Bragg study provides the best answers for the first set of questions regarding the costs associated with systems of care. The study documented that aggregate expenditures were three times

---

[4]There are other studies that examine the overall costs of systems of care and how those costs vary across sites (e.g., Foster, Kelsch, Kamradt, Sosna, & Yang, 2001). These studies generally lack a comparison group or any measure of the costs of services. There are other studies that examine the broader costs of mental health services, but these studies focus on managed care rather than systems of care (Libby et al., 2002; Norton et al., 1999).

higher at the demonstration than at the comparison sites (Foster et al., 1996). This gap was driven both by a large increase in the number of children served and by a 59% increase in expenditures per treated child. The latter was largely driven by longer time in treatment. For the first 6 months, mean expenditures per child were actually lower at Fort Bragg. Furthermore, expenditures at the demonstration were further inflated by the fact that children there received lower-cost services, such as day treatment, in addition to the inpatient services the former were intended to replace.

Project data also revealed that expenditures were concentrated somewhat more heavily on the most costly children. During the 3-year period, roughly 7% and 5% of treated children had expenditures in excess of $25,000 at the demonstration and comparison sites, respectively. This accounts for 73% and 63% of total expenditures during that time. The demonstration also seemed to strengthen the link between expenditures and the need for mental health services (as measured by baseline measures of functioning, symptomatology, and prior service use).

Regarding the second set of questions, however, the FBEP offers few insights because such questions were beyond the original scope of the study. In particular, three features of the study made it particularly difficult to draw any conclusions about cost shifting and cost offset. First, because the demonstration did not involve interagency coordination, the potential for examining cost offset and cost shifting was somewhat limited. Second, no administrative data were available on these other child-serving sectors. The only information on involvement in these sectors was derived from interviews with the study children and their parents. Self-reports of this sort can be a weak basis for assessing involvement in those other sectors and provide no basis for measuring costs. Parent or child reports of involvement in special education may be inaccurate; respondents also may not want to report involvement in juvenile justice or child welfare because of the stigma involved.

A third key feature of the study was methodological in nature and involved large between-site differences at baseline. Children at the comparison site were 50% more likely to report involvement in special education at study entry (Foster, 1998). A similar gap existed for involvement in juvenile justice (Bickman et al., 1995). These gaps are especially difficult to interpret because of the way children and adolescents were recruited into the study. In some instances, individuals were entering services, and in others, they were transitioning between different services. For the latter, it is difficult to know whether a baseline difference represents a preexisting difference or an outcome of the intervention. As a result, it is difficult to assess the impact of the demonstration on involvement in these sectors.

The CMHS Comparison Pairs Study

The system-of-care philosophy is being promoted around the country through the Comprehensive Community Mental Health Services for Children and Their Families Program funded by the Substance Abuse and Mental Health

Services Administration (see Chapter 22 in this book). That program is being evaluated in 67 communities (Center for Mental Health Services, 1999). As part of the evaluation, three system-of-care sites were matched with comparison sites. One pair comprises a system of care in Stark County (Canton), Ohio, and a comparison site in Mahoning County (Youngstown), Ohio.

In these two Ohio communities, 450 children were recruited to participate in a longitudinal study involving in-person interviews. As part of the evaluation, researchers at ORC Macro collected service utilization and cost data describing mental health services provided by the central community mental health centers (CMHCs) in which study participants were enrolled. As is usually the case, however, the data only describe services received at or arranged by the mental health center and provide no information on expenditures by other child-serving agencies. Information on the use of inpatient care also is not available.

As a result, information on involvement in mental health inpatient, juvenile justice, special education, and child welfare services is unavailable (Foster & Connor, 2002). To fill these gaps, service utilization and cost data were collected from the agencies and providers involved in both communities. That effort involved 18 agencies and providers and included services received between 1997 and 2000. Budgetary information from these providers was used to calculate the costs of services received. Analyses of service use and expenditures were limited to the 12 months following study entry to include as many children as possible. (Although children were enrolled at different times throughout the 4-year period, service and cost data were available for at least 12 months for all children.)

Initial analyses explored the first set of questions involving the impact of the system of care on expenditures on mental health services. Analyses of (only) management information system (MIS) data provided by the CMHCs revealed that per-child mental health expenditures were 81% higher under the system of care during the year following study entry ($3,533 vs. $1,954). Adding mental health inpatient expenditures closed the gap somewhat because fewer children in the system of care received inpatient services (9% vs. 4%). After including those expenditures, the between-site gap narrowed to $1,321 ($3,693 vs. $2,372, respectively).

Further analyses of those figures using a reward renewal model revealed that the increased costs of service use under the system of care were driven by longer treatment episodes (Foster & Xuan, 2003). This model involves the simultaneous estimation of hazard models of entering and exiting an episode of care and a model of (log-transformed) costs per episode day. Those analyses revealed that the hazard of leaving treatment among those receiving services was 68% lower under the system of care. (This difference translates into episodes of care that were roughly twice as long as those at the comparison site.) Costs per day of treatment, however, were 25% lower at the system of care, reflecting the substitution of less costly forms of inpatient care. (The system of care had no effect on the likelihood that an individual would enter or reenter services.)

Preliminary analyses shed light on other elements of the first set of questions. Those analyses, for example, suggested that the system of care did not strengthen the link between expenditures and individual characteristics. We estimated regressions of log-transformed costs on age, gender, race and ethnicity, family demographics (family structure and income, as well as caregiver education and employment), and baseline symptomatology and functioning (including school performance). Predictive power was measured using the R^2, which was identical across sites (.17). Furthermore, the system of care had a small effect on the distribution of expenditures across children. In particular, 43% versus 38% of all mental health expenditures for Mahoning and Stark Counties, respectively, were devoted to the top decile of children in each of the samples.

Additional analyses of these data have focused on the effects of a system of care on expenditures in other child-serving agencies. Community data for the 12 months following study entry revealed that children at the comparison site were more likely to have been involved in juvenile justice (19% vs. 14%). Incorporating expenditures in juvenile justice, special education, and child welfare reduced the between-site difference in expenditures to $868 ($5,796 vs. $4,929 for the system of care and comparison sites, respectively). Further exploration of the agency data, however, revealed that past involvement with community agencies was substantially greater for youth at the comparison site, especially for juvenile justice and inpatient mental health services. To adjust for these differences, the authors used propensity score matching methods. When the comparisons were properly adjusted, the between-site difference actually turns in favor of the system of care ($102). This estimate is very imprecise because of limited statistical power. Nonetheless, the figures imply that there was a 65% chance that the system of care actually reduced public expenditures as measured (Foster & Connor, 2002).

The study of these two sites in Ohio sheds further light on the first two sets of questions dealing with the costs of systems of care. Like any study limited to a single community and one system of care, however, it offers no insight into the third question regarding how community-level variations affect costs. Indeed, the expenditures on mental health services reported for Stark County seem rather low compared to cost data reported elsewhere. Foster et al. (2001) reported that per-child expenditures exceeded $13,000 for a 6-month period at three CMHS sites (Milwaukee, Santa Barbara, and Hawaii). Because of methodological differences, this figure is not strictly comparable to that for Stark, but this average dwarfs the figures reported in this section. For that reason, it is unclear how readily the data from Ohio generalize to other sites, where the number and types of children served or the services and policy infrastructure might differ.

WHY ARE WE SO FAR FROM WHERE WE NEED TO BE?

Current research provides few answers to the three sets of questions posed earlier and offers little basis for policy making. This sad state of affairs reflects a variety of problems, such as problems with data access and quality and methodological problems. These problems are amplified as we move from expenditures on mental health services to broader measures of expenditures and, concomitantly, a wider array of agencies. Analyses of data from multiple sites complicate matters still further.

A first set of barriers to assessing expenditures on mental health services involves problems with data access and quality. For collecting data on services and expenditures, several options are available. One option is self- or caregiver report. Such reports are often inadequate for assessing costs, however. Respondents may suffer from poor recall or may never have known the magnitude of payments from public or other sources. A preferred alternative is to rely on the MIS maintained by community mental health providers. Such data, however, pose special challenges. First, the MIS may not include expenditures for services that are nonbillable, such as some elements of the intake and assessment processes. Such omissions are particularly problematic when they involve expensive services or case management, which is central to the system-of-care philosophy. In addition, administrative expenses can represent a significant portion of the costs of serving children but may not be included in the MIS.

MIS data provided by public agencies may suffer from even more fundamental problems of data quality. In their analyses of data from three sites in the CMHS evaluation, Foster et al. (2001) found that as many as 20% of study participants had no records in the agency MIS. This omission is surprising and particularly troubling, given that the agencies themselves recruited the study participants. Still other problems relate to data access. Obtaining appropriate authorization from the client or his or her caregiver may be difficult.

A second set of challenges are methodological: These include issues related to statistical power and to adjusting between-site comparisons for pre-existing differences (unrelated to the system of care per se). Regarding the former, sample sizes for studies of systems of care often reflect planned comparisons of mental health outcomes involving measures that are normally distributed. For those outcomes, sample sizes of roughly 200 per site are adequate. Expenditure data, however, are far from normally distributed. For example, in the case of the Ohio study, expenditures during the 12 months following study entry ranged from $16 to more than $25,000. The figures are quite skewed: Mean expenditures are roughly 70% greater than median expenditures ($2,846 vs. $1,687). As a result, the power of the study to detect between-group differences is severely compromised.

As illustrated by the Fort Bragg study, one means for circumventing this problem is to conduct population-level analyses of expenditures. In that study, many of the analyses of services and expenditures involved data on all children and youth treated, not just the sample of individuals for whom interview data were available. However, such data are not useful for some issues, such as the link between level of need or other individual characteristics (available only in interview data) and expenditures.

Another methodological challenge involves the problems inherent in comparisons of communities with different service delivery systems. In the case of quasi-experimental designs (like the CMHS Comparison study and FBEP), researchers have compared communities with enhanced service delivery with other communities representing "care as usual." The two communities often differed even before one implemented a services innovation. There are various ways to adjust between-group comparisons for those differences, but the different adjustments may produce different estimates of the effect of the system of care. Reconciling the various estimates—and explaining the methods to policymakers—poses additional challenges to producing needed policy-relevant information on expenditures and costs.[5]

In addressing our second set of questions—the effect of the system of care on expenditures in multiple child-serving sectors—these problems all worsen. Issues of data quality and access are especially complicated when multiple child-serving agencies are involved. Negotiating the agreements necessary to access the data is often difficult and time-consuming. The data involved may be more sensitive than even those on the use of mental health services (e.g., child welfare). Some agencies may be reluctant to release data in an environment where lawsuits are common. Combining data from multiple agencies creates still other problems. Data from different sources must be linked, sometimes using imperfect identifiers.

Methodological problems may also be thornier in analyzing broader expenditures. Issues of statistical power, for example, likely will be worse because only some children will be involved in the other child-serving sectors. In the Ohio costs data, for example, 83% of respondents had no juvenile justice costs during the 12 months following study entry. For those youth who did, costs ranged from $63 to $44,601 per child. Expenditures were even more skewed than for mental health services (mean expenditures [$6,738] were more than five times the median [$1,262]).

Comparing expenditure data across sites complicates matters still further. The problems experienced with measuring expenditures at each site remain, but cross-site comparisons raise important issues concerning comparability of methodology. For example, the coverage of different data sources may vary by sites: Child welfare data may include family preservation services at one site but not the other. Unless some effort is made to estimate the costs of the missing services at the latter, between-site comparisons of expenditures will reflect differences in data availability. (Of course, another option is to discard the data on those services where they are available, but doing so may hide a potential impact of the system of care.)

Problems of comparability are particularly pronounced in the calculation of costs per unit of service. Our discussion presumes that per-unit costs will represent reimbursements or expenditures per unit of service. Those rates

---

[5] This problem is also conceptual; in particular, ambiguity often surrounds the term *preexisting*. This problem exists because the system of care may predate the study, and as a result, children and youth may have had involvement with the system prior to baseline data collection. As a result, between-site differences at baseline are difficult to interpret. As discussed earlier, this problem was present in the Fort Bragg study, and data for Stark County revealed that substantial portions of children enrolled in that study had contact with the system prior to study entry.

may differ dramatically across communities, however. One community may include facility costs in the cost per day spent in a youth detention center; in another, those costs may be excluded. (The facility in the former might be new, and that community still may be retiring the resulting debt. The facility in the latter may have been constructed long ago.) Given a focus on expenditures, the resulting differences in per-unit costs are sensible: Expenditures in the two communities do actually differ. However, interpreting those differences is difficult, especially as they relate to the system of care and mental health services. Juvenile justice costs may be lower in one community not because of a change in individual behavior but because of differences in the age of the juvenile justice facility.[6]

CONCLUSION: NEXT STEPS ON THE JOURNEY

Although this chapter has focused on the problems associated with economic research on systems of care, our intention is not to discourage such research. In fact, the environment has never been better for work in this area. CMHS has widely funded systems of care, and policymakers are keenly interested in the cost implications. In addition, although many challenges exist with data collection, agency MIS have never been more sophisticated and continue to improve. Similarly, positive developments are occurring in other systems in response to national initiatives to improve data on children at risk and in public systems (e.g., child welfare; Waldfogel, 2000).

However, the terminus of our journey is to provide policymakers with the data they need for allocating society's resources efficiently and fairly. A fair assessment of progress to date is that we still have a long way to travel. Two steps would move us in the right direction. The first involves improving both the data and methodology used to gauge the impact of systems of care on expenditures. The second involves broadening the scope of our inquiry beyond public expenditures to include a broad array of outcomes for individual served, their families, and society more generally.

Better Answers to Questions About Public Expenditures

As the discussion in the previous section makes clear, the next step is continued improvement in the quality of data provided by public agencies and systems. More powerful computers and more complex software alone, however,

---

[6] This problem points to the reason economists focus on the societal perspective in gauging costs. In the case at hand, the resources used in constructing the juvenile justice facility have opportunity costs. Those costs exist regardless of whether and how the local government is actually paying for the facility. Those opportunity costs are the basis for the societal perspective.

will not solve problems of data availability and quality. The fundamental problem is that researchers often need providers and agencies to collect data in a format and with a level of detail other than what are currently available. Data systems within agencies currently reflect (and constrain) the ways in which those agencies use information. An example involves the services for which agencies pay contracted providers a fixed amount or an amount that depends on the number of beds or slots reserved for that agency's clients. Because payments are not tied to specific children and the time they spend in that facility, neither the provider nor the agency has much incentive to record this information accurately. Such information, however, is vital for answering many of the questions posed previously (e.g., which children are the most costly?).

To solve these problems, researchers and providers need to become partners in developing better data systems. When asking providers or agencies to collect additional data, researchers need to provide a sense of why the information is valuable and how it will be used. Researchers must generate analyses of those data that are useful to the providers as well. Furthermore, researchers may need to scale back their requests for data, especially when the potential size of the expenditures involved is small. Requests for new or additional data need to be assessed in light of the benefits relative to the costs of assembling that information.

Partnerships between researchers and community agencies need to be initiated early in the life of a project and need to be ongoing. As these mutually beneficial relationships develop, the trust that results may eliminate many problems researchers face in gaining access to necessary data. These partnerships also will provide researchers with a better sense of how agencies use the data they collect and of its quality. Only in the context of these partnerships will the potential of large, multisite initiatives like the CMHS system-of-care evaluation be realized.

A second way in which analyses of expenditures can be improved involves methodology. As the discussion has made clear, serious methodological challenges impede the development of a solid research base. In some instances (e.g., developing per-unit costs for services), research on adults or on physical illnesses may provide some guidance. In other instances (e.g., estimating the costs of special education), researchers may have to rely on researchers outside of health policy (e.g., experts in special education finance; Chambers & Hartman, 1983; Hartman, 1983). The good news is that progress is ongoing in many of these areas.

The answers to some methodological issues will emerge only over time. For some issues, researchers in other fields have not agreed on good solutions to the problems involved. In the short term, one useful strategy would be to develop a common economic framework that researchers could use in evaluating systems of care. Even (and especially) in cases where no standard technique or procedure exists, such a framework could specify the approach that researchers agree to use to maximize between-study comparability. To some extent, the basis for that framework has been established in health services research by the Panel on Cost-Effectiveness in Health and Medicine (Gold et al., 1996). The work of that panel establishes a reference case that guides researchers in reporting the results of cost-effectiveness analyses. It addresses a variety of issues around which substantial variability has existed in research practice (e.g., the proper estimate of costs to include in calculating cost-effectiveness ratios). Many of these issues have yet to be addressed in research on systems of care, but the relatively underdeveloped state of research represents an opportunity of sorts. Standards could be established before a wide range of practices develop.

For research on systems of care, that framework would need to cover problems and issues specific to mental health and to areas of overlap with nonhealth sectors. Such a framework might include specific recommendations for calculating the costs of mental health services delivered under capitation or of special education services. The team of researchers establishing these standards clearly would have to be interdisciplinary.

Other methodological problems in this area are not specific to analyses of expenditures and costs per se. As noted previously, comparisons of different communities are essential to understanding the economic implications of systems of care. Better methodological techniques, such as propensity score matching methods (Dehejia, 1998; Heckman, Ichimura, & Todd, 1998; Rosenbaum & Rubin, 1983), are being developed to adjust between-site comparisons for preexisting differences.

Expanding the Scope of Inquiry

Clearly, more and better research on expenditures on mental health services is needed, but expenditures cannot be the only basis for evaluating mental health services (Sturm, 2001). Indeed, it may be rather unrealistic to think that the system of care can reduce total public expenditures. At best, reduced expenditures in juvenile justice, child welfare, special education, and other sectors may only offset a portion of greater expenditures on mental health services. More generally, few, if any, public programs could be justified solely on the basis of short-term savings on other services. Public education, for example, likely would not pass such a stringent test. Clearly, in many realms of public policy, the best way to lower public expenditures is to do nothing.

A complete economic analysis therefore must reflect client outcomes, such as school performance and delinquency. Those outcomes have long-term consequences for employment, receipt of disability services and payments, and future involvement in the criminal justice system, to name just a few. A full assessment of the impact of systems of care also must consider these effects and others, such as the impact on families. The latter may involve lost leisure time or reduced productivity at work.

This discussion highlights the limitations of an economic analysis based on the public (or taxpayer) perspective. A full assessment of costs and benefits of better mental health services must be made from the societal perspective. That perspective incorporates the long-term effects of mental health problems and treatment on family members and other members of society, such as victims of crime.

These effects (and the associated opportunity costs) are difficult to measure and interpret apart from an understanding of the way families adjust their resources to deal with a child's emotional and behavioral problems. As a result, a full economic analysis would be complemented by consideration of the broader range of topics outlined in this chapter's introduction. For example, a full economic analysis would capture the impact of improved mental health services on parental employment. A broad model of household resource allocation would offer some insight into how parents balance their own employment with their children's need for their time. The estimation of the parameters of such a model involving data from one study could be used to estimate effects of a service or intervention in another study where the available data were more limited (e.g., no data were available on parental employment). Indeed, the impact of some changes to service delivery could be simulated even before those changes were implemented.

In sum, the possibilities and potential benefits of the economic analysis of systems of care are large. Our hope is that more research teams will engage economists as collaborators, both to examine questions related to expenditures and to consider broader issues surrounding household production and children's emotional and behavioral problems.

AUTHORS' NOTE

Thanks to Elizabeth Gifford, the staff at ORC Macro International, and the editors for helpful feedback on earlier drafts. Note that all working papers referenced in the chapter are available at www.personal.psu.edu/emf10/

REFERENCES

Angold, A., Costello, E. J., Burns, B. J., Erkanli, A., & Farmer, E. M. Z. (2000). Effectiveness of nonresidential specialty mental health services for children and adolescents in the "real world." *Journal of the American Academy of Child and Adolescent Psychiatry, 39*(2), 161–168.

Banks, S. M., & Pandiani, J. A. (2002). *Mental health and criminal justice caseload overlap in five counties.* Paper presented at the annual meeting of the Research and Training Center for Children's Mental Health, Tampa, FL.

Bickman, L., Andrade, A. R., & Lambert, E. W. (2002). Dose response in child and adolescent mental health services. *Mental Health Services Research, 4*(2), 57–70.

Bickman, L., Guthrie, P. R., Foster, E. M., Lambert, E. W., Summerfelt, T. W., Breda, C., et al. (1995). *Evaluating managed mental health services: The Fort Bragg experiment.* New York: Plenum Press.

Center for Mental Health Services. (1999). *Annual report to Congress on the evaluation of the Comprehensive Community Mental Health Services for Children and Their Families Program.* Atlanta: ORC Macro.

Chambers, J. G., & Hartman, W. T. (1983). A resource-cost-based approach to the funding of educational programs: An application to special education. In J. G.

Chambers & W. T. Hartman (Eds.), *Special education policies: Their history, implementation and finance* (pp. 193–240). Philadelphia: Temple University Press.

Courtney, M. E. (2000). Managed care and child welfare services: What are the issues? *Children and Youth Services Review, 22*(2), 87–91.

Davis, M., & Foster, E. M. (in press). Parental preferences and the mental health of children: Structural estimation analysis. *International Economic Review.*

Dehejia, R. H., & Wahba, S. (1998). *Propensity score matching methods for non-experimental causal studies* (National Bureau of Economic Research Working Paper Series 6829). Cambridge, MA: National Bureau of Economic Research.

Embry, R. A., Buddenhagen, P., & Bolles, S. (2000). Managed care and child welfare: Challenges to implementation. *Children and Youth Services Review, 22*(2), 93–116.

Evans, M. E., & Banks, S. M. (1996). The Fort Bragg managed care experiment. *Journal of Child and Family Studies, 5*(2), 169–172.

Foster, E. M. (1998). *Final report: Benefit-cost analysis of the Fort Bragg longitudinal evaluation.* Nashville, TN: Vanderbilt University, Center for Mental Health Policy.

Foster, E. M. (2000). Is more better than less? An analysis of children's mental health services. *Health Services Research, 35*(5), 1135–1158.

Foster, E. M. (2002). How economists think about family resources and child development. *Child Development, 73*(6), 1904–1914.

Foster, E. M. (2003). Is more better than less? An application of propensity score analysis. *Medical Care, 41*(10), 1183–1192.

Foster, E. M., & Connor, T. (2002). *The public costs of improved mental health services for children and adolescents.* Manuscript submitted for publication.

Foster, E. M., Dodge, K. A., & Jones, D. (2003). Issues in the economic evaluation of prevention programs. *Applied Developmental Science, 7*(2), 74–84.

Foster, E. M., Kelsch, C. C., Kamradt, B., Sosna, T., & Yang, Z. (2001). Expenditures and sustainability in systems of care. *Journal of Emotional and Behavioral Disorders, 9*(1), 53–62.

Foster, E. M., Summerfelt, T. W., & Saunders, R. (1996). The costs of a continuum of care: The lessons of the Fort Bragg demonstration. *Journal of Mental Health Administration, 23*(1), 92–106.

Foster, E. M., & Xuan, F. (2003). *Reward renewal analyses of mental health expenditures.* Manuscript in preparation.

Friedman, R. M. (1996). The Fort Bragg study: What can we conclude? *Journal of Child and Family Studies, 5*(2), 161–168.

Gold, M. R., Russell, L. B., Siegel, J. E., & Weinstein, M. C. (1996). *Cost-effectiveness in health and medicine.* New York: Oxford University Press.

Hargreaves, W. A., Shumway, M., Hu, T. W., & Cuffel, B. (1998). *Cost-outcome methods for mental health.* New York: Academic Press.

Hartman, W. T. (1983). Projecting special education costs. In J. G. Chambers & W. T. Hartman (Eds.), *Special education policies: Their history, implementation and finance* (pp. 241–288). Philadelphia: Temple University Press.

Heckman, J. J., Ichimura, H., & Todd, P. E. (1998). Matching as an econometric evaluation estimator. *Review of Economic Studies, 65,* 261–294.

Kingdon, D. W., & Ichinose, C. K. (1996). The Fort Bragg managed care experiment: What do the results mean for publicly funded systems of care? *Journal of Child and Family Studies, 5*(2), 191–195.

Libby, A. M., Cuellar, A. E., Snowden, L. R., & Orton, H. D. (2002). Substitution in a medical mental health carve-out: Services and costs. *Journal of Health Care Finance, 28*(4), 11–23.

Manning, W. G., Newhouse, J. P., Duan, N., Keeler, E. B., & Leibowitz, A. (1987). Health insurance and the demand for medical care: Evidence from a randomized experiment. *American Economic Review, 77*(3), 251–277.

Marketing Department Practice Directorate, American Psychological Association. (2002). *Medical cost offset.* Retrieved April 20, 2002, from http://www.apa.org/practice/offset3.html

Mechanic, D. (1999). *Mental health and social policy* (4th ed.). Boston: Allyn & Bacon.

Morrisey, M. A. (1994). *Cost shifting in health care: Separating evidence from rhetoric.* Washington, DC: AEI Press.

Norton, E. C., Lindrooth, R. C., & Dickey, B. (1999). Cost-shifting in managed care. *Mental Health Services Research, 1*(3), 185–196.

Rosenbaum, P. R., & Rubin, D. B. (1983). The central role of the propensity score in observational studies for causal effects. *Biometrika, 70*(1), 41–55.

Simpson, J., Jivanjee, P., Koroloff, N., Doerfler, A., & Garcia, M. (2001). *Promising practices in early childhood mental health* (Systems of Care: Promising Practices in Children's Mental Health, 2001 Series, Vol. 3). Washington, DC: Center for Effective Collaboration and Practices, American Institutes for Research.

Sturm, R. (2001). The myth of medical cost offset. *Psychiatric Services, 52,* 738–740.

Waldfogel, J. (2000). Child welfare research: How adequate are the data? *Children and Youth Services Review, 22*(9/10), 705–741.

Weisbrod, B. A., Test, M. A., & Stein, L. I. (1980). Alternative to mental hospital treatment. *Archives of General Psychiatry, 37,* 400–405.

Weisz, J. R., Han, S. S., & Valeri, S. M. (1996). What we can learn from Fort Bragg. *Journal of Child and Family Studies, 5*(2), 185–190.

Wolff, N. (1998a). Designing economic evaluations to measure social costs. In M. H. Epstein, K. Kutash, & A. Duchnowski (Eds.), *Outcomes for children and youth with emotional and behavioral disorders and their families* (pp. 385–424). Austin, TX: PRO-ED.

Wolff, N. (1998b). Measuring costs: What is counted and who is accountable? *Disease Management and Clinical Outcomes, 1*(4), 114–128.

Wolff, N., & Helminiak, T. W. (1993). The anatomy of cost estimates—The "other" outcome. *Advances in Health Economics and Health Services Research, 14,* 159–180.

Wolff, N., Helminiak, T. W., & Diamond, R. J. (1995). Estimated societal costs of assertive community mental health care. *Psychiatric Services, 46*(9), 898–906.

Wolff, N., Helminiak, T. W., Morse, G. A., Calsyn, R. J., Klinkenberg, W. D., & Trusty, M. L. (1997). Cost-effectiveness evaluation of three approaches to case management for homeless mentally ill clients. *American Journal of Psychiatry, 154*(3), 341–348.

Zerbe, R. O. Jr., & Dively, D. D. (1994). *Benefit–cost analysis in theory and practice.* New York: HarperCollins.

The *Service Assessment for Children and Adolescents* (SACA)

CHAPTER 11

A Review of Reliability, Validity, and Adult–Child Correspondence[1]

Arlene Rubin Stiffman, Sarah McCue Horwitz, and Kimberly Hoagwood

This chapter describes the *Service Assessment for Children and Adolescents* (SACA), an instrument that assesses the types of mental health services children use, the treatments they receive within service settings, the reasons for service use, and the quality of services (Hoagwood et al., 2000; Horwitz et al., 2001; Stiffman et al., 2000). The SACA was developed in response to a need for an instrument that would assess child and adolescent use of mental health services. The concept behind its development was to formulate an instrument that could examine service use in multiple settings and the pathways from setting to setting so as to be able to understand episodes of care. The SACA was constructed as a new instrument, modifying the *Child and Adolescent Services Assessment* (CASA; Farmer, Angold, Burns, & Costello, 1994), with additions from the *Services for Children and Adolescents Adult Interview* (SCA–PI; Arnold et al., 1997), the *Referral Sequence and Problem Interview* (RSPI; Weisz, 1996), and the *Service Utilization and Risk Factors* (SURF; Leaf et al., 1996). The instrument was constructed in modules by individual service setting, with questions taken from each of the four adult instruments just listed.

REVIEW OF UNADDRESSED ISSUES, NEED FOR INSTRUMENT

Although the distribution and prevalence of children's mental, emotional, and behavioral disorders in U.S. communities can now be estimated with some precision (Brandenburg, Friedman, & Silver, 1990; Costello, 1989), information about the kinds of services used by children has been largely absent. This gap has posed significant obstacles to the planning and development of

---

[1] Copyright reproduction permission obtained for sections previously published in Hoagwood et al. (2000); Horwitz et al. (2001); Stiffman et al. (2000). Copies of the SACA may be obtained from NIMH, Consortium on Child and Adolescent Research, Room 7167, MSC 9630, Bethesda, MD, 20892-9630.

national, state, and even local service programs. In the absence of information about the kinds of services that are needed or are used, matching of treatment needs and services is attempted in almost complete ignorance.

A thorough review of the mental health services literature identified several uninvestigated issues concerning the measurement of children's utilization of mental health services. First, to examine the predictors of onset and cessation of utilization, services data must be collected in meaningful units (Kessler, Steinwachs, & Hankin, 1980). Episodes of care are considered to be the boundaries for summing all inputs to the care process by specifying beginning and ending points and the course of services used (Hornbrook & Berki, 1985). Second, the literature review revealed the need to examine the predictors of and pathways into, between, and out of mental health services (Burns et al., 1995; Farmer, Stangl, Burns, Costello, & Angold, 1999; Stiffman et al., 2001; Weisz & Weiss, 1991). Third, instruments measuring service use should address the intensity, content (specific treatments), and coordination of care received (Bickman, 1996; Glisson & Hemmelgarn, 1998; Weisz, Donenberg, Han, & Weiss, 1995). Fourth, because few studies have examined how racial identity, acculturation, and cultural mistrust affect help-seeking patterns, these questions need to be addressed in any measurement development (Costello, Farmer, Angold, Burns, & Erkanli, 1997). Finally, the literature review emphasized the need to include both adult and child perspectives, assess lifetime and 1-year use, and disaggregate types of services from provider and setting.

Review of Extant Instruments

To determine whether key information about children's use of mental health services could be obtained via currently available instruments, we evaluated instruments used in recent studies on the features identified in the literature review. The Methods for the Epidemiology of Child and Adolescent Mental Disorders (MECA) service-use questions (the SURF), sponsored by the National Institute of Mental Health (NIMH), could not identify episodes, provide any information on pathways, or disaggregate provider from setting, content, or assessment of care (Leaf et al., 1996). The CASA demonstrated good to excellent adult and child 3-month test–retest reliability (Ascher, Farmer, Burns, & Angold, 1996; Farmer et al., 1994), but in the form reviewed, did not examine the most recent episode of care, disaggregate type of provider from place of service, or examine pathways into care. The SCA–PI, which was developed for use in the Multisite Treatment Study for Attention-Deficit/Hyperactivity Disorder, had no child version, and its 3-month time frame could not address either lifetime or 1-year use. The RSPI details the process of entry into mental health services (Weisz, 1996), but it was not designed to disaggregate type of service from provider and setting or assess the duration, intensity, or content of services received. There are no reliability and validity data available for the RSPI. Finally, no instrument contained a barriers section that covered both lack of any services and unused additional services.

Issues in Assessing Reliability, Validity, and Adult–Child Correspondence

Policymakers and planners are often most interested in those children who use many services. However, it is often difficult to obtain reliable estimates of service for those who are high service users. Without appropriate reminder cues, it is easy to mistakenly include or exclude some of the services received within the assessed time frame or to omit some received for brief periods, thus reducing the reliability figures. The distress consequent to caregivers' attempts to obtain necessary treatments for their child's problems, the pressure on them as caregivers (Angold et al., 1998), and the sensitivity of questions associated with mental health conditions may either sharpen or impede recall of certain services (Fendrich, Johnson, Wislar, & Nageotte, 1999).

Issues of accuracy or concurrent validity in health services research (operationally defined herein as the correspondence between adult reports of child mental health service use and inpatient medical records, outpatient medical records, and school administrative records) have been troubled by the absence of a gold standard or objective referents against which to calibrate self-reports. Assessing child mental health services via adult reports also poses a special challenge. Adults do not participate directly in many of the services for their child, so they may not know about them other than through hearsay. To the extent that adults learn about the services from their children, the reports may not be accurate because their children may not fully understand what services they received or why; the children may have understood what they received at one point in time but may not remember well or may not have the language skills to describe what happened to them.

INSTRUMENT

The SACA begins with a module that gathers data on lifetime and past year use of 30 service settings grouped in broad areas: inpatient, outpatient, and school. Following the initial section, 30 individual modules ask more specific questions about each of the settings. Figure 11.1 shows exemplar questions from the initial module and an individual module. Figure 11.2 shows the flow between modules. Once the order of use of services in the past 12 months has been ascertained in the initial section, the specific individual modules are arranged in order of use (beginning 12 months prior to the interview) to facilitate the unfolding of the respondent's story. The initial section can also be used independently as well as in conjunction with the individual modules. Because the instrument was developed for use across the United States, general service setting terminology is used. To avoid an excessively long

Initial Mode: (first questions only)

Has [child] ever stayed overnight at an inpatient facility such as a (read each and code):

	No	Yes	DK	Col. B Age First Used	Col. C Used Past Year No	Col. C Used Past Year Yes	Col. D Past Year Use Start Month	Col. D Past Year Use Stop Month
SV1. Psychiatric hospital	0	1	9	___ ___	0	1	___ ___	___ ___
SV2. Psychiatric unit in a general hospital	0	1	9	___ ___	0	1	___ ___	___ ___

Individual Module, selected questions only (subcategories and response categories not included here):

1. During the past 12 months, how many different times was [child] admitted to a psychiatric hospital where (he or she) stayed overnight? _____

   A. What was the name and address of the psychiatric hospital [child] was in during the past 12 months (starting with the most recent)? _____

2. How many nights altogether has [child] stayed overnight in any psychiatric hospital since [date 12 months ago]? _____

3. What were the most important behavioral or emotional reasons [child] was admitted to [place in 1A]? _____

4. Who referred [child] or told you to take (him or her) to [place in 1A]? _____

5. Now I am going to read a list of the types of treatments, services, and counseling programs that might be provided in a psychiatric hospital. We realize that you may or may not know whether [child] received some of these. In those cases, it is fine to say you don't know. In (his or her) most recent admission to a psychiatric hospital, did [child] _____

6. Was a set of treatment goals outlined at the start of [child's] treatment? _____

7. You mentioned that [child] is no longer in a psychiatric hospital. Is this because (read all and code) _____

8. Thinking about this most recent hospitalization:

   A. How well do you think the treatment chosen for [child] matched (his or her) needs?
   _____

9. What is the total charge for [child's] most recent stay in [place in 1A]? _____

FIGURE 11.1. Example questions from the *Service Assessment for Children and Adolescents.*

instrument, the amount of information asked varied, with the most detail asked only of the specialty mental health settings and school counseling. The SACA has parallel adult and child versions focusing solely on the service use of the child.

In the individual modules, queries about reasons for seeking service are designed to elicit specific problems rather than global descriptions (e.g., depression) or life events (e.g., a divorce). Questions about specific treatments ask respondents about child-related interventions such as therapy or counseling, medications, case management and evaluation or testing, and family-oriented services.

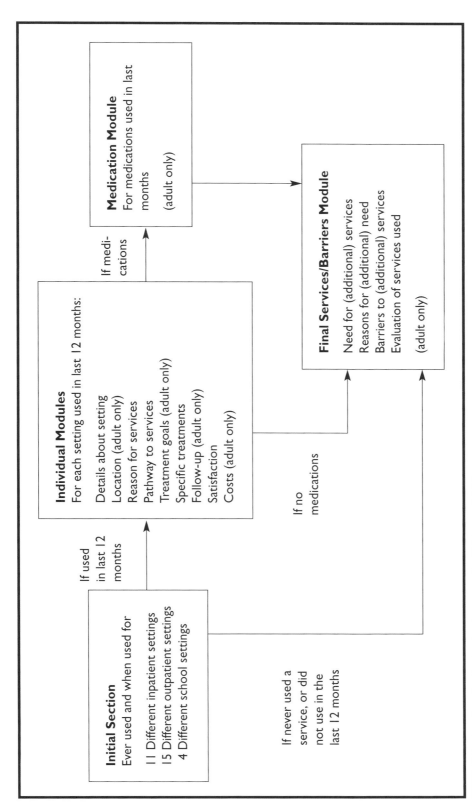

FIGURE 11.2. Flowchart for the *Service Assessment for Children and Adolescents*.

The SACA also contains two specialized modules for barriers and medications. The final services module (barriers) is asked of everyone, regardless of whether he or she reported using services. For those who report using services, a series of questions ascertains the most and least beneficial services, whether additional services were felt to be needed, and why any additional services were not accessed. For those respondents who reported no service use, questions are asked about whether the respondent thought the child needed services, the reason for needing services, and why services were not accessed. The Medications Module, designed for adult report only, elicits information about prescription psychoactive medications used in the previous month, as well as the dose, duration, and insurance coverage for any psychoactive medications.

The SACA child version is constructed in the same manner as the adult version but with fewer detailed questions in the individual modules and without the medication or final services modules. To avoid asking the child about factual items likely to be known only or best by the adult, the individual modules in the child version omit questions on costs, communication of treatment goals, treatment follow-up, or location of care.

New Versions/Uses/Modifications

In the years since the SACA was first developed, many adaptations have been made to the instrument to accommodate the needs of various researchers. It has been translated into Spanish for use in Puerto Rico (Canino et al., 2002), modified for assessing services of very young children by Horwitz, adapted to assess care from informal providers and traditional healers in American Indian populations (Stiffman, Striley, Brown, Limb, & Ostmann, 2003), and modified into a brief three-page version for use as a repeated measure by Stiffman. The adaptation for informal providers simply adds categories of informal providers to the categories of residential care, outpatient care, and school care. The brief forms assess use only within a contained time period (such as 3 months) and add a final column with a checklist of potential treatments received at that service setting (see Figure 11.3). In addition, Stiffman modified the format (but not the questions) of the Medications Module into a single form so that interviewers do not have to switch back and forth between the two original forms, one for the questions and one for answers. No additional reliability, validity, or correspondence analyses have been done on any of these various revisions or versions.

METHOD

Procedures

Data on the SACA were collected in two sites: in St. Louis by investigators from the Department of Psychiatry at Washington University and in Ventura

(*text continues on p. 256*)

Briefest SACA: Answer the next section at each report:

I. In the last 3 months, has (youth) stayed overnight in a hospital, treatment center, group or foster home, juvenile justice facility, or emergency shelter for problems with drugs or alcohol, behaviors, or feelings?

Yes.
No ... Go to II.

Has (youth) stayed overnight in a (read each and code)? If "yes," answer Cols. A and B.

				If Yes: Col. A No. Nights in Last 3 Mos.	If Yes: Col. B Check Types of Services Given:
1. Hospital for problems with drugs or alcohol, behaviors, or feelings	No	Yes	DK	___ ___ ___ nts.	__assessment __individual treatment/therapy __group treatment __family/parent treatment/ed __medication __education/training
2. Drug or alcohol treatment unit	No	Yes	DK	___ ___ ___ nts.	__assessment __individual treatment/therapy __group treatment __family/parent treatment/ed __medication __education/training
3. Residential treatment center	No	Yes	DK	___ ___ ___ nts.	__assessment __individual treatment/therapy __group treatment __family/parent treatment/ed __medication __education/training
4. Group home	No	Yes	DK	___ ___ ___ nts.	__assessment __individual treatment/therapy __group treatment __family/parent treatment/ed __medication __education/training
5. Foster home	No	Yes	DK	___ ___ ___ nts.	__assessment __individual treatment/therapy __group treatment __family/parent treatment/ed __medication __education/training
6. Detention center/prison or jail	No	Yes	DK	___ ___ ___ nts.	__assessment __individual treatment/therapy __group treatment __family/parent treatment/ed __medication __education/training
7. Emergency shelter for problems with behaviors or feelings	No	Yes	DK	___ ___ ___ nts.	__assessment __individual treatment/therapy __group treatment __family/parent treatment/ed __medication __education/training
8. Other: describe _____	No	Yes	DK	___ ___ ___ nts.	__assessment __individual treatment/therapy __group treatment __family/parent treatment/ed __medication __education/training

(continues)

FIGURE 11.3. Briefest *Service Assessment for Children and Adolescents.*

II. In the last 3 months, has (youth) received outpatient help (not overnight) from a
(if yes, answer Cols. A and B):

				If Yes: Col. A No. Hours or Days of Service	If Yes: Col. B Check Types of Services Given:
9.	Community mental health center or other outpatient mental health clinic	No Yes DK		_ _ _ hrs. _ _ _ days	_ assessment _ individual treatment/therapy _ group treatment _ family/parent treatment/ed _ medication _ education/training _ case management
10.	Professional like a psychologist, psychiatrist, social worker, or family counselor not part of a service or clinic already mentioned	No Yes DK		_ _ _ hrs.	_ assessment _ individual treatment/therapy _ group treatment _ family/parent treatment/ed _ medication _ education/training _ case management
11.	Partial hospitalization or day treatment center	No Yes DK		_ _ _ hrs. _ _ _ days	_ assessment _ individual treatment/therapy _ group treatment _ family/parent treatment/ed _ medication _ education/training
12.	Drug or alcohol clinic	No Yes DK		_ _ _ hrs. _ _ _ days	_ assessment _ individual treatment/therapy _ group treatment _ family/parent treatment/ed _ medication _ education/training
13.	Therapist or counselor or family preservation worker who came to your home	No Yes DK		_ _ _ hrs. _ _ _ days	_ assessment _ individual treatment/therapy _ group treatment _ family/parent treatment/ed _ medication _ education/training _ case management
14.	Emergency room for problems with behaviors or feelings	No Yes DK		_ _ _ hrs.	_ assessment _ individual treatment/therapy _ family/parent treatment/ed _ medication
15.	Pediatrician or family doctor for problems with behaviors or feelings	No Yes DK		_ _ _ hrs.	_ assessment _ individual treatment/therapy _ group treatment _ family/parent treatment/ed _ medication _ education/training
16.	Probation or juvenile corrections officer or court counselor	No Yes DK		_ _ _ hrs.	_ assessment _ individual treatment/therapy _ group treatment _ family/parent treatment/ed _ medication _ education/training

(continues)

FIGURE 11.3. *Continued.*

II. *Continued.*

					If Yes: Col. A No. Hours or Days of Service	If Yes: Col. B Check Types of Services Given:
17.	Priest, minister, or rabbi for problems with behaviors or feelings	No	Yes	DK	_ _ _ hrs.	_assessment _individual treatment/therapy _group treatment _family/parent treatment/ed _education/training
18.	Acupuncturist/chiropractor	No	Yes	DK	_ _ _ hrs.	_assessment _individual treatment/therapy _group treatment _family/parent treatment/ed _medication _education/training
19.	Crisis hotline	No	Yes	DK	_ _ _ hrs.	
20.	Any self-help group like Alcoholics Anonymous or peer counseling	No	Yes	DK	_ _ _ hrs.	
21.	Other: describe _____	No	Yes	DK	_ _ _ hrs.	

III. Has (youth) received the following types of help in school (if yes, answer Cols. A and B):

					If Yes: Col. A No. Hours or Days of Service	If Yes: Col. B Check Types of Services Given:
22.	Being placed in a special school for students with problems with behaviors or feelings	No	Yes	DK	_ _ _ days	_assessment _individual treatment/therapy _group treatment _family/parent treatment/ed _medication
23.	Being placed in a special classroom for problems with drugs or alcohol, behaviors, or feelings	No	Yes	DK	_ _ _ hrs. _ _ _ days	_assessment _individual treatment/therapy _group treatment _family/parent treatment/ed
24.	Getting special help (such as tutoring or training) in the regular classroom for problems with behaviors or feelings	No	Yes	DK	_ _ _ hrs. _ _ _ days	_assessment _individual treatment/therapy _group treatment _family/parent treatment/ed
25.	Other counseling or therapy in school, related to problems with drugs or alcohol, behaviors, or feelings	No	Yes	DK	_ _ _ hrs.	_assessment _individual treatment/therapy _group treatment _family/parent treatment/ed
26.	Other: describe _____	No	Yes	DK	_ _ _ hrs.	_assessment _individual treatment/therapy _group treatment _family/parent treatment/ed _medication _education/training

FIGURE 11.3. *Continued.*

County by investigators from the University of California, Los Angeles, and the RAND Corporation. The field-testing was conducted to determine the reliability of the SACA (Horwitz et al., 2001), the differences between adult and child responses (Stiffman et al., 2000), and rates of false negative reporting of service utilization (Bean et al., 2000).

Sample

The study population in the two sites differed in their ethnic composition, the marital status of the respondents, and employment status and income, but they were similar in respondents' gender, relationship to the index child, age, and education (Horwitz et al., 2001).

At the St. Louis site, clinical participants were recruited from inpatient ($n = 88$) and outpatient ($n = 443$) psychiatric clinics of a local hospital. A list of children ages 4 to 17 who had been treated within the previous 12 months was compiled, and all children with diagnoses of mental retardation were excluded. Two other lists were also obtained: a list of children from public school classes and a list of children from a local day care facility ($n = 320$). A letter inviting participation in the study was sent to the caregivers of all of these children. Because a goal was to interview approximately 50% African American children, 26 families were recruited by asking African American study participants to volunteer friends and neighbors. One hundred forty-six adult–child dyads completed the test and retest interviews. Trained lay interviewers administered interviews, and, during the field period, randomly selected interviews (10%) were audited.

At the UCLA site, recruiters hired through Ventura County Mental Health (VCMH) were provided with lists of addresses of households with children between the ages of 4 and 17 selected from the VCMH management information system who had used mental health services within the previous 12 months. The service-using households were approached, screened for eligibility (i.e., language and ethnicity), and, if eligible, recruited into the study. If the service-using household was successfully recruited, the recruiter attempted to recruit a non–service-using household, matched for ethnicity and age group, in the surrounding neighborhood, according to a random approach schedule.

For service-using households, a total of 470 households were approached; 159 were eligible and 94 (59%) agreed to participate. For non–service-using households, a total of 527 were approached, 108 were eligible, and 51 (47%) agreed to participate. One hundred six adult–child dyads completed the first interview and 91 adult–child dyads completed the retest interview. Two interviewer-training sessions were held: one in St. Louis and one in Los Angeles. Training was developed collaboratively and implemented by personnel at the two sites who were experienced in the development and use of the instruments. To ensure complete independence of reports at Time 1 and Time 2 interviews, four different interviewers conducted the interviews for each adult and child pair.

Analyses

To evaluate correspondence between categorical data and to correct for chance associations, kappa (κ) statistics (Fleiss, 1981) were calculated. Kappa values over .75 represent excellent correspondence, those in the .40 to .75 range indicate good correspondence, and values <.40 indicate poor correspondence (Fleiss, 1981). Because kappas are sensitive to small sample sizes and low base rates (skewed distribution of marginal probabilities; Spitznagel & Helzer, 1985), we only interpreted kappas when at least 20 participants reported use of the service. Reliability of continuous data was evaluated with the intraclass correlation coefficient (ICC; Bartko, 1966).

Reliability Analyses

In addition to analyzing data concerning use of individual settings, we aggregated information on use of specific service settings to develop information about *any* residential, *any* outpatient, and *any* school settings, as well as specific types of residential or outpatient services, such as specialty mental health.

Validity Analyses

All contacts with service agencies to collect services data occurred after completion of interviews with the participants. For inpatient services, trained research staff abstracted records of admission and discharge summaries. Research staff also searched outpatient agency records for participants in the study. Data on use of services within schools were obtained through mailing a questionnaire to school personnel, who were asked to complete a brief questionnaire asking about the participant's receipt of specific school-based services.

Adult–Child Correspondence Analyses

Analyses for adult–child correspondence were restricted to adult–child pairs in which the child was 11 or older, because children younger than 11 had difficulty responding to items in the SACA (Horwitz et al., 2001). The reported analyses on these dyads were also restricted to the Time 1 interview (Time 2 data were analyzed, and the pattern was parallel).

RESULTS

Sample Characteristics

Adult Sociodemographic and Psychosocial Characteristics

The study samples in the two sites differed in their ethnic composition, the marital status of the respondents, employment status, and poverty status but appeared similar in respondents' gender, relationship to the index child, age, and education. Ninety-one percent of the informants were women, and 84% were the biological mother of the indexed child. Sixty-four percent were between 21 and 40 years of age. The respondents were almost equally African American (48%) and Caucasian (51.3%). Approximately two-thirds of the adult respondents had more than a high school education, and household incomes spanned the range from extreme poverty (less than $10,000 per year for 20% of the sample) to greater than $40,000 per year (37.3%). The majority of the respondents were married (57.3%), and another 25% were separated or divorced. The mean household size was four persons, and approximately 79% of the respondents were employed.

Child Sociodemographic and Psychosocial Characteristics
The child sample was approximately equally split between the two genders, with 45.3% being girls. Forty-seven percent of the sample were 10 years old and younger and 53% were between 11 and 17 years of age. As was true for the adult respondents, the sample was almost equally divided between African Americans (47.3%) and Caucasians (49.3%).

General Service Use
Of the 237 adult respondents, 164 (69.2%) reported receiving at least one service at some time in the child's life. The majority of contacts were in outpatient settings ($T_1 = 61\%$; $T_2 = 60\%$), with mental health clinics and private practitioners accounting for 67% and 68%, respectively, of all reported outpatient settings in the two administrations. Interestingly, school-based services only accounted for 28% of the settings used in both administrations. The same pattern exists for settings used in the past year, with outpatient settings accounting for the majority of reports of services use ($T_1 = 61\%$; $T_2 = 59\%$).

Reliability

Test–Retest Reliability
There was little change in reports of settings used between the Time 1 and Time 2 administrations (retests were conducted within a range of 4 to 14 days). Further, with the exception of the four outpatient settings (mental health clinics, in-home services, private mental health practitioners, and medical doctors) and two school settings (special classroom and counseling in school), the individual settings for the past 12 months are reported too infrequently to calculate the kappa statistic reliably (Spitznagel & Helzer, 1985). Therefore, all analyses are reported combined across the two sites and in five superordinate categories: any inpatient use; any specialty mental health inpatient use (psychiatric hospital, psychiatric unit in a general hospital, drug or alcohol unit, residential treatment center); any outpatient use, any specialty mental health outpatient use (mental health clinic, day treatment, drug or alcohol clinic *or* psychologist, social worker, counselor); and any school use.

Adult Initial Section Reliability

For adults, both lifetime and past 12-month test–retest reliability figures were excellent, with kappas for data combined across the two sites ranging from .82 to .94 for services ever used and .75 to .86 for use within the past year (see Table 11.1). The initial section showed that the reliability of the overall pathways question was moderate to excellent for the person spoken to prior to using services, but it was poor for the advice that person gave.

Child Initial Section Reliability

Children's test–retest reliability increases by age, with children 11 years and older demonstrating moderate to excellent reliability. Kappas for services ever used, as reported by older children, ranged from .64 to .96, and for use within the past year, from .63 to .77 (see Table 11.2). The results for younger children

TABLE 11.1

Test–Retest Reliability: Adult Respondents' Reports
of Mental Health Services Used by Their Children ($n = 237$)

Use of Mental Health Services	Test		Retest		κ	95% CI
	n	%	n	%		
Ever						
Any use	164	69	164	69	.94	.89 to .99
Any inpatient	40	17	37	16	.92	.86 to .99
Specialty inpatient[a]	26	11	27	11	.94	.86 to 1.0
Any outpatient	158	67	157	66	.94	.89 to .98
Specialty outpatient[b]	147	62	148	62	.87	.90 to .93
Any school	91	38	95	40	.82	.75 to .90
Previous 12 months						
Any use	140	59	140	59	.86	.79 to .93
Any inpatient	17	7	17	7	.75	.58 to .91
Specialty inpatient[a]	12	5	10	4	.82	.63 to .99
Any outpatient	130	55	129	54	.84	.77 to .91
Specialty outpatient[b]	118	50	117	49	.86	.79 to .92
Any school	78	33	82	35	.79	.71 to .87

Note. From "Measuring Youths' Use for Mental Health Services: Reliability of the SACA—Services Assessment for Children and Adolescents," by S. Horwitz, K. Hoagwood, A. R. Stiffman, T. Summerfelt, J. Weisz, E. J. Costello, et al., 2001, *Psychiatric Services, 52,* pp. 1088–1094. Copyright 2001 by American Psychiatric Publishers, Inc. Reprinted with permission.

[a] Specialty inpatient includes psychiatric hospital/unit, drug/alcohol treatment, and residential treatment.

[b] Specialty outpatient includes mental health clinic, day treatment, drug or alcohol clinic, or psychologist, social worker, and counselor.

TABLE 11.2
Test–Retest Reliability: Children's (≥11 years) Reports
of Their Own Mental Health Services Use (*n* = 133)

Use of Mental Health Services	Test		Retest		κ	95% CI
	n	%	*n*	%		
Ever						
Any use	101	76	95	71	.77	.64 to .89
Any inpatient	35	26	33	25	.96	.91 to 1.00
Specialty inpatient[a]	21	16	18	14	.91	.81 to 1.00
Any outpatient	91	68	90	68	.78	.66 to .89
Specialty outpatient[b]	79	59	82	62	.64	.50 to .77
Any school	59	44	50	38	.68	.55 to .80
Previous 12 months						
Any use	80	60	76	57	.72	.60 to .84
Any inpatient	18	14	17	13	.77	.61 to .93
Specialty inpatient[a]	13	10	9	7	.70	.48 to .93
Any outpatient	71	53	68	51	.74	.63 to .86
Specialty outpatient[b]	58	44	54	41	.63	.50 to .76
Any school	37	28	32	24	.63	.48 to .78

Note. From "Measuring Youths' Use for Mental Health Services: Reliability of the SACA—Services Assessment for Children and Adolescents," by S. Horwitz, K. Hoagwood, A. R. Stiffman, T. Summerfelt, J. Weisz, E. J. Costello, et al., 2001, *Psychiatric Services, 52,* pp. 1088–1094. Copyright 2001 by American Psychiatric Publishers, Inc. Reprinted with permission.

[a] Specialty inpatient includes psychiatric hospital/unit, drug/alcohol treatment, and residential treatment.

[b] Specialty outpatient includes mental health clinic, day treatment, drug or alcohol clinic, or psychologist, social worker, and counselor.

were lower, with kappas for lifetime use ranging from .41 to .64, and for past year use at .64. For children, understandably there was a tendency to confuse closely related service settings with one another (e.g., psychiatric hospitals and psychiatric units in general hospitals).

Specialized Individual Module Reliability

Modules are only used for services in the last 12 months. Adult reports of *reasons for use of services* were highly reliable, indicating that people who access services do so for well-developed reasons. Adults' reasons for use reliability figures were κ = 1.00 for psychiatric hospital, κ = .89 for mental health clinics, and κ = .87 for mental health professionals.

Reliability of adults' reports for *intensity of services,* as measured by the number of inpatient admissions and the number of visits for the most recent

TABLE 11.3
Reliability: Adult Reports on Queries in the Individual SACA Modules ($n = 237$)

	Test		Retest		κ	95% CI
	n	%	n	%		
Treatments in psychiatric hospital						
Child therapy	7	3	4	2	.72	.41 to 1.0
Case management	6	3	3	1	.66	.30 to 1.0
Medications	6	3	4	2	.80	.52 to 1.1
Evaluation or testing	3	1	4	2	.86	.58 to 1.1
Family therapy	4	2	1	.4	.40	−.15 to .94
Treatments in mental health clinic						
Child therapy	65	27	69	29	.69	.59 to .79
Case management	32	14	41	17	.60	.45 to .74
Medications	55	23	54	23	.80	.71 to .89
Evaluation or testing	55	23	58	25	.66	.55 to .78
Family therapy	43	18	41	17	.57	.43 to .70
Treatments by mental health professional						
Child therapy	48	20	46	19	.47	.33 to .61
Case management	14	6	13	6	.10	−.09 to .29
Medications	37	16	31	13	.55	.40 to .71
Evaluation or testing	19	8	20	8	.30	.10 to .51
Family therapy	42	18	30	13	.54	.40 to .69
Benefit of treatment						
Psychiatric hospital	1	.4	2	.8	.67	.05 to 1.3
Mental health clinic	39	17	45	19	.77	.66 to .88
Mental health professional	13	6	5	2	.20	−0.6 to .46
Medication use	90	39	90	39	.96	.93 to .99

Note. From "Measuring Youths' Use for Mental Health Services: Reliability of the SACA—Services Assessment for Children and Adolescents," by S. Horwitz, K. Hoagwood, A. R. Stiffman, T. Summerfelt, J. Weisz, E. J. Costello, et al., 2001, *Psychiatric Services, 52,* pp. 1088–1094. Copyright 2001 by American Psychiatric Publishers, Inc. Reprinted with permission.

outpatient mental health clinic use, was uneven, with the number of hospital admissions moderately reliable (ICC = .44) but the number of clinic visits unreliable (ICC = .03).

Testing the reliability of reports on the *types of treatments* received within any one setting was limited, as few respondents endorsed any one setting and even fewer endorsed any one treatment type. Kappas were generally moderate to excellent for treatments offered by mental health clinics (kappas ranging from .57 to .80) and poor to moderate for treatments offered by mental health professionals (kappas ranging from .10 to .55; see Table 11.3).

The kappa for adults' assessments of the *benefits* of mental health clinic use, the only benefit question with a sample size large enough for analysis, was good ($\kappa = .77$ for mental health clinic use). The numbers for reports of *follow-up services* and *cultural sensitivity* were too small for gauging reliability. The *financial questions* showed very poor reliability (ICC = .00–.25 for out-of-pocket costs).

Older children's reliability figures for *reasons for seeking treatment* were as follows: psychiatric hospital, $\kappa = .70$; mental health clinics, $\kappa = .80$; and mental health professionals, $\kappa = .75$. Reliability for younger children (9 and 10 years of age) was only moderate ($\kappa = .50$); they infrequently reported reasons for seeking care at psychiatric hospitals or mental health clinics. Reliability of older children's reports was poor for both inpatient psychiatric hospital *admissions* and *number of visits* to mental health clinics (ICCs of .27 and .24, respectively).

The number of children reporting specific *types of treatments* in any one setting was generally too low to gauge reliability, with the exception of treatments from a mental health professional. Here, the reliability of older children's reports of *child therapy, medication, evaluation/testing,* and *family therapy* was low to moderate at .38 to .54.

Medications Module Reliability

The medications module asked about medications only in the last month. Overall, when asked about *any use of medications* within the last month, adult respondents were very reliable reporters ($\kappa = .96$). Methylphenidate was the single most prevalent medication named (41/149, or 27.5%) with central nervous system (CNS) stimulants and antidepressants about equally represented. Adults were able to name the same drugs on the second administration about 87% of the time.

The percentage of correspondence was excellent as to whether the child was *still taking* the medication. The correspondence was also excellent for knowing if health insurance paid for all or part of the cost of medications ($\kappa = 1.00$ and .73 for one and two medication groups), *amount paid out of pocket* (ICC = .96 and .96), the *dose* of medications given (ICC = .88 and .99), and the *times per day* child takes medications (ICC = .86 and .85). The reliability of the *number of days* in the last month the child took medications was poor (ICC = .41 and .06). Questions on *dosage schedules,* particularly the questions attempting to capture drug "holidays" or varying weekly or daily schedules, were problematic.

Validity

Four types of service use in the past 12 months were assessed: (a) global service use for any service, (b) inpatient care, (c) outpatient care, and (d) school services. Within the latter three settings, adult reports of specific types of services were matched against service records. Inpatient care included child therapy, family therapy, medication therapy, and treatment planning. Outpatient care included child therapy, case management, family therapy, medication, and treatment planning. For the schools, the specific services included special classrooms, special help in the general education classroom, and receipt of individual counseling.

Validity of Adult Reports

Adult reports of *any service use* in inpatient settings, outpatient settings, or schools were matched against medical or administrative records at the specific service site reported. Overall, the kappa between adult report and agency records was .76, indicating high correspondence (see Table 11.4).

There was perfect correspondence between respondent reports and records for *any inpatient* service use ($\kappa = 1.00$). It should be noted, however, that the sample size was very small (ns ranged from 2 to 4). Similarly, there

TABLE 11.4
Validity: Accuracy of Adult Reports

	Medical Record		Adult Report		κ	95% CI
	n	%	*n*	%		
Any service	62	42.31	61	40.7	.76	.66 to .87
Inpatient						
Any inpatient	4	2.7	4	2.7	1.00	1.0 to 1.0
Child therapy	3	2.0	3	2.0	.66	.22 to 1.1
Case management	0		2			
Family therapy	1	0.7	3	2.0	.50	−.1 to 1.1
Medication	4	2.7	4	2.7	1.00	1.0 to 1.0
Treatment plan	4	2.7	2	1.3	.66	.22 to 1.1
Outpatient						
Any outpatient	58	39.5	55	37.4	.67	.55 to .79
Child therapy	56	38.1	44	29.9	.52	.38 to .66
Case management	2	1.4	18	12.2	.08	−.09 to .25
Family therapy	8	5.4	39	26.5	.09	−.05 to .22
Medication	37	25.2	45	30.6	.66	.53 to .80
Treatment plan	54	36.7	33	22.5	.54	.40 to .68
School						
Any school	42	31.1	26	19.3	.31	.13 to .48
Special classroom	20	14.8	7	5.2	.48	.25 to .7
Special help	20	14.8	10	7.4	.19	−.03 to .40
Counseling	17	12.6	17	12.6	.33	.00 to .56

Note. From "Concordance Between Parent Reports of Children's Mental Health Services and Service Records: The Services Assessment for Children and Adolescents (SACA)," by A. R. Stiffman, J. Weisz, D. Bean, D. Rae, W. Compton, L. Cottler, et al., 2000, *Journal of Child and Family Studies, 9,* pp. 315–331.

was perfect correspondence between respondent reports of the use of medications and medical records of such use ($\kappa = 1.00$). Moderate correspondence was found for receiving *child therapy* (.66) and for *treatment planning* (.66). Receipt of *family therapy* within the inpatient setting yielded a moderate kappa of .50.

Reports of *outpatient* service use yielded moderate levels of correspondence with medical records ($\kappa = .67$). *Medication use* yielded similar levels of correspondence, with a kappa of .66. Receipt of *child therapy* and of *treatment planning* were slightly lower (.52 and .54, respectively). There was very little correspondence between respondent reports and records for the receipt of *case management* services (.08) and receipt of *family therapy* (.09).

Reports of receipt of *any school* services for behavioral or emotional problems corresponded weakly to school records, yielding a kappa of .31. Slightly higher levels of correspondence were found for receipt of *services within a special classroom* ($\kappa = .48$). Receipt of *counseling* and of *special help in the general education classroom* matched school records poorly, yielding kappas of .33 and .19, respectively.

Validity of Child Reports

Only the St. Louis site reviewed service records to assess accuracy of child reports. Accuracy (for children over 11) was assessed by review of the last year's service records from Washington University inpatient and outpatient psychiatric services and public school records in St. Louis, Missouri (see Hoagwood et al., 2000, for more details). Information was abstracted concerning specialty residential care, specialty outpatient care, and school services. Despite the small sample size for *specialty residential service* ($n = 6$), there was excellent correspondence (97%) between child reports and records. Reports of any *specialty outpatient service* use yielded fair-to-good levels of correspondence with records ($n = 30$, 73%, $\kappa = .44$). Reports of receipt of *any school services* for behavioral or emotional problems corresponded weakly ($n = 14$, 69% correspondence) to school records.

Adult–Child Correspondence

Lifetime information on service use in each of 25 specific settings listed in the child version was aggregated to produce estimates for any service use across two time spans: lifetime and in the last year. Adults and children showed good correspondence on use of *any services in the child's lifetime,* 85% for a kappa of .57 (see Table 11.5). An examination of use of the three major venues for services (residential, outpatient, and school) elucidated differences in correspondence. Correspondence was better for *any residential services* in a lifetime or for any outpatient services in a lifetime than for any school services in a lifetime. Correspondence on *mental health specialty residential* or *specialty outpatient services* was excellent and good, respectively. Adults were more likely to report outpatient mental health specialty treatment than were children, but no other lifetime service use demonstrated any significant patterns.

TABLE 11.5

Adult–Child Concordance: Types of Service Settings Used Ever and Past Year ($n = 145$)

Service	Ever Used					Used in Previous 12 Months				
	Adult *n*	Child *n*	% Agreement	κ	95% CI	Adult *n*	Child *n*	% Agreement	κ	95% CI
Any service	112	112	.85	.57	.41 to .73	95	88	.83	.63	.50 to .76
Any residential	40	40	.94	.86	.77 to .96	18	22	.94	.77	.62 to .92
Any outpatient	108	101	.87	.68	.77 to .96	89	79	.79	.58	.45 to .71
Any school	69	66	.72	.43	.29 to .58	56	42	.75	.45	.30 to .60
Any mental health speciality inpatient[a]	27	26	.95	.84	.72 to .96	13	17	.94	.70	.51 to .90
Any mental health speciality outpatient[b]	100	88	.78	.52	.38 to .66	77	65	.74	.48	.34 to .62

Note. From "Adult and Child Reports of Mental Health Services in the Service Assessment for Children and Adolescents (SACA)," by A. R. Stiffman, S. M. Horwitz, K. Hoagwood, W. Compton, L. Cottler, W. Narrow, et al., 2000, *Journal of the American Academy of Child and Adolescent Psychiatry, 39*(8), pp. 10032–10039. Copyright 2000 by Journal of the AACAP. Reprinted with permission.

[a] Specialty inpatient includes psychiatric hospital/unit, drug/alcohol treatment, and residential treatment.

[b] Specialty outpatient includes mental health clinic, day treatment, drug or alcohol clinic, or psychologist, social worker, and counselor.

Correspondence on *any service use in the last year* was 83%, or κ = .63. Within that aggregated category, the pattern of relative correspondence levels was similar to that for any lifetime use. Correspondence on *residential services* or *outpatient services* in the last year was better than that for *school services* in the last year. Correspondence was also better for *specialty mental health in-patient services* in the last year than for *specialty mental health outpatient services* in the last year. Adults were more likely than children to report both school services in the last year and mental health specialty outpatient services in the last year.

The samples of 145 adult–child pairs yielded enough cases to examine correspondence for only some of the 25 *specific service settings* (see Table 11.6). Correspondence on lifetime use and on last year use was parallel within types of settings.

Correspondence levels on *lifetime use of a psychiatric hospital or unit in a general hospital* were excellent, whereas correspondence rates on *lifetime use of outpatient settings* ranged from 62% to 84%. Adult–child correspondence was poor for *community mental health settings* and for use of a *private therapist*. In contrast, correspondence on use of *family preservation services* in a lifetime was good. Correspondence on lifetime use of the two school settings that met sample size criteria (*a special classroom in a general education school*, or *counseling in school*) was poor to fair.

Correspondence was poor for *last year use* in the only two outpatient settings that met the sample size criteria: *community mental health center* and

TABLE 11.6

Specific Settings Used: Ever and Past Year ($n = 145$)

Setting	Ever Used					Used in Previous 12 Months				
	Adult n	Child n	% Agreement	κ	95% CI	Adult n	Child n	% Agreement	κ	95% CI
Inpatient										
Psychiatric hospital or unit in general hospital	25	24	.95	.83	.71 to .95					
Outpatient										
Community mental health center	74	39	.62	.25	.11 to .39	58	26	.67	.24	.10 to .39
Family preservation	26	31	.84	.50	.32 to .68					
Psychologist, social worker, or marriage or family therapist	62	74	.64	.29	.13 to .44	37	54	.70	.32	.17 to .48
School										
Special classroom in regular school	53	47	.79	.35	.17 to .53					
Counseling in school	53	47	.74	.42	.27 to .58	40	27	.79	.41	.24 to .58

Note. From "Adult and Child Reports of Mental Health Services in the Service Assessment for Children and Adolescents (SACA)," by A. R. Stiffman, S. M. Horwitz, K. Hoagwood, W. Compton, L. Cottler, W. Narrow, et al., 2000, *Journal of the American Academy of Child and Adolescent Psychiatry, 39*(8), pp. 10032–10039. Copyright 2000 by Journal of the AACAP. Reprinted with permission.

private therapist, with κ = .24 and κ = .32, respectively. Correspondence concerning last year's use of *counseling in school* was fair at κ = .41.

Within the individual modules, adults and children tended to agree on at least one of the behavioral or emotional reasons that they used particular services. For settings where at least 16 individuals responded, kappas for reasons for using any outpatient service, any school service, and any mental health specialty outpatient service were good at .72, .70, and .71, respectively.

DISCUSSION

Test–Retest Reliability

The SACA demonstrated that the adult interview had uniformly excellent reliability for both lifetime and 12-month service use. The instrument takes between 2 and 45 minutes to administer, with the initial section ranging between 2 and 15 minutes ($M = 8$ minutes).

Comparing the adult test–retest reliability data to those reported for the CASA, the 12-month reliability of the SACA documents that reasonable recall over a longer time period can be achieved. The brevity of the initial section of the SACA appears to prevent attenuation of responses, an important problem in instruments with repetitive formats (Piacentini et al., 1999). Further, an examination of test–retest results stratified by the length of recall period (≤ 1 week vs. > 1 week) indicates consistently high correspondence over the two time periods.

The child data present a more varied picture. For children 11 years and older, the kappas for lifetime and 12-month use were in the good to excellent range, demonstrating that adults and children 11 years of age and older can report both lifetime and 12-month use of mental health services with adequate reliability. These results are consistent with the findings from child reports using the CASA (Farmer et al., 1994). The reliability figures for 9- and 10-year-old children were considerably lower than those for children at least 11 years of age. A careful examination of the children's responses suggested considerable confusion about several of the settings; thus, we question whether children under 11 years of age are reliable reporters of their own use of mental health services.

Within the individual modules, types of treatments, with the exception of case management and other support services (help with rent, food, etc.) achieved excellent test–retest reliability for adults and children, suggesting that clearly demarcated services are reported reliably. Similarly, adults and children usually reported assessments of benefit and follow-up quite reliably. Adults and children too infrequently answered questions on cultural sensitivity to warrant firm conclusions. The questions on out-of-pocket costs showed poor reliability.

The Medications Module demonstrated that dose, form, and frequency of use, as well as whether insurance paid for the medications, can be reliably reported. Detailed information about dosages on different days was difficult to report reliably and was very time-consuming to collect. The start date for medications appeared to cause some confusion, but an added question regarding length of time the child had been on medications in months and years may elicit more reliable duration information.

Validity

The investigation of validity demonstrates that reasonable levels of correspondence between adult reports and medical or administrative records can be obtained with the SACA. Despite the small sample size for inpatient use, perfect concurrence between adult reports and service records was obtained for inpatient care and medication use in that setting. Outpatient services can be reported with moderate levels of correspondence, but school service reports by adults correspond poorly with school records.[2]

Wide variation was found, however, in the correspondence between SACA reports of specific types of treatments in inpatient, outpatient, or school settings and the evidence obtained from records reviews. In inpatient settings, medication use was reported with perfect accuracy, whereas family therapy, child therapy, and treatment planning were reported with moderate levels of correspondence. In outpatient settings, medication use, child therapy, and treatment planning were reported with moderate levels of accuracy, whereas reports of case management or family therapy displayed no relationship to records. In school settings, only placement in a special classroom for help with emotional or behavior problems was reported with a moderate level of correspondence to school records, and adult reports of the use of other specific types of schools services (e.g., special help in a general education classroom or counseling) had almost no association with school records.

These variations are likely due to a number of factors. As has been found in other studies (e.g., Ascher et al., 1996), the more restrictive the service, the more likely it is to be recalled. Similarly, the use of medications is likely to be a memorable and repeated action; medication use requires both ongoing adult action and physician monitoring. Furthermore, recall may be increased by either the extremity of the service or its concreteness (e.g., a pill bottle exists).

Discrepancies between adult reports and service records may also arise because of confusion surrounding the terminology used by service providers. Although the SACA was administered by trained interviewers, contained a glossary of terms, and was developed after incorporating suggestions from adults who participated in focus groups, adults and providers may very well lack a shared terminology. A prime example of this may be case management—a service well known by service providers but largely unrecognized by families.

---

[2] Although not reported here, child reports also appear to be acceptably accurate in their correspondence with service reports. Levels of record/SACA child report correspondence are highest for residential and lowest for school services (Hoagwood et al., 2000).

Finally, variations in accuracy across services may have arisen because there is variation in the visibility of services. School mental health services are largely invisible to children who receive them, and, perhaps to their adult care-givers as well. This may occur in part because adults are not in school to ob-serve their children receiving services and in part because of the terminology used in schools to avoid stigmatizing children or services. For example, school counseling may be called "guidance," children with emotional or behavioral problems may be sent to a resource room to help them with their "special needs," and therapies may be called "related services."

Other reasons for variations in the ability of adults to report accurately about their child's service use center on the problems inherent in secondhand reporting. If children poorly understand the nature of the services they are re-ceiving, their adults' ability to respond to detailed questions about types of services is compromised. In circumstances of strain, distress, or frustration, commonly faced by families whose children require mental health care, the accuracy of such reports may be further compromised. Finally, of course, variations might also be a consequence of inaccuracies or incompleteness in service records.

Adult–Child Correspondence Conclusions

The SACA shows a correspondence rate between adults and children that is higher than that reported for the only other service use instrument with such data for children (Leaf et al., 1996). Further, its correspondence rate is as high or higher than that reported for either diagnostic status or behavior symptom checklists. Leaf et al. (1996) reported that their highest kappa for generic cate-gories of service use on the MECA was .45. In contrast, the SACA kappas for lifetime services range from a low of .43 to a high of .86. Similarly, the SACA shows a fair to excellent correspondence for generic categories of services used in the last year.

The adult–child correspondence for specific service settings in the SACA is also higher than that reported for other instruments, with half of the kappas at good to excellent for lifetime use. Correspondence for specific set-tings used in the last year was less adequate, which may be a consequence of the smaller sample size for the 12-month reports.

There are some explanations for any high adult–child correspondence in the SACA, and for any lack of correspondence. The specific structured questions about each type of service appear to prompt good recall, whereas discrepancy may relate to perception. Because different informants contrib-ute different information, discrepancy is not equivalent to lack of interrater reliability but relates to differing experiences, priorities, and perceptions (Verhulst & van der Ende, 1992). Child and adult reports each add new or dif-ferent information, but each agrees well with the other. The utility of obtain-ing both adult and child reports lies in the personal perspectives each gives concerning the treatment received.

Limitations

The most serious limitation of the pilot study on the SACA concerns the sample size. Because the SACA asks questions about so many different settings, a large sample is required to analyze all specific settings and specific experiences or treatments within particular settings. Because the number of participants using any one setting and any one treatment in most settings was so low, it is harder to draw specific conclusions from reliability estimates for the individual module questions. One would need an even larger sample to examine the joint or interactive impact of gender, child age, race, and mental health status on reliability, validity, and parent–child correspondence. Also, the samples were drawn only from two cities with large visible services. Rural samples might respond differently. Rates of correspondence may also have been affected by higher proportions of service users than one would find in a random sample. Although report/record correspondence is discussed as a means of assessing accuracy, validity remains elusive, as there are no objective referents for calibrating self-reports (see Fendrich et al., 1999). Medical and school service records are notoriously incomplete, and all possible extant records were not reviewed.

Clinical Implications

Clinicians may be aided by understanding the areas where reliability or validity is low or where adult and child reports differ. An interesting issue concerns how children's understanding that they are being treated for a mental health problem affects their treatment cooperation or progress. Adults and children appear to be unaware that they are receiving some mental health services, because the service is couched within another context (even labeled with terminology designed to blur the mental health emphasis). They may not know that special classrooms are directed toward their mental health or that outpatient clinics are offering specialty mental health services. Misconceptions may raise dropout rates. Also, the stigma of receiving certain services, particularly in school, may lead to lower satisfaction or compliance.

Although the SACA was developed for use in a population-based study, it can be used in any number of differently designed studies, including clinical trials, and can be adapted for use as a repeated measure (as are the brief versions). It might potentially be used in any study or evaluation of service access, service pathways, or treatment modalities. Particular service providers, such as schools or school systems, might choose to use the SACA in whole or in part to monitor the way their own service provision fits into the larger picture of services received by youth. Case managers might want to use a brief version to track their clients, the actual use of their referrals, and the service provided by those referred sites. It may also be used for treatment planning by national, state, and local mental health administrators to help calibrate children's treatment needs against service availability and use.

Research Implications

The SACA is capable of collecting some of the information about mental health services that has been missing in previous research and, therefore, can greatly expand the knowledge base in children's mental health services. The modular format of the SACA, with an initial service overview section, makes it highly adaptable for differing research modalities. The initial section of the SACA, which obtains information on the use of generic settings (without going into detailed modules), might be most appropriate to use alone in studies with smaller sample sizes, or as adapted to a brief version. Furthermore, researchers might modify the specific modules for generic types of settings rather than for specific settings. That is, the modules for therapists and outpatient mental health could be aggregated into a module for any specialty mental health outpatient services (see Tables 11.1 and 11.2).

The SACA's ability to elicit answers with high correspondence between adult and child reports is also important for service researchers. The findings indicate that it is not necessary to do both adult and child service assessments in all research on mental health services. This is especially encouraging news for those researchers working with high-risk child populations, where an adult figure who knows the history of the child is often not available. Adults are the only appropriate reporters when the children are young, and they are also more appropriate as the source of information likely to be known only to the adult, such as financing, marital therapy, or adult education. In contrast, the child report is as adequate or better if the researcher wants to learn about residential services or a child's understanding of the services he or she received.

Conclusions

This study has demonstrated that adults can report the use of mental health services by their children in ways that are reliable, correspond closely to service records, and are in agreement with their children's reports. Given that the time frame for reporting in the SACA was 1 year and that the instrument was embedded in a much lengthier interview, strategies for shortening the time frame or reducing respondent burden need to be examined. The results indicate that researchers must decide upon the type of information that they desire and use the initial section, the modules, the adult or child reports, a brief version, or some combination thereof to obtain the most relevant information. The SACA allows the researcher to choose cost-effective approaches to data collection.

AUTHORS' NOTE

This work is a product from the multisite study of Mental Health Services Use, Needs, Outcomes, and Costs in Child and Adolescent Populations (UNOCCAP), supported by the National Institute of Mental Health (NIMH); the Administration for Children, Child, and Families (ACYF); the Center for Mental Health Services (CMHS); the National Institute of Child Health and Human Development (NICHD); and the U.S. Department of Education (DOE). Four independent research teams in collaboration performed the UNOCCAP study with staff from NIMH and ACYF. The four sites' principal investigators are Linda B. Cottler (U01 MH/HD54293), Benjamin B. Lahey (U01 MH/HD 54282), Philip J. Leaf (MH/HD54280), and Mary Jane Rotheram-Borus (U01 MH/HD54278). The NIMH principal collaborators are Kimberly E. Hoagwood, Peter S. Jensen, William E. Narrow, and Grayson S. Norquist. NIMH project officers are Darrel A. Regier and Thomas Lalley. ACYF principal collaborators are Michael Lopez and Louisa Tarullo.

REFERENCES

Angold, A., Messer, S. C., Stangl, D., Farmer, E. M. Z., Costello, E. J., & Burns, B. J. (1998). Perceived parental burden and service use for child and adolescent psychiatric disorders. *American Journal of Public Health, 88,* 75–80.

Arnold, L. E., Abikoff, H. B., Cantwell, D. P., Conners, C. K., Elliott, G., Greenhill, L. L., et al. (1997). National Institute of Mental Health collaborative multimodal treatment study of children with ADHD (the MTA): Design challenges and choices. *Archives of General Psychiatry, 54,* 865–870.

Ascher, B. H., Farmer, E. M. Z., Burns, B. J., & Angold, A. (1996). The Child and Adolescent Services Assessment (CASA): Description and psychometrics. *Journal of Emotional and Behavioral Disorders, 4,* 12–20.

Bartko, J. J. (1966). The intraclass correlation coefficient as a measure of reliability. *Psychological Reports, 19,* 3–11.

Bean, D. L., Leibowitz, A., Rotherman-Borus, M. J., Duan, N., Horwitz, S., Jordan, D., et al. (2000). False-negative reporting and mental health services utilization: Parents' reports about child and adolescent services. *Mental Health Services Research, 2,* 239–248.

Bickman, L. (1996). A continuum of care: More is not always better. *American Psychologist, 51,* 689–701.

Brandenburg, N. A., Friedman, R. M., & Silver, S. E. (1990). The epidemiology of childhood psychiatric disorders: Prevalence findings from recent studies. *Journal of the American Academy of Child and Adolescent Psychiatry, 29,* 76–83.

Burns, B. J., Costello, E. J., Angold, A., Tweed, D., Stangl, D., Farmer, E. M., et al. (1995). Children's mental health service use across service sectors. *Health Affairs, 14,* 147–159.

Canino, G., Shrout, P. E., Alegria, M., Rubio-Stipec, M., Chavez, L. M., Ribera, J. C., et al. (2002). Methodological challenges in assessing children's mental health services utilization. *Mental Health Services Research, 4*(2), 97–108.

Costello, E. J. (1989). Developments in child psychiatric epidemiology. *Journal of the American Academy of Child and Adolescent Psychiatry, 28,* 836–841.

Costello, E. J., Farmer, E. M. Z, Angold, A., Burns, B. J., & Erkanli, A. (1997). Psychiatric disorder among American Indian and white youth in Appalachia: The Great Smoky Mountains study. *American Journal of Public Health, 87,* 827–832.

Farmer, E. M. Z., Angold, A., Burns, B. J., & Costello, E. J. (1994). Reliability of self-reported service use: Test–retest consistency of children's responses to the Child and Adolescent Services Assessment (CASA). *Journal of Child and Family Studies, 3,* 307–325.

Farmer, E. M. Z., Stangl, D. K., Burns, B. J., Costello, E. J., & Angold, A. (1999). Persistence and intensity: Patterns of care for children's mental health across one year. *Community Mental Health Journal, 35,* 31–46.

Fendrich, M., Johnson T., Wislar, J. S., & Nageotte, C. (1999). Accuracy of adult mental health service reporting: Results from a reverse record-check study. *Journal of the American Academy of Child and Adolescent Psychiatry, 38,* 147–155.

Fleiss, J. L. (1981). *Statistical measures for rates and proportions* (2nd ed.). New York: Wiley.

Glisson, C., & Hemmelgarn, A. (1998). The effects of organization climate and interorganizational coordination on the quality and outcomes of children's service systems. *Child Abuse and Neglect, 22,* 1–21.

Hoagwood, K., Horwitz, S. M., Stiffman, A. R., Weisz, J., Bean, D., Rae, D., et al. (2000). Concordance between parent reports of children's mental health services and service records: The Services Assessment for Children and Adolescents (SACA). *Journal of Child and Family Studies, 9,* 315–331.

Hornbrook, M. C., & Berki, S. E. (1985). Practice mode and payment method: Effects on use, costs, quality, and access. *Medical Care, 23,* 484–511.

Horwitz, S. M., Hoagwood, K., Stiffman, A. R., Summerfelt, T., Weisz, J., Costello, E. J., et al. (2001). Measuring youths' use of mental health services: Reliability of the SACA (Services Assessment for Children and Adolescents). *Psychiatric Services, 52*(8), 1088–1094.

Kessler, L. G., Steinwachs, D. M., & Hankin, J. R. (1980). Episodes of psychiatric utilization. *Medical Care, 18,* 1219–1227.

Leaf, P. J., Alegria, M., Cohen, P., Goodman, S. H., Horwitz, S. M., Hoven, C. W., et al. (1996). Mental health service use in the community and schools: Results from the four-community MECA study. *Journal of the American Academy of Child and Adolescent Psychiatry, 35,* 889–897.

Piacentini, J., Roper, M., Jensen, P., Lucas, C., Fisher, P., Bird, H., et al. (1999). Informant-based determinants of symptom attenuation in structured child psychiatric interviews. *Journal of Abnormal Child Psychology, 6,* 417–428.

Spitznagel, E. L., & Helzer, J. E. (1985). A proposed solution to the base rate problem in the Kappa statistic. *Archives of General Psychiatry, 42,* 725–728.

Stiffman, A. R., Horwitz, S. M., Hoagwood, K., Compton, W., Cottler, L., Bean, D. L., et al. (2000). The Service Assessment for Children and Adolescents (SACA): Adult and child reports. *Journal of the Academy of Child and Adolescent Psychiatry, 39,* 1032–1039.

Stiffman, A. R., Striley, C. W., Brown, E., Limb, G., & Ostmann, E. (2003). American Indian youth: Southwestern urban and reservation youths' need for services and whom they turn to for help. *Journal of Child and Family Studies, 12,* 319–333.

Stiffman, A. R., Striley, C. W., Horvath, V., Hadley-Ives, E., Polgar, M., Elze, D., et al. (2001). Organizational context and provider perception as determinants of mental health service use. *Journal of Behavioral Health Services and Research, 28*(2), 1–17.

Verhulst, F., & van der Ende, J. (1992). Agreement between adults' reports and adolescents' self-report of problem behavior. *Journal of Child Psychology and Psychiatry and Allied Disciplines, 33,* 1011–1023.

Weisz, J. R. (1996). *Studying clinic-based child mental health care: Research in progress.* Los Angeles: University of California.

Weisz, J. R., Donenberg, G., Han, S. S., & Weiss, B. (1995). Bridging the gap between laboratory and clinic in child and adolescent psychotherapy. *Journal of Consulting and Clinical Psychology, 63,* 688–701.

Weisz, J. R., & Weiss, B. (1991). Studying the "referability" of child clinical problems. *Journal of Consulting and Clinical Psychology, 59,* 266–273.

Cultural Diversity

A Challenge for Evaluating
Systems of Care

CHAPTER 12

Nirbhay N. Singh

A number of systems of care for children and adolescents with emotional and behavioral disorders (EBD) have been initiated over the last decade. As defined by Stroul and Friedman (1986, p. 3), a system of care is "a comprehensive spectrum of mental health and other necessary services which are organized into a coordinated network to meet the multiple and changing needs of severely emotionally disturbed children and adolescents." Although overlapping in many respects, the systems of care in many states and localities vary in terms of their conceptual models, as well as in their service delivery systems. The systems of care in North Carolina (Behar, 1996), the four-county California systems of care (Attkisson, Dresser, & Rosenblatt, 1996), the Fort Bragg managed-care experiment (Bickman, Heflinger, Lambert, & Summerfelt, 1996), the Robert Wood Johnson Foundation's Mental Health Services Program for Youth (Saxe, Cross, Lovas, & Gardner, 1996), and the various wraparound models (Clark & Clarke, 1996; VanDenBerg & Grealish, 1996) provide specific examples of systems of care for integrating services for children and adolescents with EBD.

The proliferation of systems of care suggests that policymakers and service providers do not believe that any one model fits the needs of all children in all settings. Indeed, models of systems of care vary along several dimensions, including conceptual and service goals, target populations, service delivery systems, degree and types of interagency collaboration, governance structures, state and local financing of services, and outcomes. Given that most of these models have been initiated within the last few years, we have minimal information regarding how well these models are implemented in different localities and the nature of the outcomes for children with EBD who are provided the services. However, the current political and fiscal policies mandate that the service delivery process, as well as outcomes for children with EBD and their families, be evaluated empirically. Thus, evaluation of current practices and outcomes is critical in the future development of systems of care.

PROGRAM EVALUATION

The nature and functions of program evaluation have grown substantially since this field emerged in the 1960s. The early models of program evaluation were developed from quantitative research methods emphasizing robust experimental designs, standardized data collection methods, objective and reliable data from large samples, and statistical analyses of the data. These early models were intended to provide information on the relationship between service programs and their outcomes. The recognition that these models did not account for the unique characteristics, contexts, and processes of individual programs as perceived by the programs' developers, the recipients of the program services, and the various stakeholders of the programs led to the development of evaluation models that replaced quantitative with naturalistic, qualitative research methods. Although these qualitative models were useful in the evaluation of specific programs, they were of limited value in terms of generalizing the findings across programs or for comparative evaluations of different programs. More recently, program evaluation models have begun to use both quantitative and qualitative approaches, depending on the nature of the questions being asked.

Along with the development of different methods for evaluating programs, there was a growing recognition that program evaluations served an increasing number of functions. For example, program evaluation data could be used in a dynamic fashion as formative information to facilitate the modification and refinement of program structures, processes, and functions or as summative information to judge a program's accomplishments. Further, evaluation data could be used by policymakers and funding agencies to ensure accountability of the program. A related development was the recognition that the role of the evaluator varied, depending on the proposed use of the evaluation findings. Although a general discussion of these issues is beyond the scope of this chapter, Table 12.1 presents a brief summary of different approaches to program evaluation, the specific role of the evaluator, the particular emphasis of each approach, and the issues that are most pertinent for each approach. In addition, Table 12.1 also includes a summary of specific types of information needed to undertake each type of program evaluation.

All of the approaches to evaluation presented in Table 12.1 provide an overall framework for gathering pertinent information for any system of care. The needs of the stakeholders (e.g., funding agencies, service providers, service recipients), the program objectives, and the evaluator's role often combine to determine the specific nature of the information to be collected. However, regardless of the particular approach chosen, most program evaluations provide data on five key aspects of a service delivery system. First, the evaluation must describe the characteristics of the context in which the services are delivered, because context provides the framework or constraints within which the program's services and outcomes must be evaluated. For example, sociopolitical, financial, and program-specific factors play critical roles in determining not only the nature of the services delivered within a program but also the outcomes of the services provided. Second, the evaluation must describe the characteristics of the service recipients because these variables are correlated to outcomes. Third, a description of the process for implementing the program goals is necessary because it provides the basis for comparison with other programs that may have similar goals. Fourth, the evaluation must document the extent to which the goals of the program are achieved. Fifth, and finally,

TABLE 12.1

Approaches to Program Evaluation

Approach	Evaluator's Role	Emphasis	Focusing Issues	Information Needed
Experimental	Expert/scientist	Research design	What effects result from program activities, and can they be generalized?	Outcome measures Client characteristics Variation in treatments Other influences on clients Availability of control groups
Goal oriented	Measurement specialist	Goals and objectives	What are the program's goals and objectives, and how can they be measured?	Specific program objectives Criterion-referenced outcome measures
Decision focused	Decision support person	Decision making	Which decisions need to be made, and what information will be relevant?	Stage of program development Cycle of decision making Data gathering and reporting routines
User oriented	Collaborator	Information users	Who are the intended information users, and what information will be most useful?	Personal and organizational dynamics Group information needs Program history Intended uses of information
Responsive	Counselor/facilitator	Personal understanding	Which people have a stake in the program, and what are their points of view?	Variation in individual and group perspectives Stakeholder concerns Program history Variation in occasions and sites

Note. From *How to Focus an Evaluation,* by B. M. Stecher and W. A. Davis, 1987, Thousand Oaks, CA: Sage. Copyright 1987 by B. M. Stecher and W. A. Davis. Adapted with permission.

the evaluation must include an analysis of the program in terms of financial, human, and time costs. The evaluation may include data from cost–benefit, cost-effectiveness, cost-utility, and cost-feasibility analyses (Levin, 1983).

In this chapter, I will discuss selected aspects of cultural diversity as they affect services and program evaluation in systems of care. I will focus primarily on three of the five key aspects of program evaluation—namely, context, participants, and outcomes. Although they are equally important, less emphasis will be placed on process and costs because of space limitations. Readers interested in costs should consult an excellent review by Ruiz, Venegas-Samuels, and Alarcon (1995). Finally, I will briefly discuss issues related to the competencies in cultural diversity needed by program evaluators to ensure appropriate program evaluations in the future.

CONTEXT

In terms of program evaluation, *context* may be defined in a number of ways. For example, it has been referred to as the web of experience that includes thoughts, acts, and the past (Kuhns & Martorana, 1982) and as the general framework that influences a person's current decision making about specific issues (Welshimer & Earp, 1989). Miles and Huberman (1984) defined *context* as the immediately relevant aspects of a situation in which a person functions. Context provides the framework for the prediction, explanation, and understanding of the phenomenon of interest. However, the use of context in program evaluation ranges from nonuse, as in context stripping, to extensive use, as in the assessment and interpretation of the findings. Context stripping is used in quantitative research when the researcher is interested in the misguided notion of discovering universal, context-free laws of human behavior. In program evaluation, context stripping assumes that the context of the participant's life and well-being is irrelevant to his or her current functioning. Typically, contextual aspects of systems of care have been described as the background or backdrop to the program evaluation, and the impact of the context subsequently is not considered in terms of the evaluation methodology or the interpretation of the findings; the context is divorced from the process and outcomes of the evaluation. However, nothing in systems of care is acontextual, and a program evaluation makes sense only when the process and outcomes of a service delivery system are understood within its context.

CULTURAL CONTEXT OF SYSTEMS OF CARE

Differences in the culture of the service recipients, the service providers, and the program evaluators can have a profound impact on the outcome of systems of care. The rapidly changing demographic composition of the United States will be reflected in the children and adolescents with EBD and their families in systems of care across this country. Cultural differences in values, approaches to child rearing and education, views of mental illness, and the seeking of services for their children undoubtedly influence many aspects of the involvement of families in systems of care. Further, the cultural competence and sensitivity of service providers will affect not only the nature of the services sought and received by these families but also the level of their involvement with different sectors of the service system. Finally, how well our program evaluations truly reflect the well-being and improvements in the quality of life of diverse children with EBD and their families is dependent on the evaluators understanding and valuing the cultural worldviews of the families served within the systems of care being evaluated.

CULTURE

No single definition of culture is likely to be universally accepted; it is a dynamic conceptual abstraction that has been socially constructed by groups of people, and it is continually modified and transmitted across generations. Broadly defined, *culture* is "the shared values, traditions, arts, history, folklore, and institutions of a group of people that are unified by race, ethnicity, nationality, language, religious beliefs, spirituality, socioeconomic status, social class, sexual preference, politics, gender, age, disability, or any other cohesive group variable" (Singh, 1995b). Clearly, this definition recognizes that all of us simultaneously belong to more than one cultural group and that each person is in a complex dynamic relationship with other individuals from overlapping cultural traditions.

The components of a culture can be classified across several dimensions. For example, aspects of a culture can be classified as objective, which refers to its tangible or observable aspects, or subjective, which refers to its invisible or mental aspects (Triandis, 1977). The objective aspects of a culture, which include such things as its members' clothing, food, and artifacts, are relatively easily seen, understood, and accepted by people of other cultures. Although the basis of many cultural stereotypes originates at this level, few cross-cultural misunderstandings occur at the objective cultural level. The subjective aspects of a culture, which refer to values, ideals, attitudes, roles, and norms, are less easily understood by people of other cultures and provide the basis for much misunderstanding between people of different cultures. Understanding and appreciating the subjective aspects of another culture often pose the greatest challenge to service providers and evaluators in systems of care, because this requires a nonjudgmental acceptance of the nuances of that culture.

CULTURAL AWARENESS, SENSITIVITY, AND COMPETENCY

As with the term *culture,* there are many definitions of cultural awareness, sensitivity, and competency. *Cultural awareness* is a general term used to indicate that a person is conscious of the similarities and differences within, between, and among cultures. Awareness is a necessary but not sufficient condition for a person to behave in a culturally appropriate manner toward others from different cultures. *Cultural sensitivity* is a more specific term used to indicate that a person not only has an awareness of the nuances of one's own culture as well as those of other cultures but also does not assign a negative or positive value to the differences within, between, and among cultures. Sensitivity means that the person accepts cultural differences nonjudgmentally. *Cultural competency* is a term used to indicate that a person has "knowledge and skills that enable him or her to appreciate, value and celebrate similarities and differences within, between and among culturally diverse groups of people" (Singh, 1996, p. 124). Competency is a dynamic concept and does not imply that a person ever reaches a state of being universally culturally competent; rather, it implies that the person has the knowledge and skills for displaying and increasing his or her understanding and appreciation of the changing nature and nuances of his or her own culture as well as those of others.

DIVERSITY IN THE UNITED STATES

In 1990, the population of the United States consisted of 75% Anglo Americans (non-Hispanic White), 12% African Americans, 9% Hispanics, 3% Asians and Pacific Islanders, and 0.8% Native Americans (American Indian; U.S. Bureau of the Census, 1992a). In 1990, the U.S. Department of Health and Human Services also predicted that by the year 2000, African Americans would constitute 13.1% of the total population, Hispanics 9.4%, Asians and Pacific Islanders 3.5%, and Native Americans 1%. By the year 2050, the composition of the different ethnic groups in the United States will change dramatically. The percentage of Anglo Americans will decrease to 52.7%, and African Americans, Hispanics, Asians and Pacific Islanders, and American Indians will increase to 16.2%, 21.1%, 10.7%, and 1.2% of the population, respectively (O'Hare, 1992; U.S. Bureau of the Census, 1992b). The largest proportional increase will be seen in the Hispanic and Asian and Pacific Islander groups.

Although the U.S. Bureau of the Census and the Office of Civil Rights officially recognize five racial/ethnic groups (i.e., American Indian, Asian, Hispanic, Black, and White), there is great diversity within these groups. For example, African Americans may differ in terms of cultural heritage, ethnic identity, family structure, religious affiliation and spirituality, and socioeconomic status. Hispanics may have different ancestral heritage, originating from Mexico, Puerto Rico, Central or South America, or Cuba. Asian Americans include the Chinese, Filipinos, Japanese, Koreans, Asian Indians, Vietnamese, Cambodians, and Laotians. Pacific Islanders include those who come from the dozens of countries and thousands of islands in the Pacific Ocean. Native Americans include people from more than 200 tribes who speak one or more of the 200 tribal languages (LaFromboise, 1988). Finally, there is additional diversity within each of these groups. As diversity increases in our society, the diversity of children and adolescents with EBD and their families in our systems of care will inevitably increase.

DIVERSITY IN SYSTEMS OF CARE

The prevalence of EBD in school children has been estimated to be anywhere between 2% and 12% (Office of Technology Assessment, 1986). However, Kauffman (1997) has suggested that 3% to 6% of students in our schools probably have emotional and behavioral disorders that require some form of intervention. Although the data are limited, there is a good general indication that children with EBD form a culturally diverse group. For example, an analysis of nine recent studies on the characteristics of children in systems of care showed that on average, the age of the children ranges from about 8 to 16 years; about 70% to 75% of them are boys; and between 50% and 75% are Caucasians, followed by about 25% to 30% African Americans, and 10% Hispanic Americans and others, including Native Americans, Asians, Pacific Islanders, and those of mixed races (Barber, Rosenblatt, Harris, & Attkisson, 1992; Cullinan, Epstein, & Quinn, 1996; Epstein, Cullinan, Quinn, & Cumbald, 1994, 1995; Landrum, Singh, Nemil, Ellis, & Best, 1995; Quinn et al., 1996; Quinn, Newman, & Cumbald, 1995; Silver et al., 1992; Singh, Landrum, Donatelli, Hampton, & Ellis, 1994).

These data indicate that even when only three indicators of cultural diversity (age, gender, and ethnicity/race) are taken into account, there is a broad spectrum of children with EBD who are being served in various systems of care in this country. Of course, virtually no data are available on some of the other aspects of cultural diversity in these children and their families, such as their nationality, language, religious beliefs, spirituality, socioeconomic status, social class, sexual preference, politics, and disability status, among others. The reporting of these data will be crucial in future research because it may well be that some of these variables will be found to correlate highly not only with the nature of the services needed or sought by children with EBD and their families but also with the types of services that are most appropriate.

A related issue is the lack of similar data reported in outcome studies from various systems of care. First, such data provide an indication of cultural diversity of the sample being provided services. Second, the reporting of these data indirectly indicates that evaluators and, perhaps, the service providers are aware of the unique needs of children and families from different cultural groups. For example, it is well established that evaluators may need to use assessment instruments and diagnostic methods that are culturally appropriate for children from different racial and ethnic groups. Further, children from diverse cultural backgrounds may need additional interventions that are different from the generic programs used with White, middle class children and their families (Singh, Ellis, Oswald, Wechsler, & Curtis, 1997; Singh, Williams, & Spears, 2002). Third, these data alert the reader to look for cultural influences on the research methods and statistics used in the outcome analysis.

The changing cultural demographics of our society are reflected in the demographics of children with EBD and their families in systems of care. As the numbers of children from culturally diverse families increase in systems of care, the context in which services are being delivered is also changing. This change has immense implications for the nature and effectiveness of the services delivered in systems of care.

PARTICIPANTS

Data on the participants or the recipients of the services are of prime importance to both the service providers and the evaluators. Depending on the program evaluation model chosen (see Table 12.1), the evaluator may either simply access the data on the characteristics of the participants from the service providers or collaborate with the service providers in setting up the process for obtaining the information on the participants. In either case, the information to be collected will include the customary sociodemographic data as well as assessment and diagnostic data.

SOCIODEMOGRAPHIC AND INTAKE INFORMATION

The sociodemographic and intake data will include the contextual information already discussed, with the caveat that data are collected on only those variables that are directly relevant to service delivery and outcomes. Service providers and evaluators should remember that collecting data, even on sociodemographic variables, is an intrusive process that affects the children as well as their family members. The degree of intrusiveness experienced by families is dependent on a number of factors, including their cultural heritage, social customs, and expectations of outcome.

Children with EBD and their families participate in the intake interview and data collection process because they view their participation as serving a legitimate purpose—that is, in return for providing the requested data, they will receive needed services. Given that initial interviews are used not only to gather factual sociodemographic data and to determine the nature of the services sought but also to establish a working relationship with the children and their families, the information provided by the families is contextually grounded and jointly constructed by the families and the interviewer. That is, the child and the family are strongly influenced by the interviewer and, at the same time, the interview is strongly influenced by the child and his or her family.

Inherent in the transactional relationship between the participants and the service providers or evaluators are potential iatrogenic effects of the data collection that are akin to the demand characteristics (Orne, 1962) and experimenter expectancies (Rosenthal, 1969) in participant–researcher interaction systems. We know, for example, that the interviewer's age, demeanor, gender, race/ethnicity, professional experience, and interpersonal style, among other variables, may affect the subjective responses of the participants. Further, some service recipients, particularly those from holistic cultures, such as American Indian, African American, Asian, and Puerto Rican (see Singh et al., 1997), may experience embarrassment or distress in revealing intimate aspects of their family to a complete stranger, especially in view of the fact that it is a one-sided exchange of personal and family information. Participants from cultures in which telling others about disruptions in one's family life or mental illness in a family member is seen as a loss of face (Zane, 1991) may provide information that is sanitized for public consumption. Finally, participants from the dominant Anglo-American culture may also have an acute emotional response to answering seemingly innocuous questions, such as those about one's social networks and social support (Anglin, 1996).

The impact of collecting participant sociodemographic and intake data on the well-being of children with EBD and their families has not been considered in the evaluation of systems of care. In the context of family therapy, it has been shown that the mere asking of questions is a form of intervention because it invariably results in some change in family transactions (Bussell, Matsey, Reiss, & Hetherington, 1995). The situation is further complicated when cultural variables interact with the need to collect data regarding the child with EBD and his or her family. Service providers and program evaluators need to be aware of the obvious conflict between gathering enough data on which to base appropriate interventions and protecting the participants' welfare, particularly if the participants are from cultures that are sensitive to some of the questions being asked. We need to have a better understanding of culturally diverse participants' reactions to questions typically asked in sociodemographic and related questionnaires. At the very least, we will need to understand the data collection experience from the perspective of the participants (Singh, 1995a).

Finally, we need to consider whether the standard questions in our sociodemographic forms and intake interviews tap into the issues and experiences of culturally diverse families. Most of the questions typically included in these forms and interviews are based on our experiences with Anglo-American children with EBD and their families, or they are based on a priori notions of inquiry into areas that will lead to more detailed assessments on standardized instruments. It is unlikely that these questions will include the experiences of culturally diverse families that they deem important to their child and to themselves. A more compelling alternative would be to use "client-based" methodologies (Kuehl, Newfield, & Joanning, 1990) and ethnographic interviews (Lincoln & Guba, 1985), which would enable the participants and service providers to collect information needed to collaboratively construct the service needs and culturally appropriate interventions for the child with EBD and his or her family.

When service providers and evaluators collaborate with the service recipients to construct a family's sociodemographic profile, the contour of the cultural characteristics of the family is very rich. In addition to the standard demographic variables traditionally highlighted in Western system-of-care evaluations, many families will include information on their family origins, migration patterns, and location of significant family members in this country and in their country of origin. These data can used by service providers to determine the availability, as well as the strength, of the family's support systems, a major moderating variable in intervention outcome.

Other issues that families will raise include the social roles of extended family members, general health status of each member, their holistic perspective on what constitutes illness, their attitudes and responses to illness, and help-seeking behavior with regard to health and mental health services. Rosado (1980) has suggested that the following variables be discussed with families because they provide the basis for assessing their mental health needs: their perceptions of the etiology of psychiatric and psychological problems, psychological support systems, verbal and nonverbal communication patterns within the extended family, the language spoken most often in the family home, time orientation (linear vs. circular), spiritual resources, and their conceptions of physical and mental well-being.

Finally, the coping experiences of people from cultures that have traditionally been marginalized in this country also have a bearing on their mental health and help-seeking behavior. Thus, information on their adaptation to a majority Anglo-American culture that has different values and practices discrimination is very important. This type of information can be obtained in terms of a family's assimilation, acculturation, biculturalism, and multiculturalism (Dana, 1993). Clearly, culturally sensitive sociodemographic information can be gathered only through collaborative constructions with the family members. The critical importance of sociocultural information in the planning of culturally sensitive services and in minimizing institutional barriers in service provision cannot be overstated.

ASSESSMENT

In systems of care, service providers and program evaluators use the assessment process as a systematic method for learning about the characteristics and needs of children with EBD and their families. In the psychiatric model, one of the anticipated outcomes of clinical assessment is that it will lead to a diagnosis of psychopathology, if present. Diagnostic assessment has been seen as an important part of the process for providing services because there is an assumption that the better the goodness-of-fit between the assessment and the proposed interventions, the better the outcomes (Meyer, 1989).

Assessment of Ability and Achievement

Standardized tests of ability and achievement are used with children for a number of reasons. For example, the results of these tests may be used by teachers for making curricular decisions; that is, they can determine in which subject areas the child needs instructional attention. Similarly, the test data may be used for placing students in special programs, such as special education or gifted programs. Further, the same test data may be used within the context of accountability to assess the effectiveness of teachers, schools, and school districts. Although ability and achievement tests are not standard components of an intake assessment in systems of care, often the test data are requested from the school system and incorporated in the child's profile. In many cases, children are referred to different service agencies depending on the grouping in which they have been placed in school as a consequence of their performance on these tests.

One of the assumptions in standardized testing is that, regardless of their personal life experiences, all children taking the test understand the meaning of a question or test item in exactly the same way. However, this assumption ignores contextual factors and is not supported by data (Glick, 1985). Research has not produced any evidence for a generalized cognitive processor in children or adults that operates across knowledge domains; rather, the data strongly support the notion that learning is predominantly context specific (Scribner & Cole, 1981). As most tests have culture-specific items, tests of ability and achievement are context specific with culture-specific items. In addition, there are other, more general, factors that may affect test outcome. For example, when compared to the normative sample for a test, factors such as language differences, urban and rural subcultures, exposure to specific test materials or test formats, cultural differences in a testing situation, socioeconomic status, and social desirability, among others, will affect test outcome (Bond, 1990; Brescia & Fortune, 1989; Groth-Marnat, 1990; Neisser et al., 1996). The critical issue for service providers and evaluators is that if ability and achievement test data are to be used for the purpose of determining any aspect of service provision, they must be aware of the fact that sociocultural contexts significantly influence cognitive performance.

Assessment Methodology

There are few standardized assessment instruments that may have universal application—that is, they can be used with all children or adults, regardless of their cultural heritage and personal life experiences. Typically, the assessment instruments used in assessing children with EBD in various systems of care have been developed in this country from an Anglo-American perspective. Although the developers of some instruments have attempted to include normative samples that contain participants from diverse cultures, rarely have these instruments fulfilled the methodological requirements for a valid instrument that can be used with participants from different cultures. For example, few developers of instruments have factor analyzed their normative samples separately for the different subgroups to see if they all have the same factor structure.

Service providers and program evaluators may begin with a choice between an emic (indigenous) or an etic (universal) orientation in their assessment methods if they are at all aware of the methodological problems inherent in participant populations that involve multiple cultures. In cross-cultural research, *emic* refers to the perspective of the people within the culture, and *etic* refers to a universal perspective that applies across cultures. In working within the emic perspective, the service providers or evaluators elicit meaning, experiences, and perceptions from the participant's, rather than from their own, point of view. Thus, they are more interested in understanding the participant's beliefs and values that underlie the psychopathology or psychological distress rather than imposing their own beliefs and theoretical perspectives on the assessment data. Clearly, the emic perspective is closely aligned with qualitative methods of inquiry because these methods focus on understanding phenomena from the viewpoint of the participants; that is, these methods of inquiry emphasize understanding the transactional processes between the participants and their environments rather than in controlling and predicting outcomes.

Etic methodologies require the use of instruments that are valid and reliable, and the data are evaluated and interpreted by the evaluator in terms of current theories of the phenomena of interest. Thus, the etic perspective is closely aligned with quantitative methods of inquiry that are based on accepted conceptual frameworks and hypothesis testing. Further, quantitative methods are based on a deductive approach in which the meaning of the phenomena of interest is not understood until the data collection is complete and the data are statistically analyzed. In contrast, qualitative methods rely on inductive analyses of the data, letting the meaning of the phenomena emerge as the evaluator interacts with the participants. Thus, in this approach, the meaning of the phenomena is socially constructed by the participants and the evaluator.

What is the implication of the emic–etic distinction for program evaluation in systems of care? The main implication is that data based on the etic method of inquiry do not provide a complete understanding of the participants if the assessment and outcome instruments used are not valid and reliable for the participant's culture. A related issue is that hardly any clinical assessment instruments have been developed from an emic perspective. The traditional solution to this problem has been to translate and adapt standard Western assessment instruments and structured interviews to different cultures using the forward–back translation format. Thus, for example, a standardized rating scale in English is translated into Japanese and then back-translated into English. The accuracy of the Japanese version is assessed by correlating the back-translated English version with the original English version. However, this is not a satisfactory solution because it presumes universality of symptom patterns across cultures (Fegert, 1989), an assumption that is clearly at variance with the research data (Mezzich, Kleinman, Fabrega, & Parron, 1996). Further, the manner in which psychiatric or psychological problems or distress is expressed varies within, between, and among cultures, and this is not reflected in the instruments constructed in this manner.

Another solution has been to develop assessment instruments and structured interviews de novo for a specific culture using Western concepts of psychopathology, psychological distress, and behavior disorders. The new scale is assumed to be valid if its factor structure is similar to those found in Western cultures (Elton, Patton, Weyerer, Diallina, & Fichter, 1988). One assumption of this method of developing new instruments is that similar factor structures will emerge in different cultures only if similar behaviors or beliefs exist in these cultures. Thus, the similarity of the factor structure of a rating scale in two or more cultures is assumed to be evidence for the cross-cultural utility of the scale. However, this approach also has its problems, including the fact that it does not take into account culture-specific disorders (Mezzich et al., 1996).

Selecting Culturally Appropriate Instruments

Flaherty et al. (1988, p. 258) have suggested that instruments intended for use across cultures can be selected according to the following priorities: (a) instruments already proven to be cross-culturally equivalent, (b) instruments that have been extensively tested and found to be psychometrically sound in one culture but have not been tested in other cultures, and (c) instruments that have high face validity but require further psychometric testing in the country of origin followed by cross-cultural validation. Of course, a fourth option is to develop a new instrument if none are available to measure the phenomenon of interest. The likelihood of finding an instrument that has already been proven to be cross-culturally equivalent is very slim at the present time. The second option, to use an extensively tested and well-validated instrument from one culture and test it in another, has been chosen most often in cross-cultural research in mental health and psychological distress. Typically, these instruments are translated into the language of another culture, if necessary, and tested for their usefulness in the second culture. This option has had negligible use in program evaluation in systems of care.

When working in Peru with a Spanish translation of the National Institute of Mental Health's diagnostic interview schedule, Gaviria et al. (1984) detected five kinds of validity problems in using a forward–back translated instrument. These included content validity, semantic validity, technical validity, criterion validity, and conceptual validity. These five psychometric dimensions of cultural equivalence can be used as the basis for testing an existing instrument with participants from another culture or for developing and evaluating an instrument for assessing in a new culture a phenomenon that exists in another culture. An instrument is culturally equivalent in two cultures if it meets the criterion on one or more of the five dimensions of validity. Thus, an instrument can be considered to have content equivalence if its items are relevant to the phenomena in the two cultures.

Flaherty et al. (1988) have developed a taxonomy of issues that need to be considered in assessing instruments for cross-cultural validation in psychiatric research. However, their taxonomy applies equally well to system-of-care evaluations. In their taxonomy, each dimension of cultural equivalence is mutually exclusive of others, and the best instrument would possess equivalence on all five dimensions. For content equivalence, each item included in the scale being assessed must describe a phenomenon that is present and relevant in the culture that the instrument is to be used in. In the development of an instrument by forward–back translation, each item from the original instrument must be checked by a team of content raters for its relevance to the new culture. Only those items that are culturally relevant are kept; new, culture-specific items may be added, and then the new scale is subjected to psychometric examination, including internal consistency, reliability and validity, and factor structure.

For semantic equivalence, the meaning of each item in the scale must remain the same after translation into the language of the new culture. Simply translating a well-validated scale from one culture into the language of another does not guarantee that the translated scale will be reliable or valid. Semantic equivalence can be achieved through the forward–back translation method. The three-phase development of the scale consists of the following: (a) forward translation from the language of Culture A to the language of Culture B by a bilingual person or a team of bilingual translators, (b) back translation of the scale from the language of Culture B to the language of Culture A by a second bilingual person or another team of bilingual translators, and (c) ratings by a panel of bilingual experts on the concordance in meaning between the original and back translated versions. Items must not only retain the same meaning as in the original scale but also use the idiom (i.e., the characteristic forms of expression) of the culture in which it is to be used or else a response bias may be evident. If an instrument is translated into more than two languages, semantic concordance among the different language versions of the scale is critical.

Technical equivalence requires demonstration of the fact that the mode of data collection has not differentially affected the participants' responses in the two cultures. This can be somewhat problematic because many oral cultures are not proficient at using pencil-and-paper tests (Vernon & Roberts, 1981). In some cultures, one-on-one interviews with women or girls is proscribed, particularly if the interviewer is a man. The repetitious questions and probing typical of semistructured interviews and questionnaires commonly used in Western research are seen as coercive in developing countries (Flaherty et al., 1988). Further, in some Asian and Native American cultures, people do not ask known-answer questions and do not take kindly to being asked such questions. One method for assessing technical equivalence requires the demonstration of concurrent validity when data on the same phenomenon in a culture are collected through two different modes (e.g., a paper-and-pencil test and an interview format) by different data collectors. Further, the technical equivalence of an instrument may be compromised if the participants from different cultures have differing response tendencies (e.g., need for social approval, trait desirability, acquiescence).

Criterion equivalence requires the demonstration that responses to similar items on an instrument relate to the same normative concept or independent criteria in the two cultures. According to Flaherty et al. (1988), *criterion equivalence* refers to "the instrument's capacity to assess the variable (i.e., phenomenon) in both cultures studied and to the fact that the interpretation of the results from the instruments is the same in both cultures" (p. 261). This means that an instrument with a high degree of sensitivity and specificity in one culture would show similar rates of sensitivity and specificity in the second culture. If not, it may be an indication that the cutoff scores for the instrument in the second culture may need recalibration. If recalibration does not solve the problem, the most likely interpretation is that either the instrument does not measure the target phenomenon in the same manner or the target phenomenon does not exist in a similar manner in the two cultures. However, it must be remembered that the critical issue in criterion equivalence is "not whether the phenomena or symptoms occur, but whether the diagnostic criteria actually measure the same phenomena" (Flaherty et al., 1988, p. 262) in the two cultures.

Conceptual equivalence is demonstrated if an instrument measures the same basic construct or concept in two or more cultures. In systems of care, it would be expected that conceptually equivalent instruments would measure the same psychiatric disorders, psychiatric distress, or emotional problems across cultures. This would presume that the disorders are conceptualized and quantified in a similar manner across target cultures.

Finally, service providers and evaluators need to understand that even if cross-cultural equivalence of instruments has been satisfactorily resolved, there is the issue of *intracultural diversity,* which increasingly poses problems in assessment. For example, intergenerational differences in assimilation, acculturation, language use, and worldviews pose assessment problems within a culture similar to those posed by differences between cultures. That is, we do not know much about how multiple generations within a culture formulate their expressions of psychiatric or psychological distress, nor do we know if standard assessment measures of mental health are reliable and valid across multiple generations within a culture.

Clearly, the adequacy of the assessment instruments and methodology are at the heart of any program evaluation. In current systems of care, the majority of the instruments being used were developed for Anglo-Americans, and few, if any, of the instruments were developed from the service recipients' perspectives. The assessment instruments reflect the cultural bias of the Anglo-American culture and may not be totally appropriate as measures of psychiatric illness or psychological distress in children from other cultures.

DIAGNOSIS

Recent studies of children and adolescents in systems of care show that they suffer from a wide range of psychiatric disorders (Barber et al., 1992; Epstein et al., 1995; Quinn, Epstein, Cumbald, & Holderness, 1996; Singh et al., 1994). Of the many diagnostic issues that are important, two deserve special attention. The first issue is whether the *DSM–IV* nosology (American Psychiatric Association [APA], 1994) provides a valid formulation of the mental health of children and adolescents who are not Anglo-American. The second issue stems from the fact that psychiatric disorders, psychological distress, and behavior problems occur in the context of the child's family, friends, and community. Thus, the issue is whether we should be using a relational nosology in addition to the individually focused system of *DSM–IV.*

Culturally Formulated Diagnosis

There is extensive evidence to show that people from diverse cultures are more frequently misdiagnosed than Anglo-Americans (Good, 1993; Lin, 1996). Some of the reasons for the misdiagnosis include problems of language, cultural nuances, and biases of the clinicians. Further, until the publication of the *DSM–IV,* clinicians did not have the benefit of cultural formulation guidelines for psychiatric diagnosis. The *DSM* has always been about treating mental disorders rather than about the people who have these disorders (Strauss, 1992), and when the focus is on people, it is clear that their culture has a tremendous impact not only on the experience and manifestation of a mental disorder but also on its assessment, course, and response to treatment (Fabrega, 1987; Hooper, 1991; Kleinman, 1988; Rogler, 1989). The recent addition of cultural formulation guidelines has increased the cultural validity and suitability of the *DSM–IV* (see Table 12.2).

Although current research with children and adolescents with EBD has not focused on the cultural aspects of their psychiatric disorders and emotional problems, extrapolation from the adult literature suggests that non–Anglo-American children may well be misdiagnosed. Further, we know from recent descriptive and epidemiological research on children with EBD in systems of care that a large percentage of them are on psychotropic medication for their psychiatric problems (Epstein et al., 1995; Landrum et al., 1995; Singh et al., 1994). However, research also has shown that no attention has been paid to the fact that there are cross-ethnic and cross-national variations in the dosing and side-effect profiles of psychotropic medications (Lin, Anderson, & Poland, 1995). In addition, recent work in pharmacokinetics, pharmacogenetics, and pharmacodynamics has indicated that culture and ethnicity greatly influence the disposition and effects of many psychotropic drugs that these children are prescribed (Lin, Poland, & Nakasaki, 1993). Service providers and program evaluators must be cognizant of these findings because culturally diverse children may be (a) misdiagnosed and therefore may be receiving inappropriate treatment and (b) on doses of psychotropic medication that are not optimal for them. Both of these scenarios may lead to negative outcomes for the children.

Relational Diagnosis

The focus of the *DSM* as a nosological system has always been on the individual's mental disorders. In the *DSM–IV,* it is stated quite clearly that "each of

TABLE 12.2

The *DSM–IV* Cultural Formulation Guidelines

The following outline for cultural formulation is meant to supplement the multiaxial diagnostic assessment and to address difficulties that may be encountered in applying *DSM–IV* criteria in a multicultural environment. The cultural formulation provides a systematic review of the individual's cultural background, the role of the cultural context in the expression and evaluation of symptoms and dysfunction, and the effect that cultural differences may have on the relationship between the individual and the clinician…. In addition, the cultural formulation suggested below provides an opportunity to describe systematically the individual's cultural and social reference group and ways in which cultural context is relevant to clinical care. The clinician may provide a narrative summary of the following categories:

Cultural Identity of the Individual

Note the individual's ethnic or cultural reference groups. For immigrants and ethnic minorities, note separately the degree of involvement with both the culture of origin and the host culture (where applicable). Also, note language abilities, use, and preferences (including multilingualism).

Cultural Explanations of the Individual's Illness

The following may be identified: the predominant idioms of distress through which symptoms or the need for social support are communicated (e.g., "nerves," possessing spiritus, somatic complaints, inexplicable misfortune), the meaning and perceived severity of the individual's symptoms in relation to norms of the cultural reference group, any local illness category used by the individual's family and community to identify the condition, the perceived causes or explanatory models that the individual and the reference group use to explain the illness, and current preferences for and past experiences with professional and popular sources of care.

Cultural Factors Related to Psychosocial Environment and Levels of Functioning

Note culturally relevant interpretations of social stressors, available social supports, and levels of functioning and disability. This would include stresses in the local social environment and the role of religion and kin networks in providing emotional, instrumental, and informational support.

Cultural Elements of the Relationship Between the Individual and the Clinician

Indicate differences in culture and social status between the individual and the clinician and problems that these differences may cause in diagnosis and treatment (e.g., difficulty in communicating in the individual's first language, in eliciting symptoms or understanding their cultural significance, in negotiating an appropriate relationship or level of intimacy, in determining whether a behavior is normative or pathologic).

Overall Cultural Assessment for Diagnosis and Care

The formulation concludes with a discussion of how cultural considerations specifically influence comprehensive diagnosis and care.

Note. From *Diagnostic and Statistical Manual of Mental Disorders* (4th ed., pp. 843–844), American Psychiatric Association, 1994, Washington, DC: Author. Copyright 1994 by the American Psychiatric Association. Adapted with permission of the author.

the mental disorders is conceptualized as a clinically significant behavioral or psychological syndrome or pattern that occurs in an individual…. It must currently be considered a manifestation of a behavioral, psychological, or biological dysfunction in the individual" (APA, 1994, pp. xxi–xxii). However, as family members and service providers, we know that the emotional and behavioral disorders of children and adolescents are associated more with interpersonal problems than with intrapsychic distress. When the cultural context is overlaid on the relational nature of children's emotional and behavioral disorders, it makes sense to diagnose a child's problems in terms of the context in which they occur.

Further, children and adults from holistic cultures view themselves as being a part of the whole; they see themselves in relational terms. That is, they are interdependent and interconnected with all others in their family, community, and the cosmos (Singh, 1995b, 1995c). They are a part of an interpenetrated collective that is defined by kinship, and they tend to value harmony with their environment, holistic thinking, group identity, cooperation, and cohesiveness above mastery of and control over their environment, dualistic thinking, individualism, and competition. Further, people from holistic cultures value the relational context in their lives, and they find comfort in extended family relationships. They are likely to place the well-being of the extended family above their own; when one member of their family has a problem, the problem is seen as belonging to the entire family.

Service providers and evaluators must be cognizant of the worldviews of children and families from different cultures. Thus, using a linear diagnosis that is focused clearly on an individual may not sit well with people who come from holistic cultures and who see the problem as affecting all members of the family rather than just the child with EBD. With all families, service providers should use an emic perspective and view the problem from the perspective of the family members. Thus, if a diagnosis is to be made, it must be relational rather than individualistic. Similarly, an emic perspective should be taken for developing a treatment program. In the absence of family involvement and ownership of the treatment program, there is an excellent chance that the prescribed treatment will be assessed by the family as being inappropriate and subsequently will prove to be ineffective. Indeed, service providers may wish to use group and family modes of treatment because these methods may be culturally aligned with the family's strong sense of the interconnectedness of all family members.

OUTCOMES

In systems of care, the measures used to determine the need for services as well as baseline assessments of psychopathology, psychological distress, and behavior problems are also used to provide data on outcomes. With the exception of an instrument to measure consumer satisfaction with the services, additional instruments are rarely needed just for evaluating outcomes. Nonetheless, if additional instruments are needed, the principles enumerated for selecting assessment instruments will apply. In addition to the appropriate choice of measures, an appreciation of cultural influences on methods, data analysis, and interpretation of the findings is of prime importance.

CONSUMER SATISFACTION

The general issues involved in assessing consumer satisfaction in systems of care have recently been reviewed by Young, Nicholson, and Davis (1995). Perhaps the only critical issue that they did not include was a cultural perspective in understanding and evaluating consumer satisfaction. Current consumer satisfaction measures assume that the participant belongs to a homogeneous group called "consumers" and that all consumers behave in the same way and have the same expectations of outcome. The emic perspective suggests that consumer satisfaction may be affected to a large extent by the participant's explanatory models of causation and symptomatology of illness, experiences of the illness, preference for different forms of treatment (e.g., allopathy vs. folk healing), view of the therapist or healer, and expected outcomes. These issues are rarely, if ever, considered in the selection or design of a measure of consumer satisfaction.

A cultural perspective suggests that to fully assess the consumer's satisfaction with the services, we need an insider's view or, in the parlance of anthropology, we need the "native point of view" (Geertz, 1983). A culturally valid consumer satisfaction instrument must be based on the participant's personal perspective, and there are a number of issues that will determine the nature of the items that should be included in such an instrument.

Cultural Identity

The participant's cultural identity (e.g., ethnicity, religious and spiritual beliefs) provides the context within which the illness or disorder is viewed. For example, Asian Indian Hindus believe in karma, destiny, and fate, and this provides the context within which they view their illness and its outcome. Believing that their illness is karmic, they may not have any expectations regarding either the treatment or the outcome of such treatment. Thus, they may rate their satisfaction with the services as high regardless of the nature or quality of the services offered. The ethnomedical context of Navajo Indians provides another example of the importance of cultural identity. Navajo Indians identify illnesses by the agents that cause them, rather than by symptom identification, as in Western culture (Adair & Deuschle, 1970). Thus, they may rate satisfaction with services in a Western system of care as low because they would have a hard time understanding why a therapist would spend hours taking down their history or giving them a physical examination prior to treatment. Knowing the cultural identity of the participant will help the service providers and evaluators understand how that person will react to the services offered.

Cultural Idioms

Cultural factors that are pertinent to the participant's psychiatric disorder or psychological distress will have an impact on his or her rating of consumer satisfaction. These cultural factors may include culture-specific illnesses, explanatory models for their disorders, cultural significance of the symptoms, and patterns and rates of seeking services. Hallucinations provide an excellent example of the cultural significance of symptoms. For example, it is a normative experience for Plains Indians to hear the voices of recently deceased family members calling them from the spirit world (Kleinman, 1996). If the same experience is reported by someone from a Western culture, the experience would be considered hallucinatory, and the person would be deemed in need of mental health services.

Differential rates of help-seeking behavior have been found to be related to culture and ethnicity (Snowden & Cheung, 1990). Asians, Pacific Islanders, and Hispanics appear to seek the services of mental health providers at lower rates than Anglo-Americans because it is customary in these cultures to maintain the mentally ill family member at home. They use Western mental health services only when all traditional/folk measures have failed, and they will do so with some degree of shame because of the stigma that is attached to having a family member with mental illness. In such cases, services are sought only when the family feels that the problem is intractable, and their satisfaction with the services will be influenced by this context.

Participant's Relationship and Expectations of the Therapist

There are great cultural variations in consumer–therapist relationships, and issues associated with these relationships influence consumer satisfaction with the overall services. For example, Italians place a much greater emphasis on the therapist's character and humanitarian attitude than on his or her medical or psychiatric skills, especially for physicians (Zborowski, 1969). In contrast, Jewish patients place a greater emphasis on the therapist's quality of training and professional experience than on personal qualities (Zborowski, 1969). Thus, in addition to other variables, consumer satisfaction ratings will differ depending on the patient–therapist relationship desired and achieved by the consumers.

Other cultural variables that influence consumer satisfaction with services include, but are not limited to, cultural expectations of clinical decision making (Schreiber & Homiak, 1981), the therapist's understanding of the consumer's language and his or her ability to communicate clearly with the consumer, cultural variations in levels of symptom reporting, degree of rapport and confidentiality established with the therapists, and cultural expectations of treatment outcome. The implication for service providers and evaluators is that no single global measure will encompass these variables or provide a reliable and valid measure of consumer satisfaction. The use of a simple, unidimensional rating scale, as is popular in the mental health field today, is probably an indication of our ignorance of or insensitivity to cultural perspectives in consumer satisfaction in systems of care.

CULTURAL INFLUENCES ON METHODS, DATA ANALYSIS, AND INTERPRETATION OF FINDINGS

Standard program evaluation methods may be used when the evaluator, service providers, and participants in a service delivery system are all from the same ethnic and racial group. However, even belonging to the same racial and ethnic group does not preclude differential cultural influences within the group. Thus, cultural influences need to be considered whenever differences between two groups of people are being investigated.

Cultural Influence of the Evaluator

The nature of the questions asked in a program evaluation is determined by a number of factors, including the cultural background of the evaluator. Formulation of the questions is dictated, in part, by the personal experiences and cultural bias of the evaluator and others who are involved in determining the evaluation methodology. From an emic perspective, it is reasonable to assume that not all recipients of the services, or even the service providers, will view the program evaluation questions as equally important or relevant to them as they may be to the evaluator, because there will be cultural and personal differences in how issues regarding evaluation are viewed.

In many cases, because of their presumed importance, the evaluation questions are simply imposed on the service recipients and the service providers. The evaluator makes the decision regarding what and how to assess. In a practical sense, the evaluator's level of rapport with the participants will affect their responses, especially if they are from socioeconomically disadvantaged groups (Fuchs & Fuchs, 1986). Further, culturally relevant feedback provided by the evaluator typically improves performance, particularly on achievement and ability tests (Groth-Marnat, 1990). Interpretation of test results and other data are strongly influenced by the evaluator's cultural attitudes, traditions, ideals, subjective predisposition, and personal and moral convictions (Kaplan & Saccuzzo, 1989).

Sampling of Participants

Typically, the evaluator has no control over sampling issues, unless the evaluation is driven by a research hypothesis and the participants are randomly assigned to predetermined conditions. In such cases, evaluators have the opportunity to decide whether the sample included in the program evaluation will be representative of a given culture or will be based on other considerations, such as the participant's need for services and availability. Evaluators need to be aware that in the absence of some formal sampling procedures, the service recipients in most systems of care typically do not constitute a representative sample of their cultures, and that findings of intergroup differences in such samples should not necessarily be ascribed to cultural differences.

In many program evaluations, the pool of service recipients from different cultures is not large enough to analyze in terms of the cultural influences on outcome. Further, even if the numbers of service recipients from each culture are large enough, the evaluator may still not be able to make intercultural judgments because the samples across cultures may not be equivalent. That is, just because there are 100 African American children and 100 Anglo-American children in a wraparound program (VanDenBerg & Grealish, 1996) does not necessarily mean that the two samples are equivalent. For example, the children in the two samples could differ on a number of variables, including socioeconomic status, educational achievement, disability status, social experiences, exposure to technology, resilience to life stressors, and social support. Thus, program evaluators must consider not only differences arising from culture but also other plausible variables that may account for the observed differences between the two groups.

Cultural Influences on Data Analysis

Many instruments used in program evaluations include some form of rating for each item (e.g., 1 = *strongly disagree;* 5 = *strongly agree*). Cross-cultural research shows that there is a tendency in some cultures to respond in terms of a "cultural response set" to such items in rating scales. For example, when requested to rate consumer satisfaction on a 7-point scale, service recipients from Culture A may rate either 6 or 7 and those from Culture B may rate either 4 or 5. The evaluator may interpret these data as showing that consumers from Culture A are generally more satisfied than those from Culture B. All things being equal, this is a reasonable interpretation of the data. However, what if further research shows that people from Culture B actually rate everything a few points lower than the people from Culture A? This cultural response set in people from Culture B means that they have a cultural tendency to use the middle part of the scale most often. When the cultural response set is taken into account, the program evaluator may now conclude that people in the two cultures are generally equally satisfied with the services.

Program evaluators should be aware of the possibility that cultural response sets may confound the cultural differences in the data. In addition, they need to be aware of the possibility that there may be cultural differences as well as cultural response sets, or either may be present by itself. Finally, it should not be forgotten that cultural response sets are also a part of cultural differences.

Cultural Influences on Interpreting the Data

As in life itself, data from program evaluations are open to multiple plausible interpretations. For example, the data may reflect true cultural differences, cultural response sets, or an interaction of the two. In many cases, other alternative interpretations will also be possible. Because program evaluation deals with people in the context of their lives and few, if any, intervening variables are controlled, the data may be only suggestive of a cultural difference. This ambiguity in the data leaves open the possibility for biased interpretation by the evaluator. For example, if the evaluator is looking for cultural differences, the ambiguity may allow him or her to interpret the data as showing a cultural difference. Indeed, we all interpret our data through our own cultural lenses. Further, as consumers of program evaluation data, we should not forget that regardless of their nature, all data are biased in some way.

In summary, we need to be aware of the importance of cultural influences on the nature and conduct of program evaluations. These influences are in addition to those that are inherent in the manner service providers deliver services to culturally diverse children with EBD and their families.

CULTURAL COMPETENCIES

It is almost de rigueur in any discussion of cultural diversity to refer to the need for training in cultural competency. The seminal work of Cross, Bazron, Dennis, and Isaacs (1989) on culturally competent systems of care for children with EBD from diverse cultures provided the guiding principles for cultural competency training. Concurrently, researchers and policy analysts noted that there was a significant underutilization of mental health and related services by culturally diverse families, especially those with low incomes, when compared to Anglo-American families (Ruiz et al., 1995). The lack of cultural competency in service delivery systems was viewed as a major barrier to accessing services by culturally diverse families.

Although a small cottage industry has developed to enhance cultural competency in systems of care, there is little evidence to suggest that these efforts have had a major impact on our service delivery system, including program evaluation. Nonetheless, some progress has been made. For example, we now have a number of tools that can be used to measure the cultural competency of agencies (e.g., Dana, Behn, & Gonwa, 1992) as well as that of individual service providers (e.g., Sodowsky, Taffe, Gutkin, & Wise, 1994). These tools can be used to determine training needs as well as progress made in cultural competency by both agencies and individual service providers.

Several investigators have enumerated a number of guidelines and principles regarding cultural competencies that service providers and therapists should possess (e.g., Hinkle, 1994; Kalyanpur & Harry, 1997; Sue, Arredondo, & McDavis, 1992). These guidelines and principles are broad enough that they could also be useful for program evaluators.

Further, program evaluators can go through a series of steps to ensure that their evaluations are culturally competent. First, they must ensure that they have a good understanding of program evaluation models and methods that transcend particular cultures. Second, this knowledge must be complemented with competency training in their own culture as well as in other cultures. Third, because one cannot have a good grasp of the cultural nuances of all cultures in our society, program evaluators will need to collaborate with informed people from the target cultures, including the service recipients, service providers, representatives from funding agencies, and other professionals. This collaborative effort should yield the basic design, choice of culturally appropriate instruments, methods, and the process of program evaluation for a particular culture. Fourth, the planned evaluation should be tested in a pilot project and extensive feedback obtained from the service recipients, service providers, collaborators, and other significant personnel (e.g., funding agency staff, program evaluation experts). The feedback would be used to revise and strengthen the evaluation plans. Fifth, the evaluation should be undertaken and data-analytic plans developed that take into account potential cultural influences in data analysis and interpretation. Sixth, the data should be analyzed and informed members of the target culture, as well as of different cultures, should provide feedback on the data analysis and interpretation of the findings. Finally, the program evaluation findings should be revised in accordance with the feedback. In summary, culturally competent program evaluation is a complex endeavor that should be performed by those who are trained in program evaluation and have some degree of cultural competency.

CONCLUSIONS

Cultural influences are pervasive in human society and need to be taken into account when we provide and evaluate mental health and related services. Regardless of whether our own definitions of culture are narrow or broad, we all belong to multiple cultures and, therefore, we all have to transcend overt or covert cultural barriers in our daily lives. One of the most important things we can do as people is to develop cultural self-awareness so that we are aware of the hidden cultural assumptions that influence our interactions with others. Further, such awareness will assist us in clarifying our own biases and prejudices, which we may have tacitly accepted as a part of who we are.

In this chapter, I have raised some issues that deal explicitly with cultural influences on service delivery and its evaluation. The broad definition of culture that I have used is derived from our understanding of the complexity of human society as viewed by social scientists.

Issues of culture go well beyond the mere enumeration of race, creed, and gender; they encompass the breadth of diversity witnessed in our world today. However, because of space considerations, the focus of this chapter has been limited to issues that deal mainly with race and ethnicity. Even with issues regarding race and ethnicity, I have not covered some essential ground (e.g., biracial, multiracial, and multiethnic people) for the same reason. Other issues of diversity (e.g., age, gender, sexual orientation, socioeconomic status, religion) are equally important and no less worthy of our attention.

The focus of this chapter has been the cultural influences on assessment of children and adolescents with EBD. And, although the issues that arise in the assessment of their families are similar, numerous assessment issues that are specific to the culturally appropriate assessment of families need to be addressed. Issues regarding cultural influences on service delivery, and the wider context of culturally responsive systems of care, need to be addressed as well.

Given the pervasive effects of culture on human behavior, the prospect of accounting for the influence of all cultural variables in every facet of program evaluation can be quite daunting. Obviously, the effects of even the major cultural variables can neither be assessed meaningfully nor controlled in any one program evaluation. Indeed, it would be folly to attempt to do so, not only because of the size of the task but also because of the dynamic nature of cultural influence in the lives of the service recipients, service providers, and program evaluators. Our energies may be better directed at finding program evaluation principles and methods that are universal, that would apply across cultures, and that are specific to different cultural groups.

REFERENCES

Adair, J., & Deuschle, K. (1970). *The people's health: Medicine and anthropology in a Navajo community.* New York: Appleton-Century-Crofts.

American Psychiatric Association. (1994). *Diagnostic and statistical manual of mental disorders* (4th ed.). Washington, DC: Author.

Anglin, J. P. (1996). Eureka! Bathed in transformation. In L. Heshusius & K. Ballard (Eds.), *From positivism to interpretivism and beyond* (pp. 19–25). New York: Teachers College Press.

Attkisson, C. C., Dresser, K. L., & Rosenblatt, A. (1996). Service systems for youth with severe emotional disorder: System-of-care research in California. In L. Bickman & D. J. Rog (Eds.), *Children's mental health services* (pp. 236–280). Thousand Oaks, CA: Sage.

Barber, C. C., Rosenblatt, A., Harris, L. M, & Attkisson, C. C. (1992). Use of mental health services among severely emotionally disturbed children and adolescents in San Francisco. *Journal of Child and Family Studies, 1*, 183–207.

Behar, L. B. (1996). State-level policies in children's mental health: An example of system building and refinancing. In L. Bickman & D. J. Rog (Eds.), *Children's mental health services* (pp. 21–41). Thousand Oaks, CA: Sage.

Bickman, L., Heflinger, C. A., Lambert, E. W., & Summerfelt, W. T. (1996). The Fort Bragg managed care experiment: Short term impact on psychopathology. *Journal of Child and Family Studies, 5*, 137–160.

Bond, L. (1990). Understanding the black/white student gap on measures of qualitative reasoning. In F. C. Serafica, A. I. Schwebel, R. K. Russell, P. D. Isaac, & L. B. Myers (Eds.), *Mental health of ethnic minorities* (pp. 89–107). New York: Praeger.

Brescia, W., & Fortune, J. C. (1989). Standardized testing of American Indian students. *College Student Journal, 23*, 98–104.

Bussell, D. A., Matsey, K. C., Reiss, D., & Hetherington, M. (1995). Debriefing the family: Is research an intervention? *Family Process, 34*, 145–160.

Clark, H. B., & Clarke, R. T. (1996). Research on the wraparound process and individualized services for children with multi-system needs. *Journal of Child and Family Studies, 5,* 1–5.

Cross, T. L., Bazron, B. J., Dennis, K. W., & Isaacs, M. R. (1989). *Towards a culturally competent system of care* (Vol. 1). Washington, DC: CASSP Technical Assistance Center, Georgetown University Child Development Center.

Cullinan, D., Epstein, M. H., & Quinn, K. P. (1996). Patterns and correlates of personal, family, and prior placement variables in an interagency community based system of care. *Journal of Child and Family Studies, 5,* 299–321.

Dana, R. H. (1993). *Multicultural assessment perspectives for professional psychology.* Boston: Allyn & Bacon.

Dana, R. H., Behn, J. D., & Gonwa, T. (1992). A checklist for the examination of cultural competence in social service agencies. *Research on Social Work Practice, 2,* 220–233.

Elton, M., Patton, G., Weyerer, S., Diallina, M., & Fichter, M. (1988). A comparative investigation of the principal component structure of the 28-item version of the General Health Questionnaire (GHQ). *Acta Psychiatrica Scandinavica, 77,* 124–132.

Epstein, M. H., Cullinan, D., Quinn, K. P., & Cumbald, C. (1994). Characteristics of children with emotional and behavioral disorders in community-based programs designed to prevent placement in residential facilities. *Journal of Emotional and Behavioral Disorders, 2,* 51–57.

Epstein, M. H., Cullinan, D., Quinn, K. P., & Cumbald, C. (1995). Personal, family, and service use characteristics of young people served by an interagency community-based system of care. *Journal of Emotional and Behavioral Disorders, 3,* 55–64.

Fabrega, H., Jr. (1987). Psychiatric diagnosis: A cultural perspective. *Journal of Nervous and Mental Disease, 175,* 383–394.

Fegert, J. M. (1989). Bias factors in the translation of questionnaires and classification systems in international comparative child and adolescent psychiatric research. *Acta Paedopsychiatrica, 52,* 279–286.

Flaherty, J. A., Gaviria, F. M., Pathak, D., Mitchell, T., Wintrob, R., Richman, J. A., et al. (1988). Developing instruments for cross-cultural psychiatric research. *Journal of Nervous and Mental Disease, 176,* 257–263.

Fuchs, D., & Fuchs, L. S. (1986). Test procedure bias: A meta-analysis of examiner familiarity effects. *Review of Educational Research, 56,* 243–262.

Gaviria, M., Pathak, D., Flaherty, J., Garcia-Pacheco, C., Martinez, H., Wintrob, R., et al. (1984). *Designing and adapting instruments for a cross-cultural study on immigration and mental health in Peru.* Paper presented at the annual meeting of the American Psychiatric Association.

Geertz, C. (1983). *Local knowledge.* New York: Basic Books.

Glick, J. (1985). Culture and cognition revisited. In E. D. Neimark & R. De Lisi (Eds.), *Moderators of competence* (pp. 99–144). Hillsdale, NJ: Erlbaum.

Good, B. J. (1993). Culture, diagnosis and comorbidity. *Culture, Medicine and Psychiatry, 16,* 427–446.

Groth-Marnat, G. (1990). *Handbook of psychological assessment* (2nd ed.). New York: Wiley.

Hinkle, J. S. (1994). Practitioners and cross-cultural assessment: A practical guide to information and training. *Measurement and Evaluation in Counseling and Development, 27,* 103–115.

Hooper, K. (1991). Some old questions for the new cross-cultural psychiatry. *Medical Anthropology, 5,* 299–330.

Kalyanpur, M., & Harry, B. (1997). A posture of reciprocity: A practical approach to collaboration between professionals and parents of culturally diverse backgrounds. *Journal of Child and Family Studies, 6*(4), 487–509.

Kaplan, R. M., & Saccuzzo, D. P. (1989). *Psychological testing: Principles, applications, and issues.* Pacific Grove, CA: Brooks/Cole.

Kauffman, J. M. (1997). *Characteristics of emotional disorders of children and youth* (6th ed.). Upper Saddle River, NJ: Merrill.

Kleinman, A. (1988). *Rethinking psychiatry: From cultural category to personal experience.* New York: Free Press.

Kleinman, A. (1996). How is culture important for DSM–IV? In J. E. Mezzich, A. Kleinman, H. Fabrega, & D. L. Parron (Eds.), *Culture and psychiatric diagnosis: A DSM–IV perspective* (pp. 15–25). Washington, DC: American Psychiatric Press.

Kuehl, B. P., Newfield, N. A., & Joanning, H. (1990). A client-based description of family therapy. *Journal of Family Psychology, 3,* 310–321.

Kuhns, E., & Martorana, S. (1982). *Qualitative methods for institutional research.* San Francisco: Jossey-Bass.

LaFromboise, T. D. (1988). American Indian mental health policy. *American Psychologist, 43,* 388–397.

Landrum, T. J., Singh, N. N., Nemil, M. S., Ellis, C. R., & Best, A. M. (1995). Characteristics of children and adolescents with serious emotional disturbance in system of care: Part II. Community-based services. *Journal of Emotional and Behavioral Disorders, 3,* 141–149.

Levin, H. M. (1983). *Cost-effectiveness: A primer.* Thousand Oaks, CA: Sage.

Lin, K. M. (1996). Cultural influences on the diagnosis of psychotic and organic disorders. In J. E. Mezzich, A. Kleinman, H. Fabrega, & D. L. Parron (Eds.), *Culture and psychiatric diagnosis: A DSM–IV perspective* (pp. 49–62). Washington, DC: American Psychiatric Press.

Lin, K. M., Anderson, D., & Poland, R. E. (1995). Ethnicity and psychopharmacology. *Psychiatric Clinics of North America, 18,* 635–647.

Lin, K. M., Poland, R. E., & Nakasaki, G. (1993). *Psychopharmacology and psychobiology of ethnicity.* Washington, DC: American Psychiatric Press.

Lincoln, Y. S., & Guba, E. G. (1985). *Naturalistic inquiry.* Thousand Oaks, CA: Sage.

Meyer, R. G. (1989). *The clinician's handbook: The psychopathology of adolescence and adulthood.* Needham Heights, MA: Allyn & Bacon.

Mezzich, J. E., Kleinman, A., Fabrega, H., & Parron, D. L. (1996). *Culture and psychiatric diagnosis: A DSM–IV perspective.* Washington, DC: American Psychiatric Press.

Miles, M., & Huberman, A. (1984). *Qualitative data analysis: A sourcebook of new methods.* Thousand Oaks, CA: Sage.

Neisser, U., Boodoo, G., Bouchard, T. J., Boykin, A. W., Brody, N., Ceci, S. J., et al. (1996). Intelligence: Knowns and unknowns. *American Psychologist, 51,* 77–101.

Office of Technology Assessment. (1986). *Children's mental health: Problems and services* (Background paper; Pub. no. OTA-BP-H-33). Washington, DC: U.S. Government Printing Office.

O'Hare, W. P. (1992). America's minorities: The problem of diversity. *Population Bulletin, 47*(4), 1–47.

Orne, M. T. (1962). On the social psychological experiment: With particular reference to demand characteristics and their implications. *American Psychologist, 17,* 776–783.

Quinn, K. P., Epstein, M. H., Cumbald, C., & Holderness, D. (1996). Needs assessment of community-based services for children and youth with emotional or behavioral disorders and their families: Part 2. Implementation in a local system of care. *Journal of Mental Health Administration, 23,* 432–446.

Quinn, K. P., Epstein, M. H., Dennis, K., Potter, K., Sharma, J., McKelvey, J., et al. (1996). Personal, family, and service utilization characteristics of children served in an urban family preservation environment. *Journal of Child and Family Studies, 5,* 469–486.

Quinn, K. P., Newman, D. L., & Cumbald, C. (1995). Behavioral characteristics of children and youth at risk for out-of-home placements. *Journal of Emotional and Behavioral Disorders, 3,* 166–173.

Rogler, L. H. (1989). The meaning of culturally sensitive research in mental health. *American Journal of Psychiatry, 146,* 296–303.

Rosado, J. W., Jr. (1980). Important psychocultural factors in the delivery of mental health services to lower-class Puerto Rican clients: A review of recent studies. *Journal of Community Psychology, 8,* 215–226.

Rosenthal, R. (1969). Interpersonal expectations: Effects of the experimenter's hypothesis. In R. Rosenthal & R. L. Rosnow (Eds.), *Artifact in behavioral research* (pp. 181–227). New York: Academic Press.

Ruiz, P., Venegas-Samuels, K., & Alarcon, R. D. (1995). The economics of pain: Mental health care costs among minorities. *Psychiatric Clinics of North America, 18,* 659–670.

Saxe, L., Cross, T. P., Lovas, G. S., & Gardner, J. K. (1996). Evaluation of the mental health services program for youth: Examining rhetoric in action. In L. Bickman & D. J. Rog (Eds.), *Children's mental health services* (pp. 206–235). Thousand Oaks, CA: Sage.

Schreiber, J., & Homiak, J. (1981). Mexican Americans. In A. Harwood (Ed.), *Ethnicity and medical care* (pp. 264–337). Cambridge, MA: Harvard University Press.

Scribner, S., & Cole, M. (1981). *The psychology of literacy.* Cambridge, MA: Harvard University Press.

Silver, S. E., Duchnowski, A. J., Kutash, K., Friedman, R. M., Eisen, M., Prange, M. E., et al. (1992). A comparison of children with serious emotional disturbance served in residential and school settings. *Journal of Child and Family Studies, 1,* 43–59.

Singh, N. N. (1995a). In search of unity: Some thoughts on family–professional relationships in service delivery systems. *Journal of Child and Family Studies, 4,* 3–18.

Singh, N. N. (1995b, June). *Living from our center: Consciousness, spirituality and exceptionality.* Paper presented at the Colloquium on Spirituality, Consciousness and Exceptionality, Sugarloaf Conference Center, Temple University, Chestnut Hill, PA.

Singh, N. N. (1995c, October). The quest for wholeness: Personal growth in daily life. In C. R. Ellis & N. N. Singh (Eds.), *Children and adolescents with emotional and behavioral disorders: Proceedings of the Fifth Annual Virginia Beach Conference* (p. 150). Richmond: Virginia Commonwealth University, Medical College of Virginia, Commonwealth Institute for Child and Family Studies.

Singh, N. N. (1996). Cultural diversity in the 21st century: Beyond E Pluribus Unum. *Journal of Child and Family Studies, 5,* 121–136.

Singh, N. N., Ellis, C. R., Oswald, D. R., Wechsler, H. A., & Curtis, W. J. (1997). Value and address diversity. *Journal of Emotional and Behavioral Disorders, 5*(1), 24–35.

Singh, N. N., Landrum, T. J., Donatelli, L. S., Hampton, C., & Ellis, C. R. (1994). Characteristics of children and adolescents with serious emotional disturbance in system of care: Part I. Partial hospitalization and inpatient psychiatric services. *Journal of Emotional and Behavioral Disorders, 2*, 13–20.

Singh, N. N., Williams, E., & Spears, N. (2002). To value and address diversity: From policy to practice. *Journal of Child and Family Studies, 11*, 35–45.

Snowden, L. R., & Cheung, F. K. (1990). Use of inpatient mental health services by members of ethnic minority groups. *American Psychologist, 45*, 347–355.

Sodowsky, G. R., Taffe, R. C., Gutkin, T. B., & Wise, S. L. (1994). Development of the Multicultural Counseling Inventory: A self-report measure of multicultural competencies. *Journal of Counseling Psychology, 41*, 137–148.

Stecher, B. M., & Davis, W. A. (1987). *How to focus an evaluation.* Thousand Oaks, CA: Sage.

Strauss, J. S. (1992). The person—Key to understanding mental illness: Towards a new dynamic psychiatry, III. *British Journal of Psychiatry, 161*(Suppl. 18), 19–26.

Stroul, B. A., & Friedman, R. M. (1986). *A system of care for severely emotionally disturbed children and youth.* Washington, DC: CASSP Technical Assistance Center, Georgetown University Child Development Center, National Technical Assistance Center for Children's Mental Health.

Sue, D. W., Arredondo, P., & McDavis, R. J. (1992). Multicultural counseling competencies and standards: A call to the profession. *Journal of Counseling and Development, 70*, 477–486.

Triandis, H. C. (1977). *Interpersonal behavior.* Pacific Grove, CA: Brooks/Cole.

U.S. Bureau of the Census. (1992a). *Census of population and housing—Summary tape file 1: Summary population and housing characteristics.* Washington, DC: U.S. Government Printing Office.

U.S. Bureau of the Census. (1992b). *Current population reports, P25-1092: Population projections of the United States by age, sex, race, and Hispanic origin: 1992–2050.* Washington, DC: U.S. Government Printing Office.

U.S. Department of Health and Human Services. (1990). *Healthy people 2000* (PHS 91-50213). Washington, DC: U.S. Government Printing Office.

VanDenBerg, J. E., & Grealish, E. M. (1996). Individualized services and supports through the wraparound process: Philosophy and procedures. *Journal of Child and Family Studies, 5*, 7–21.

Vernon, S. W., & Roberts, R. E. (1981). Measuring nonspecific psychological distress and other dimensions of psychopathology: Further observations on the problem. *Archives of General Psychiatry, 38*, 1239–1247.

Welshimer, K., & Earp, J. (1989). Genetic counseling within the context of existing attitudes and beliefs. *Patient Education and Counseling, 13*, 237–255.

Young, S. C., Nicholson, J., & Davis, M. (1995). An overview of issues in research on consumer satisfaction with child and adolescent mental health services. *Journal of Child and Family Studies, 4*, 219–238.

Zane, N. (1991, August). *An empirical examination of loss of face among Asian Americans.* Paper presented at the annual meeting of the American Psychological Association, San Francisco.

Zborowski, M. (1969). *People in pain.* San Francisco: Jossey-Bass.

Programs and Evaluations

SECTION III

Wraparound Milwaukee
Program Description and Evaluation

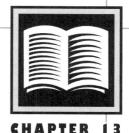

CHAPTER 13

Bruce Kamradt, Stephen A. Gilbertson, and Nancy Lynn

Wraparound Milwaukee is an innovative system of care for children with serious emotional, behavioral, and mental health needs and their families. It uses an approach that places an emphasis on developing and delivering services to families that are strength based, highly individualized, and community focused. The Wraparound Milwaukee philosophy stresses that the family, the community, and the service system must work together to support the youth and his or her family to achieve healthy functioning (Burns & Goldman, 1998). Operationally, the program can be described as a unique public managed-care entity, responsible for meeting all the mental health, substance abuse, social service, and other supportive needs of the most complex youth in the Milwaukee community. The term *wraparound* is usually defined as a philosophy of care that includes a definable planning process involving the child and family that results in a set of community services and natural supports individualized for that child to obtain a set of positive outcomes. These services are said to be "wrapped" around the specific needs of that child and family (Burchard & Clarke, 1990). Wraparound Milwaukee adheres to essential core elements common to all wraparound approaches. These core elements are presented in Table 13.1.

The dissemination and evolution of the wraparound process owes much to the groundbreaking work of the Child and Adolescent Service System

TABLE 13.1

Core Elements of Wraparound Approaches Used in Wraparound Milwaukee

- Community-based care
- Individualized services based on the needs of the client
- Adherence to culturally competent services and supports
- Family involvement in the design and delivery of services
- Team-driven planning process
- Flexible funding
- Balance of formal and informal services to support families
- Collaboration among child-serving systems
- Unconditional care (never giving up on a child)
- Presence of an ongoing evaluation process

Program (CASSP), which laid out many of these core elements in its implementation in the late 1980s and early 1990s. Ira Lourie, the "founding father" of CASSP, has described the system of care and wraparound process as the foundation of CASSP (Katz-Leavy, Lourie, Stroul, & Zeigler-Dendy, 1992). The principles of CASSP were further implemented through recent demonstration grants from the U.S. Department of Health and Human Services Center for Mental Health Services (CMHS), administered by the Substance Abuse and Mental Health Services Administration (SAMHSA). In 1994, Wraparound Milwaukee was one of the first communities to receive funding through this initiative to develop a comprehensive system of care for youth with serious emotional needs and their families.

WHO IS SERVED IN THIS PROGRAM?

Wraparound Milwaukee serves children and adolescents through age 18 who have a serious emotional, behavioral, or mental health disturbance and are referred to the program by a court order from the county's juvenile court system. To qualify as having a severe emotional disturbance under Wisconsin state Medicaid guidelines requires that a child have a mental or emotional disturbance listed in the fourth edition of the American Psychiatric Association's *Diagnostic and Statistical Manual of Mental Disorders* (*DSM–IV;* American Psychiatric Association, 1994). Further, the child's condition must have persisted for 6 months and be expected to persist for a year or more. The child must have either functional symptoms or impairments that place him or her at immediate risk of residential treatment, psychiatric hospitalization, or juvenile correctional placement. Finally, the child must be receiving services from two or more of the following child-serving systems: mental health, social services, child welfare, juvenile justice, or special education (Integrated Services Programs for Children with Severe Disabilities, 1999–2000).

WHAT IS THE RATIONALE FOR SERVING THIS TARGET GROUP?

The group of youth served by Wraparound Milwaukee has the highest service costs of children seen in child welfare, mental health, and juvenile justice agencies in the Milwaukee area. Before the development of Wraparound Milwaukee, these youth received traditional mental health services, such as residential or inpatient placements. Evaluation studies by the Planning Council of Milwaukee showed that these placements were ineffective with this difficult-to-treat population. In the planning council's 1994 study, Milwaukee County youth with serious emotional needs placed in residential treatment centers were found to have high rates of failure (e.g., dropping out of the program). Of those placements deemed successful by these residential facilities, nearly 60% were referred back to either the child welfare or juvenile justice systems within 6 months of discharge from residential facilities. These discouraging findings led the child welfare and juvenile justice agencies to search for alternatives to residential treatment that could control costs and improve outcomes.

Although Wisconsin's Medicaid program does not pay for residential treatment for children, it does pay for psychiatric hospital care. Medicaid was expending large amounts of money for the care of youth with serious mental health disturbance who fell into two categories: (a) youth who were in inpatient psychiatric facilities prior to placement in a residential treatment center and (b) youth who dropped out of these residential centers and returned to a psychiatric hospital. Medicaid was aware, as the Surgeon General's report pointed out, that there were few, if any, studies that demonstrated the long-term effectiveness of inpatient psychiatric care on the lives of children with serious emotional and mental health needs (U.S. Department of Health and Human Services, 1999). Similar to the child welfare and juvenile justice systems in Wisconsin, Medicaid was searching for a better system to control costs in the area of inpatient psychiatric care for children.

RESPONDING TO THE CHALLENGE OF THESE YOUTH

The poor outcomes of these youth, together with the high costs of providing services through the existing service structures, set the stage for a new approach. In 1995, shortly after Milwaukee County received federal funding to develop a new system of care for youth with serious emotional disturbance, the director of children's mental health services and key program staff approached the health and human services director, child welfare director, chief probation officer for the county, and chief juvenile court judge to assist in designing a pilot project. This project would utilize the wraparound approach to serve 25 youth currently in residential treatment centers. The "25 Kid Project," as it was called, targeted 25 youth selected by child welfare and juvenile justice who had been in residential treatment centers for 6 months or longer (one child had been placed in the center for 10 years) with no immediate discharge plan. There would be no "eject or reject" of any youth in the pilot effort, meaning no child would be excluded from participating or be expelled from the program. The goals of the program were to determine if (a) these youth could be returned home or to their community, (b) they could be kept safe and the community kept safe upon their return, and (c) the cost of community placement would be equal to or less than the cost of a residential treatment placement (Kamradt, 1999).

Although system representatives expressed some initial skepticism, 17 of the 25 youth (68%) were returned to the community within 120 days. Over the course of a year, 24 of the 25 youth were returned to the community. Recidivism rates were very low for these children (only 3 children returned to institutional-based care within 1 year), and the average cost of keeping these youth in the community was under $3,000 per month per child—much less than the $5,000 per month or more for residential treatment costs (Kamradt, 1999).

As a result of the success of the 25 Kid Project, Wraparound Milwaukee began to incrementally enroll two groups of youth: (a) all remaining youth in residential treatment centers and (b) all newly identified youth who were at risk of residential treatment placement. Rather than youth being court-ordered by juvenile justice or child welfare into a specific residential treatment center, the youth are court-ordered to the Wraparound Milwaukee Program, provided that their parent(s) are amenable to participating in the program. The wraparound team working with the child and his or her family determines the necessity of placement, specific placement resources, or preferably an alternative placement in the youth's own home or community with a comprehensive array of services to support and meet the child's treatment needs. Even after the child has returned home, the court order for Wraparound Milwaukee services and supports stays in place until the family can meet the child's needs without wraparound services.

A "flexible" court order issued by children's court gives Wraparound Milwaukee the authority to determine the level of placement and placement location. This flexible court order allows Wraparound Milwaukee to make short-term residential placements for 24- to 48-hour crisis/respite care or for 30 to 90 days for stabilization. In addition, this type of court order allows the program to move a child to a less restrictive level of care without having to obtain a new court order—for example, from residential treatment placement to a treatment foster home and then to the child's natural home. Wraparound Milwaukee care coordinators exercise a "Change of Placement" to notify and gain approval from the court for plans to change a child's placement.

THE DEMOGRAPHICS OF THE POPULATION WRAPAROUND MILWAUKEE SERVES

Wraparound Milwaukee primarily serves a male population (71% are boys). The average age for enrollees in the program is 13.2 years, with the majority (85%) between the ages of 12 and 17. There are large numbers of minorities in the population served, with African Americans (63%) making up the largest sub-population, followed by Caucasians (29%). The average income of nearly half (47%) of enrollees is at or below the federal poverty level of $15,000 per year. In 2001, Wraparound Milwaukee served 869 children and their families. The average daily enrollment was 560 families.

THE STRUCTURE OF WRAPAROUND MILWAUKEE

Wraparound Milwaukee is best described as a publicly operated care management organization (CMO). Although they use many managed-care business techniques and strategies, CMOs differ from traditional managed-care organizations in that they focus on providing enrollees with a broad range of mental health, substance abuse, and other supportive services. Services from multiple sectors are combined into a single system of care for the defined group of youth and their families. Enrollees in a CMO usually have high levels of service needs, which contrasts with enrollees of traditional managed-care arrangements, many of whom have very low service needs and low utilization rates.

County governments operate most health and human services in Wisconsin. Governance of Wraparound Milwaukee is under the auspices of the Milwaukee County Department of Health and Human Services (DHHS). The Milwaukee County Behavioral Health Division (BHD) is the division within DHHS that is the designated administrative entity for the provision of public mental health services for adults and children. Wraparound Milwaukee is the care management organization for children's mental health services that was developed by BHD to manage the delivery of mental health services to the defined group of youth with serious emotional and mental health needs and their families.

The key child-serving agencies in Milwaukee County collaborating with Wraparound Milwaukee to fund the services provided to the defined target group include the following: (a) the Bureau of Milwaukee Child Welfare, a state-administered, privately operated system overseeing all child protection services in Milwaukee County; (b) Milwaukee County Delinquency and Court Services, a county-operated probation service for delinquent youth; (c) Division of Health Care Financing, a state agency administering all Medicaid services, including all special managed-care programs; and (d) Milwaukee County Behavioral Health Division, Children's Branch, a county agency responsible for overseeing public mental health services for children in Milwaukee and designated to operate Wraparound Milwaukee.

There are other key local- and state-level cooperating agencies that do not provide program funding but provide in-kind services and supports through existing programming. These agencies include (a) Milwaukee public schools and the 27 other school districts in Milwaukee County; (b) the Adult Service Division within Milwaukee County that provides alcohol and other substance abuse resources, as well as transition services for young adults; and (c) the State Bureau of Mental Health, which provides technical assistance and other services.

BLENDED FUNDING

A trademark of Wraparound Milwaukee is the pooled funding that was created to meet the comprehensive needs of children with serious emotional needs and their families. Funds from various child-serving systems and Medicaid are blended using case rates and a capitation arrangement to create maximum flexibility and the most sufficient funding base possible (see Figure 13.1).

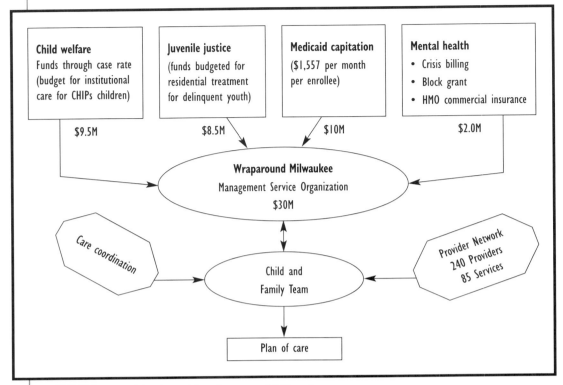

FIGURE 13.1. Pooled funds used by Wraparound Milwaukee.

The Bureau of Milwaukee Child Welfare, the state agency responsible for the operation of child welfare services in Milwaukee, pays Wraparound Milwaukee a monthly case rate of $3,535 per month per child for each child welfare case enrolled in Wraparound Milwaukee. Child welfare authorities have viewed this rate as advantageous, because this agency would otherwise have to pay nearly $7,300 per month per child for a residential placement. This case rate is based on actuarial studies done by Wraparound Milwaukee to identify the child welfare costs, which were approximately $9.5 million in 2001. The case rate is paid for the duration of the child's court order into Wraparound Milwaukee, which is generally 12 months, as that was the average length of residential placement before the Wraparound Milwaukee model was initiated. It should be noted, however, that Wraparound Milwaukee has recently reduced the average placement time to 4 months or less.

The Department of Juvenile Justice initially paid the same case rate but now provides about $8.5 million per year in funding to Wraparound Milwaukee through a $\frac{1}{12}$ per month allocation of their budgeted out-of-home funds. Wraparound enrolls approximately 260 youth who would otherwise be placed in residential treatment centers or state correctional facilities for the duration of the court order. Children with dual juvenile justice and child welfare court orders receive a 50% monthly split in funding between child welfare and juvenile justice.

Because Medicaid was concerned about reducing high-cost inpatient psychiatric hospitalizations for the target population, they negotiated a separate contract with Wraparound Milwaukee to arrange for the provision of mental health and substance abuse services to these youth. Wraparound Milwaukee was designated as a special managed-care project by Medicaid in 1997. As a type of HMO, Wraparound Milwaukee receives a monthly capitation payment of $1,557 per child for each Medicaid-eligible child (approximately 85% of enrollees), in addition to the case rates paid by child welfare or the fixed rate paid by juvenile justice. This capitation payment rate was determined by the state's health-care financing division and was based on the mental health/substance abuse costs of the defined population. Wraparound Milwaukee receives 95% of the mental health and substance abuse costs for these youth as determined by actuarial analysis performed by the state. Total Medicaid payments in 2001 were approximately $10 million.

Wraparound Milwaukee also bills Medicaid directly for crisis services, such as the operation of the mobile crisis team and crisis mentors, which were not in the original actuarial study. Other funds come in through a mental health block grant, Social Security Insurance (SSI), and insurance companies. These other funds totaled about $2 million in 2001.

The pooled funds are managed by Wraparound Milwaukee, which serves as the administrative service organization. Funds are available to the family through the child and family team process, which is overseen by a care coordinator, who, with the family, determines service needs. Vendors bill Wraparound Milwaukee for the costs of providing services to families. Payments to vendors are made once each claim is adjudicated based on the units of service authorized.

THE WRAPAROUND VALUE BASE DICTATES CARE AND TREATMENT

Critical to the success of Wraparound Milwaukee is the values base underlying its operation and its approach to the delivery of services to families. The principal values and philosophy of Wraparound Milwaukee include the following:

1. *Build on strengths to meet needs.* Historically, mental health programs have been designed around the deficits and problems of the child and his or her family. Wraparound Milwaukee's philosophy is centered on identifying the strengths of the child and family. Those personal, family, and community strengths become resources around which to develop an effective care plan.

2. *One family—one plan.* A single care plan is developed among all agencies serving that family. There are no separate education plans, child welfare plans, mental health agency plans, and so forth, that guide treatment. Care is delivered in a seamless fashion.

3. Best fit with culture and preferences. An emphasis is placed on understanding the culture and heritage of the family to ensure that staff are better able to understand the needs of that family.

4. Community-based responsiveness. Wraparound Milwaukee believes children are best served when cared for in their own community rather than in institutions. Institutional placements are unnatural settings for the treatment of children. Wraparound Milwaukee places emphasis on the development of a range of community services as an alternative to institutionalization.

5. Increase parent choice and family independence. The care plan developed by the family and the services delivered are designed to help strengthen and enable the family to make their own choices. A long-term goal of the program is for families to function independently.

6. Care for children in the context of families. Families are seen as the best judge of what their children and family need. Family involvement is seen as integral to the care-planning process.

7. Never give up. Care is provided in an unconditional manner. When a case plan is not working, the child is not blamed; rather, the plan is modified to meet the changing needs of the child and family.

CARE AND TREATMENT IN WRAPAROUND MILWAUKEE

The cornerstone of the wraparound system is the care coordinator. The care coordinators facilitate the wraparound process by conducting strengths/needs assessments, facilitating the team planning, identifying and obtaining treatment resources and supports for the child and family, and monitoring and evaluating the care plan. Care coordinators work with small caseloads of no more than eight families. They are mostly bachelor's-level workers who are intensively trained and certified in the wraparound process by Wraparound Milwaukee.

Care coordinators meet with the child and family within the first week of referral. The initial visit focuses on establishing rapport, hearing the family tell their story, discovering child and family strengths, determining immediate needs, and formulating the crisis safety plan. Within the first 30 days of enrollment, the care coordinator works with the family to develop the Child and Family Team. This team consists of individuals who provide support, either formally or informally, to that child and family. These typically include the care coordinator, family members, relatives, church members, friends, counselors, teachers, mentors, and a probation worker or child welfare worker. The team may also include a family advocate or a staff psychologist for complex cases, such as juvenile sex offenders or fire starters.

A care plan is developed by the Child and Family Team through a process that incorporates the family's vision, strengths, and needs. Needs are prioritized and strategies developed to meet those needs, including assigning roles and tasks to team members. Wraparound Milwaukee uses a domain-based plan of care. Required domains include the family, crisis/safety/legal, psychological, and educational/vocational aspects of the child's life. Other domains that are routinely addressed include the child's living arrangement, medical, cultural/spiritual, social, and recreational needs.

The care plan includes short-and long-term goals and must be approved by the family and by a psychologist/psychiatrist who understands the wraparound process and is credentialed to provide such services in the Wraparound Milwaukee Provider Network. From the plan developed by the Child and Family Team, the care coordinator generates a monthly service authorization request (SAR), which authorizes payment to providers for any paid services that are identified as needed in the care plan. Providers are notified through the Internet-based information system employed by Wraparound Milwaukee of the type of service, rate, and units to be provided for the month covering each authorization.

MOBILE URGENT TEAM

The Mobile Urgent Team supports the care plan developed by the Child and Family Team by intervening in crisis situations at times when a care coordinator is not available or when the situation requires clinical assessment and intervention beyond what a care coordinator could reasonably be expected to provide. The team used by Wraparound Milwaukee consists of three psychologists and five social workers with specific training and expertise in crisis intervention and trauma response. This team of eight professionals is available 24 hours per day, and all Wraparound Milwaukee participants are automatically enrolled in this crisis service.

The Mobile Urgent Team also reviews all requests for inpatient psychiatric hospital admissions. This team operates an eight-bed group home and several foster homes capable of providing short-term crisis stabilization (of up to 14 days) while the crisis team and care coordinator work with the family toward the goal of returning the child to his or her home. The availability of the crisis team has allowed Wraparound Milwaukee to nearly eliminate the use of inpatient psychiatric care for most children enrolled in the project. Annual hospital inpatient days decreased from 5,000 days in 1996 to less than 200 days in 2001.

PROVIDER NETWORK

A key to the success of Wraparound Milwaukee has been its ability to individualize services based on each youth's need. That requires the availability of a comprehensive array of services to respond to the specific needs identified by the Child and Family Team. It has meant moving away from creating slots in preexisting services or other forms of categorical funding for services. The one-size-fits-all approach is the antithesis of the Wraparound Milwaukee model.

Wraparound Milwaukee has built and developed an array of more than 80 different services. They are provided on a fee-for-service basis, with Wraparound Milwaukee setting the unit price for each type of service. Rather than traditional contracts, vendors apply to provide one or more of the services as part of a provider network. No provider is guaranteed a certain volume of service or a fixed contract minimum. Providers must agree to provide services within the wraparound philosophy and values. The provider network now includes more than 230 individual providers and agencies. This design allows for more diversity in the types of providers and services available as well as increased choice for families, who may choose their preferred providers from the network.

INFORMAL SERVICES AND NATURAL SUPPORTS

Wraparound Milwaukee offers a remarkable array of formal services to youth and their families. However, the informal services identified by the care coordinator and Child and Family Team during the strength-based assessment are often just as valuable as the formal services. For example, families may identify a friend or relative who has a positive relationship with the youth and may be willing to become a mentor to the child or who can provide respite care to the parents. These informal supports often remain with the family even after discharge from the program. Other examples of informal supports include a neighbor willing to provide transportation, a local church that provides a peer support group, and a YMCA program that offers recreation and a summer camp program. These services can often be initiated at little cost and offer the advantage of always being there for the child and family in their own community.

FAMILY ADVOCACY AND SUPPORT

Families are involved in all aspects of the Wraparound program. Families United of Milwaukee was created in 1998 as a vehicle for family input and participation in the program. This organization has taken on several valuable roles in its support of families. The Families United of Milwaukee program offers many services, including providing one-to-one client/family advocacy on the Child and Family Teams, operating support groups, conducting family satisfaction surveys of Wraparound Milwaukee, helping to train and orient new care coordinators and other service providers, sponsoring family activities in the evenings and on weekends, and assisting other parents in various activities and in crises. The Families United coordinator and assistants are part of the Wraparound management group and serve on all agency committees.

EVALUATION OF WRAPAROUND MILWAUKEE

Wraparound Milwaukee has, from its onset, prioritized program evaluation and the dissemination of the results to key stakeholders. These findings are also used to inform the policies and practices of Wraparound Milwaukee. As part of the administrative and program processes, Wraparound Milwaukee staff continuously review program goals, examine program activities, and track and disseminate information on multiple outcomes. This evaluative and strategic work is a collaborative and evolving process. Families, care coordinators, wraparound administrative staff, evaluation consultant(s), children's court staff, and other community partners all contribute to the program evaluation.

Wraparound Milwaukee uses an evaluation consultant who serves as a database manager and statistical analyst. Research assistants from local universities assist with data collection and entry. Demographic, clinical, community safety, education, and service information are all included in the analyses. Data-based reports are regularly generated and serve to promote program review and development activities.

WRAPAROUND MILWAUKEE OUTCOMES

The outcomes of most interest to stakeholders have been in the areas of demographics, consumer satisfaction (caregiver and youth), service utilization, cost, education, youth behavior changes, and community safety. Each of these outcomes is discussed in this section.

Demographics

In an effort to examine outcomes of Wraparound Milwaukee over time, data on youth at enrollment in Wraparound Milwaukee during 1999, 2000, and 2001 were compared. The total sample size was 1,031 youths (1999, $n = 330$; 2000, $n = 334$; 2001, $n = 367$). Statistical analyses of the demographics of youth and families across years yielded no significant differences in age, gender, income, or race/ethnicity.

Caregiver Satisfaction

The *Family Quality Improvement Questionnaires,* a set of four surveys developed and administered through the Wraparound Milwaukee Quality Assurance Department in collaboration with Families United of Milwaukee, are currently being used to measure caregiver satisfaction at specific points in time. These surveys are aimed at obtaining caregivers' perceptions of and satisfaction with the wraparound process as facilitated by their care coordinator. Surveys are sent to caregivers at 1 week after enrollment, 6 months, 1 year, 2 years, and at disenrollment. Table 13.2 details the results of the most recent survey of caregivers at disenrollment. The results show that the majority of caregivers surveyed were satisfied with the services they received. However, they were less certain of their ability to access needed services after leaving the program.

TABLE 13.2

Results from Caregiver Satisfaction Survey

Question	N	Very Much So	Somewhat	Not at All
1. Did you and your child and family team adequately plan for disenrollment?	94	63.8%	25.5%	10.6%
2. Did you feel the needs you identified in your plan of care were met by your child and family team?	95	55.8%	33.7%	10.5%
3. Do you think there is an adequate crisis/safety plan in place for your child and family?	83	79.5%	6.0%	14.5%
4. Are you comfortable with your child's school placement?	77	76.6%	11.7%	11.7%
5. Do you think your child and family will need community services/support of some kind in the future?	93	44.1%	35.5%	20.4%
5a. Will you know how to find those services in the community?	68	48.5%	23.5%	27.9%
6. Do you feel your child/family was treated with respect while you were enrolled in Wraparound Milwaukee?	99	90.9%	6.1%	3.0%
7. Do you feel Wraparound Milwaukee staff were sensitive to your cultural/ethnic/religious needs?	97	91.8%	4.1%	4.1%
8. Overall, do you believe that your Wraparound Milwaukee care coordinator was helpful to you and your family?	97	89.7%	7.2%	3.1%
9. Do you believe that the other services provided by Wraparound Milwaukee were helpful?	87	75.9%	20.7%	3.4%
10. Overall, do you feel that Wraparound Milwaukee has helped to empower you to handle challenging situations that you and your family may face in the future?	94	61.7%	30.9%	7.4%

Youth Satisfaction

In 2001, a State of Wisconsin Bureau of Community Mental Health performance improvement project titled "Assessing Youth Perceptions of Wraparound Milwaukee" was completed. One hundred twenty-seven youth between the ages of 13 and 17 who had been enrolled in the program between 6 and 9 months were surveyed. Overall, 78% of the respondents gave Wraparound Milwaukee a grade of A or B. The majority of youth reported that they liked the services they received and would recommend the program to a friend or family member. In addition, a majority of youth noted that they were better able to deal with daily life, felt better about themselves, and were getting along better with others.

Service Utilization and Cost

It has been the aim of Wraparound Milwaukee to promote the development and utilization of community-based and family-focused services. Table 13.3 depicts the proportion of youth using services offered within the Wraparound Milwaukee continuum of care during the first 6 months of program enrollment. This table allows for comparison across years 1999, 2000, and 2001.

TABLE 13.3

Percentage of Wraparound Services Used for 3 Consecutive Years of Admissions

Service	1999[a] (n = 327)	2000[a] (n = 332)	2001[a] (n = 329)	%Δ 1999–2001
Mentoring	58%	41%	24%	−34%
Respite	14%	14%	17%	+3%
Individual therapy	21%	21%	27%	+6%[*]
In-home therapy	34%	41%	51%	+17%[*]
Group counseling	3%	7%	9%	+6%[*]
Day treatment	21%	21%	23%	+2%
1:1 crisis stabilization	7%	23%	45%	+38%[*]
Regular foster care	5%	5%	8%	+3%
Group home	11%	14%	19%	+8%
Treatment foster care	5%	11%	11%	+6%[*]
Residential treatment center	61%	52%	41%	−20%[*]
Psychiatric hospital	5%	5%	6%	+1%
Average monthly cost*	$3,872	$3,843	$3,427	

[a]First 6 months of enrollment only.

[*] Significant increases at the $p < .05$ level.

Through a series of chi-square analyses, it was determined that there were significant increases in the proportion of service use during the first 6 months of program enrollment in the following areas: individual therapy, in-home therapy, group counseling, one-to-one crisis stabilization, and treatment foster care. Significant decreases were evident in the use of residential treatment centers. Analyses of trends have indicated significant decreases in average monthly cost for the first 6 months of program enrollment, from $3,872 in 1999 to $3,427 in 2001, $F(2, 984) = 4.232, p < .05$.

Utilization of community-based treatments such as in-home, outpatient individual, and group therapies consistently rose over time, whereas institution-based care significantly declined. The shift away from standard mentoring toward one-to-one crisis stabilization appears to reflect a shift in program policy aimed at promoting a higher level of accountability and training among providers of individualized paraprofessional youth support and guidance. Cost comparisons over time reflect a consistent downward trend, particularly evident after the first 6 months of enrollment. This statistically significant finding is most reflective of the replacement of increasingly costly institutional placements with more cost-effective community-based care.

Education

Youth enrolled in Wraparound Milwaukee often come to the program with an extensive history of truancy and academic failure. The average Wraparound Milwaukee youth is in seventh grade at the time of enrollment. Fifty-four percent of Wraparound Milwaukee youth had been placed in special education prior to their enrollment. At intake, Wraparound Milwaukee youth on average had a grade point average of 1.1 on a 4.0 scale. According to baseline scores on the *Wide Range Achievement Test* (WRAT–3; Wilkinson, 1993), 70% of youth were found to be below grade level in reading and 87% were below grade level in math at the time of enrollment. Analyses to identify significant changes in WRAT scores have not yet been completed.

During the year prior to enrollment, the average enrollee attended 65% of the possible school days. During the first 6 months of enrollment in the program, this number increased to 84%. When compared to the first 6 months, a slight decrease was seen in attendance for the second 6 months of enrollment in the program (79% of possible school days), but this number remains higher than attendance rates seen preenrollment. Future analyses will include youth report cards, which will allow for a more comprehensive examination of education outcomes.

Youth Behavior/Mental Health Concerns

Standardized clinical measures—the *Child Behavior Checklist* (CBCL; Achenbach & Edelbrock, 1991); *Youth Self-Report* (YSR; Achenbach, 1991); and the *Child and Adolescent Functional Assessment Scale* (CAFAS; Hodges & Wong, 1996)—are used to assess outcomes. For each of these measures, higher numbers reflect greater problems.

The CBCL and YSR are both used to assess behavioral and emotional problems of youth as reported by the parent and the youth, respectively. For these two measures, a *T*-score above 63 is considered in the "clinical range" of emotional and behavioral functioning. Youth enrolled during 1999, 2000, and 2001 all had similar levels of behavior problems at intake according to total problem CBCL scores (well within the clinical range of the CBCL) and YSR scores (see Figures 13.2 and 13.3). As is apparent for each of the years, youth

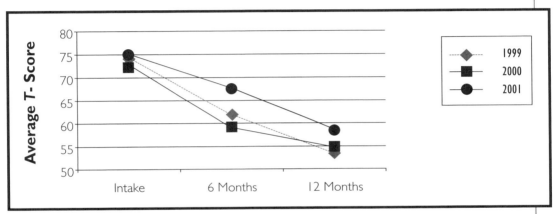

FIGURE 13.2. Trends in *Child Behavior Checklist* (Achenbach & Edelbrock, 1991) scores for youth enrolled in 1999 (*n* = 142), 2000 (*n* = 158), and 2001 (*n* = 83).

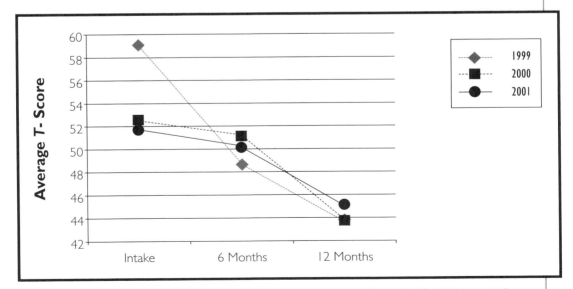

FIGURE 13.3. Trends in *Youth Self-Report* (Achenbach, 1991) scores for youth enrolled in 1999 (*n* = 104), 2000 (*n* = 118), and 2001 (*n* = 56).

rated themselves or were perceived by their parents as experiencing significantly fewer behavioral problems during the course of their first year within Wraparound Milwaukee: YSR, $F(2, 273) = 18.013, p < .01$, and CBCL, $F(2, 379) = 52.774, p < .01$.

The CAFAS evaluates the level of the youth's current functional impairment, in this case, as rated by the care coordinator. The CAFAS yields a total score composed of eight subscale scores (range of possible total score is 0–240). For each subscale, a score of 20 or 30 (out of a possible 30 points) is considered in the moderate to severe range of impairment. As with the CBCL and YSR, at enrollment in Wraparound Milwaukee, there were no significant differences among the three groups on CAFAS ratings by the care coordinator, $F(4, 1,080) = 1.390$, *ns* (see Figure 13.4). However, significant improvement was evident during the first year of enrollment in Wraparound Milwaukee for youth enrolled in 1999, 2000, and 2001, $F(2, 539) = 119.816, p < .01$.

Community Safety

Youth referred to Wraparound Milwaukee have often endured harsh conditions. Intake assessments of enrolled youth suggest a high incidence of known family risk factors, including poverty (75%), parental substance abuse (44%), physical abuse (38%), parental abandonment (36%), parental incarceration (31%), and domestic violence (29%). Correspondingly, the rate of legal reoffense has been of keen interest to stakeholders. Youth often evidence a serious legal offense history, including sexual assault (17%) and battery (19%), and they are referred to Wraparound Milwaukee as a condition of their probation. As is consistent with prior reports regarding the program (Seybold, Gilbertson, & Edens, 2002), the rates of offenses and adjudications have decreased significantly during enrollment and have continued to decline during the year following disenrollment, $F(2, 178) = 32.751, p < .01$. Figure 13.5 shows the

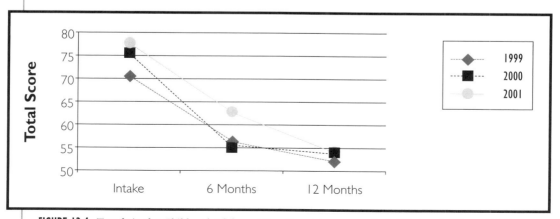

FIGURE 13.4. Trends in the *Child and Adolescent Functional Assessment Scale* (Hodges & Wong, 1996) scores for youth enrolled in 1999 ($n = 208$), 2000 ($n = 227$), and 2001 ($n = 108$).

proportion of youth referred to Wraparound Milwaukee due to an offense, as well as rates of adjudication prior to and during enrollment and following disenrollment. Figure 13.6 illustrates the types of offenses committed by youth referred due to an offense prior to and during enrollment and following disenrollment.

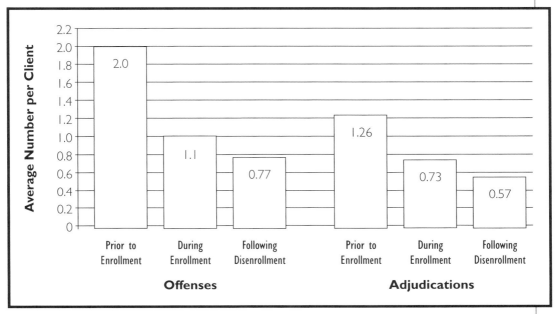

FIGURE 13.5. Trends in the average number of youth offenses and adjudications ($N = 490$; data through December 31, 2001).

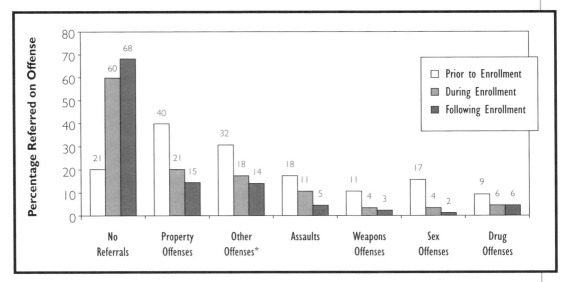

FIGURE 13.6. Percentage of youth referred for offenses by type ($N = 490$; data through December 31, 2001). *Note.* "Other offenses" primarily consist of disorderly conduct.

It should be noted that a recent comparison examining the rates of re-offense during and after enrollment for youth enrolled during 1999 and 2000 revealed no statistically significant differences between program years, thus demonstrating the consistency of this outcome over time. This finding again highlights the fact that valued outcomes can be sustained with more cost-effective and less restrictive care.

Wraparound Milwaukee was the recipient of a U.S. Department of Justice grant (1999–2002) aimed at implementing a comprehensive and community-based approach to serve youth with sexual behavior problems. Using this collaborative approach, which is central to Wraparound Milwaukee, is consistent with emerging best practice notions of what is effective with high-risk youth (Righthand & Welch, 2001). Treatment and level of supervision decisions are now a product of holistic assessment of the youth's and family's strengths, needs, and risks (Gilbertson, Storm, & Fischer, 2001). Within Wraparound Milwaukee, 88 and 100 adjudicated juvenile sex offenders were provided comprehensive services during 2000 and 2001, respectively. Public expenditure during 2001 was $400,000 less than in 2000, despite the increase in the number of families served. This change was largely due to the implementation of front-end specialized assessment and corresponding collaboration between the mental health and legal agencies, which resulted in more appropriate utilization of expensive and restrictive residential treatment versus community-based alternatives. In addition, very low levels of sexual offense recidivism occurred despite the utilization of less institution-based treatment and supervision and more community-based care of families.

CHALLENGES TO IMPLEMENTING PROGRAMS LIKE WRAPAROUND MILWAUKEE

The challenges for other communities to implement programs like Wraparound Milwaukee are not insurmountable. The following are lessons learned along the road to development and implementation of this program.

1. *Trust among stakeholders.* Collaboration among child welfare, juvenile justice, mental health, Medicaid, and education requires that the leadership in those child-serving systems have a stronger belief in helping children achieve better outcomes than in protecting their own "turf." There has to be willingness to share and pool resources, as well as a willingness to change those policies and procedures that are barriers to collaboration and to create and use methods of conflict resolution when disagreements occur. Communication channels must be open so that when a potential crisis occurs, the systems can more easily work with one another to resolve the issue.

2. *Belief in the values.* Wraparound has a strong values base emphasizing strength-based plans, family involvement, creation of resources based on needs,

and individualized service plans. These concepts must be embraced by all system partners. This can be difficult if juvenile court looks at children in their system as needing to be punished for their misdeeds and looks at parents as responsible for their child's problems; if mental health professionals focus on identifying deficits and problems in children rather than strengths; or if child welfare seeks to protect and remove children at the expense of working with a parent or parents to identify resources that may allow them to keep their children. Wraparound Milwaukee has been fortunate that the child-serving systems have supported the Wraparound values base through cross-system training, changes in policies and procedures, and articulation of the values base in joint concept papers to their staff. This has resulted in a greater voice for families in the court process as well as more shared roles for care coordinators, probation workers, and child welfare staff.

3. *Pooled funding.* No single child-serving system can meet the needs of children with complex mental health and emotional needs. The only way to adequately meet these needs is through flexible pooling of funding of all systems or through flexible services. This, again, requires other systems to give up some control of these funds to get back something in return—fewer children being institutionalized and better overall outcomes through community-based care. No child-serving system in Wraparound Milwaukee has actually had to increase expenditures since the program began serving the target group of youth. In 1995, the contribution of child welfare and juvenile justice was $18.5 million for residential treatment care of 375 youth; today, $18 million of the same funding serves 850 or more youth each year (a daily average of about 560 youth). Institutional funding has been shifted to community-based funding, and all of these systems are now actually fiscally ahead due to the pooled funding approach.

4. *Information sharing.* It is critically important to share information among all system partners. This has been achieved in various ways in Wraparound Milwaukee. There is now a single release of information for all children in Wraparound Milwaukee. All system partners—child welfare, special education, juvenile justice, and mental health—use a single-page release of information signed by the parent or legal guardian. Another example of how Wraparound Milwaukee is sharing information is through an Internet-based management information system that allows care coordinators, providers, and families to use one system for care plans, progress notes, service authorization, vendor invoicing, and all statistical reporting. Additionally, Wraparound Milwaukee provides a monthly newsletter, annual report, and online policies and procedures to enhance communication and information exchange.

5. *Ability to achieve and disseminate program outcomes.* The improved outcomes achieved by youth in Wraparound Milwaukee have been a powerful force in sustaining the investment of key stakeholders. This has been particularly true for the judicial system. The judges have been keenly interested in the reduction of recidivism rates for delinquent youth while enrolled in Wraparound Milwaukee and after discharge from the program. Due to these improvements, the judges seem to have a greater trust in Wraparound Milwaukee

and are more willing to give the program greater latitude in determining the child's placement. Because of the influence of the judicial system, support from the courts is critical to maintaining and expanding these types of programs.

6. *Maintaining community safety.* Wraparound Milwaukee works with a large number of high-risk juvenile sex offenders, fire setters, and other youth who have committed serious crimes. These are seriously emotionally disturbed youth needing treatment. The court and probation agency demand that these children not reoffend or hurt themselves or others if placed in the community. This requires care coordinators to have well-developed crisis safety plans for each child. It only takes one negative incident to destroy an entire program the size of Wraparound Milwaukee. This has been avoided so far through careful attention and planning around the most high-risk youth.

7. *Strong and identifiable organizational structure.* The creation of a separate care management organization, whether public or private, appears to be key to the success of this type of endeavor. The other child-serving systems recognize the ability of Wraparound Milwaukee to effectively manage the pooled funding through unique managed-care techniques, fiscal operations, information technology, quality assurance/utilization control, and other measures. Wraparound Milwaukee's Medicaid status as its own type of HMO or special managed-care entity is unique. The other child service systems have come to rely on Wraparound Milwaukee's expertise in managing the care of their most complex youth. That would not have been as easily done without a separate organizational structure.

8. *Effective leadership.* There is no question that strong leadership of all child-serving systems, not just in Wraparound Milwaukee, needs to be present. Leaders need to have a vision and passion for this type of work that can be articulated to staff. Within the care management organization, leadership must extend throughout the entire organization. It is also helpful if there is a consistency among team members from the beginning of the project through to implementation and operation. The leadership and staff must be creative, flexible, patient, and perhaps most importantly, they must embrace the Wraparound values.

9. *Good parent—professional partnerships.* Wraparound Milwaukee has made great efforts to involve families in all aspects of the program. It is critical to build trust among families, who often have felt betrayed or ignored by the traditional service system. Families are involved with all committees and program structures. Family members are always involved with cross-system training in order for system partners and providers to gain a better understanding of the perspectives that families offer. Wraparound Milwaukee and Families United continue to emphasize the partnership that needs to be present to achieve the best outcomes for the children and families.

In summary, it is reasonable to assume that implementation of Wraparound Milwaukee has contributed to desired outcomes for families and other stakeholders. Youth and families enrolled in Wraparound Milwaukee clearly are improving on measures of positive and desired outcomes. Although direct causality cannot be scientifically defended on the basis of the current evaluation, logic would suggest that Wraparound Milwaukee's model of providing strength-based, comprehensive, flexible, and cost-effective alternatives to institutional care has contributed significantly to broad-based and valued outcomes for youth and families.

REFERENCES

Achenbach, T. M. (1991). *Manual for the Youth Self-Report and 1991 Profile.* Burlington: University of Vermont, Department of Psychiatry.

Achenbach, T. M., & Edelbrock, C. (1991). *Manual for the Child Behavior Checklist/ 4–18 and 1991 Profile.* Burlington: University of Vermont, Department of Psychiatry.

American Psychiatric Association. (1994). *Diagnostic and statistical manual of mental disorders* (4th ed.). Washington, DC: Author.

Burchard, J., & Clarke, R. (1990). The role of individualized care in a service delivery system for children and adolescents with severely maladjusted behavior. *Journal of Mental Health Administration, 17*(1), 48–60.

Burns, B. J., & Goldman, S. K. (1998). *Promising practices in children's mental health* (Vol. 4). Washington, DC: Center for Effective Collaboration and Practice, American Institutes for Research.

Gilbertson, S., Storm, H., & Fischer, E. (2001). *Evaluating the families of juvenile sex offenders in Milwaukee County, Wisconsin.* Poster presented at the annual meeting of the Association for the Treatment of Sexual Abusers, San Antonio, Texas.

Hodges, K., & Wong, M. M. (1996). Psychometric characteristics of a multidimensional measure to assess impairment: The Child and Adolescent Functional Assessment Scale. *Journal of Child and Family Studies, 5,* 445–467.

Integrated Services Programs for Children with Severe Disabilities, Wis. Stat. § 46.56 (1999–2000).

Kamradt, B. (1999). *The 25 Kid Project: How Milwaukee utilized a pilot project to achieve buy-in among stakeholders in changing the system of care for children with severe emotional problems.* Unpublished monograph.

Katz-Leavy, J., Lourie, I., Stroul, B., & Zeigler-Dendy, C. (1992). *Individualized services in a system of care.* Washington, DC: CASSP Technical Assistance Center, Georgetown University Child Development Center.

Planning Council of Milwaukee. (1994). *Study of residential treatment placements in Milwaukee County.* Unpublished manuscript.

Righthand, S., & Welch, C. (2001). *Juveniles who have sexually offended: A review of the professional literature* (Office of Juvenile Justice and Delinquency Prevention Report, U.S. Department of Justice). Washington, DC: Office of Justice Programs.

Seybold, E., Gilbertson, S., & Edens, S. (2002). Reductions in legal offenses of delinquent youth enrolled in the Wraparound Milwaukee Program: One year follow-up. In C. Newman, C. Liberton, K. Kutash, & R. M. Friedman (Eds.), *The 14th Annual Research Conference proceedings, A system of care for children's mental health: Expanding the research base* (pp. 247–249). Tampa: University of South Florida.

U.S. Department of Health and Human Services. (1999). *Mental health: A report of the Surgeon General.* Rockville, MD: National Institute of Mental Health, Substance Abuse and Mental Health Services.

Wilkinson, G. S. (1993). *The Wide Range Achievement Test* (3rd ed.). Wilmington, DE: Wide Range.

Santa Barbara County Multiagency Integrated System-of-Care Project

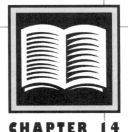

CHAPTER 14

An Overview of Its Service Model, Evaluation Approaches, and Legacy

Michael J. Furlong, Michelle W. Woodbridge, Todd Sosna, and Annie Chung

In the late 1970s, Santa Barbara County had a rich continuum of services for children with emotional and behavioral disorders (EBD), albeit based on more traditional mental health models. An array of residential, inpatient, and outpatient services were available to youth. For example, the County Mental Health Department at that time actually provided weekly psychiatric consultation to the school-based Center for Therapeutic Education. However, with the 1978 passage of California's Proposition 13 (an initiative that significantly reduced property tax revenues to California counties), public funds to support children's mental health became scarce, and service options were severely restricted. By the early 1990s, among the 58 counties in California, the expenditures for children's mental health services in Santa Barbara County were among the lowest per capita in the entire state. With a past history of quality children's mental health services, pressing unmet needs, and an interest in developing collaborative services models, Santa Barbara County was eager to seek and to be a part of the Center for Mental Health Service's (CMHS) federally funded system-of-care initiative (Lourie & Hernandez, 2003; Vinson, Brannan, Baughman, Wilce, & Gawron, 2001).

The Santa Barbara County Multiagency Integrated System of Care (SB–MISC) project received federal grant support from October 1994 through September 2000. A detailed final report of this project is available for review (Furlong et al., 2000). The goals of this chapter are to provide (a) an overview of the principles that guided the development and implementation of SB–MISC for youth with EBD and their families, (b) an example of a specialized local study that shows how evaluation resources were used to better inform local service planning for juvenile probation involved youth, and (c) a perspective on the legacy of the SB–MISC project to children's mental health services in Santa Barbara County.

SB–MISC CONTEXT, GOALS, AND SERVICES

Santa Barbara County Setting

Santa Barbara County is located 100 miles north of Los Angeles, California. Approximately 400,000 ethnically diverse individuals populate this coastal region. Of the estimated 95,000 youth living in the county, 52% are Caucasian, 40% are Latino (predominantly Mexican and Central American), 5% are Asian/Pacific Islander, and 3% are African American. Due to the high cost of living (the median price of homes in the Santa Barbara city area is more than $650,000) and the largely agrarian employment opportunities (agriculture produces the most revenue in the county), 29% of Santa Barbara County's families meet federal poverty criteria (Damery, Furlong, Casas, DeVera, & Soliz, 2002). The county has three primary population centers that are separated by 30 to 60 miles of open space (mostly farmland and national forests). Each community has unique economic and population characteristics. As a result, services in the county must be distributed across communities so that (a) families have access to them and (b) they are provided in a culturally appropriate manner. Professionals charged with implementing SB–MISC made a critical early decision to establish one-stop service centers in each community that collocated staff from all referring public agencies. This gave families, for the first time, access to services in a convenient and organized manner. It also facilitated communication between the family case manager and staff from other agencies who were working with the family.

SB–MISC Program Description

SB–MISC is a delivery system based on the tenets of mutual interagency benefit and precision-of-fit services that was established to serve children who show a serious emotional or behavioral disorder. Premised on the principles outlined by Stroul and Friedman (1986), SB–MISC is characterized by structures that promote multiagency collaboration, individualized strength-based care, and partnership with families.

SB–MISC Principles

Critical to SB–MISC is adherence to a set of 16 principles. These principles, with a brief description of the structures that were established to ensure authentication of the related practices, are listed in Table 14.1.

Interagency Collaboration

The SB–MISC is designed to serve 1,350 children countywide at any one time, with a staff of 137 from 11 public and private agencies operating out of three

TABLE 14.1

System-of-Care Operating Principles and Their Implementation
in the Santa Barbara Multiagency Integrated System of Care (SB–MISC)

Principle	SB–MISC Implementation
Shared responsibility for solutions	A collaborative of agencies is jointly responsible for partnering with families in completing assessments, developing a plan of care, and providing services.
Genuinely integrated services	Enrolled children and their families are eligible to receive services offered by any of the partner agencies based on unmet needs and promotion of their goals.
Child-centered, family-focused, and autonomy-enhancing services	All SB–MISC staff are trained in establishing partnership with children and their families and developing strength-based, child-centered, and family-focused care plans. The child, family, or provider may call for a wraparound meeting to ensure consensus among all involved.
Culturally appropriate services delivery	All staff are trained in the importance of culture in partnering with families, developing care plans, and providing services. Outcome data are analyzed to assess the degree of relationships among culture and access, level of care, and attainment of child and family goals.
Readily accessible services	Care coordinators from the enrolling agencies have the authority to authorize specific services and supports for a child or his or her family to ensure quick access to care.
Comprehensive multi-need services	An expanded array of intensive community-based services is available to children and their families, in addition to any and all services funded by any of the enrolling agencies prior to SB–MISC.
Universal individualized service plan	A single plan of care that includes cross-system goals and services is developed for each child and his or her family.
Community-based alternatives to group home care	Therapeutic foster care and intensive home- and school-based approaches were expanded through contracts with local private nonprofit agencies.
Clinical expertise	SB–MISC staff receive quarterly outcome evaluation reports to promote quality improvements. Outcome reports present data on the child and his or her family, level of care provided, and attainment of child and family goals.
Unconditional perseverance	Once enrolled, children retain eligibility for services until they achieve their goals, their families relocate their permanent residence, the children turn 18, or the children/families choose to end their participation in SB–MISC.
Continuity into adulthood	Agreements are established with the adult mental health system to ensure smooth transition to adult services, when needed.
Accountability	Outcome data are routinely collected and shared. Outcome reports include information about children and families, levels of care, and attainment of child and family goals. Reports are disseminated quarterly to families, staff, and administrators. Information from reports is used to improve client care and program administration through regular meetings to discuss its implications.

(continues)

TABLE 14.1 *Continued.*
System-of-Care Operating Principles and Their Implementation
in the Santa Barbara Multiagency Integrated System of Care (SB–MISC)

Principle	SB–MISC Implementation
Rational management of services	Services are strength based, individualized, and intended to build skills and social support networks. Care coordinators have the authority to develop care plans in partnership with children and their families. However, care coordinators have a responsibility to seek input from the collocated cross-agency interdisciplinary team to ensure that services are authorized that are most likely to be effective.
Customer-centered services	Children and their families are customers, regardless of the circumstances that bring them into care. Staff are trained to provide services that are respectful.
Policy of reinvestment of funds	SB–MISC is expected to attain both short-term and long-term outcomes resulting in rapid and sustained cost avoidance and savings; therefore, agencies have agreed to reinvest savings in discretionary funds attributable to the system of care.
Self-correction	Outcome data reports are used to inform families, staff, and administrators about the success of the SB–MISC and to promote self-correction, when needed.

regional sites. The SB–MISC collaboration includes public mental health, child welfare, juvenile probation, public health, county office of education, two school districts, and five private child- and family-serving agencies. The collaboration among these agencies is voluntary, premised on mutual benefit. Mutual benefit is achieved when the responsibilities of each agency to its consumers and the community are better met through the partnership. Mutual benefit in SB–MISC is promoted through eight key agreements.

Enrollment Decisions
Enrolling agencies (e.g., mental health, child welfare, juvenile probation, public health, and schools) independently select children for enrollment based on the use of criteria established by each agency to identify children with EBD and the greatest levels of need. As a consequence, each of the public agency partners is assured that the children of greatest need for which their agency is responsible will be able to benefit from the SB–MISC.

Commitment of Resources
Enrolling agencies redirect personnel, equipment, and financial resources to support the SB–MISC. Redirection of resources is proportional to the level of resources that that agency would have dedicated to serving the children being

enrolled into SB–MISC if it had not been established. Accordingly, SB–MISC builds on the existing service base, and all partner agencies are assured that supplanting or cost shifting will not occur. Agencies that redirect staff and resources create a "doorway" to enroll children into the system of care as just described. SB–MISC built on the county's existing children's mental health program, which included about 15 clinicians. The redirection was substantial and grew over time as the SB–MISC expanded. For example, in the fifth year of operation, about 200 staff from 10 public and private agencies were collocated in SB–MISC, which had a total budget of just over $12 million. Nine probation officers, three child welfare workers, and one public health nurse were redirected, along with almost $2 million in funding from probation and child welfare.

Collocation of Personnel

All redirected staff and resources are collocated in regional cross-agency, interdisciplinary sites. All contracted private agency staff and additional public agency staff (originally funded by the grant) are also collocated in the three regional SB–MISC sites. As a consequence, communication and collaboration are greatly enhanced. Moreover, collocated sites support the development of a unique SB–MISC identity.

Access to a Full Continuum of Community-Based Care

A full continuum of community-based services is provided through a collaboration of all the enrolling agencies and five private child- and family-serving agencies. The private agencies all have contracts with county mental health to provide one or more flexible services in the home, school, and community settings. All of the staff funded under SB–MISC private provider contracts are collocated along with the public agency personnel in regional cross-agency, interdisciplinary sites. As a result, all children enrolled by the partner agencies have access to a full continuum of care in their local communities.

Coordination of Care

A single care coordinator is assigned to each child and his or her family. Care coordinators may be mental health caseworkers, child welfare social workers, probation officers, public health nurses, or school caseworkers. The enrolling agency is responsible for care coordination; assignments are made accordingly. Care coordinator workloads varied from a low of 1:8 for an intensive probation and child welfare worker, to 1:15 for a public health nurse, to a high of 1:30 for a mental health case manager. All children enrolled by the partner agencies have care that is coordinated, preventing fragmentation and duplication. Moreover, coordinated and individualized care promotes achievement of strong, enduring outcomes.

A Single, Strength-Based Plan of Care

The care coordinator has the responsibility to partner with each child and his or her family to develop a single (cross-agency) strength-based, individualized plan of care. The care coordinator has the authority to broker any and all system-of-care services available through the partner agencies, a private network of providers, and a flexible fund. The care coordinator, child, family member, or provider can initiate wraparound meetings as needed. As a consequence, all children enrolled by the partner agencies have a single plan of care developed in partnership with each child and his or her family and coordinated by a single point of contact.

Shared Information

All SB–MISC cross-agency staff have access to assessment and treatment information. Access to this information is achieved through a cross-agency release of information consent that is voluntarily provided by the child's parent or legal guardian. Information is accessed only as needed and only to promote achievement of the child and family's goals.

Shared Training and Supervision

All SB–MISC staff received common training to promote authentication of program principles and practices. Training topics included SB–MISC principles, family partnership, cross-agency collaboration, care planning, and outcome evaluation. Moreover, supervisors from each of the partner agencies are collocated along with their direct service staff. The cross-agency supervisors work as a team to ensure fidelity to SB–MISC principles and practices and to resolve any interagency obstacles. Consequently, staff approach their work from a shared framework. Prior to SB–MISC, typical interagency obstacles included restricted access to information, disagreements over which services to offer and which agency was financially responsible, and decisions about the need for out-of-home care. The SB–MISC cross-agency supervisors now work as a team to promote individualized, strength-based care. They facilitate sharing of information, accessing needed services, sharing costs, and settling disagreements about recommendations for out-of-home care.

Precision-of-Fit Service Delivery

The SB–MISC is premised on the understanding that the best outcomes for children and their families, for the community, and in terms of cost are directly related to the precision of fit between child/family strengths and needs and the level of care provided. In the absence of an appropriate and precise fit, a child will be over- or underserved. This perspective is similar to the principles of effectiveness, efficiency, and equity discussed by Rosenblatt and Woodbridge (2003). Imprecision or mismatch is directly related to unachieved outcomes and financial waste. The adverse consequences of overserving and underserving are significant. Overserving exposes a child and family to unnecessarily intrusive and restrictive interventions, fosters dependence on service providers, undermines child and family autonomy, and results in inefficient use of expenditures. In contrast, underserving fails to achieve child and family outcomes, diminishes hope, reduces confidence in the effectiveness of future interventions, and results in expenditures being misdirected. The combination of the two can result in a paradoxical situation characterized by diminished hope and participation in services coupled with dependence on and "demandingness" for services.

Family Partnership

Achieving authentic partnership with children and their families is critical to achieving optimal outcomes. Family partnership is needed to identify strengths and needs, articulate family goals, develop individualized care plans, build on strengths, and promote social support networks. The defining feature of family partnership is shared decision making in the development of a plan of care and delivery of services. SB–MISC promotes family partnership through the care-planning process, training of staff, and the implementation of a family mentor program.

Care plans for each child are developed in a partnership of the child, his or her family, and the care coordinator. The care coordinator has the responsibility of developing a plan with full input and agreement from the child's family; he or she also has the authority to immediately authorize services. When agreement is not achieved, a wraparound meeting involving family, friends and support persons, and other providers is convened. The goal of the wraparound meeting is to develop a consensus-based plan.

All staff are trained in establishing partnership with children and their families. The training addresses why partnership is important and the process for achieving shared decision making. A team of parents and providers teach the course.

A family mentor program was developed to promote family partnership. The program consists of 15 full-time family partners who are collocated at the SB–MISC sites. Family partners are parents or family members who have had responsibility for raising a child with an EBD who has been the recipient of public services. Family mentors work directly with families and staff to promote partnership, individualized and strength-based plans, and effective services.

DESCRIPTION OF THE SB–MISC PROGRAM OUTCOMES

From the outset, the SB–MISC evaluation component was integrated into the program's guiding principles and practices. However, the evaluation design did not allow for controlled studies and, given the requirement to collect data intensively as part of the national evaluation, a different approach was taken in Santa Barbara County. It was recognized early on that the practical constraints placed on the evaluation design did not facilitate definitive global outcome studies. Consequently, SB–MISC adopted a formative evaluation model integrating two approaches. First, assessment data were rapidly processed so that they could be disseminated to the SB–MISC partners (see Woodbridge, Furlong, Casas, & Sosna, 2001, for examples of this). Second, analyses were completed that had high interest to the collaborative partners—ones designed to better understand who was being served, what services were provided, what child- and family-level goals had been achieved, and how those who responded to care differed from those who did not. This led to a series of studies that intensively examined SB–MISC participants—who they were and what types of improvement they were showing (Casas, Furlong, Alvarez, & Wood, 1997; Casas, Pavelski, Furlong, & Zanglis, 1999–2000; Flam, Furlong, & Wood, 1997; Robertson et al., 1998; Rosenblatt et al., 1998; Wood, Chung, et al., 1998; Wood, Furlong, Casas, & Sosna, 1998; Wood et al., 1997; Zanglis, Furlong, & Casas, 2000). Information about these studies and the final SB–MISC evaluation report are available online at www.education.ucsb.edu/ school-psychology.

Specialized Local Project Outcomes—Probation Gateway: Reducing Juvenile Recidivism

As SB–MISC evolved, the probation department became the second most common gateway into services. This partnership highlights how participation in SB–MISC may be associated with the reduction of juvenile crime recidivism. This concern became the topic of a specialized local study, and its results influenced subsequent probation practices and service options. As such, the evaluation study provides an example of how local data collection and analysis can support local policy and program decisions.

Purpose of the Local Study of Juvenile Recidivism

The purpose of the probation-focused study was to ascertain which youth and family characteristics, as well as intervention strategies, contribute to differential juvenile justice outcomes after 1 year of participation in SB–MISC. With the intent of better understanding the mechanisms associated with youth outcomes, Hoagwood, Jensen, Petti, and Burns (1996) introduced a conceptual model of treatment efficacy research involving children. They emphasized the need to address the multiplicity of factors associated with youth outcomes by proposing that researchers focus on examining symptoms/ diagnoses, overall functioning, consumer satisfaction, environmental conditions, and system-level factors in their investigative efforts. Borrowing from this efficacy research model, this study (a) describes the juvenile justice involvement trends of these youth from their first contact with the juvenile justice system and throughout their first year of SB–MISC participation; (b) describes the sociodemographic characteristics, risk profiles, presenting problems, and emotional/behavioral functioning of these youth upon entry into SB–MISC; and (c) identifies and describes the service configurations (type and frequency) provided to these youth and their families. To address public policy and community safety concerns on a global level, this research inquiry served as a foundation for answering the daunting question of what works in decreasing youth involvement in criminal activities, and more specifically, what works for the youth being cared for in Santa Barbara County. Evidence of success in reducing juvenile recidivism at the local level is needed to validate probation's intensive investment in SB–MISC.

Probation Participants

This subset of 178 SB–MISC juvenile probation–involved youth (131 boys, 47 girls) entered services between January 1995 and December 1997. They had histories of multiple arrests at intake, thus representing youth who have already entered a trajectory of reoffending. Their mean age at first referral to probation was 13.0 years ($SD = 1.65$), and their mean age at service entry was 14.8 years ($SD = 1.4$ years). They represented the following ethnic backgrounds: 53% Latino, 27% Caucasian, 13% African American, 2.3% Asian American, and 1.7% Native American. Thus, Latino and African American youth were overrepresented in this juvenile offender sample in comparison to the ethnic composition of Santa Barbara County's youth population.

The criteria used by juvenile probation for SB–MISC participation included the following risk factors: (a) history of out-of-home placement; (b) physical, emotional, or sexual abuse; (c) substance abuse by the youth; (d) substance abuse by family members; (e) violent/sexual offense by the youth; (f) serious emotional disturbance or mental disorder; (g) caregiver with a mental disorder; and (h) gang involvement. Thus, youth referred to the project by juvenile probation represent a population with multiple risks, current behavioral difficulties, and numerous needs.

Tables 14.2 and 14.3 present data showing sociodemographic and early juvenile offending profiles of the youth by total study sample and 1-year recidivism status. To explore the nature of differential recidivism outcomes in this study, the number of rearrests after 1 year of SB–MISC involvement determined the participants' general recidivism status as the following: *Abstainers* were those youth who were not rearrested during this follow-up period and abstained from any further criminal activity; youth who were rearrested only one time during the follow-up period were identified as *desisters,* as their reoffense profiles suggested attenuation of delinquent behaviors. Youth who were arrested two or more times were grouped as *persisters* because their reoffense profiles supported high levels of continued delinquent behaviors.

TABLE 14.2

Sociodemographic Characteristics by Total Sample and Post-1-Year Recidivism Status

Variable		Total (N = 178)	Abstainers (n = 66)	Desisters (n = 41)	Persisters (n = 71)
			Recidivism Status		
Age at					
First probation referral	M	13.04	13.04	13.30	12.88
	SD	1.65	1.91	1.58	1.41
SB–MISC entry	M	14.78	14.92	15.02	14.49
	SD	1.41	1.69	1.08	1.24
Gender (%)					
Male		73.6	69.7	65.9	81.7
Female		26.4	30.3	34.1	18.3
Ethnicity (%)					
Caucasian		26.4	27.3	20.5	29.6
Black		12.5	16.7	15.4	7.0
Latino/a		56.8	50.0	61.5	60.6
Other		4.0	6.0	2.6	2.8
Risk factors (%)					
Physically abused		39.1	33.9	50.0	38.3
Sexually abused		14.1	16.4	6.7	16.0
Suicide attempt		19.9	18.8	15.8	23.2
Substance use		90.2	80.0	94.9	97.1
Parent conviction		31.5	28.3	37.8	30.9
Family violence		70.9	67.8	74.3	71.9
Family substance abuse		83.0	75.0	86.1	89.2
Income ≤$15,000		56.2	51.9	51.5	62.3

Note. Frequencies are presented for each variable except age. SB–MISC = Santa Barbara multiagency integrated system of care.

Procedure

Data collection and analyses for this local study included three processes: (a) conducting an archival review of Santa Barbara County's juvenile probation database to ascertain the participant's offense history prior to program entry and from program entry to the annual follow-up; (b) obtaining demographic variables and risk factors, as well as participant's level of emotional and behavioral functioning, from his or her comprehensive individualized assessment, which had been conducted upon service entry; and (c) synthesizing service utilization information from Santa Barbara County's mental health database to identify the amounts and types of services utilized from entry to the annual follow-up.

The standard SB–MISC intake assessment procedures were followed. Data at intake and the annual follow-up were collected by trained assessment staff using a multitrait, multimethod approach. This procedure involved clinicians, youth, and caregivers, who completed sociodemographic, family

TABLE 14.3

Early Offending Profiles at Intake by Total Sample and Post-1-Year Recidivism Status

			Recidivism Status		
Variable		Total (N = 178)	Abstainers (n = 66)	Desisters (n = 41)	Persisters (n = 71)
Juvenile justice contacts					
No. sustained petitions	M	3.51	3.06	3.73	3.79
	SD	2.86	2.78	2.56	3.08
No. arrests	M	2.98	2.43	3.00	3.49
	SD	2.53	1.91	2.62	2.88
No. institutional commitments	M	0.34	0.29	0.39	0.37
	SD	0.88	0.76	1.12	0.83
Most serious offense (%)					
Felony		41.6	43.9	39.0	40.8
Misdemeanor		48.3	48.5	53.7	45.1
Truancy/runaway		10.1	7.6	7.3	14.1
Type of offense (%)					
Violent		27.5	36.4	17.1	25.4
Property		43.8	34.8	63.4	40.8
Drug		4.5	6.1	4.9	2.8
Other felony/misdemeanor		14.1	15.1	7.3	16.9
Status		10.1	7.6	7.3	14.1

Note. Frequencies are presented for each variable except for juvenile justice contacts.

history, youth functioning, and service satisfaction questionnaires. For the purposes of this specialized local study, data were derived from the sources and instruments described next.

Measures

CLIENT INFORMATION WORKSHEET (CIW). This 139-item instrument was a modified version of one designed by national system-of-care evaluators in conjunction with federal funding agencies to collect comprehensive historical information about participants. Items address sociodemographic, child and family risks, presenting problems, *DSM* diagnoses, and educational and health information. This instrument was completed by the assessment coordinator, who retrieved this information from existing client files and, when necessary, from caregivers or other service providers.

CHILD BEHAVIOR CHECKLIST (CBCL). This 113-item parent report instrument measures the competencies and problem behaviors of youth ages 4 to 17 across nine syndrome scales: Withdrawn, Somatic Complaints,

Anxious, Depressed, Social Problems, Thought Problems, Attention Problems, Sex Problems, and Delinquent Behavior (Achenbach, 1991). Derived from these syndrome scales are the Internalizing and Externalizing summary composites. The Internalizing composite includes the Withdrawn, Somatic Complaints, and Anxious/Depressed scales; the Externalizing composite consists of the Delinquent Behavior and Aggressive Behavior scales. The Total Problem Score index is the composite based on all syndrome scales. Across research and clinical practice settings, the CBCL is the most frequently used assessment tool to measure caregivers' perceptions of children's problem behaviors (Furlong & Wood, 1998).

JUVENILE JUSTICE INVOLVEMENT. Data on the number and severity of contacts with law enforcement were collected from juvenile probation records for tracking the recidivism of youth from prior to program entry through the annual follow-up. Specific items from the juvenile probation database included (a) number of sustained petitions; (b) number of arrests; (c) most serious offense type (status, property, and violent); (d) offense seriousness (felony, misdemeanor, other); (e) number of institutional commitments ("any court order, confining the minor to the California Youth Authority, county juvenile hall, ranch, or camp"); and (f) length of institutional commitments (coded by time period: 1 = *3 months or less;* 2 = *3 to 6 months;* 3 = *6 months to 1 year;* and 4 = *more than 1 year*).

SERVICE UTILIZATION. With the inception of SB–MISC, all service providers were introduced to service accountability protocols. This was managed by County Mental Health in its billing data management system. Thus, all services were documented in this database for billing purposes. Service type, frequency, and cost variables were synthesized from participants' service entry and through the annual follow-up. The following service categories were utilized in the data analyses:

1. *Assessment*—encompassed a comprehensive examination of the youth and family's historical and present level of emotional and behavioral functioning, their needs, and their strengths.
2. *Case management*—included care coordination services that match the youth/family needs to the available resources in the project and served as the basis for interagency communication about participants.
3. *Flexible services*—included a compilation of innovative resources such as family mentors, after-hours outreach, intensive behavioral intervention, and alcohol and drug services.
4. *Medication/crisis intervention*—encompassed two separate services that were collapsed into one category because of the low frequency of usage. Medication services included providing prescriptions, scheduling follow-up appointments, and disseminating information about medications for all general physical health and psychiatric needs.

Crisis intervention referred to providers who were designated to evaluate risk of, and provide services to prevent imminent risk of, harm to self or others.

5. *Therapy*—constituted individual, group, or family modalities of psychotherapy, as well as intensive in-home interventions and intensive in-school interventions.

Comparing Abstainers, Desisters, and Persisters

Combinations of demographic, risk, behavioral, and service variables were examined via juvenile offenders' recidivism status (abstainers, desisters, persisters) following 1 year of SB–MISC involvement. Those variables significantly differing ($p < .05$) across recidivism status from univariate analyses of variance (ANOVAS) and chi-square tests (not shown in this chapter, but available upon request), as well as predictor variables strongly supported by previous juvenile delinquency research, were included in a stepwise discriminate analysis. The purpose of this stepwise discriminant function analysis was (a) to determine the combination of predictor variables that discriminate among the recidivism status groups, (b) to determine the strength of the association between predictor variables and group membership, and (c) to ascertain how reliably and adequately the predictor variables classify youth by their recidivism status (e.g., greater than the chance rate weighted for group size) at the annual SB–MISC follow-up.

It was thought that combinations of the aforementioned variables would reliably assess recidivism group status (abstainers, desisters, persisters) of juvenile offenders after 1 year of participation in SB–MISC. To test this idea, predictor variables meeting the previously discussed inclusion criteria were included in a stepwise discriminant analysis (p to enter $= .05$, p to remove $= .10$). These predictors included age at first referral to probation, age at SB–MISC entry, gender, substance use, in-home placement, total number of family risk factors, CBCL Internalizing, CBCL Externalizing, number of arrests at SB–MISC entry, most serious violation for a violent offense, most serious violation for a property offense, most serious violation for a status offense, number of assessment sessions received, case management sessions received, flexible service sessions received, and therapy sessions received.

Of the 178 cases in this sample, 47 were dropped from the stepwise discriminant analysis due to missing service utilization and CBCL data. The missing data were equitably distributed across recidivism status groups because there were no significant differences between those with and without service utilization data, $\chi^2(2, N = 178) = 1.26, p = .53$, and those with and without CBCL data, $\chi^2(2, N = 178) = .03, p = .99$. Thus, 131 cases (49 abstainers, 28 desisters, and 54 persisters) were used to complete this analysis. Because the total number of youth in each recidivism status group was known, prior probabilities were used to predict group membership. The results of this stepwise discriminant analysis revealed a reliable prediction of recidivism group status, $F(8, 250) = 5.53, p < .0001$. Presented in Table 14.4 are the

TABLE 14.4

Results of Stepwise Discriminant Analysis
Predicting Post-1-Year Recidivism Status

Step	Variable Entered	Wilks' λ	F	df	p
1	Substance use	.887	8.13	2, 128	<.0001
2	Case management	.812	6.95	4, 254	<.0001
3	In-home placement	.758	6.24	6, 252	<.0001
4	Age at SB–MISC intake	.722	5.53	8, 250	<.0001

Note. SB–MISC = Santa Barbara multiagency integrated system of care.

results of this analysis. There was a strong association between groups and predictors for two discriminant functions, $\chi^2(8, N = 178) = 41.23, p = .0001$, and after the removal of the first function, $\chi^2(3, N = 178) = 10.89, p = .012$. The two discriminant functions accounted for 75.1% and 24.9%, respectively, of the between-group variability in discriminating a youth's recidivism status post–1-year SB–MISC involvement. The first discriminant function maximally separated abstainers from both desisters and persisters, while the second discriminant function showed a large separation between desisters and persisters, with abstainers falling closer to persisters.

Collectively, substance use, amount of case management, in-home placement status, and age at SB–MISC intake were the strongest predictors contributing to the resulting two discriminant functions (loadings of .50 or higher; Tabachnick & Fidell, 1989). The loading matrix of correlations between predictors and discriminant functions (see Table 14.5) suggests that substance use history and the amount of case management utilization were the strongest predictors distinguishing abstainers from the other groups on Function 1. Thus, abstainers are less likely to be substance users and receive fewer case management services than desisters and persisters. Additionally, there are two strong predictors, in-home placement and age at SB–MISC intake, that distinguish desisters from persisters and abstainers on Function 2. It appears that desisters are more likely to live in their family home and to be slightly older than either abstainers or persisters at SB–MISC intake. Thus, these results partially support the hypothesis that a demographic variable (age at SB–MISC referral), child risk factors (positive substance use history, in-home placement), and a service utilization variable (case management) all contribute to the reliable prediction of juvenile offenders' recidivism group status post–1-year SB–MISC entry.

The accuracy of the predictor variables to classify youth by their recidivism status groups post–1-year SB–MISC entry (a practical consideration of great interest to the probation department) was evaluated using prior probabilities weighted for group size (37.4% for abstainers, 21.4% for desisters, and 41.2% for persisters). Results of this stepwise discriminant analysis yielded two discriminant functions that correctly classified 53.3% of the youth. However, persisters (75.8%) and abstainers (55.6%) were more likely to be classi-

TABLE 14.5

Loading Matrix of Correlations Between
Predictor Variables and Discriminant Functions

Predictor Variables	Function 1	Function 2
Substance use	.678	.148
Case management	.485	−.310
In-home placement	.171	.716
Age at SB–MISC intake	−.167	.602
Gender	−.106	−.105
No. family risk factors	.083	−.045
CBCL internalizing	.080	−.067
CBCL externalizing	.177	−.146
Age at first probation referral	−.047	.325
No. arrests at SB–MISC intake	−.024	.124
Most serious—violent offense	−.064	.130
Most serious—property offense	−.028	.060
Most serious—status offense	.076	−.180
Assessment	.110	−.135
Flexible services	.351	−.061
Therapy	.078	−.054

Note. SB–MISC = Santa Barbara multiagency integrated system of care. CBCL = *Child Behavior Checklist* (Achenbach & Edelbrock, 1991).

fied correctly than were desisters (8.8%). This suggests that other factors not included in this analysis differentiate desisters from persisters and abstainers.

Utility of Differentiating Juvenile Offenders by Recidivism Status

The results from this local study showed that reliably assessing juvenile offenders' propensity to discontinue (abstainers), reduce (desisters), or continue (persisters) their delinquency involvement using demographics, youth risk factors, and service utilization after 1 year of system-of-care interventions is possible. Identifying youth by their recidivism status provided not only statistically significant but also clinically meaningful information regarding juvenile offenders' characteristics. Furthermore, including system-of-care interventions in the study expanded upon previous research and illustrated how service utilization is related to youth recidivism outcomes.

Implications and Impacts of the Local Recidivism Study

In Santa Barbara's implementation of a system-of-care model, the juvenile probation department has been a primary contributor and supporter. The findings from this local study indicate that many of the juvenile offenders involved in the SB–MISC project experienced decreases in their delinquency involvement after 1 year of system-of-care interventions (60.1%; 37.1% had no new arrests, and another 23.0% had only one new arrest, predominantly for probation violations). These results are indeed promising, given that a 10% reduction in recidivism has been viewed as clinically meaningful (Lipsey, 1995), and the findings reinforce and encourage the involvement of the probation department in SB–MISC.

Using the findings from this local evaluation study, the probation department began to invest more resources into service delivery founded on a strength-based system-of-care model. They used this to successfully obtain a California State Board of Corrections grant ($5 million) to implement a comprehensive continuum of service (truancy prevention, early intervention, family caseloads, and aftercare) in the Santa Maria community of northern Santa Barbara County (see www.education.ucsb.edu/school-psychology for this project's final reports).

The probation department also took notice of these juvenile offenders' high rates of substance abuse, especially among the persisters, their moderate rates of clinically significant emotional problems at intake, and their differential recidivism profiles following 1 year of system-of-care interventions. These reinforced local perceptions that juvenile offenders have substantial mental health needs, which is consistent with other research (e.g., Armistead, Wierson, Forehand, & Frame, 1992; Kempton & Forehand, 1992). On the basis of the findings of the local study, the probation department implemented a new service delivery model based on family/neighborhood contexts and more focused on the impact of substance abuse on recidivism. This led to another successful application for funding to implement a family-focused program based on system-of-care principles for probation youth with substance-related conditions (see www.education.ucsb.edu/school-pscyhology for information about this project).

SB–MISC: THE CONTINUING STORY

As the presentation of the specialized study demonstrated, the effective use of local evaluation resources can reinforce commitment to the system-of-care model, inspire agencies to embrace more fully the system-of-care philosophy, and lead to concrete actions that create more appropriate resources for children and their families. In this section of the chapter, we present reflections on the integration and evolution of SB–MISC through the eyes of veteran agency staff and administrators who have been partners in this system of care since its inception. Interviews were conducted approximately 2 years after the termination of federal funding—when the SB–MISC project had a life of about 8 years in the county—and with staff from major public agencies, as well as community-based organizations (CBOs). In a semistructured, informal environment, we asked these colleagues to reflect on the benefits, challenges, and legacy of the SB–MISC. Their perspectives suggest a system of care that greatly influenced the practice and philosophy of care provision, cultivating collaborative arrangements for planning, implementation, and evaluation of child and family services. In the wake of funding limitations, however, priorities have shifted and cost management seems to have defined care management—despite the documented cost-effectiveness of fully operationalized systems of care. The story of this evolution is told in their words next.

The Legacy of SB–MISC

Service providers and administrators attributed many accomplishments to SB–MISC that left a legacy in the county service delivery system, namely, providing strengths-based, individualized services; family partnership; and interagency collaboration.

Current System-of-Care Options in Santa Barbara County

According to interviewed system veterans, the current status of the SB–MISC project may be defined as a smaller, specialized, *fiscal* system of care with more traditional service delivery and referral systems. That is, the SB–MISC is serving a subpopulation and is smaller in scope, although "its principles are throughout the system." Staff described the current service delivery as "more medical model focused and more problem focused," with the comprehensive assessment determining the services for the child and family. One administrator claimed that although the county is expanding the use of family conferencing in its service planning, the broader scope of SB–MISC has ended: "Since the funding stopped, many services had to be dismantled or refined. They simply can't offer the complete menu of services for every family," she said. Another administrator admitted that the county's overall goal is to "reshape SB–MISC to keep it effective but also to fit it in what we can pay for." In fact, a director of a CBO described the system's evolution with the following adage: "Before, when we had a family with a need, we asked, 'How will they be served?' Now we ask, 'How will they be paid for?'" Still, the following system-of-care structural attributes continue to exist:

- collocation of system-of-care staff to share information, resources, and space
- subcontracts with nonprofit community-based organizations for innovative services (such as intensive in-home care and therapeutic foster care)
- one treatment plan and one assessment per child

To maintain the collaboration, agencies and organizations must go "treasure hunting for funding streams." This has led to "cooperative and creative funding," with all of the partner agencies working together to maintain the primary SB–MISC structures, staffing, and contracts. Despite the challenges and the bumps in the road, those interviewed continue to view the system of care as a critical component of county services that should be maintained: "It's such a good model. We have learned so many good lessons from it," confirmed one agency administrator. Another affirmed the sustainability of the SB–MISC culture: "There has been some regression, but we now have a better idea about how agencies can work together. We are sharing clients, sharing space, and sharing resources. That's not going away."

Strength-Based Individualized Care

Rather than fitting families into service categories prefabricated on the basis of available resources, service providers in the system of care tailored supports around the families' strengths and needs. "SB–MISC put words and placed values in the strengths-based model," attested one community-based provider. "That attitude has permeated [our organization]. Our rigid, clinic-based model has evolved into community and home-based services. SB–MISC gave us confidence to put therapists in the community, our satellite offices, and the families' homes. It really changed the way we do business." Another public agency administrator characterized this change in focus and assessment practice as the "critical and major difference contributing to a reduction in placements; increases in keeping children in their homes and in the community; and increases in other outcomes, such as school performance and clinical improvements."

Family Partnership

This innovative delivery system bred new partnerships among the gateway agencies, community-based organizations, and family members. Because families were included in service planning meetings, the service providers became more sensitive in their language and use of terminology. One administrator reflected on this change in the county service providers: "Talking differently has led them to thinking differently."

Interagency Collaboration

SB–MISC facilitated the development of new relationships between government and community agencies, and the system provided the impetus for achieving a high degree of collaboration among various county departments. One public administrator affirmed that the federal grant was a "springboard to move us from being in our own worlds to working together." As a testament to this, he described how all of the partner agencies met on a monthly basis—and continue to do so to this day—to provide a forum for sharing issues of mutual concern, including information about clients, coordination of services, and funding mechanisms. Another director of a community-based organization declared, "With our role in SB–MISC, this was the first time as a CBO that we felt like we were included. Our organization became an integral part of the county mental health effort." She believes the system of care helped service agencies across the county to (a) gain perspective about the community impact and legal constraints of each agency or organization, (b) gain access to personnel and collegial services, and (c) share ownership and decision making.

One hallmark of this collaborative approach was an innovative cross-system training and mentoring model developed by the system's development specialist in partnership with the University of California, Santa Barbara's (UCSB) Gevirtz Graduate School of Education. Key features of the training included use of family members as trainers, cross-system job shadowing, hands-on skills building and case review, coaching, conflict resolution, and service plan development (Meyers, Kaufman, & Goldman, 1999). System-of-care staff across the board cited the job-shadowing experiences as having the most memorable and lasting impact on them and their practices. "Although everyone thought they knew what each other's responsibilities were, this experience showed providers the daily challenges and requirements too complex to describe," said one administrator.

Another essential element of the collaborative approach was the SB–MISC's collocation of cross-agency staff in three regional offices across the county. One mental health supervisor claimed, "The collocation blurred the departmental lines and approaches to cases"; another CBO provider believed it "helped to cement personal relationships and co-agency collaboration." An administrator in social services asserted, "My idea of success over the last 4 to 5 years was taking people to the collocated SB–MISC sites. And when I did, if you didn't know people there, you could not identify who was from probation, who was a social worker, who was a nurse, who worked for alcohol, drugs, and mental health. An outsider cannot identify who comes from what background. There's been an acculturation so people are all on the same page about service delivery. All of them have the same mind-set, the same approach. This was *absolutely* not true before we started SB–MISC."

Problems and Suggested Solutions in Implementation

Despite its innovation and lasting legacy, administrators and service providers with a history in SB–MISC also cited critical ongoing problems and hurdles. Describing these challenges may provide guidance to other communities.

Administrative Infrastructure Needs To Be Strong, Sustainable, and Collaborative

One of the basic problems that continued to challenge the Santa Barbara system-of-care model was, according to a number of administrators, the "failure to provide for the necessary and fundamental infrastructure support." This problem included administrative assistance, clerical functions, and data collection and tracking. Because a majority of the federal funds went into staff enhancements and direct purchasing of services, the "nuts and bolts" of the operations were left inadequately supported. One provider claimed, "This really held us back. Having money in the system hid the need … but it was obvious that certain fundamentals were not there." Inevitably, these administrators believed that morale and productivity were compromised by this oversight.

Those interviewed also cautioned that you "can't look at SB–MISC devoid of the challenges of the Department of Alcohol, Drugs, and Mental Health Services," because this was the lead agency charged with development and implementation of the system. They cited economic concerns of the department as well as major shifts in personnel at the administrative levels that affected the confidence, competence, and fiscal soundness of SB–MISC implementation and sustainability—especially when federal funding subsided.

In addition, community-based organizations questioned the authenticity of the parternship's authority structure during early implementation of SB–MISC. One director said, "We were at the table, but we clearly knew where the power and authority really was. Unfortunately, that was in a department that was in disarray…. There was more a promise of full partnership than what it really was. We were not naive to the fact that decisions were made behind closed doors." At the same time, county agencies viewed the CBOs' position as one lacking equal voice because they avoided assuming risk. One administrator said the CBOs were viewed as benefactors of "sweetheart contracts that covered their service costs without risk. They were protected, so agencies felt that they could tell them what to do since [the county agencies] were assuming the risks." Ultimately, frustrations ensued as agencies criticized the CBOs' sense of "entitlement," and the CBOs felt less and less integrated as true partners.

Administrators and providers suggested that more time be spent discussing and implementing a clear governance structure, fiduciary responsibilities, administrative infrastructure, and the concept of partnership. One staff member advised, "We needed to talk more about 'Who's in charge?' and 'Who's making decisions?' " Additionally, a CBO partner reflected that "continued dynamism and excitement needs a strong core to cultivate a sense of purpose and passion. That needs nurturing!" She suggested that the leadership of the system of care "must be healthy and whole to maintain the dream." The vision and mission of the system of care must be embedded in an institutional history and in the system's providers and leadership to carry the underpinnings of a program with such scale. Suggested solutions included (a) nurturing solid, consistent leaders who can instill dedication and enthusiasm in a system of care while also maintaining a stable level of infrastructure and (b) maintaining a consistent forum for discussions about leadership and governance.

A New Culture of Service Delivery Takes Time, Patience, and Persistence

Administrators admonished that you must expect that some people will be unable to make a complete "culture change" that embraces the principles and values of a system of care. The skills needed for collaborative service delivery are different from what is taught to professionals. One staff member characterized participation in SB–MISC as "a process of self-selection: those willing to learn the new skills remained in the service delivery system." Administrators quickly realized, according to an administrator in top management, that the "best workers were in SB–MISC: the progressive, human service-oriented professionals." Unfortunately, this often led to their promotions outside of the system of care.

Simultaneously, family members were at the table during this process of change within the Santa Barbara mental health service delivery system. The culture previously shared by some service providers is encapsulated in the statement "the professional knows best." Relationships with families, however, could not take this tenor or be adversarial for the model to be effective. Therefore, not every professional could remain in the children's system of care. A new accountability structure and a new culture evolved based on partnerships with families.

Professionals may be resistant to a new and tighter accountability structure, and turf issues can make shared ownership difficult—if not impossible. As staff are asked to assume wider, collaborative roles and to partner with families, the stress and strain of role change and greater oversight can be taxing. Services might still lack the essential coordination on which the system is founded due to the complexity of scheduling and organization. In this wake, "people fall back on what they are used to doing before," cautioned one administrator, "and collaboration can break down a fair amount."

To offset these "bad habits," professionals who know the system-of-care model and culture need to be those staff who are intimately connected to the work in the community. In addition, training programs at the university level should be well aligned to community-based work. Most staff and administrators also suggested that systems invest wisely and generously in evaluation: "Santa Barbara County benefited from data collected and analyzed by UCSB—a credible evaluator. The data showed outcomes of importance to the community, and they were the reason for much of probation's success in receiving state challenge grants for future funding."

Funding Demands Constant Attention
Despite Evidence of Positive Outcomes

One administrator stated, "There is a mandate for collaboration, but there are no coordinated funding streams to support collaboration." As a result, system-of-care agency staff and administrators "spend an enormous amount of time trying to bring in new funds, and the public service agencies must still fight it out for general fund allocations" to serve children and their families. Therefore, suspicions about funding intentions and sharing monies arise even in healthy collaboratives, making partnership and flexible funding real challenges. Furthermore, in the case of the SB–MISC, one CBO administrator believes that there has been a shift in priority to serve children who have Medi-Cal rather than those with the greatest need (many of whom have no insurance or ability to pay for mental health care), because there is funding available for the former but not the latter.

At the outset, SB–MISC was implemented on the assumption that demonstrated outcomes would result in sustainability. Although strong outcomes were found and cost savings realized, sustainability was affected by new program priorities, state funding reductions, and a move back toward core mandated services. Administrators and system developers quickly learned from inception that the system of care had to build in sustainable funding streams, for example, Medi-Cal billing mechanisms, and had to demonstrate strong outcomes. However, when general fund dollars from the state and county are limited, the service delivery system can be pressured to move away from system-of-care principles toward a system in which finances drive care decisions.

SUMMARY

The goal of this chapter was to provide the reader with an overview of the SB–MISC, ideas about how local evaluation resources were used to reinforce agencies and affect local planning, and a perspective on the future of system of care in Santa Barbara County. SB–MISC is an evolving system of care, one that is affected by fluctuations in resolve and access to resources. This is natural and expected. Its history provides a very realistic picture of what other communities might anticipate as they seek to implement a principle-based system-of-care model. The spirit of family partnership; strength-based, individualized care; and interagency collaboration made palpable in the SB–MISC have enduringly shaped the way services are provided throughout the county. Further, the formative evaluation model that was established at the inception of the SB–MISC was a critical component of the system of care and a catalyst for other significant innovations in services for children and families. Moreover, the basic structure, staffing, and contracts initiated in the SB–MISC have been retained 3 years after the end of federal grant funding. The spirit of collaboration garnered by SB–MISC also motivated county agencies to seek additional funding sources based on cross-agency service delivery. This produced two large state-funded delinquency prevention grants, a state-funded truancy prevention program, and a federally funded safe school/ healthy students initiative grant. Despite these continuing successes, the challenges associated with these accomplishments have been and continue to be substantial. Strong leadership and a sound collaborative infrastructure are critical. Despite positive outcomes and demonstrated cost savings, financial pressures, funding requirements, and political realities can result in shifts in priorities and a diminished adherence to system-of-care principles and practices. It is unrealistic to assume that leadership will remain constant across all agencies. With new leadership there is often new vision, priorities, and funding decisions.

Systems of care could consider several strategies, based on Santa Barbara's experience, to ensure that children's mental health delivery systems provide effective, enduring services. First, training in the principles and practices needs to be widespread. Systems of care are often small programs within large systems. They are vulnerable to being discounted if they are not understood. Second, outcome data concerning achievement of child and family goals and corresponding costs need to be clearly reported and broadly disseminated. Policymakers and decision makers need to fully understand the outcomes achieved, the cost of care, and the costs associated with no or inadequate care to make sound decisions about programs and appropriations. Third, and most important, consumers (youth and their families) need to organize and be empowered to join policymakers in program and appropriations decisions. Consumer and family member groups can become the constant that persists across changes in leadership, economics, and politics.

AUTHORS' NOTE

A copy of the SB–MISC project final report is available online at www.education.ucsb.edu/school-psychology. SB–MISC was originally funded by a grant (No. 6-HS5SM51592-01) from the Centers for Mental Health Services, a principle operating component of the Substance Abuse Mental Health Services Administration, within the U.S. Department of Health and Human Services. The contents of this chapter are the responsibility of the authors and do not necessarily represent the official views of the Centers for Mental Health Services; the Santa Barbara County Alcohol, Drug, and Mental Health Services; or other public or private agencies in Santa Barbara County.

REFERENCES

Achenbach, T. M. (1991). *Manual for the Child Behavior Checklist/4–18 and 1991 Profile.* Burlington: University of Vermont, Department of Psychiatry.

Armistead, L., Wierson, M., Forehand, R., & Frame, C. (1992). Psychopathology in incarcerated juvenile delinquents: Does it extend beyond externalizing problems? *Adolescence, 27,* 309–314.

Casas, J. M., Furlong, M. J., Alvarez, M., & Wood, M. (1997, February). ¿Qué dice? Initial analyses examining three Spanish translations of the CBCL. In C. Liberton, K. Kutash, & R. Friedman (Eds.), *The 10th Annual Research Conference proceedings: A system of care for children's mental health, expanding the research base* (pp. 459–464). Tampa: University of Southern Florida, Louis de la Parte Florida Mental Health Institute, Research and Training Center for Children's Mental Health.

Casas, J. M., Pavelski, R., Furlong, M. J., & Zanglis, I. (1999–2000). Addressing the mental health needs of Latino youth with emotional and behavioral disorders: Practical perspective and policy implications. *Harvard Journal of Hispanic Policy, 12,* 47–70.

Damery, H., Furlong, M. J., Casas, J. M., DeVera, Z., & Soliz, A. (2002). *Ninth annual Santa Barbara children's scorecard.* Santa Barbara, CA: KIDS Network.

Flam, C., Furlong, M. J., & Wood, M. (1997). *Evaluating the fidelity of wraparound service planning: Are we practicing what we preach?* Unpublished manuscript, University of California, Santa Barbara.

Furlong, M. J., Casas, J. M., Zanglis, I., Pavelski, R., & Turner, J. (2000). *Santa Barbara County MISC final report.* Santa Barbara, CA: Alcohol, Drug, and Mental Health Department.

Furlong, M. J., & Wood, M. (1998). *Review of the Child Behavior Checklist.* Lincoln, NE: Buros Mental Measurement Yearbook.

Hoagwood, K., Jensen, P. S., Petti, T., & Burns, B. J. (1996). Outcomes of mental health care for children and adolescents: I. A comprehensive conceptual model. *Journal of the American Academy of Child and Adolescent Psychiatry, 35,* 1055–1063.

Kempton, T., & Forehand, R. (1992). Suicide attempts among juvenile delinquents: The contribution of mental health factors. *Behavior Research and Therapy, 30,* 537–541.

Lipsey, M. W. (1995). What do we learn from 400 research studies on the effectiveness of treatment with juvenile delinquents? In J. McGuire (Ed.), *What works: Reducing reoffending: Guidelines from research and practice* (pp. 63–78). Chichester, England: Wiley.

Lourie, I. S., & Hernandez, M. (2003). A historical perspective on national child mental health policy. *Journal of Emotional and Behavioral Disorders, 11,* 5–10.

Meyers, J., Kaufman, M., & Goldman, S. (1999). *Promising practices: Training strategies for serving children with serious emotional disturbance and their families in a system of care (Systems of care: Promising practices in children's mental health, 1998 series,* Vol. 5). Washington, DC: Center for Effective Collaboration and Practice, American Institutes of Research.

Robertson, L., Bates, M., Wood, M., Rosenblatt, J., Furlong, M., Casas, J., et al. (1998). The educational placements of students with emotional and behavioral disorders served by Probation, Mental Health, Public Health, and Social Services. *Psychology in the Schools, 35,* 333–346.

Rosenblatt, J. A., Robertson, L. M., Bates, M. P., Wood, M., Furlong, M. J., & Sosna, T. (1998). Troubled or troubling? Characteristics of youth referred to a system of care without system-level referral constraints. *Journal of Emotional and Behavioral Disorders, 6,* 42–54.

Rosenblatt, A., & Woodbridge, M. W. (2003). Deconstructing research on systems of care for youth with EBD: Frameworks for policy research. *Journal of Emotional and Behavioral Disorders, 11,* 27–38.

Stroul, B. A., & Friedman, R. (1986). *A system of care for children and youth with severe emotional disturbances.* Washington, DC: Georgetown University Child Development Center, CASSP Technical Assistance Center.

Tabachnick, B. G., & Fidell, L. S. (1989). *Using multivariate statistics* (2nd ed.). New York: HarperCollins.

Vinson, N. B., Brannan, A. M., Baughman, L. N., Wilce, M., & Gawron, T. (2001). The system-of-care model: Implementation in 27 communities. *Journal of Emotional and Behavioral Disorders, 9,* 30–42.

Wood, M., Chung, A., Furlong, M. J., Casas, J. M., Holbrook, L., & Richey, R. (1998). What works in a system of care? Services and outcomes associated with a juvenile probation population. *UC Davis Journal of Juvenile Law and Policy, 2,* 63–71.

Wood, M., Furlong, M., Casas, J., & Sosna, T. (1998). A system of care for juvenile probationers. *UC Davis Journal of Juvenile Law and Policy, 2,* 5–9.

Wood, M., Furlong, M., J., Rosenblatt, J., Robertson, L., Scozzari, F., & Sosna, T. (1997). Understanding the psychosocial characteristics of gang-involved youth in a system of care: Individual, family, and system correlates. *Education and Treatment of Children, 20,* 281–294.

Woodbridge, M., Furlong, M. J., Casas, J. M., & Sosna, T. (2001). Santa Barbara's multiagency integrated system of care. In M. Hernandez et al. (Eds.), *Developing outcome strategies in children's mental health* (pp. 63–80). Baltimore: Brookes.

Zanglis, I., Furlong, M. J., & Casas, J. M. (2000). Case study of a community mental health collaborative: Impact on identification of youth with emotional or behavioral disorders. *Behavioral Disorders, 25,* 359–371.

The Bridges Project

Description and Evaluation of a School-Based Mental Health Program in Eastern Kentucky

CHAPTER 15

Vestena Robbins and Beth Jordan Armstrong

Kentucky has more than a decade of experience in designing and implementing community-based systems of care for youth with severe emotional disabilities (SED) and their families. This rich history began when the Kentucky Department for Mental Health and Mental Retardation Services (KDMHMRS) responded to the national call to action to better meet the needs of youth with SED through the development of the Child and Adolescent Service System Program (CASSP) initiative. In 1986 the KDMHMRS received monies directed toward developing a CASSP office in the Division of Mental Health (DMH) within the KDMHMRS. This office was instrumental in providing technical assistance related to children's mental health services, creating a Children and Youth Services Branch within the DMH and developing an interagency task force aimed at crafting a statewide framework for delivering services to youth with SED in a manner consistent with CASSP principles.

These initial efforts led to the procurement of a Robert Wood Johnson Foundation grant in the late 1980s that facilitated the development and implementation of a service coordination model, known as Bluegrass IMPACT, in central Kentucky. In addition to establishing a coordinated interagency approach to service delivery, this model provided funding for services not traditionally available, such as mentoring, school-based services, and intensive in-home therapy. The success of the Bluegrass IMPACT model raised the awareness of the Kentucky General Assembly regarding the plight of the children's mental health system in the state and led to the passage of legislation in 1990 that defined Kentucky IMPACT. This plan codified into law the statewide replication of the Bluegrass IMPACT model and established the State Interagency Council and 18 Regional Interagency Councils to provide oversight and coordination of program implementation (see Illback, Nelson, & Sanders, 1998, for a comprehensive discussion of program features).

Simultaneous reform efforts were occurring in education, with the creation of a multidisciplinary task force that studied and revised state guidelines for identifying students with emotional and behavioral disabilities as well as the passage of the Kentucky Educational Reform Act (KERA) in 1990. Although KERA mandated significant changes in financing, governance, and curriculum to improve the learning and achievement of all of Kentucky's students, some initiatives directly affected students with mental health issues, such as the creation of Family Resource and Youth Service Centers and the development of extended school services for students at risk.

With statewide implementation of the IMPACT model, Kentucky also instituted a comprehensive program evaluation effort incorporating both process and outcome data collection to assess the effectiveness and quality of the system of care. A 5-year evaluation of the program revealed significant reductions in the psychiatric hospitalization of children and thus service costs; clinical gains in behavioral functioning; and improvements in family support, placement stability, and family satisfaction with services (Illback, Sanders, & Birkby, 1995). The evaluation also revealed limited coordination and integration between education and other child-serving agencies, the continued underidentification of students with emotional problems, and less positive school-related outcomes for these youth. To that end, the Kentucky DMH applied for and received a 6-year Comprehensive Community Mental Health Services for Children (CMHSC) and Their Families Program grant to expand its system of care for youth with SED and their families, with particular emphasis on developing and promoting school-based interventions and family involvement. This school-based mental health initiative, the Bridges Project, is being implemented in 20 schools within the Appalachian region of the state. This chapter describes the Appalachian region and key features of the program. Program outcomes are reported; implementation realities and future system-of-care expansion efforts are discussed.

SETTING: CHARACTERISTICS OF THE APPALACHIAN REGION

Much of eastern and southeastern Kentucky is located in the Appalachian Mountains. The three regional Mental Health/Mental Retardation Boards with which the DMH contracts for services through the Bridges Project fall within this geographical area of the state. The characteristics of this area differ dramatically from the rest of the state. Counties in this region ranked among the lowest in the state with respect to child well-being (Kentucky KIDS Count Consortium, 2000). High rates of poverty, unemployment, and illiteracy further contribute to increased risk for mental health and academic problems of children in this area. Compounding these risk factors are barriers to effective service delivery, such as lack of transportation, limited community services and resources, and a shortage of qualified human services staff.

PROGRAM FEATURES: MOVING FROM COEXISTENCE TO COLLABORATION

Given the predominately rural nature of Kentucky, many CMHCs operate as the primary providers of behavioral health services for youth and their families within each of the 14 mental health service areas of the state. The CMHC has become the agency to which school districts most frequently refer youth with emotional and behavioral needs. Regional children's mental health services directors report school-based mental health as one of the fastest growing program areas in the state.

Consistent with national trends (Center for Mental Health in Schools, 2001), a variety of school mental health service delivery mechanisms are being implemented to address the mental health needs of students across Kentucky. These delivery mechanisms range from school personnel referring and encouraging families to seek services at the local CMHC or with state agency or private providers to the expanded school-based mental health model available through the Bridges Project in the southeastern portion of the state. The Bridges Project extends school-based mental health services beyond the traditional mental health consultation model to a comprehensive three-tiered model of mental health service delivery that focuses on providing prevention, early intervention, and intensive services to all children and youth in the school.

Within the Bridges Project, the delivery of school-based mental health services is accomplished through a partnership with school personnel, families, and a Student Service Team (SST). The SST is composed of a service coordinator, a family liaison, and an intervention specialist, all of whom are employees of the regional CMHC but are housed on the school campus. The service coordinator serves as a case manager for children and youth identified with severe emotional and behavioral disabilities by facilitating wraparound team meetings and linking the family with natural supports and formal resources in the community. These individuals are bachelor's-level service providers who receive training in service coordination and team facilitation strategies. The family liaison, the parent of a youth with an emotional or behavioral disability, serves in a professional role by providing peer-to-peer mentoring to family members and building local and regional family support networks. There are no formal educational requirements for this position; however, these individuals must complete a certification process through Opportunities for Family Leadership, the state office for family leadership. The intervention specialist is a mental health clinician with a master's degree or the professional equivalent who has received additional training in functional behavioral assessment and the development of behavior intervention plans and school-based supports. Each school also has access to a regional behavior consultant, who provides assistance to schools in the implementation of schoolwide strategies and supports and consultation on individual and group behavioral interventions. Fifteen SSTs and three behavior consultants serve 20 campuses throughout the three participating regions, including prekindergarten through high school and alternative school settings.

Providing a Continuum of Mental Health Services and Supports

The implementation of a continuum of mental health services and supports is based upon a positive behavior support (PBS) framework. Defined as a "broad range of systemic and individualized strategies for achieving important social and learning outcomes while preventing problem behavior" (Turnbull et al., 2002, p. 377), PBS has expanded from a focus on individual children to a systemwide intervention approach for schools (Dwyer & Osher, 2000; Scott & Hunter, 2001). This proactive data-based approach focuses on providing multiple levels of intervention to address the academic and mental health needs of all youth, not just those with the most challenging behaviors. The assumption underlying PBS is that a continuum of effective behavior supports is required to meet the needs of all youth in a school (Sugai, Sprague, Horner, & Walker, 2000).

Based on a three-tiered prevention model, PBS is a research-based approach for promoting prosocial behavior of all students (universal interventions and supports), both those at risk for or beginning to exhibit problem behavior (targeted interventions and supports) and those with chronic and severe emotional and behavioral problems (intensive interventions and supports). The application of schoolwide PBS can enhance system-of-care approaches for students with intensive needs by providing an environment of proactive interventions across all students and a schoolwide systems approach to prevention and early intervention (Eber, Sugai, Smith, & Scott, 2002).

Universal Interventions

Universal interventions constitute a form of primary prevention and focus on promoting the mental health and prosocial behavior of all students. Universal approaches are typically effective at preventing problem behavior for the majority (80%–90%) of students. These strategies focus on enhancing protective factors in the school, home, and community while preventing the development of problems through the efforts of all school personnel and caregivers. Essentially, universal interventions are focused on creating a positive school climate that increases school safety and positive student–adult relationships.

Coordination and oversight of universal interventions rests with the Positive Behavior Support Team, which includes full representation of school personnel (i.e., administration, teachers at all grade levels, certified staff, specialized support staff), mental health, families, and the community. Through their attendance at ongoing trainings and monthly meetings, the Positive Behavior Support Team members are responsible for planning, monitoring, and maintaining the schoolwide intervention program (Lewis, 2001; Scott & Nelson, 1999). Regional behavior consultants are available to "coach" teams as they move through this process. Schoolwide interventions might include developing a set of clearly defined schoolwide rules and expectations for student behavior; establishing schoolwide approaches for teaching and reinforcing expected prosocial behaviors; and redesigning routines, schedules, and environments to prevent, minimize, or eliminate disruptive behavior. Schoolwide initiatives specific to mental health promotion may include mental health education and awareness activities (e.g., the inclusion of a mental health column in the school newsletter, S.O.S. Suicide Prevention Program); mental health promotion (e.g., Red Ribbon Week; Child Abuse Prevention Month;

Baby, Think It Over); and parent networking and parent education (e.g., library of mental health resources for parents, parent education and support groups).

BUILDING THE FOUNDATION FOR STUDENT SUCCESS: AN EXAMPLE

A small elementary (K–5) school participating in the Bridges Project has met with success in planning, designing, and implementing universal academic and mental health interventions to improve school climate and overcome barriers to student success. The Positive Behavior Support Team created the following mission statement to guide the actions of the team: "We, the staff, are committed to providing a positive learning environment where students are encouraged to reach their full potential." The following Guidelines for Success were established to meet the school's mission: Be Responsible, Always Try, Do Your Best, Cooperate with Others, and Treat Everyone with Dignity and Respect. These guidelines are posted throughout the school, and lesson plans are developed to teach students the skills necessary to behave in accordance with the guidelines. For example, a schoolwide kick-off was held in which students and staff designed and performed skits illustrating the guidelines. Students are reinforced for following the guidelines through activities, such as "Caught Ya Being Good" tickets that can be exchanged for incentive items at the school store. The Positive Behavior Support Team continues to meet on a monthly basis to review existing interventions and to design additional schoolwide strategies and supports aimed at enhancing student academic performance and promoting mental health.

Targeted Interventions

The establishment of effective universal strategies and supports will likely result in a significant reduction in student discipline problems. Not all students, however, are responsive to universal interventions, and an estimated 5% to 10% require interventions targeted specifically for their unique needs (Sprague, Sugai, & Walker, 1998). Targeted interventions are designed for youth who are at risk or who are beginning to exhibit signs of emotional or behavioral problems; they are administered individually or in small groups.

Within the Bridges Project, school-based screening committees have been established to review referrals and determine whether youth require targeted or intensive services. The composition of this team varies from school to school, depending upon the level of behavioral expertise of individual members, but typically includes a school administrator, an intervention specialist, a family liaison, and a special educator. These individuals meet on an as-needed basis to review referrals and collect necessary data to determine the level of service intensity required for a student. For example, behavioral observations may be conducted or school discipline records may be reviewed to gather needed information. If deemed in need of a targeted intervention, the team uses a strengths-based problem-solving process to develop a behavioral intervention or treatment plan to address the targeted problem area. Targeted interventions may include, for example, mentoring, tutoring or other academic support, or the development of a positive behavior plan.

 A TARGETED INTERVENTION IN ACTION: HOMEWORK HELPERS

A review of referrals to the Bridges school-based screening committee revealed a group of five elementary-age boys who were having difficulty with homework completion. Through a problem-solving process, the screening committee determined that a small-group intervention would be implemented as a first step to address this issue. The intervention specialist sent caregivers an information packet including tips for setting up an effective study environment at home and assisting children with homework. On Monday mornings, the students met with the intervention specialist to receive their weekly homework tracking form and participate in skill-building sessions related to organization, study habits, and goal setting. On Fridays, students met with the intervention specialist again to conduct a progress check of homework completion, celebrate student successes, and assist those who did not meet their goals. Anecdotal evidence suggests that for some students, participation in the Homework Helpers group led to improved self-perception, social interactions, grades, and parent satisfaction with student progress.

Intensive Interventions

Despite implementation of effective universal and targeted interventions, there remain 1% to 5% of youth who require more intensive interventions to succeed. These students have chronic and complex emotional or behavioral needs that span home, school, and community settings and require a comprehensive multiagency treatment approach. Similar to other communities' implementing system-of-care initiatives, the Bridges Project applies a team-based wraparound process to design and implement individualized service plans (Burns & Goldman, 1999; Eber & Nelson, 1997). School-based Bridges personnel facilitate the development of an individualized wraparound team whose members can identify and build upon the unique strengths and needs of the youth and his or her family. This team is composed of the youth, his or her family, and other community members selected by the family. Other team members may include school personnel, service providers, and natural community supports that do or could potentially have a positive impact on the youth and family (e.g., extended family members, clergy, coaches, peers).

Wraparound, a promising practice for improving outcomes for this population (Burns & Goldman, 1999; Eber, Osuch, & Redditt, 1996; Malloy, Cheney, & Cormier, 1998), incorporates a family-centered and strengths-based philosophy to guide service planning. Wraparound planning generally follows an eight-step process. The first step in the planning process includes initial conversations. The team facilitator (i.e., service coordinator) meets individually with the child, the caregiver(s), school personnel, and others on the team who have knowledge of the child and family across life domains. This gives all parties a safe setting in which to share their perspectives on the strengths and barriers prior to the team's first meeting. Conversations are ended with an identification of the strengths and resources of the child, the family, the person being interviewed, and the community at large, setting the stage for the strengths-based approach utilized in the formal team meeting.

The second step is to begin the team meeting with a review of the strengths identified through the initial conversation process. Barriers and challenges are not ignored but rather are approached through a discussion of how the previously identified strengths of the youth, other team members, and the community can best be utilized to address them.

Upon listing strengths of all involved parties, developing a team mission statement is the third step. The team mission statement is positive, focused, and brief (Eber et al., 2002). Ideally, the mission statement should "fit on a bumper sticker"; for example, "Jake will live at home and succeed at school." The team mission statement identifies a goal not only for the child but also for the team as a whole and gives the team a point to which it can return if the team meeting should get disorganized or off track.

The fourth step in the process is the identification of the child and family's needs across life domains. All team members may not have had the opportunity to be involved in an initial conversation, so the team meeting may be the first time some members have a chance to identify needs. This part of the process is not a time for team members to rehash all of the barriers and challenges the child and family are experiencing; rather, it allows the team to identify current needs of child and family.

Following needs identification, the fifth step for the team is prioritization of the needs. Safety issues, if they exist, are prioritized, followed by needs that are important to the child, caregiver(s), and others who spend a large amount of time with the child (i.e., school personnel). It is important in this phase to narrow the focus to three or four areas to be addressed in the short term. As prioritized needs are met, future team meetings begin to focus on less critical areas as identified in Step 4. The sixth step is developing actions through which needs will be addressed. Team members identify existing resources or design individualized interventions using a blend of formal and informal services and supports. Step 7, typically completed in conjunction with the previous step, involves assigning tasks related to the identified actions and soliciting commitments from team members and others involved with the family to ensure that actions are completed according to timelines.

Finally, the team facilitator documents a summary of the process on a designated wraparound planning form. This document serves as the foundation for future team meetings and subsequent planning. Careful monitoring of implementation and outcomes across multiple life domains (i.e., social/emotional, medical, basic needs, academic, living environment) is ongoing and is the responsibility of all team members. If through the evaluation and monitoring process identified actions are deemed ineffective or a crisis situation arises, the team will revisit earlier steps in the process to develop an alternate plan. The wraparound process is a key component of the full continuum of PBS in the Bridges schools because it is the mechanism for ensuring that proactive, outcome-based interventions for the students with the most intensive needs and their families are developed in a creative yet efficient manner.

 SCHOOL-BASED WRAPAROUND: JAKE'S STORY

Jake is a 13-year-old middle school student being raised by his maternal grandmother. By the beginning of his fifth-grade year, he had been enrolled in five other schools across three states. Jake's family changed schools frequently as a result of the inability to address his behavior within the school system.

Jake currently attends a school that is participating in the Bridges Project. Jake is beginning his second year at the school. Since enrolling there, he has had a total of three office referrals. In the past, he averaged three office referrals a week!

In other schools, Jake worked from the time he got home until bedtime, trying to finish his homework, but he was still failing almost all classes. His family was told he would be in reform school by the time he was 12. He now completes his homework quickly in the evening, and he consistently receives As and Bs.

In other programs, professionals encouraged Jake's family to put him on medication, but they did not discuss the importance of other supportive services. His grandmother describes past school and mental health services as disjointed and prescriptive. Due to the coordinated supports provided to Jake and his family by school and mental health personnel through the Bridges Project, Jake's grandmother receives fewer calls from the school and can focus on supporting her family rather than leaving work to meet with school personnel. She reports feeling that she is now working in partnership with the school rather than fighting against them.

Through her family's involvement in Kentucky's system of care, Jake's grandmother has learned about how to survive his disability. She is always getting ideas about new things to try and how to modify them if they don't work.... She has called it a "life-changing experience." Jake and his grandmother now present at state and national level conferences to share his success story with other families and professionals. The improvements in the family's quality of life testify to the importance of providing coordinated services, focusing on strengths rather than deficits, and including the family as an equal partner at all levels of decision making.

Jake's initial involvement with Bridges began 2 years ago when his school was selected to participate in the project. Prior to that time, Jake and his family received service coordination through the Kentucky IMPACT program. Because most of his difficulties occurred in a school setting, his IMPACT team determined that the Bridges Project would more comprehensively serve his needs.

In addition to himself and his grandmother, Jake's wraparound team includes a service coordinator, intervention specialist, two teachers, and the school principal. Extended team members include his aunt, a family friend, and his coach. Initial conversations revealed that Jake is bright, is motivated, wants to succeed, and enjoys positive adult attention.

Given Jake's history and identified strengths, the team developed the following mission statement: "Jake will interact successfully with peers and succeed in the classroom." The majority of needs identified by Jake's team fell into the educational/vocational and social/recreational life domains. Due to the severity of school-related problems, the team chose to prioritize needs in the educational/vocational domain. These needs centered on classroom behavior problems and difficulty with completion of schoolwork. The primary action was the development and implementation of a 504 modification plan. All core team members accepted responsibility for ensuring that the plan was implemented as written and modified as needed to meet Jake's behavioral and academic needs.

As Jake met with success at school as evidenced through a reduction in office referrals and improved grades, the team reconvened and determined that the next priority was to improve his peer-interaction skills. To meet this need, Jake began participating in a highly structured after-school program with an emphasis upon prosocial development. Building on his strength of responding well to adult attention, Jake has also begun assisting Bridges staff with implementation of an experiential curriculum in a third-grade classroom. Currently, Jake is working with his intervention specialist to appropriately apply the skills he learned in the after-school program to school and classroom settings. Jake and his team will continue to meet to address identified needs and modify his plan toward the achievement of the team's mission statement.

EVALUATION OF SCHOOL-BASED WRAPAROUND

While studies are being conducted to evaluate the effectiveness of each of the three levels of intervention, as well as the overall system, most of the evaluation effort is focused upon assessing the outcomes of children and youth with intensive needs and their families who engage in the school-based wraparound process. For the purposes of this chapter, preliminary outcomes for children served through the school-based wraparound component of the program are described.

Data used in the current analyses included information for students who were enrolled in the project during the 1999–2000 and 2000–2001 school years. Descriptive data were gathered for all children who received school-based wraparound. Child and family outcome data were gathered for children between the ages of 5 and 17.5 years at program entry who did not have a sibling already enrolled in the evaluation and whose caregiver provided consent for participation in the outcome study. Interviews were conducted with caregivers and youth who were age 11 or older. Data were collected at intake into services and every 6 months thereafter for up to 36 months. To the extent possible, follow-up interviews were conducted with caregivers and youth who exited services (e.g., met treatment goals, changed placements, moved out of the area). Longitudinal analyses were limited to outcomes at 12 months for those caregivers and youth with complete data (intake and 6- and 12-month follow-ups).

Participants

At the time of analysis, descriptive data were available for 334 children. Children served by the project ranged in age from 4 to 20 years, with an average age of 12 years. Most (73%) were boys, and 98% were White. At intake, most lived in the custody of their biological mothers only (42%), a two-parent home (38%), or the home of a relative (12%). The remaining 8% were in the custody of their biological father, adoptive or foster parents, or the state. About 67% reported annual family incomes below $15,000, and more than 80% were eligible for Medicaid. The average household size was four persons.

Caregivers reported that 45% of the children had experienced one or more child risk factors, including physical abuse, sexual abuse, previous psychiatric hospitalization, sexual abusiveness, suicide attempt, substance use, and a history of runaway behavior. Of those children with multiple child risk factors, 13% had experienced two child risk factors prior to intake, and 13% had experienced three or more. With respect to family risk factors, 100% of the caregivers indicated that their child had experienced one or more risk factors, including a family history of mental illness, domestic violence, criminal conviction, or substance use. Almost half (49%) had experienced three or more family risk factors, whereas 27% reported only one family risk factor and 24% reported two risk factors.

Almost 83% of the youth were diagnosed with a disruptive behavior disorder, and 22% had a mood disorder. Of the sample, 39% had more than one mental health diagnosis. In addition to mental health concerns, caregivers reported that 42% of the youth experienced chronic or recurring health problems, most commonly asthma, allergies, and headaches. Of those youth with health concerns, 49% took medication for the problems. In the 6 months prior to intake, 44% took medication related to their emotional or behavioral symptoms.

Clinical and Functional Outcomes

Behavioral and Emotional Strengths

An analysis of change in emotional and behavioral strengths (*Behavioral and Emotional Rating Scale;* Epstein & Sharma, 1997) from baseline to 12 months indicated slight but statistically insignificant increases in the average strength quotient. Using a reliable change index (RCI; Jacobson & Truax, 1991) to assess individual change in strengths over time, we found that from intake to 6 months, 47% of the children ($n = 78$) displayed clinically significant improvement in strengths, 27% remained stable, and 26% deteriorated.

Problem Behavior

Figure 15.1 illustrates the significant decrease in scores on the *Child Behavior Checklist* (CBCL; Achenbach, 1991a) from intake to 12-month follow-up for the Internalizing, Externalizing, and Total Problems scales. The greatest amount of change was experienced during the first 6 months in the program. No significant differences over time were noted on the *Youth Self-Report* (YSR; Achenbach, 1991b). The RCI results ($n = 76$) indicated that 36% of children exhibited clinically significant improvement on CBCL total scores from intake to 6-month follow-up, 60% remained stable, and only 4% experienced worsened problem behavior following entry into the program. The RCI results for the YSR ($n = 53$) revealed that only 15% of the youth experienced a clinically significant improvement between baseline and 6 months. The majority (83%) remained stable, and 2% worsened.

Functioning

Children ($n = 37$) receiving school-based wraparound experienced a substantial decrease in functional impairment between entry into the program and 1 year later, as measured by the *Child and Adolescent Functional Assessment Scale* (CAFAS; Hodges, 1990). As was true with problem behavior, the greatest change in functioning occurred in the first 6 months of service delivery. An examination of categories of impairment revealed that 62% of the children had marked or severe functional impairment at baseline and 37% were in this range at 6-month follow-up. The percentage had dropped to 19% by 1 year postentry.

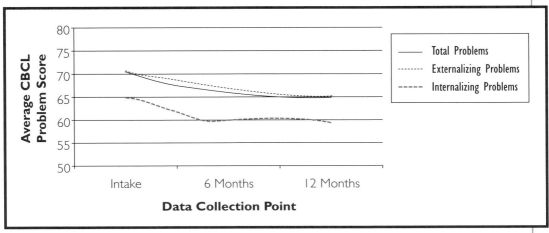

FIGURE 15.1. Average *Child Behavior Checklist* (CBCL; Achenbach, 1991a) scores at intake, 6-month, and 12-month follow-up ($N = 37$). *Note.* Internalizing scale $F(2, 37) = 8.24$, $p = .001$; Externalizing scale $F(2, 37) = 9.26$, $p = .001$; Total scale $F(2, 37) = 13.63$, $p = .000$.

Educational Performance

For children with complete data ($n = 17$), the average number of days absent during the 6 months prior to intake decreased steadily from baseline ($M = 5.5$, $SD = 10.9$), to 6 months ($M = 4.1$, $SD = 5.6$), to 1 year ($M = 3.6$, $SD = 6.9$); however, these changes were not statistically significant. The percentage of children receiving school disciplinary actions decreased over time, whereas the number achieving a C average or better increased (see Figures 15.2 and 15.3).

Substance Use

Youth age 11 and older for whom 1-year follow-up data were available ($n = 25$) reported little change in their use of cigarettes (intake: 64%; 1 year: 60%) and an increase in marijuana usage between intake (16%) and 1-year follow-up (28%). Alcohol use decreased by 16% over time (intake: 36%; 1 year: 20%).

Summary of Findings

Children and youth with serious emotional disabilities receiving school-based wraparound through the Bridges Project were demographically similar to those in other studies of this population (Cullinan, Epstein, & Sabornie,

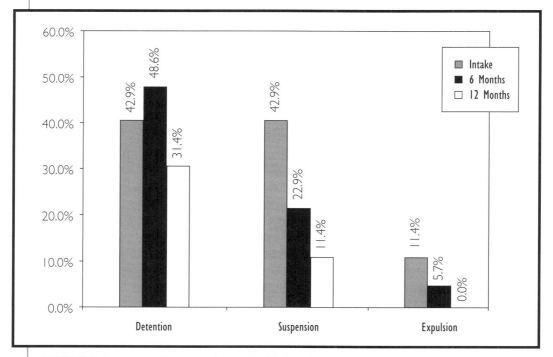

FIGURE 15.2. Percentage of students ($n = 35$) with disciplinary actions over time.

1992; Greenbaum et al., 1998). Most were boys and entered the program during early adolescence. Consistent with the racial composition of the region, almost all were White and the majority lived in poverty. In addition to poor economic conditions, these children and youth present with multiple risk factors, primarily familial in nature, such as having a biological parent with a history of mental illness or substance abuse. At program entry, most were diagnosed with disruptive behavior or mood disorders and experienced serious behavior problems and functional impairment.

At 1-year postintake, children and youth displayed significantly lower levels of problem behavior and functional impairment, with the greatest change occurring during the first 6 months of service delivery. Grades improved and school disciplinary incidents decreased. Changes in substance use varied, revealing an increase in marijuana use, a decrease in alcohol usage, and little change in cigarette smoking.

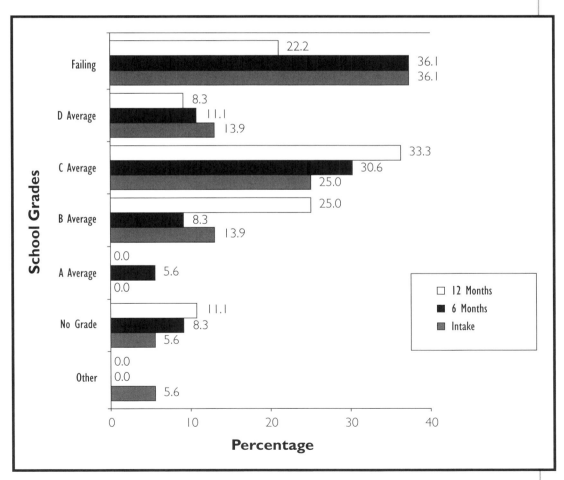

FIGURE 15.3. School grades for youth ($n = 36$) over time.

SYNTHESIS

The Bridges Project represents a significant shift in the role of mental health providers in schools. The investment of mental health resources in school-wide prevention, early intervention, and the facilitation of school-based wraparound teams expands traditional mental health models to an integrated, strengths-based approach. The application of system-of-care principles through a school-based wraparound approach has allowed schools in the Bridges Project to experience success with some of their most challenged and challenging youth in such areas as improved behavioral functioning, decreased problem behavior, and increased academic performance. Although these changes are encouraging, much work remains to determine how to positively affect other life domains, such as substance use, delinquency, and physical health.

Partnerships between mental health and education around systemic models such as PBS can provide a structure for more efficient and effective delivery of mental health services. As previously stated, this requires a significant change in the traditional delivery of mental health to include assisting with schoolwide prevention, providing early intervention, and building competencies with the system-of-care concept and related tools, such as school-based wraparound. The development of a school-based continuum of care that uses evidence-based practices commensurate with demonstrated needs of students is a concept that may be useful for other mental health providers seeking models for efficiently and effectively organizing their supports and services. Being part of the day-to-day environment of the school through a schoolwide PBS approach and assisting in improving overall learning environments for all students can be considered a long-term investment of mental health resources.

Implementation Realities

Identifying and Supporting Qualified Staff Is Critical

Staff recruitment and retention is a challenge in any human services program. Although rural mental health provides a setting for creative professional growth and development, a lack of human services providers with appropriate education and experience is a major barrier in implementation of this model. As in many rural areas having difficulty attracting new providers to their area, CMHCs in eastern Kentucky are committed to "growing their own" staff by providing postsecondary educational opportunities and professional development to staff during their employment.

Conjoint Hiring and Supervision Improves Relationships

Although the regional CMHCs employ the SST staff, regional project directors have included school administrators in the screening and selection process for SST members for their respective schools. This enables parties from both agencies to interview candidates and assess how well individuals will fit into the school culture. Additionally, the joint interviewing process assists in building trust among agencies.

Because SSTs have their offices and work in school buildings, day-to-day traditional supervision by CMHC administrators is not feasible or effective. Through collaboration with school administrators, functional supervision of Bridges staff by school personnel has been arranged. A designated school supervisor, typically the family resource/youth service center director or principal, is responsible for overseeing the daily administrative duties of Bridges staff (i.e., on-site supervision and signing timesheets). Student Service Team members have responsibility for adhering to policies and procedures of both the CMHC and the school district. This practice has increased integration of Bridges staff into the school and acceptance of the Bridges model.

Supervision Is Essential to Maintaining Model Fidelity

Maintaining high fidelity in the implementation of a continuum of positive supports and interventions is contingent upon the quality and consistency of the supervision process. Supervision must occur at all levels of program implementation. At the universal level, supervisors assist staff in identifying ongoing academic and mental health universal interventions, as well as areas for future development in prevention. At the targeted level, the supervisors assist staff in keeping interventions short term and focused on the presenting problem. Another important issue in supervision at this level is helping staff identify when services should either be terminated due to successful completion of therapeutic goals or, if chronic needs are identified, stepped up to the intensive level. At the intensive level, the supervisor assists team members in working through the steps of the wraparound process, because it can be easy for teams to forego an important step to save time or as a result of pressure to provide interventions and services. Finally, supervisors encourage staff, particularly service coordinators, to identify and use natural resources rather than to single-handedly attempt to meet the needs of the youth and family.

Training Should Be Ongoing and Focused

To develop capacity and an infrastructure to implement and sustain the model, all administrative and program staff should receive intense training prior to service delivery. System-of-care values and the wraparound process must be understood before families are served. Additionally, ongoing opportunities for postimplementation practice refinement with supervisors and consultants are essential to maintaining model integrity. Periodic reviews of best practices and new research developments in the areas of wraparound and multilevel intervention may decrease the likelihood of model drift.

Evaluation and Program Efforts Should Be Mainstreamed

Evaluation efforts should not be viewed as intrusive or external to program efforts but rather should become an integral part of day-to-day operations, with frequent examination and use of data at multiple levels (i.e., from prevention to systems levels). Such an approach ensures that practice, programs, and policies are based on the best available evidence and that quality and outcomes are monitored in an ongoing manner.

Readiness for Innovation Should Be Assessed

Many viable programs fall by the wayside due to an organization's lack of readiness for effective program implementation. The identification of key indicators of readiness serves as a first step in assessing whether an organization has the necessary requisites to effectively implement the innovation. Ongoing assessment of readiness and organizational capacity-building strategies are critical to successful program implementation. Assessing the readiness of schools and mental health agencies to provide an integrated continuum of services and supports is critical to the effective implementation and maintenance of adopted values and practices (Robbins, Collins, Liaupsin, Illback, & Call, in press).

System-of-Care Enhancements

Ongoing review of project successes and challenges suggests potential areas of program development and expansion. Exciting opportunities to meld the core values into new and existing programs have surfaced, and discussions have ensued as to how best to integrate components of the project into a statewide vision for systems change.

School-Based Mental Health and Early Childhood

The need to look at the impact of early intervention and prevention in early childhood has been realized through the implementation of the Bridges Project. Symptoms of emotional and behavioral problems are often noticed at a very early age. It is imperative that the mental health system work with early childhood service providers and parents to promote emotionally healthy environments and to teach young children to deal effectively with their emotions.

Mental Health Promotion Efforts

Although the implementation of a three-tiered service delivery model is new in the mental health arena, the model has a history in public health. Physical health professionals have been able to provide illness prevention or health promotion services, short-term therapies, and long-term treatments for years. This is possible, in no small part, because of a concerted effort to raise public awareness of the vital role that preventive medicine plays in maintaining physical wellness. Policymakers have been pushed to incorporate health promotion or illness prevention initiatives into all aspects of health-care reform. The adoption has been more difficult with mental health. Historically, payment for mental health services is often dependent on both the client having a psychiatric diagnosis and the credentials of the service provider. Additionally, limits are frequently placed on the number and type of mental health services allowable under an insurance plan. Without the availability of a funding source, it is easy for preventive activities to succumb to billable mental health services. Through implementation of universal-level academic and mental health strategies, it is hoped that barriers to mental health will be broken down and youth will be more able to reach their potential.

Expanding Interagency Partners

The Kentucky IMPACT model provides a format to identify and involve community partners and resources within the lives of the youth served by the project. As the model has matured, it has been determined that youth have challenges that require services beyond the scope of traditional community mental health. Three areas often identified are chronic health problems, substance abuse, and juvenile justice involvement. Strengths and barriers must be explored across life domains rather than limiting the discussion to mental health issues when physical health, substance abuse, and legal issues abound. The wraparound process can only be effective when youth are holistically treated through involvement by parents and partners in all child-serving agencies.

AUTHORS' NOTE

Support for this research was provided by a grant from the Substance Abuse and Mental Health Services Administration (5 HS5 SM52273-05).

REFERENCES

Achenbach, T. M. (1991a). *Manual for the Child Behavior Checklist/4–18 and 1991 Profile.* Burlington: University of Vermont, Department of Psychiatry.

Achenbach, T. M. (1991b). *Manual for the Youth Self-Report/11–18 and 1991 Profile.* Burlington: University of Vermont, Department of Psychiatry.

Burns, B. J., & Goldman, S. K. (Eds.). (1999). *Promising practices in wraparound for children with serious emotional disturbance and their families: Systems of care (Promising practices in children's mental health, 1998 Series,* Vol. 4). Washington, DC: Center for Effective Collaboration and Practice, American Institutes for Research.

Center for Mental Health in Schools. (2001). *Mental health in schools: Guidelines, models, resources, and policy considerations* (executive summary). Los Angeles: University of California, Department of Psychology.

Cullinan, D., Epstein, M. H., & Sabornie, E. J. (1992). Selected characteristics of a national sample of serious emotionally disturbed adolescents. *Behavior Disorders, 17,* 273–280.

Dwyer, K., & Osher, D. (2000). *Safeguarding our children: An action guide.* Washington, DC: U.S. Departments of Education and Justice, American Institutes for Research.

Eber, L., & Nelson, C. M. (1997). School-based wraparound planning: Integrating services for students with emotional and behavioral needs. *American Journal of Orthopsychiatry, 67*(3), 385–395.

Eber, L., Osuch, R., & Redditt, C. A. (1996). School-based applications of the wraparound process: Early results on service provision and student outcomes. *Journal of Child and Family Studies, 5,* 83–99.

Eber, L., Sugai, G., Smith, C. R., & Scott, T. M. (2002). Wraparound and positive behavioral interventions and supports in the schools. *Journal of Emotional and Behavioral Disorders, 10*(3), 171–180.

Epstein, M. H., & Sharma, J. (1997). *Behavioral and Emotional Rating Scale: A strength-based approach to assessment.* Austin, TX: PRO-ED.

Greenbaum, P. E., Dedrick, R. F., Friedman, R. M., Kutash, K., Brown, E. C., Lardieri, S. P., et al. (1998). National Adolescent and Child Treatment Study (NACTS): Outcomes for children with serious emotional and behavioral disturbance. In M. H. Epstein, K. Kutash, & A. Duchnowski (Eds.), *Outcomes for children and youth with behavioral and emotional disorders and their families: Programs and evaluation best practices* (pp. 21–54). Austin, TX: PRO-ED.

Hodges, K. (1990). *The Child and Adolescent Functional Assessment Scale.* Ann Arbor, MI: Author.

Illback, R. J., Nelson, C. M., & Sanders, D. (1998). Community-based services in Kentucky: Description and 5-year evaluation of Kentucky IMPACT. In M. H. Epstein, K. Kutash, & A. Duchnowski (Eds.), *Outcomes for children and youth with behavioral and emotional disorders and their families: Programs and evaluation best practices* (pp. 141–172). Austin, TX: PRO-ED.

Illback, R. J., Sanders, D., & Birkby, B. (1995). *Evaluation of the Kentucky IMPACT program at Year 5: Accomplishments, challenges, and opportunities.* Frankfort, KY: Cabinet for Health Services, Division of Mental Health, Children and Youth Services Branch.

Jacobson, N. S., & Truax, P. (1991). Clinical significance: A statistical approach to defining meaningful change in psychotherapy research. *Journal of Consulting and Clinical Psychology, 59,* 12–19.

Kentucky KIDS Count Consortium. (2000). *2000 Kids Count county data book.* Louisville: Kentucky Youth Advocates.

Lewis, T. (2001). Building infrastructure to enhance schoolwide systems of positive behavioral support: Essential features of technical assistance. *Beyond Behavior, 11*(1), 10–12.

Malloy, J., Cheney, D., & Cormier, G. (1998). Interagency collaboration and the transition to adulthood for students with emotional or behavioral disabilities. *Education and Treatment of Children, 1,* 303–320.

Robbins, V., Collins, K., Liaupsin, C., Illback, R. J., & Call, J. (in press). Evaluating school readiness for implementation of positive behavioral supports. *Journal of Applied School Psychology.*

Scott, T. M., & Hunter, J. (2001). Initiating schoolwide support systems: An administrator's guide to the process. *Beyond Behavior, 11*(1), 13–15.

Scott, T. M., & Nelson, C. M. (1999). Universal school discipline strategies: Facilitating positive learning environments. *Effective School Practices, 17*(4), 54–64.

Sprague, J., Sugai, G., & Walker, H. (1998). Antisocial behavior in schools. In S. Watson & F. Gresham (Eds.), *Child behavior therapy: Ecological considerations in assessment, treatment, and evaluation* (pp. 451–474). New York: Plenum Press.

Sugai, G., Sprague, J. R., Horner, R. H., & Walker, H. M. (2000). Preventing school violence: The use of office discipline referrals to assess and monitor school-wide discipline interventions. *Journal of Emotional and Behavioral Disorders, 8*(2), 94–101.

Turnbull, A., Edmonson, H., Griggs, P., Wickham, D., Sailor, W., Freeman, R., et al. (2002). A blueprint for schoolwide positive behavior support: Implementation of three components. *Exceptional Children, 68*(3), 377–402.

Description and Evaluation of Project SUPPORT

CHAPTER 16

Service Utilization To Promote the Positive Rehabilitation and Community Transition of Incarcerated Youth with Emotional Disorders

Deanne Unruh, Michael Bullis, Cindy Booth, and John Pendergrass

Youth with emotional disorders (ED) face great difficulties in their transition from adolescence into young adulthood. This reality was illustrated in the National Longitudinal Transition Study (NLTS; DeStefano & Wagner, 1992; Wagner, 1992), which (a) included a nationally representative sample of special education students and (b) was conducted prospectively to describe the transition from school and community adjustment experiences of students after leaving school. On virtually every outcome examined in the project, young people with ED demonstrated poorer outcomes compared to their peers with other types of disabilities and also fared less well in standards from other databases on peers without disabilities (Marder, 1992; Valdes, Williamson, & Wagner, 1990). The following results from that study stand out.

- Participants with ED (a) exhibited high unemployment, (b) demonstrated instability in terms of keeping a job, (c) worked fewer hours, and (d) earned lower wages as compared to participants with other special education disabilities (D'Amico & Blackorby, 1992). Two years after leaving school, 59.3% were unemployed, and 3 to 5 years after leaving school, 52.6% were unemployed. A total of 19% had lost a job between these two time points, and 23.7% had been employed at both data collection points. Of those who were employed 3 to 5 years after high school, 12.4% were working part time and 35% were working full time.
- More than half (57.8%) of the sample of participants with ED were enrolled in some type of vocational education while in school, as compared to 64.8% for all participants in the study (Valdes et al, 1990; Wagner, 1991). Various estimates suggest that roughly 20% of all adolescents without disabilities will drop out of school (Blackorby, Edgar, & Kortering, 1991). More than half, 58.6%, of the participants with ED dropped out of school—as compared to 37.1% for all participants

375

and 35.6% for participants with learning disabilities—far and away the highest dropout rate for any disability group. Less than 2 years after leaving high school, 17% of participants with ED were enrolled in postsecondary programs, whereas 3 to 5 years after leaving, 25.6% of the sample had enrolled.

- Approximately 20% of all adolescents commit an offense by age 17 that, if they were caught, would be of a magnitude for which they would be arrested, and about 17% of all arrests are of persons under the age of 18 (Dryfoos, 1990). Wagner and Shaver (1989) noted that in the NLTS, almost 50% of the participants with ED had been arrested while in high school. Wagner (1991) noted that 58% of the sample were arrested at least once 3 to 5 years after leaving school, 73% of those participants with ED who dropped out had been arrested at least once, and there was a 20.7% increase between less than 2 years and 3 to 5 years after leaving school—the highest rate of all disability groups.
- Given the multifaceted nature of ED, as well as the dismal transition achievements of this population, one would think that members of this population would receive services from a number of community-based social service agencies. However, the NLTS (Marder, Wechsler, & Valdes, 1993) revealed that only 5.7% of participants with ED received services from vocational rehabilitation and, according to parent reports regarding their son or daughter with ED, 43.9% of participants with ED had a need for personal counseling but only 27.1% received such services.

As poor as these outcomes are, there is speculation that those approximately 100,000 youths who are incarcerated yearly for extreme forms of criminal behaviors (Gallagher, 1999)—many of whom display some sort of emotional disturbance or learning disorder (Foley, 2001)—experience even worse transition outcomes than peers with ED from mainstream public schools. Further, criminality occurring during adolescence can have long-term consequences as young men and women age into adulthood in terms of work, social adjustment, and continuing criminal acts (Ensminger & Juon, 1998; McCord, 1992; Robins, 1966, 1978; Wolfgang, Thornberry, & Figilo, 1987). A recent study that we have completed on the facility-to-community transition of youth with and without disabilities on parole from the Oregon Youth Authority (OYA, Oregon's juvenile correctional system)—the TRACS Project (Transition Research on Antisocial Youth in Community Settings)—provides strong support for such a contention (Bullis & Yovanoff, in press; Bullis, Yovanoff, Mueller, & Havel, 2002).

At any given time, approximately 1,000 to 1,100 youth are committed to OYA by the courts, and another 2,000 are placed on parole in the community and supervised by that agency. In the TRACS project we randomly constructed a sample of 531 youth with and without disabilities who were remanded to OYA and gathered data on their educational, personal, and criminal histories and on the services they received while in OYA. After parole, we interviewed the youth and, if possible, a family member at 6-month intervals to profile the youth's community adjustment experiences over a 1- to 3-year period. We documented the participants' return to OYA and placement in the adult correctional systems by accessing extant state databases from those two agencies. Key findings from TRACS are summarized next (Bullis & Yovanoff, in press; Bullis et al., 2002).

- The TRACS sample displayed a 43% return to OYA custody, and 16% of the sample were placed in the adult correctional system after release from OYA.
- Twelve months after the point of parole was the point in time after which virtually all "age-eligible" youth (i.e., youth who turn 18 do not return to OYA as they "age out" of that system) did *not* return to OYA. Stated differently, if youth on parole did not return to OYA in the 12-month period following parole, it was extremely unlikely they would return after that time.
- After parole from OYA, only 35% of the TRACS sample were engaged in either school or work at different points over the data collection period.
- Participants with disabilities (most of whom had ED) had much lower engagement rates in school or work and much higher return rates to the juvenile or adult correctional systems than participants without disabilities.
- The employment rate for the TRACS sample was much lower than that found for the ED sample in the NLTS (an average of just less than 30% over 2 years after leaving OYA compared to 58% 2 to 4 years after leaving school for the NLTS sample). The TRACS sample's engagement in school or work also was much lower than that found for adolescents with disabilities in a statewide transition project for adolescents with disabilities in the public schools (an average of 35% over the first year after leaving OYA compared to 75% for the public school sample; Benz, 2000; Benz, Lindstrom, & Latta, 1999).
- Being engaged in work or school 6 months after parole from OYA was strongly associated with being engaged 12 months after parole from OYA and remaining in the community—out of OYA or the adult correctional system. Compared to participants who were *not* engaged 6 months after parole, participants who *were* engaged at that time were 2.38 times less likely to be in custody and 3.22 times more likely to be engaged in work or school 12 months after parole. Being engaged at 6 months after parole was an especially potent protective factor for youth with disabilities.
- Few TRACS participants received services from any community-based social service agencies, but those who did fared far better than those who did not. Participants who received services from mental health were 2.25 times more likely to be engaged 6 months after parole. Participants receiving services from any of a number of other community-based agencies were 1.96 times more likely to be engaged at 6-months after parole.

Clearly, youth with ED who have been incarcerated and paroled back to the community face great challenges when returning to the community. They experience difficulties securing work and returning to school, and few social service agencies—other than parole—assist them in reintegrating into society in a positive manner. Conversely, the TRACS results strongly suggest that involvement in school or work after exit from the juvenile correctional system can be a powerful protective factor for this group of young people. Such an emphasis is very much in line with other findings in the professional literature.

Lipsey and Wilson (1998), in a synthesis of research on juvenile crime prevention, found that intervention programs focused on structured learning, school achievement, and job skills can reduce recidivism among incarcerated youth who have returned to the community. Several studies have pointed to the association of earning a high school diploma or general education development (GED) diploma with lower rates of return to the correctional system (Ambrose & Lester, 1988; Brier, 1994) and higher rates of employment in the community (Black et al., 1996). Another promising line of work is related to the provision of intensive aftercare services for incarcerated youth returning to the community by employing "wraparound" service coordination coupled with a school and work emphasis (Altschuler & Armstrong, 2001). Federally funded transition projects specifically for high-risk youth with mental health or criminal backgrounds (Bullis & Cheney, 1999; Bullis & Fredericks, 2002; Bullis et al., 1994; Bullis, Moran, Todis, Benz, & Johnson, 2002) have pointed to the importance of the role of a transition specialist (TS) in the lives of these young people as an advocate and mentor (Todis, Bullis, D'Ambrosio, Schultz, & Waintrup, 2001). The TS works with the youth to secure meaningful educational and work placements by emphasizing the youth's strengths and interests in developing an Individualized Service Plan (ISP) and providing each youth with multiple opportunities to succeed in those school or work placements (Clark, 1998; Clark & Davis, 2000).

In this chapter we describe a statewide project that has been developed and implemented to assist youth with ED on parole to transition successfully from correctional facilities into their home communities: Project SUPPORT (Service Utilization to Promote the Positive Rehabilitation and Community Transition of Incarcerated Youth with Emotional Disorders). Project SUPPORT was initiated in 1999 as a statewide service effort managed by the Oregon Department of Education (ODE), the OYA, Oregon Office of Vocational Services (VR), and the University of Oregon (UO). In the following sections we discuss the (a) development and background of the project, (b) basic components of the service delivery model, (c) evaluation procedures, and (d) preliminary project results.

PARTICIPANTS

The target population for Project SUPPORT consisted of youth incarcerated in OYA possessing (a) a special education disability (e.g., emotional disturbance, learning disability), (b) psychiatric diagnosis (i.e., as defined by the fourth edition of the *Diagnostic and Statistical Manual of Mental Disorders [DSM–IV],* American Psychiatric Association, 1994), or (c) a combination of both special education and psychiatric conditions. Project referrals initially were garnered from a list of youth currently residing within OYA's correctional facilities. Once the project became established—and treatment managers, parole officers, and facility education staff became knowledgeable about the project and referral criteria—these staff persons became the primary referral sources to the project.

Table 16.1 presents basic information on the youth served thus far in Project SUPPORT: (a) demographics, (b) disability status, (c) individual barriers, (d) criminal history, and (e) education. A total of 225 participants were served from August of 1999 through December of 2002. The average age at entry into the project was 17.1 years, which means that youth are, or shortly will be, 18 when released from OYA. There were 175 (78%) boys and 50 (22%) girls. Ethnic minority status was reported for 57 (26%), with the remaining 164 (74%) identified as Caucasian. Although only 16% of those reporting a special education diagnosis ($n = 121$) were diagnosed with an emotional disturbance, 95% ($n = 208$) reported possessing a *DSM–IV* psychiatric label. The three most prevalent *DSM–IV* diagnosis categories were (a) a disorder first diagnosed in infancy through adolescence (68%; e.g., attention-deficit disorder [ADD] and attention-deficit/hyperactivity disorder [ADHD], conduct disorder, oppositional-defiant disorder); (b) a substance-related disorder (46%); and (c) a mood disorder (27%; e.g., bipolar, depressive, or manic-related disorders).

In addition to a disabling condition, project participants clearly demonstrated other high-risk characteristics. A list of 22 barriers was collected on project participants in regard to (a) employment, (b) education, (c) living status/residence, and (d) family/personal. Project participants reported on average 8.5 barriers, with a range of 1 through 16. The top three identified barriers were a history of (a) substance abuse (79%), (b) absenteeism or suspension from school (78%), and (c) running away from home or residential placement (75%). In addition, two-thirds of all participants reported prior residence in a foster care or group home and also possessed an anger management deficit. Nearly two-thirds of all participants had been adjudicated at age 14 or younger, and typically, multiple crimes contributed to the adjudication and eventual incarceration of an individual. Diverse types of crimes were demonstrated by project participants. The most prevalent adjudicated property crimes included (a) theft (36%), (b) criminal mischief (26%), (c) burglary (25%), and (d) unauthorized use of a motor vehicle (21%). Person-to-person crimes involved assault (21%) or sex-related crimes (17%). Additionally, approximately 70% of all participants had not earned a high school completion document, with 21% having earned a GED diploma and 7% having earned a regular high school diploma.

(*text continues on p. 382*)

TABLE 16.1

Demographic and Background Information
on Project SUPPORT Participants ($N = 225$)

Information	n	%
Background		
Age at entry		
Average age at entry is 17.1 years		
Gender		
Male	175	78
Female	50	22
Ethnicity		
Caucasian	164	74
Ethnic minority	57	26
OYA involvement at entry into Project SUPPORT		
Within close custody	162	76
On parole in community	37	17
In OYA camp	13	76
Disability Information		
Disability summary		
Both IDEA/*DSM–IV* diagnosis	111	49
DSM–IV only	98	44
IDEA only	10	4
Missing data	6	3
Types of IDEA disabilities[a]		
Specific learning disability	62	28
Emotional disturbance	36	16
Disorders diagnosed in childhood/adolescence	153	68
Substance related	104	46
Types of *DSM–IV* diagnoses[a]		
Mood-related disorders	61	27
Anxiety-related disorders	41	18
Personality-related disorders	21	9
Adjustment-related disorders	12	5
Impulse-control-related disorders	11	5
Total no. disabilities		
1–2	181	80
3–4	37	16
5–6	1	1
Missing data	6	3
Barriers[b]		
No. barriers per participant		
1–3	7	1
4–6	52	23
7–9	77	34
10–12	58	26
>12	28	12
Five top-ranked barriers[a]		
Substance abuse	180	80

(*continues*)

TABLE 16.1 *Continued.*
Demographic and Background Information
on Project SUPPORT Participants (*N* = 225)

Information	n	%
Barriers (continued)		
Five top-ranked barriers (*continued*)		
Absenteeism/suspension history	178	79
Ran away from home/residential placement	163	72
Anger management deficit	147	65
Previous foster care/group home placement	150	67
Criminal History		
Age at first adjudication		
<12	38	17
12–14	109	48
15–17	68	30
Types of offenses[a]		
Theft crimes	80	36
Criminal mischief	59	26
Burglary	56	25
Unauthorized use of motor vehicle	48	21
Assault	48	21
Sex-related crimes	39	17
Possession of controlled substance	19	8
Education		
Education completion documents		
No completion document	162	72
Document received while in facility	55	24
Document received prior to facility	10	4
No document	162	72
Type of completion document received		
GED	48	21
High school diploma	15	7
Modified diploma	1	1
Type of educational training received while in the facility[a]		
High school diploma coursework	162	72
Social skill/anger management	112	50
GED preparation work	98	44
Basic academic skills training	86	38
Independent living skills training	81	36
Work experience training	65	29
Professional/technical education	143	64
Community college credit	23	10

Note. Percentages have been rounded and may not equal 100%. Missing data are not presented within the summary; therefore, total numbers may not equal total *N*.
OYA = Oregon Youth Authority.

[a] More than one category possible for an individual (e.g., two *DSM–IV* diagnoses); percentages therefore do not equal 100.

[b] Data collected on 22 barriers across the domains of employment, education, residential status, and family/personal. Average number of barriers is 8.6.

SETTING

The service delivery model for Project SUPPORT was initiated by three state agencies: ODE, OYA, and VR. Staff from the UO were hired to provide technical assistance to the agencies and service delivery staff and to develop and manage a data collection system that would evaluate the project's impact on the participants (Benz & Bullis, 1998). At the outset of the planning process, two broad goals were defined by the state agency staff. These goals were to (a) develop a systemwide service delivery model resulting in lower rates of recidivism and more positive rates of employment and education outcomes for incarcerated adolescents with disabilities returning to the community and (b) embed the program model within the existing community and state agencies to maintain support for this targeted population.

Project SUPPORT was funded initially through matching funds from the three state agencies. In the first 2 years of operation, VR was the fiscal agent for the project. ODE took fiscal leadership for the project beginning in the third year. Both state agencies contracted with local education service districts (ESDs) or school districts to provide education services to the state youth correctional facilities in each region and were provided an additional contract to hire Project SUPPORT staff (i.e., a TS). This contract provided needed funds to support the TS position, which is community based and requires extensive amounts of local travel, along with mobile technology (e.g., laptop, a cell phone), to complete the service delivery responsibilities associated with the position. The typical contracted budget for one TS position ranges between $60,000 and $65,000 per year. The contract rate depends on the salary rate for the transition specialist, typically a noncertified staff person (e.g., individual with an associate's degree or with a college degree not in teaching), and on job setting (i.e., in our state, urban school districts tend to pay more than rural districts; transportation costs also vary across regions, depending on the amount of travel required to visit the various youth correctional facilities and maintain contact with youth in the community).

To embed project services within the systemic structures of the three state agencies, a sustainable funding process was developed within existing fiscal structures. The initial startup funds provided by the state agencies offered the opportunity for the development of the collaborative relationships across agencies and project services (e.g., build TS caseloads) to enable the following funding strategy to be implemented.

Once Project SUPPORT was established within each region, the project would use the average daily membership (ADM) generated by the youth served within the project to maintain the TS position. All Oregon public school students generate state school support through ADM monies that follow students to the district in which they are enrolled and support educational services provided to these students. This financial support is available to all students who have not earned a standard diploma and who are (a) less than 19 years of age, or (b) through 21 years of age for a youth receiving IDEA services. Each student enrolled in a public school is allotted 1.0 ADM, which is then forwarded to the student's district of enrollment. Oregon statutes provide higher levels of state educational support through weighted ADM amounts for populations requiring additional instructional or support services. Weighted ADM monies are allowable for the following types of students: (a) special education, (b) English language learners, (c) teen parents, and (d) neglected/delinquent youth status. For example, every student meeting the criteria is allotted 1.0 ADM plus monies attached to whatever funding "weight" to which he or she is eligible. Youth involved in the juvenile justice system have an extremely high incidence of the characteristics that generate these higher-than-average levels of ADM support and thus provide a higher level of monies to the schools than typical students.

These monies, as defined through the weighted ADM formulas, provide educational support for the additional assistance juvenile corrections students, such as Project SUPPORT participants, receive to remain in school or as transition services when leaving public education. Because the TSs are ESD or school district employees and provide transition services to support a youth's educational goals and develop employability skills, their services meet the criteria for project youth to qualify for the state school support. This funding strategy allows for the project to fit within the existing state school funding model, which helps sustain the project across time.

In 1999, four regions, both rural and urban, were selected across the state as pilot sites. A fifth region was added in 2000. Four additional regions were added in the latter half of 2001, achieving geographical statewide coverage. Currently, there are nine TSs in Project SUPPORT who provide transition services to youth with disabilities (the majority of whom have ED or a significant psychiatric disorder) as they leave the youth correctional facilities across all of Oregon. Our plans are to hire four more TSs over the course of the next 4 years and to focus on locales with a high concentration of youth from racial minority groups (Bullis & Unruh, 2002).

PROGRAM FEATURES

Service Components

Project SUPPORT's service delivery components are grounded in (a) prior evidence that demonstrates that engagement in work or school immediately upon release from a youth correctional facility has a protective effect for the youth and (b) service delivery components developed and refined in other model demonstration projects (e.g., Bullis & Fredericks, 2002; Clark & Davis, 2000). Project SUPPORT features the following service delivery components:

- Direct services to each project participant are provided collaboratively and include (a) VR counselor, (b) OYA treatment manager, (c) OYA parole officer, and (d) facility and community education staff. These staff work in concert with a TS, who works directly with the youth and assumes primary responsibility for the youth's transition into school or work placements, as well as the coordination of transition services across agencies. The initial responsibility of the TS is to define the youth's strengths, needs, interests, and life goals to develop a transition plan with services aligned to the unique needs and interests of each project participant. This plan is created in concert with the requirements of the youth's parole plan. To foster close relationships between youth and the TS, caseloads are intentionally kept small ($n = 12$ to 15 per TS). The transition services provided each participant are individualized and based on the TS's ability to make decisions and connections with each youth, weighing information provided by the youth, family, and agency staff. Generally, the TS facilitates or provides services to each youth in the following domains: (a) functional skill assessment, (b) self-determination, (c) competitive job placement, (d) individualized education and support, (e) social skill instruction, and (f) service coordination. Functional skill assessments (i.e., assessments of work, living, and social skills) activities include the review and integration of existing academic and intelligence assessments for each youth. TSs use structured interviews of individual needs and strengths, as well as situational assessments (e.g., trial placement in vocational settings). Environmental assessment methods (e.g., Waintrup & Kelley, 1999) are used to appraise the requirements of the school and work settings in which participants could be placed and to focus accommodations for those placements (e.g., alternate ways to complete jobs, natural supports).

- Self-determination strategies are used to ensure that services are designed around the unique needs, interests, and strengths of each participant. Each youth, his or her PO, treatment manager, and, as appropriate, family members, are involved centrally in planning each youth's transition services. A project transition plan is developed prior to the youth's exit from custody and is based on (a) the interests and needs of the youth and (b) the guidelines prescribed on the youth's parole plan.
- Competitive job placement is central to the activities designed for the youth. Every effort is made to place youth in competitive jobs as quickly as possible after their return to the community. These placements often complement an educational component. The job placements are frequently part time and temporary, allowing youth to experience different types of jobs and develop basic employment skills (e.g., punctuality, following instructions, attendance).
- Individualized educational placement and support are defined by the educational and career goals of each project participant. Because of the project's affiliation with school districts in Oregon, the TS is knowledgeable about access to various local educational options in those programs. If the youth is enrolled in school, the TS facilitates the transfer of the youth's Individualized Education Program (IEP) to the appropriate educational placement.
- Social skills instruction for project participants is completed both informally and formally by the TS on an ongoing basis. Through placements in competitive work settings, project participants will encounter

unfamiliar persons in unfamiliar settings and under unfamiliar rules and expectations. The TSs teach transition-related social skills to support the youth in their employment and educational endeavors.

• Service coordination among the three state agencies and local service providers is critical to the success of the project participant in the community. The TS spends much of the first year of his or her position building systemic relationships with community-based agencies (e.g., vocational rehabilitation, probation and parole, mental health). Major activities of the TS include (a) identifying the necessary services for the individual and assisting the individual to access those services and (b) maintaining regular communication with those social services staff regarding participants.

Project SUPPORT's services are directed to promoting a youth's immediate engagement in school, employment, or both upon parole from custody. Figure 16.1 presents a "typical" participant's path in transitioning from the youth correctional facility to the community. The service delivery model (a) identifies targeted youth prior to parole from OYA (screening and referral); (b) develops a service plan surrounding the youth's interests, needs, and life goals (in-facility activities); (c) facilitates youth access to identified services immediately upon parole from the correctional facility (immediate pre/postrelease activities); and (d) once a youth has stabilized in the community, provides follow-up transition support as events or needs arise (e.g., finding a new apartment, completing taxes, searching for car insurance [postrelease activities]). Services are based on the TS and collaboration between and among (a) treatment managers in the correctional facilities, (b) POs, and (c) community-based education programs.

The in-facility phase is the first phase, in which the project participant begins the development of preemployment skills. These activities focus on the initiation of a positive relationship between the youth and TS. The initial

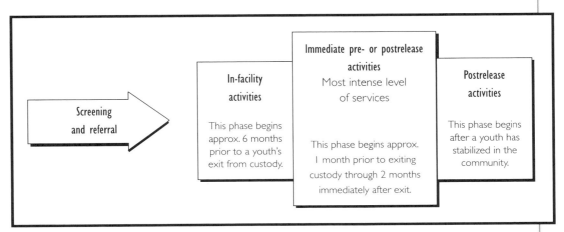

FIGURE 16.1. Phases of Project SUPPORT (Service Utilization to Promote the Positive Rehabilitation and Community Transition of Incarcerated Youth with Emotional Disorders) pattern of services.

responsibility of the TS is to help define the youth's strengths, needs, interests, and life goals and to develop a transition plan aligned with those needs and interests. During this phase, the TS works with OYA facility treatment managers and education providers and community-based POs to develop a project transition plan for the youth. Finally, the TS begins assisting the youth to develop skills to (a) complete accurate job applications, (b) practice job interviews, (c) complete financial aid paperwork to enroll in school, and (d) obtain needed identification cards (e.g., Social Security, a birth certificate).

The second phase of project services is the immediate pre/postrelease phase. Activities in this phase are critical and include the most intense level of services provided to project participants. During this phase, the TS works with the youth's PO to assist in the youth's transition to the community and completing his or her parole plans. While the youth is still in the correctional facility, the TS organizes community-based supports aligned with the youth's transition plan. These supports often include (a) choosing the educational placement for the youth and ensuring the IEP is immediately transferred to the community educational setting, (b) connecting the youth with employment agencies, and (c) making appointments with community service agencies (e.g., mental health, alcohol/drug support).

The final phase of the service delivery model is the ongoing support phase. Once a youth has stabilized in the community and is positively engaged in work or school, the TS focuses on supporting and maintaining the youth's engagement within the community. Through the earlier phases the youth has built a strong relationship with the TS and can request support or ask further questions regarding her or his transition needs in the community as needs arise. Each TS is trained to assess and identify signs of a youth returning to negative behaviors (e.g., drug use, gang activity) associated with previous criminal activity. If these signs occur, the TS and youth, along with the PO, address these issues.

Composite Case Study

The following case study, compiled by TSs of a "typical" Project SUPPORT participant, Eric, provides an example of one young man's experiences in the project. Eric first became involved with the juvenile justice system when he was 13 for being a minor in possession of tobacco. As he aged, he developed a pattern of running away from home and attending and leaving multiple schools; he also began using alcohol and drugs. Eventually, Eric was placed on probation for attempted burglary and criminal mischief. At age 16, he was committed to OYA for stealing a car and carrying a concealed weapon. He admitted to being under the influence of methamphetamine when these offenses occurred. After being incarcerated for about a year, Eric was referred to Project SUPPORT by his PO. At the time of referral to the project, Eric was scheduled to leave custody and transition back to his aunt's home in about 4 months, just prior to his 18th birthday.

After Eric was referred to Project SUPPORT, the TS providing SUP-PORT services in the community where Eric would return talked with him about his career goals and interest in participating in the project. Prior to incarceration, Eric had experienced poor grades coupled with sporadic school attendance. He had been identified for special education services in elementary school but was not on an IEP during the middle or high school years. He had been diagnosed with ADD, and while in OYA he was diagnosed with three *DSM–IV* disorders: (a) polysubstance abuse, (b) dysthymic disorder, and (c) conduct disorder requiring medication. On the basis of these various conditions, he was found eligible for the project and for VR services.

To initiate services, the TS met with Eric to further assess his educational and career interests. Eric shared that it would not be good for him to go back to a traditional high school. He explained that work was often too difficult; his typical pattern was to feel hopeless and then give up. Other educational options he considered included a high school completion program at a local community college or trying to take his GED exam. He also talked about going directly to work and had several ideas about potential employment. He stated that he wanted to pursue a career in a construction trade, possibly as an electrician or installing drywall or roofing. Another interest was playing in a band, because he plays the guitar. Other options included the Job Corps and the military because they would provide opportunities for job training.

Several months prior to his parole, Eric participated in a parole transition screening to help identify educational placement and his mental health needs and to establish his parole agreement. Eric's Project SUPPORT TS, PO, and facility education and treatment staff all participated in this process. Eric's PO identified Eric's aunt's home as where he would live upon returning to the community on parole. The aunt had been involved in his treatment while he was incarcerated and was committed to helping Eric transition back to the community.

The TS researched various community programs, job training programs, and educational programs aligned with his career interests in construction or music. Through several meetings, Eric and the TS narrowed his options to a high school completion program at a local community college close to where he would live. The community college also provided certification programs in the construction trades. The TS and Eric completed the necessary financial aid paperwork to enroll in the construction job training program along with the high school completion program. Eric was paroled to his aunt's house but had to wait 2 weeks for the new term at the community college to begin. During this time, Eric met with a VR counselor, and an employment plan was written. VR paid for items Eric would need for work and school, including (a) a monthly bus pass that would be his only source of transportation and (b) steel-toed boots and a tool belt, which were requirements for the construction program. The TS also helped Eric enroll in the state's health plan, which would ensure that he could continue his medications. As part of his parole agreement, Eric had to follow up his alcohol treatment in the facility by attending community Alcoholics Anonymous (AA) meetings. He and the TS located an AA meeting close to his aunt's house. Eric was unfamiliar with his aunt's community and riding the public transit system. Together, Eric and the TS practiced using the bus route from his aunt's house to his AA meeting and then also to the community college. Eric and the TS also visited the public employment office to introduce him to available job hunt services.

Eric began attending the high school completion program and construction job training program and continued to attend the local AA meetings. The TS checked in with Eric on a regular basis to see how things were going and to talk through problems that may have arisen in school or at the job site. Eric shared that he had met new friends in his construction classes and had started to do things socially with them. At the end of the term, Eric, his VR counselor, and TS met to assess the last quarter and plan the next term. At the meeting, the staff found that Eric had begun to frequently miss his high school coursework and that he had "blown up" a couple of times during a work project and had left class. The class instructor said that he thought Eric was hanging with a group in the class that were using drugs. The TS noted that Eric had begun to check in less frequently and was not interested in meeting with her to catch up on his progress in the community.

The TS was concerned and spoke with Eric's PO about the situation. When they spoke with Eric about these concerns, he at first was defensive. He finally shared that the school coursework was very hard for him, but he really did enjoy the construction program. At this point, Eric broke down and shared that he had been using drugs again and that his angry outbursts were because he was using again and that he had gone off his medications. The PO ordered that Eric begin attending a community-based drug treatment center. The group discussed investigating Youthbuild, a program in which youth attend school and get paid for learning the construction trade by the companies whose products are built in the program. An appointment was made for the next day for Eric and the TS to visit the program and enroll, if he was interested. Eric did not make it to the appointment, and when the TS called his house, his aunt shared that he had not come home the previous night. Eric disappeared for 3 weeks and then returned to his aunt's house and made contact again with the TS and PO. At that time, the PO decided to place Eric in a local residential drug treatment center. Eric understood that if he did not make progress in treatment, he would be incarcerated for a parole violation.

After 90 days, Eric was released from the drug treatment facility and returned to his aunt's house. Eric continued to attend the construction program and maintained his drug treatment aftercare appointments. He found a part-time job in the evenings doing construction cleanup work and began saving money from his earnings from his school program to get an apartment with a friend he had met in the program. Six months later, Eric continued to check in with his PO and TS. His urine analysis tested clean and his parole was terminated because he had met all his parole agreement terms. He graduated from Youthbuild a couple of months later and began searching for full-time employment. He used the public employment office and his VR counselor for job tips. Eric and the TS visited the HUD housing office to apply for low-income housing and also checked out some thrift stores for furniture and basic kitchen items for his future apartment. The TS and Eric completed his first tax return papers together.

After graduating, Eric was hired full time with benefits at a local construction company. With his second paycheck he was able to make a deposit and together with a friend move into an apartment that was located through the housing program. Eric only checked in with his TS on occasion, and they agreed that he did not need any further transition services, so he exited successfully from the project.

EVALUATION

Evaluation Procedures

One unique aspect of Project SUPPORT is that it includes a strong and ongoing evaluation component. Data collection activities are fully integrated into the TSs' service delivery activities, and a regular review of project results by the project managers informs and guides systemic, policy-related decisions. Staff from the University of Oregon's Institute on Violence and Destructive Behavior were contracted to develop these procedures, supervise data collection, manage the project's database, and produce regular reports on the project's impact. Both process and participant outcome evaluation strategies have been used throughout the development and implementation of Project SUPPORT.

The process evaluation consisted of multiple activities to assess the fidelity of project implementation, along with needed information to adjust project services to meet the needs of the project participants. First, a comprehensive needs assessment was completed in each region. Multiple stakeholder groups for the needs assessment included (a) parole youth with disabilities; (b) parents, foster parents, or residential care providers; (c) POs; (d) facility education providers; (e) facility treatment managers; (f) community education providers; and (g) community agency members (e.g., VR, mental health, alcohol and other drug treatment). The needs assessment was completed in a community forum of stakeholder participants using a group processing procedure (nominal group technique) defining both existing supports and barriers present within the communities of project implementation. Youth with disabilities who had exited custody but who had reoffended also were interviewed for their perspective on barriers in the community and what might support them effectively when they are released from custody again. Findings from this needs assessment were useful in developing and implementing a "tailored" service delivery model that addressed the specific needs of each community.

Second, ongoing stakeholder surveys were completed to assess both project fidelity and the collaborative development process of the project. A theme of needing to develop communication and collaboration strategies across agencies was identified as a barrier in the needs assessment, and strategies to circumvent this barrier were measured. Third, evaluation surveys were conducted of all training sessions and training materials created for the project.

This information was used to develop and refine additional project training needs and also to ensure that training procedures and products were sufficiently detailed for replication purposes.

The project's "process" evaluation focuses on the transition outcomes achieved by the project participants. Participant outcome data are collected to (a) assist in the development of a service delivery model that addresses the needs of project participants and (b) monitor whether participants are being engaged in education, employment, and community support services. A data collection process and management information system (MIS) were developed. TSs were trained in data collection procedures and were responsible for completing the data collection forms. The entry form (completed when each youth enters the project) collects extensive personal, educational, social, and family data on project participants, along with baseline measures on the key outcomes. This information provides an introduction to an individual participant's barriers to transition and also an aggregate "snapshot" of project participants. The update form is completed on every participant every 2 months while the youth is actively involved in the project. This form collects information on the key outcome measures. The information is summarized to demonstrate the sample's rates on key outcomes at 2-month intervals after participants are paroled to the community. The exit form is completed once a youth has completed his or her transition plan goals and collects information on key outcome measures. A follow-up form is completed every 3 months for a total of 2 years after a youth leaves the project to document the long-term impact of project services on each individual's community adjustment.

Key outcome measures examined in the project across the data collection instruments were identified from the three transition outcome constructs identified in the IDEA: education, employment, and personal/social experiences. We also examined a fourth—and more global—outcome construct: engagement. DeStefano and Wagner (1992) stated that many young adults may be involved in a number of activities and not fully integrated into a lifelong vocation, suggesting that a more accurate index of success in the community can be reached by examining young adults' involvement in school and work. We developed an outcome index called "engagement" (engaged = *competitively employed full time* or *enrolled in a school program full time,* or *working part time and going to school part time* and *not arrested or institutionalized*). Engagement rates are summarized at the 2-, 4-, and 6-month intervals to understand the rates of engagement of youth immediately upon their exit from custody in the youth correctional facility. These data assist the state managers and project staff in determining if project activities are focused toward project goals of maintaining a youth's positive engagement in employment and educational enrollment in the community.

Participant Outcomes

Key outcomes measures on the rates of (a) overall engagement, (b) educational enrollment, (c) employment, and (d) recidivism are monitored as part of the ongoing process evaluation and are presented in Table 16.2. Measures are collected at 2-, 4-, and 6-month intervals after a youth exits custody. Overall engagement (employed or enrolled and not incarcerated) at 2 months after exit was demonstrated by 63% of all project participants in the community. This overall engagement rate remained consistent at both 4 and 6 months, with 68% engaged at 4 months and 61% at 6 months. We also examined individual engagement rates of both employment and enrollment in a school/training program. Of those participants in the community, approximately 50% were employed in some type of paid employment. Enrollment in school was lower, at 32% at 2 months, 26.6% at 4 months, and 17.9% at 6 months. Of the employed youth, almost 31% were earning $7.50 per hour or more and about 40% were working 35 hours a week or more. Project services focus on connecting youth with various employment supports. Various work-related services were accessed by participants: (a) Approximately 47% of project participants were involved in VR services, (b) nearly 25% of participants visited the public employment office for services, and (c) 13% used the Workforce Investment Act (WIA) agencies.

TABLE 16.2

Engagement Outcomes in the Community

Outcome	2 Months (n = 117)		4 Months (n = 79)		6 Months (n = 56)	
	n	%	n	%	n	%
Enrolled and/or employed and not reincarcerated[a]	74	63.2	54	68.4	34	60.7
Education engagement status in community: enrolled and not reincarcerated[a]	37	31.6	21	26.6	10	17.9
Employment engagement status in community: employed and not reincarcerated[a]	56	47.9	42	53.2	28	50.0
Returned to custody (adult/juvenile)	2	1.7	5	6.3	5	8.9
Services used in community[a]						
VR	54	47.0	41	55.4	22	43.1
Mental health services	25	21.7	19	25.7	14	27.5
Alcohol and other drug services	41	35.7	27	36.5	16	31.4
Welfare	2	1.7	3	4.1	2	3.9
Social Security Administration	7	6.1	3	4.1	1	2.0
Public employment office	27	23.5	16	21.6	8	15.7
WIA/JTPA/One-Stop	15	13.0	13	17.6	5	9.8

Note. Percentages have been rounded and may not equal 100%. Missing data are not presented within the summary; therefore, total numbers may not equal total *N*. This information summarizes only those youth who are *actively* involved within Project SUPPORT. These percentages do not capture the youth who exited successfully/unsuccessfully from the project. This information provides a snapshot of project services. These data indicate that program services are focused on program goals such as (a) remaining in community, (b) education status, (c) employment status, and (d) services utilized in community. VR = Oregon Office of Vocational Services; WIA = Workforce Investment Act; JTPA = Job Training and Partnership Act.

[a] Data summarized only for youth who have entered the community during the pattern of services.

Support services used in the community by participants were also examined to understand whether these services were aligned with primary barriers associated with mental illness and substance abuse—two barriers identified at entry into the project. Alcohol and other drug treatment services were used by more than 35% of all participants within 2 months of their exit from the youth correction facility. This rate was maintained at 4 months and slightly declined (31.4%) at 6 months. The use of mental health services was maintained across time at a rate between 22% and 28% of use by project participants during the first 6 months in the community.

Table 16.3 presents information on participants who have exited the project. Exit criteria for the project are defined as (a) being positively engaged in either school or a job that is related to the youth's overall career goal for at least 90 days and (b) exhibiting no need for further transition support (e.g., independent living skill development, etc.). On the basis of these exit criteria, 29 (26%) project participants out of 112 total exits have exited successfully.

TABLE 16.3
General Exit Information

		n	%
Reason for exit	Closed successfully	29	26
	Moved/unable to contact	22	20
	Ran away	18	16
	Lack of follow-through	13	12
	Charged with adult crime	12	11
	Other	10	9
	Participant declined further services	8	7
Hourly wage at exit	<$6.50/hour	0	0
	$6.50 to $7.49	14	52
	$7.50 to $8.49	3	11
	$8.50 to $9.49	2	7
	>$9.50/hour	5	19
Hours worked per week at exit	<10 hours/week	1	4
	10–20 hours/week	3	11
	21–34 hours/week	4	15
	>35 hours/week	15	56
Living status at exit	With parents/family	40	36
	On the run	16	14
	OYA corrections	8	7
	Homeless	6	5
	Adult corrections	10	9
	With roommates	5	7
	Alone	6	5
	Residential treatment facility	2	2
	With spouse/partner	2	2
	Foster care	2	2

Note. Percentages have been rounded and may not equal 100%. Missing data are not presented within the summary; therefore, total numbers may not equal total N. N = 112. OYA = Oregon Youth Authority.

Other reasons for exiting the program have included (a) moved/unable to contact (20%), (b) did not follow through (12%), (c) ran away (16%); (d) declined further services (7%), and (e) charged with adult crime (11%). Of youth who exited successfully, 37% earned more than $7.50 per hour and 71% worked between 21 and 40 hours per week.

SYNTHESIS

Service Delivery and Participant Outcomes

In this first review of the participant outcome results, Project SUPPORT is assisting youth with ED to achieve positive transition outcomes related to employment and education. It must be remembered that no comparison group or control group was used to provide a standard comparison against which to compare Project SUPPORT participants. Currently, the OYA is in the process of negotiating with other state agencies to access long-term employment, adult corrections, and education data to provide a comparison group with Project SUPPORT participants over a further extended time period.

To date, it is evident that project services have been focused on assisting incarcerated youth with ED to become engaged in the productive endeavors of employment and school. Review of the participant outcomes demonstrates that the overall engagement rates (63%), specifically, the competitive employment rates, are in alignment with project activities focusing on engaging the youth in employment opportunities. Transition specialists have been trained to support the youth in becoming competitively employed immediately upon exit from the youth correction facility. This employment focus is critical for youth who are returning to the community at the age of 18 to further support their transition goals of working toward living independently. Education and employment engagement may also serve as protective factors that help a youth maintain his or her status in the community without returning to juvenile custody or being sentenced to adult corrections (Bullis et al., 2002).

One area of concern noted is the low incidence of involvement with alcohol and drug services and mental health services (approximately 25% and 35%, respectively). These rates are disturbingly low, considering that 95% of these youth have a mental health diagnosis. Evaluation strategies are currently being designed to help determine if these low engagement rates in mental health and alcohol and other drug services are indicative of (a) the target population, (b) a systemic barrier causing lack of access by these youth to local community services, or (most likely) (c) a combination of both. These findings will help provide a springboard for the project's state managers to adjust the service delivery model to increase the engagement rates of these two services—mental health support and drug treatment—to project participants. Examining this process will shed light on (a) the reasons for this nonengagement in these support services and (b) whether, if these support services were accessed, such involvement would have a positive impact on increasing the overall employment and educational engagement rates.

The results from the TRACS study provide a comparison standard by which to judge the effect of the project's services. We should note, however, that only 73% of the TRACS participants had a special education or *DSM–IV* disability, whereas all of the youth in Project SUPPORT have such a condition. Moreover, in TRACS, youth with disabilities fared far more poorly than youth without disabilities in terms of their community engagement. In TRACS, only 46.7% of the respondents were engaged 6 months after exiting the youth correctional facility. The Project SUPPORT engagement rate was higher, at 61% at 6 months after leaving custody. This increase in engagement is notable—especially in light of the disability differences between the two groups—and offers evidence that Project SUPPORT services do provide positive assistance to youth with ED as they leave the juvenile correctional system and return to the community.

Through Project SUPPORT services, youth are demonstrating positive engagement in school and employment. Also, for *each* youth not returned to a youth correctional facility, a savings of approximately $51,000 per year in reincarceration costs is achieved. This cost of incarceration far exceeds the expense of one transition specialist (approximately $60,000–$65,000) who works with approximately 30 to 35 youth per year to maintain the youths' community status. Moreover, this comparative cost saving does not take into account the long-term cost benefits regarding the potential to positively affect the life course of this high-risk population and the overall increase in public safety while reducing victim, restitution, and court costs.

Implementation Process

Although the focus of this chapter was not the description of the implementation process for the multistate agency collaboration of Project SUPPORT, several aspects of this process deserve mention. We must admit that neither (a) developing a collaborative multistate agency project nor (b) providing services to this very-high-risk population was easy, and neither happened without major setbacks. It is an *extremely* arduous and time-consuming process to develop a program implemented across multiple state agencies. The challenges we faced included (a) sharing youth information across multiple agencies; (b) defining roles of the TS and the local agency staff (e.g., PO, treatment manager, and community agency staff); (c) combining vocabularies of three state agencies; and (d) developing a knowledge base within each agency of Project SUPPORT. As we met, a collaborative network slowly developed as each region began to gain experience in the nuances of service delivery at systemic and individual service delivery levels. State-level strategies were developed to encourage this process, but it typically was the individual experiences of the TS, PO, and treatment managers working collaboratively to support the transition of a project participant that really provided a clear understanding and support of the project by the agency staff.

It also must be recognized that adjudicated youth with ED constitute a *very*-high-risk population and often demonstrate dismal transition outcomes.

For TSs who become involved with the lives of these individuals, it is often frustrating to watch amazing progress made by a youth with whom they have worked closely and then—seemingly without warning—one incident may cause the youth to lose his or her job, run from a residential placement, or even return to a correctional setting. Additionally, to support a youth's involvement within an employment or educational setting requires a whole host of other activities for many youth to succeed in those targeted placements. For example, TSs often find themselves helping a youth navigate the health-care system to ensure that the youth can remain on her or his medications, find housing, shop for interview clothes, figure out the transit system to get to work on time, file tax returns, or attend their first local Alcoholics Anonymous meeting.

Undoubtedly, the keystones of this project are the painstaking collaborative process developed across agencies and the relationship fostered between the TS and the youth. This relationship is key but expensive to maintain, considering the small caseloads ($n = 12$–15 participants per TS) that Project SUPPORT maintains. The relative expense of this collaborative project, however, is placed into perspective when we consider the cost of incarcerating a youth for 1 year: approximately $51,000—and this figure does not include the court and victim costs for a youth's continued involvement within the justice system. The cost of the project is further put into perspective when we consider the long-term positive contributions that can be made by these high-risk youth *if* they are assisted to access and gain their employment and education goals. We are optimistic that the project has potential and that positive outcomes will continue to be realized as Project SUPPORT continues. It is our hope that Project SUPPORT will prompt the development of similar projects to facilitate transition for adjudicated youth with ED.

AUTHORS' NOTE

We want to thank all transition specialists, vocational rehabilitation counselors, parole officers, and youth correctional facility education and treatment staff who helped to start Project SUPPORT. Special thanks for their endless collaborative assistance and encouragement they extended to the youth participating in the project in their transition into the community.

REFERENCES

Altschuler, D. M., & Armstrong, T. L. (2001). Intensive aftercare for the high-risk juvenile parolee: Issues and approaches in reintegration and community supervision. In T. L. Armstrong (Ed.), *Intensive interventions with high-risk youths: Promising approaches in juvenile probation and parole* (pp. 45–84). Monsey, NY: Criminal Justice Press.

Ambrose, D., & Lester, D. (1988). Recidivism in juvenile offenders: Effects of education and length of stay. *Psychological Reports, 63,* 778.

American Psychiatric Association. (1994). *Diagnostic and statistical manual of mental disorders* (4th ed). Washington, DC: Author.

Benz, M. (2000). *Youth Transition Project decade report: 1990–2000.* Eugene: University of Oregon, Institute on the Development of Educational Achievement.

Benz, M., & Bullis, M. (1998). *Technical assistance and evaluation of facility-to-community transition programs for incarcerated youth.* (State contract to the Institute on the Development of Educational Achievement, University of Oregon, from the Oregon Division of Vocational Rehabilitation)

Benz, M., Lindstrom, L., & Latta, T. (1999). Improving collaboration between schools and vocational rehabilitation: The Youth Transition Program model. *Journal of Vocational Rehabilitation, 13,* 55–63.

Black, T., Brush, M., Grow, T., Hawes, J., Henry, D., & Hinkle, R. (1996). Natural bridge transition program follow-up study. *Journal of Correctional Education, 47,* 4–12.

Blackorby, J., Edgar, E., & Kortering, L. (1991). A third of our youth? A look at the problem of high school dropout among students with mild handicaps. *The Journal of Special Education, 25,* 102–113.

Brier, N. (1994). Targeted treatment for adjudicated youth with learning disabilities: Effects on recidivism. *Journal of Learning Disabilities, 27,* 215–222.

Bullis, M., & Cheney, D. (1999). Vocational and transition interventions for adolescents and young adults with emotional or behavioral disorders. *Focus on Exceptional Children, 31*(7), 1–24.

Bullis, M., & Fredericks, H. D. (Eds.). (2002). *Providing effective vocational/transition services to adolescents with emotional and behavioral disorders.* Champaign-Urbana, IL: Research Press.

Bullis, M., Fredericks, H. D., Lehman, C., Paris, K., Corbitt, J., & Johnson, B. (1994). Description and evaluation of the Job Designs program for adolescents with emotional or behavioral disorders. *Behavioral Disorders, 19,* 254–268.

Bullis, M., Moran, T., Todis, B., Benz, M., & Johnson, M. (2002). Description and evaluation of the ARIES project: Achieving rehabilitation, individualized education, and employment success for adolescents with emotional disturbance. *Career Development for Exceptional Individuals, 25,* 41–58.

Bullis, M., & Unruh, D. (2002). *Project SUPPORT: Service utilization to promote positive outcomes in the community-based rehabilitation and transition of youth with disabilities on parole.* Funded grant proposal to the Institute on Violence and Destructive Behavior, University of Oregon, from the Office of Special Education Programs, Model Demonstration Projects to Support Quality Educational and Transition Programs in the Justice System for Youth with Disabilities.

Bullis, M., & Yovanoff, P. (in press). The importance of getting started right: Examination of the community engagement of formerly incarcerated youth. Manuscript submitted for publication, *The Journal of Special Education.*

Bullis, M., Yovanoff, P., Mueller, G., & Havel, E. (2002). Life on the "outs"—Examination of the facility-to-community transition of incarcerated adolescents. *Exceptional Children, 69,* 7–22.

Clark, H. B. (1998). *Transition to independence process: TIP operations manual.* Tampa: University of South Florida, Florida Mental Health Institute.

Clark, H. B., & Davis, M. (Eds.). (2000). *Transition to adulthood: A resource for assisting young people with emotional or behavioral difficulties.* Baltimore: Brookes.

D'Amico, R., & Blackorby, J. (1992). Trends in employment among out-of-school youth with disabilities. In M. Wagner, R. D'Amico, C. Marder, L. Newman, &

J. Blackorby (Eds.), *What happens next? Trends in postschool outcomes of youth with disabilities* (pp. 4.1–4.47). Menlo Park, CA: SRI International.

DeStefano, L., & Wagner, M. (1992). Outcome assessment in special education: What lessons have we learned? In F. Rusch, L. DeStefano, J. Chadsey-Rusch, L. Phelps, & E. Szymanski (Eds.), *Transition from school to adult life* (pp. 173–207). Sycamore, IL: Sycamore.

Dryfoos, J. (1990) *Adolescents at risk.* New York: Oxford University Press.

Ensminger, M., & Juon, H. (1998). Transition to adulthood among high-risk youth. In R. Jessor (Ed.), *New perspectives on adolescent risk behavior* (pp. 365–391). Cambridge, England: Cambridge University Press.

Foley, R. (2001). Academic characteristics of incarcerated youth and correctional education programs: A literature review. *Journal of Emotional and Behavioral Disorders, 9,* 248–259.

Gallagher, C. A. (1999, March). Juvenile offenders in residential placement, 1997. *OJJDP Fact Sheet.* Washington, DC: U.S. Department of Justice, Office of Juvenile Delinquency Prevention.

Lipsey, M. W., & Wilson, D. B. (1998). Effective intervention for serious juvenile offenders: A synthesis of research. In R. Loeber & D. P. Farrington (Eds.), *Serious and violent juvenile offenders* (pp. 313–345). Thousand Oaks, CA: Sage.

Marder, C. (1992). *Secondary students classified as seriously emotionally disturbed: How are they being served?* Menlo Park, CA: SRI International.

Marder, C., Wechsler, M., & Valdes, K. (1993). *Services for youth with disabilities after secondary school.* Menlo Park, CA: SRI International.

McCord, J. (1992). The Cambridge-Somerville Study: A pioneering longitudinal-experimental study of delinquency prevention. In J. McCord & R. Tremblay (Eds.), *Preventing antisocial behavior* (pp. 196–208). New York: Guilford Press.

Robins, L. (1966). *Deviant children grown up.* Baltimore: Williams & Wilkens.

Robins, L. (1978). Sturdy childhood predictors of adult antisocial behavior: Replications from longitudinal studies. *Psychological Medicine, 8,* 611–622.

Todis, B., Bullis, M., D'Ambrosio, R., Schultz, R., & Waintrup, M. (2001). Overcoming the odds: Qualitative examination of resilience among adolescents with antisocial behaviors. *Exceptional Children, 68,* 119–139.

Valdes, K., Williamson, C., & Wagner, M. (1990). *The National Longitudinal Transition Study of special education students—Statistical almanac (Vol. 3): Youth categorized as emotionally disturbed.* Menlo Park, CA: SRI International.

Wagner, M. (1991). *The benefits associated with secondary vocational education for young people with disabilities.* Menlo Park, CA: SRI International.

Wagner, M. (1992). Analytic overview: NLTS design and longitudinal analysis approach. In M. Wagner, R. D'Amico, C. Marder, L. Newman, & J. Blackorby (Eds.), *Trends in postschool outcomes of youth with disabilities* (pp. 2-1–2-14). Menlo Park, CA: SRI International.

Wagner, M., & Shaver, D. (1989). *Educational programs and achievements of secondary special education students: Findings from the National Longitudinal Transition Study.* Menlo Park, CA: SRI International.

Waintrup, M., & Kelley, P. (1999). Environmental assessment. In M. Bullis & C. Davis (Eds.), *Functional assessment in transition and rehabilitation for adolescents and adults with learning disorders* (pp. 47–66). Austin, TX: PRO-ED.

Wolfgang, M., Thornberry, T., & Figilo, R. (1987). *From boy to man, from delinquency to crime.* Chicago: University of Chicago Press.

Outcomes for Experimental and Quasi-Experimental Studies

Multisystemic Therapy with Youth Exhibiting Significant Psychiatric Impairment

CHAPTER 17

Melisa D. Rowland, Colleen A. Halliday-Boykins, and Sonja K. Schoenwald

O riginally developed to address serious antisocial behavior in juvenile offenders (Henggeler & Borduin, 1990; Henggeler et al., 1986), multisystemic therapy (MST) is an intensive home- and community-based intervention grounded in social ecological theories of behavior (Bronfenbrenner, 1979). MST interventions are designed to target the known determinants (Elliott, Huizinga, & Ageton, 1985; Loeber & Farrington, 1998) of youth antisocial behavior in the natural ecology. Substantial evidence supports the effectiveness of MST for delinquent youth. Three randomized trials established the short- and long-term effectiveness of MST in reducing youth antisocial behavior, arrests, and incarceration (Borduin et al., 1995; Henggeler, Melton, Brondino, Scherer, & Hanley, 1997; Henggeler, Melton, & Smith, 1992; Henggeler, Melton, Smith, Schoenwald, & Hanley, 1993). Since then, several studies of the effects of MST on youth antisocial behavior have been conducted by independent researchers (Leschied & Cunningham, 2001; Satin, 2000). Central to MST-related research, the Family Services Research Center (FSRC) at the Medical University of South Carolina (Scott Henggeler, director) has been conducting federally funded programmatic research on MST and other community-based interventions since 1992. The foci of current projects within the FSRC are the transportability and dissemination of empirically validated treatments, including—but not limited to—MST, and modifications of MST for populations of youth presenting other serious problems. Subsumed under the latter category are randomized trials of MST modified to treat youth with (a) delinquency and substance use disorders (SUDs) (Randall, Henggeler, Cunningham, Rowland, & Swenson, 2001), (b) insulin-dependent diabetes complicated by poor medication compliance (Ellis, Naar-King, Frey, Rowland, & Gregor, 2003), (c) abusive and neglectful families (Kolko & Swenson, 2002), (d) sexual offending behaviors (Swenson, Henggeler, Schoenwald, Kaufman, & Randall, 1998), and (e) serious mental health problems (Henggeler, Schoenwald, Rowland, & Cunningham, 2002).

OVERVIEW OF MST

Basic Contours of the Treatment Model

Grounded in social–ecological (Bronfenbrenner, 1979) and systems (Haley, 1976; Minuchin, 1974) theory, MST is broadly specified by nine treatment principles (see Table 17.1). These principles serve as anchors for the design and implementation of MST interventions, MST supervision, and the quality assurance mechanisms designed to support clinician fidelity to the model. Using these principles, MST therapists strive to empower caregivers to address the challenges of parenting teenagers engaged in delinquent behavior and to empower the youth to function more adaptively in family, school, peer, and community contexts. The intervention strategies used by MST therapists are evidence based and include cognitive–behavioral, behavioral, functional, and behavioral family systems, as well as pharmacological interventions. Importantly, these interventions are integrated into a comprehensive social–ecological understanding of the youth and his or her family context and individualized to the strengths and weaknesses in that context. In contrast with "combined" (Kazdin, 1996) and multicomponent approaches to treatment

TABLE 17.1
Multisystemic Therapy Treatment Principles

Principle 1: The primary purpose of assessment is to understand the fit between the identified problems and their broader systemic context.

Principle 2: Therapeutic contacts should emphasize the positive and should use systemic strengths as levers for change.

Principle 3: Interventions should be designed to promote responsible behavior and decrease irresponsible behavior among family members.

Principle 4: Interventions should be present focused and action oriented, targeting specific and well-defined problems.

Principle 5: Interventions should target sequences of behavior within and between multiple systems that maintain the identified problems.

Principle 6: Interventions should be developmentally appropriate and fit the developmental needs of the youth.

Principle 7: Interventions should be designed to require daily or weekly effort by family members.

Principle 8: Intervention efficacy is evaluated continuously from multiple perspectives, with providers assuming accountability for overcoming barriers to successful outcomes.

Principle 9: Interventions should be designed to promote treatment generalization and long-term maintenance of therapeutic change by empowering caregivers to address family members' needs across multiple system contexts.

Note. From *Serious Emotional Disturbance in Children and Adolescents: Multisystemic Therapy,* by S. W. Henggeler, S. K. Schoenwald, M. D. Rowland, and P. B. Cunningham, 2002, New York: Guilford. Copyright 2002 by Guilford Press. Reprinted with permission.

(Liddle, 1996), MST interventions are not delivered as separate elements. Instead, they are strategically selected and integrated in ways intended to maximize the benefits of synergistic interaction for a particular youth and family (Henggeler, Schoenwald, Borduin, Rowland, & Cunningham, 1998).

Implementation of MST with Juvenile Offenders

Master's-level therapists using a home-based model of service delivery implement MST. Advantages of the home-based model of service delivery include the removal of barriers to service access (i.e., transportation, childcare, conflicts with work schedule) and increased ecological validity of the assessment and intervention process. MST teams typically consist of four therapists, each of whom works with four to six families at a time. Treatment is intense, averaging approximately 60 hours of direct (i.e., face-to-face) and substantial indirect (i.e., telephone, collateral) contact over a 3- to 5-month period (Henggeler, Mihalic, Rone, Thomas, & Timmons-Mitchell, 1998). The number and duration of sessions is functionally driven; that is, sessions occur as often as needed to ensure the youth and family are able to make concrete progress toward the achievement of desired treatment goals. Thus, the frequency of sessions generally decreases over time but may increase temporarily in response to problems with an ineffective intervention or the emergence of predictable or unpredictable crises. An experienced, preferably doctoral-level, mental health professional trained in MST and in MST supervision procedures supervises each team. MST supervisors are an active and integral part of the treatment team, providing weekly group supervision, field-based assistance, and ongoing promotion of therapist skill development. MST supervisors are, in turn, supported by MST consultants. These consultants are doctoral-level clinicians who work with therapists, supervisors, and administrators to facilitate adherence to the treatment model at all levels of the organization in which the treatment team is embedded. Most MST consultants are housed in a university-affiliated training organization (MST Services, Limited Liability Corporation) and provide weekly team and supervisor consultation, as well as the 5-day initial training, quarterly booster training, and ongoing assistance with implementation difficulties that may arise across or within systems.

DATA SUPPORTING THE EFFECTIVENESS OF MST WITH SERIOUS ANTISOCIAL BEHAVIOR IN YOUTH

The first controlled study of MST with juvenile offenders was published in 1986 (Henggeler et al., 1986). Compared to youth in the control condition, youth who received MST evidenced significant decreases in conduct problems, association with delinquent peers, and individual psychopathology, and their families experienced significant improvement in functioning. Subsequently, two federally funded trials (Henggeler et al., 1992; Henggeler, Melton, et al., 1997) evaluated the effectiveness of MST with chronic and violent juvenile offenders served by therapists based in community mental health centers. Simultaneously, a university-based trial with chronic juvenile offenders was conducted (Borduin et al., 1995). Across these three projects, more than 400 youth and families were randomly assigned to treatment conditions and evaluated 1.7 to 4 years following treatment. To summarize results from these studies, youth and families who received MST demonstrated (a) 25% to 70% reductions in long-term rates of rearrest, (b) 47% to 64% reductions in out-of-home placements, (c) extensive improvements in family functioning, and (d) decreased adolescent mental health problems. Collectively, more than 50% of the youth evaluated in these studies were African American, and a majority reported low socioeconomic status. Importantly, the effects of MST were not moderated by youth ethnicity (African American vs. Caucasian), age, or socioeconomic status (Henggeler, Mihalic, et al., 1998).

As a result of the documented clinical effectiveness and cost savings associated with MST (Washington Institute for Public Policy, 1998), numerous state agencies and service provider organizations sought to establish MST programs in their communities. Currently, 200 sites in 36 states and 7 countries are implementing MST with delinquent youth. MST Services (http:www.mstservices.com) is a university-affiliated organization that serves as headquarters for this dissemination process. Forty-one of these programs are participating in a federally funded study of the workforce, organizational, and extra-organizational factors associated with adherence to MST and child outcomes in diverse communities (Schoenwald, Sheidow, & Letourneau, 2004; Schoenwald, Sheidow, Letourneau, & Liao, 2003).

The establishment of MST programs in numerous communities within North America and Europe has increased consumer, provider, researcher, and policymaker interest in delivering this treatment to other populations of youth. The remainder of this chapter focuses on completed and current efforts to evaluate the appropriateness and effectiveness of MST for youth at risk of out-of-home placement due primarily to psychiatric impairment.

ADAPTING MST FOR YOUTH WITH SERIOUS PSYCHIATRIC IMPAIRMENT

The modification of MST for youth demonstrating significant psychiatric impairment was prompted primarily by the system-of-care movement, health-care finance reform, the lack of data to support the effectiveness of psychiatric hospitalization, and MST's strong track record in treating serious juvenile offenders. In 1995, the National Institute of Mental Health (NIMH) funded a randomized trial comparing MST and psychiatric hospitalization for youth in psychiatric crises (Henggeler et al., 1999). The remainder of this chapter describes lessons learned during the process of adapting and implementing MST with these youth and families and discusses research directions inspired by those lessons.

Rationale for Additions and Adaptations

In contrast with the extensive multivariate longitudinal research that documents the multidetermined nature of adolescent antisocial behavior and substance abuse (neighborhood, peer, school, family, and individual determinants; see, e.g., Elliott et al., 1985; Loeber & Farrington, 1998), research on the correlates and predictors of child psychiatric disorders has traditionally focused on individual cognitive and biological factors. Evidence that contextual factors contribute to the development and maintenance of a diverse array of mental health problems in children has been accruing for the last decade, however. Recent research on internalizing conditions, such as depression (Birmaher et al., 1996), suicidal behavior (Wagner, 1997), anxiety and post-traumatic stress disorder (Saigh, Yasik, Sack, & Koplewicz, 1999), and on disorders with an externalizing component, such as attention-deficit/hyperactivity disorder (ADHD; Barkley, 1998) and bipolar affective disorder (American Academy of Child and Adolescent Psychiatry, 1997; Geller et al., 2002), suggests the salience of various caregiver, family, peer, and school factors in predicting and sustaining mental health problems in youth. The documented pertinence of such contextual factors is consistent with the social–ecological theoretical framework and comprehensive focus of MST. At the same time, the literature suggests that several characteristics might distinguish youth with psychiatric impairments and their families from youth referred primarily for serious antisocial behavior and their families. Specifically, youth referred for stabilization of psychiatric crises are expected to show a greater prevalence of depression, anxiety, and other internalizing problems; they are more often girls and younger children; and their parents show a prevalence of psychiatric disorders relative to youth referred primarily for externalizing and serious antisocial behavior problems. Thus, MST treatment principles, the rules governing the assessment and intervention process, the integration of empirically tested treatment techniques, and the MST social–ecological framework were retained, but several aspects of the model were modified to anticipate the needs of youth referred for psychiatric hospitalization and their families.

Modifications of MST

Adapting MST to serve youth experiencing significant psychiatric impairment was a dynamic process that was especially intensive during the earliest phase of the study of MST as an alternative to psychiatric hospitalization (Henggeler, Rowland, et al., 1997); the adaptation process continued throughout the 4 years of project implementation. The modifications can be broadly categorized as administrative or clinical and are summarized in Table 17.2 (see Henggeler et al., 2002, for more detail).

Administrative Adaptations and Additions

Psychiatrists were formally incorporated into the delivery of MST for the first time in the hospitalization study. A child psychiatrist with substantial MST clinical experience served as the MST supervisor for the team. Another child psychiatrist (25% effort) and an adult psychiatrist (10% effort) helped to ensure the delivery and management of appropriate psychiatric services for

TABLE 17.2

Modifications of Multisystemic Therapy (MST) for Youth with Serious Emotional Disturbance

Type	Traditional MST	Modified MST
Administrative Modifications		
Psychiatrists	Consulted as needed	Integrated into team clinical structure
Crisis caseworkers	None required	Two per team of 4 therapists, provide crisis intervention and case management
Supervisory-level time for systems intervention	Varies, approximately 5–10 hours/week	Approximately 15–20 hours/week
Therapist education	Master's level preferred	Master's level required
Respite resources	None required	Access to array of MST respite placements, such as shelter, foster care, and inpatient, required
Supervision frequency	One group supervision a week One group consultation a week	Two group supervisions a week One group consultation a week
Caseload	4–5 families per therapist	3–4 families per therapist
Treatment fidelity	Therapist adherence measure—one per family monthly	Therapist adherence measure—one per family monthly Therapist audiotaped adherence measure—one per therapist weekly
Clinical Modifications		
Training	5-day initial MST training Quarterly booster training Supervisor training	5-day initial MST training Quarterly booster training Supervisor training Crisis intervention training Community reinforcement approach training for adult and youth substance use disorders Psychopharmacologic and psychotherapeutic training to enhance treatment of attention-deficit/hyperactivity disorder and internalizing disorders Evidence-based skill training techniques for working with borderline personality disorder

MST youth. The day-to-day psychiatric care of youth and their family members was carried out by university-based physicians training in a psychiatry residency program and supervised by the team supervisor. Thus, MST youth, families, and therapists had 24-hour access to psychiatry residents and faculty trained in the treatment model. This availability stands in contrast with procedures followed in early randomized trials of MST for juvenile offenders and in dissemination sites, where consultation from psychiatrists in the community was obtained as needed by the MST team and family.

The role of the crisis caseworker was developed to enhance the therapist's ability to achieve treatment goals with families despite the often overwhelming needs of youth and families experiencing multiple crises. The crisis caseworkers were bachelor's-level mental health professionals with experience serving youth with emotional disturbance in the community. These individuals served two functions: assisting with specific crisis interventions and providing practical, clinical, and administrative support of therapist interventions. To assist with crisis intervention, the caseworkers performed safety assessments, coordinated access to crisis services (e.g., police, ambulance), and provided clinical support to therapists during crisis situations (e.g., calming siblings, monitoring youth). Caseworker support of therapists was best categorized as case management activities (i.e., transport, finding housing and employment resources) undertaken to free therapist time for clinical interventions. The psychiatrists and caseworkers operated within the same clinical and administrative structure of MST that characterized previous clinical trials. That is, the MST therapist continued to be the primary interventionist, working with families to design and implement effective clinical interventions. The MST supervisor retained ultimate responsibility for the team's performance.

Early in the implementation of MST as an alternative to hospitalization, it became apparent that youth in psychiatric crisis and their families required substantially more time, clinical acumen with respect to psychiatric disorders in adults and children, and systems intervention (i.e., school, probation, and social services) than had been necessary in previous MST trials. Thus, administrative changes were made to accommodate these realities. The changes included (a) increased frequency of supervision (i.e., from one to three times a week), (b) reduced caseload (from four to three families), (c) allocation of more supervisor-level administrative time for system-level interventions, and (d) enhancement of techniques to facilitate therapist adherence to MST. Treatment adherence was enhanced by having trained coders rate audiotapes of therapist interventions for their adherence to the nine MST principles on a weekly basis. Feedback was then supplied to the MST supervisor, who in turn utilized this information to promote therapist adherence. This process was so helpful in facilitating and maintaining treatment integrity that it is now used in many ongoing clinical trials of MST.

Clinical Adaptations and Additions

To better equip therapists to address the needs of youth in psychiatric crisis and their families, salient aspects of research on the predictors, prevention, and treatment of youth and adult suicidal, homicidal, and psychotic behaviors were incorporated into the MST treatment model. This information was integrated into a crisis intervention protocol that provides information and tools to facilitate safety assessment and intervention, was used to train the clinical team, and appears in a recently published book (Henggeler et al., 2002).

Even after safety had been established, and in the absence of crisis, the treatment team found that helping families of youth with psychiatric impairment to achieve their treatment goals was more difficult than helping families of adolescent offenders to do so. The subjective experience of the team was that effecting change required more effort, with youth experiencing high levels of both internalizing and externalizing symptoms and caregivers experiencing significant psychiatric and substance abuse difficulties. Thus, the difficulties encountered by many families previously referred for MST, such as school expulsion, low social support, poverty, and iatrogenic effects of service system involvement, were compounded by the more extensive psychiatric symptomatology apparent in both the youth and caregivers in the hospital study. Additional training was required to better equip therapists to recognize and intervene more effectively with these difficulties. Booster training sessions focused on empirically supported assessment and intervention techniques for the following: child and adult depression and bipolar disorder, trauma symptoms in children, ADHD and posttraumatic stress disorder (PTSD) in adults and youth, anxiety disorders, borderline personality disorder, and adult substance abuse and dependence. Therapists were trained to work with psychiatrists to determine whether psychiatric evaluation and psychopharmacologic treatment were needed in conjunction with cognitive–behavioral individual therapy for adult caregivers. Substance abuse or dependence among caregivers was generally treated utilizing the community reinforcement approach and voucher system (CRA; Budney & Higgins, 1998). CRA is a manualized intervention in which therapists utilize behavioral and systemic interventions to treat adult drug dependence. This treatment was selected because an extensive favorable evidence base supports its effectiveness with adults, and its principles and procedures are highly compatible with MST.

Thus, over the 4-year implementation of MST with youth experiencing psychiatric crises and their families, all members of the treatment team—supervisor, therapists, psychiatrists, crisis caseworkers, and investigators—implemented a more extensive and comprehensive array of clinical tools than had been necessary in MST implementation with juvenile offenders and their families. In addition, respite placements were essential to stabilize some youth out of their home and family contexts. Thus, extensive efforts were invested in establishing a core set of placement resources spanning the spectrum of restrictiveness from respite foster home or shelter to inpatient psychiatric hospitalization. In each of these placement settings, the MST team maintained clinical responsibility for the youth, thus facilitating the maintenance of clinical gains and transition back to less restrictive services when the youth and family were ready.

MST AS AN ALTERNATIVE TO PSYCHIATRIC HOSPITALIZATION: OUTCOMES

Two publications have described the posttreatment outcomes for youth in the hospitalization study (Henggeler et al., 1999; Schoenwald, Ward, Henggeler, Rowland, & Brondino, 2000). The articles detailed the placement, clinical, and preliminary cost outcomes of the study's first 113 youth approximately 4 months after study intake. A summary of the participants and these outcomes is provided in Table 17.3.

Fifty-seven youth were randomly assigned to MST, and 56 were assigned to the comparison condition. The average age of the youth was 13.0 years, with 65% boys, 64% African American, 34% White, 1% Asian American, and 1% Hispanic. The majority (58%) of the youth lived in single-parent households that included at least one biological or adoptive parent, 22% lived in two-parent households with at least one biological or adoptive parent, and 20% lived with someone other than a biological or adoptive parent. The youth and families were relatively economically disadvantaged, with 75% receiving Medicaid, 72% receiving federal financial assistance, and a median monthly family income from employment of $250. Data derived from structured diagnostic interviews and records of previous mental health and juvenile justice involvement indicated that 96% of youth met criteria for more than one *DSM–III–R* diagnosis, 86% had received previous psychiatric treatment, 38% had been hospitalized for psychiatric reasons, and 38% had been involved with juvenile justice. Research assessments were conducted for all youth within 24 hours of enrollment in the project (T1), shortly after youth in the

TABLE 17.3

Multisystemic Therapy (MST) as an Alternative to Psychiatric Hospitalization: Outcomes

Study	Population	Comparison	Follow-Up	MST Outcomes
Henggeler et al. (1999) $N = 13$ (Final sample =156)	Youths presenting psychiatric emergencies	Psychiatric hospitalization	None	Decreased externalizing problems (CBCL) Improved family relations Increased school attendance Higher consumer satisfaction
Schoenwald et al. (2000)	Same sample			75% reduction in days hospitalized 50% reduction in days in other out-of-home placements
Henggeler et al. (2003)	Same sample		1 year	Initial favorable outcomes gradually dissipated by 12 months posttreatment

Note. CBCL = *Child Behavior Checklist* (Achenbach, 1991).

hospitalization condition were discharged (T2), and at the completion of MST home-based services (T3, an average of 4 months postenrollment). A multi-respondent, multimethod assessment battery composed of validated measures was used to assess youth diagnoses, including substance use and dependence; symptoms of youth and caregiver; youth functioning; family functioning; and consumer satisfaction at each time point. Data on hospitalization, placement, and arrest were obtained from official records.

With respect to hospitalization, 100% of youth in the comparison condition were hospitalized upon enrollment in the study, with 20% rehospitalized between T2 and T3. By comparison, 25% of youth in the MST condition were hospitalized during the T1–T2 period, and a total of 44% of the youth in MST were hospitalized at some point during the T1–T3 period. Length of hospital stay was significantly shorter for youth in the MST condition (3.78 vs. 6.06 days), and they experienced a 72% decrease in days hospitalized and a 50% decrease in days in other out-of-home placements relative to youth in the comparison group. The youth in the MST condition experienced significantly fewer placement changes and fewer changes to a more restrictive placement relative to their counterparts who were hospitalized for initial crisis stabilization (Schoenwald et al., 2000).

With respect to clinical posttreatment outcomes, youth in the MST condition evidenced significant improvements in externalizing symptoms as reported by caregivers and teachers on the *Child Behavior Checklist* (Achenbach, 1991). Youth in the MST condition also spent significantly fewer days out of school during the 4 months between T1 and T3 (14 days for MST vs. 37 days for the comparison group). Caregiver and youth reports on the third edition of the *Family Adaptability and Cohesion Scales* (FACES–III; Olson, Portner, & Lavee, 1985) indicated that by T2, families in the MST condition had become more structured, whereas families in the comparison condition had become less structured, and that cohesion increased in the MST condition and decreased in the comparison condition between T1 and T3. MST was equally effective in reducing youth internalizing symptoms, and youth and caregivers in the MST condition were substantially more satisfied with treatment services.

Although the findings immediately posttreatment support the effectiveness of MST as a safe, viable, and potentially better treatment than psychiatric hospitalization, long-term follow-up analyses have not been as promising. In an evaluation recently accepted for publication (Henggeler et al., 2003), youth and family outcomes 10 and 16 months after study intake were analyzed. Findings from these analyses generally indicated that many of the posttreatment effects of MST diminish over time. Multiple predictors of youth outcomes over time are being evaluated and include variables such as youth and caregiver psychiatric disturbance and substance abuse. Thus, although the MST treatment model for delinquent youth is well explicated and has substantial data to support its effectiveness for 1.7 to 4 years posttreatment, MST for youth with psychiatric disturbance is still being modified and evaluated for longer term outcomes.

FUTURE DIRECTIONS

The clinical and research experiences derived from the hospitalization study have led to the reconceptualization of the delivery of effective treatment for youth who are at imminent risk of out-of-home placement due to serious psychiatric impairment. First, it is likely that youth with significant emotional disturbance will often require longer term interventions with substantial follow-up to maintain clinical gains. Second, safely stabilizing these youth in the community requires an intense level of intervention, with more face-to-face family and therapist contact time, more supervision, and additional team members (i.e., psychiatrists, crisis caseworkers) than were required to implement MST for juvenile offenders. Third, MST clinicians serving youth with psychiatric impairment require additional training in crisis interventions, psychopharmacologic treatments, and the use of CRA with caregiver substance use disorders. Finally, the ability to access temporary out-of-home respite placement sites in which the MST model can be implemented is crucial in stabilizing many youth and families who are experiencing psychiatric crises. Thus, current projects are evaluating the feasibility of establishing a spectrum of MST-informed services that incorporate the modifications developed during the hospital study (i.e., audiocoded monitoring of therapist adherence, psychiatric services, and crisis training).

Testing an MST Continuum of Care

A randomized trial currently under way in Philadelphia is an example of new MST strategies to serve youth with emotional disturbance. The product of 4 years of collaboration among multiple stakeholders in Philadelphia, investigators at the FSRC, and the Annie E. Casey Foundation, this project will ultimately involve 100 juvenile offenders aged 10 to 16 years with comorbid psychiatric illness who are about to be placed out of home. Youth and families in this project receive services for at least 1 year from an MST team configured much like the one developed for the hospitalization study (i.e., supplemented with crisis caseworkers, psychiatrists). This project is designed to ensure that the youth served by the team have access to a continuum of placement and respite services that are clinically supervised by the MST team. Thus, therapists in the Philadelphia MST continuum-of-care project can access foster families, residential treatment, and psychiatric hospital beds when these are indicated for MST youth. Regardless of where the youth is placed, however, the MST therapist continues to provide treatment to the youth and his or her family. The MST clinical supervisor also retains clinical supervision responsibility for the youth, regardless of placement setting. Thus, a youth hospitalized temporarily due to suicidal behavior does not participate in the usual individual and group treatments provided on the ward; instead, he or she has an individualized plan established and implemented by the MST therapist, supervisor, psychiatrist, and family.

Because the capacity of families to effectively stabilize and manage chronic psychiatric problems in a child often waxes and wanes, strategies are being developed within the MST continuum project to vary the intensity of treatment delivery as well as provide a continuum of placements. As noted earlier, in previous studies and community-based MST dissemination sites, an "episode" of MST has lasted 3 to 5 months and required a therapist and a home-based model of service delivery to be available at all times. As such, therapists have not been free to provide less intensive follow-up, monitoring, or "booster" treatment sessions after the 3- to 5-month treatment period ends. In the MST continuum project, as families stabilize, the youth may be stepped down to receive less intensive levels of MST and ultimately placed on a monitoring or check-in status. Yet, treatment intensity can be accelerated if indicated by youth and family functioning. Importantly, the families participate in interventions based on the MST model, by the same MST team, at all levels of treatment intensity and levels of service.

The Philadelphia project is the second attempt made by the FSRC to implement and evaluate an MST continuum-of-care treatment for youth at risk of out-of-home placement due to psychiatric impairment. The first MST continuum project was developed jointly by the FSRC and the State of Hawaii Department of Health. Created in response to urgent needs and without the benefit of the multistakeholder collaborative process, this study was implemented for 13 months before being closed by mutual agreement of the project developers. One of the primary reasons for closing the project was the inability to create a functional continuum of MST services for youth in the treatment condition. Despite implementation difficulties, 55 youth were enrolled in the randomized trial, and 26 families were served with MST home-based services. Outcomes from this study, although preliminary, were consistent with posttreatment outcomes in the hospitalization study and provide some promise for future studies of MST for youth with psychiatric impairment (Rowland et al., 2003). To highlight important features of the MST continuum project still in operation, a case example of a youth and family receiving treatment in the Philadelphia project is outlined in the next section.

CASE EXAMPLE

Background

Samal, a 16-year-old Jamaican American boy, was referred to the MST continuum for significant behavioral, emotional, and substance use problems. At intake, Samal had a history of two prior arrests, including one for aggravated assault and one for possession of cocaine with intent to deliver. His mental health background was significant for two past suicidal attempts/gestures involving superficial self-mutilation, drug use, anxiety, and depression. He had been hospitalized once and had received 10 years of intermittent outpatient treatment.

Assessment of Strengths and Barriers

In her initial assessment of the youth, family, and their ecology, the therapist discovered numerous barriers to healthy functioning. At the family level, immediate concerns included the father's health (single parent, HIV-positive, substance dependent with chronic medical problems), and Samal's 21-year-old brother's criminal behavior. This brother, Cal, served as a co-parent, providing financial resources and some instrumental supports for the father. Both Cal and his father demonstrated poor parenting skills. Samal and two younger siblings lived in the home and experienced school failure, oppositional behaviors, substance use, and mild mental retardation. When stressed, the family appeared chaotic and disorganized. Cal's criminal behavior (i.e., selling drugs to finance family and personal needs) contributed to the family's problems and was an immediate concern for the clinical team. Cal was 15 when his mother died and he dropped out of school to provide for his siblings. At that time, his father was often absent from the home. Cal worked as a mechanic at a local garage, but he seemed to be subsidizing his income with criminal activity. He had been arrested twice for possession of marijuana with intent to sell, and several unemployed peers with similar histories frequented the home. The potential for Cal's alleged criminal actions to serve as a contributing factor to Samal's antisocial behavior through modeling, introduction of deviant peers, poor monitoring, or direct involvement in crime was an immediate urgent concern for the team. The family's problems were compounded by the community in which they lived. Residing in a high-crime, socioeconomically depressed neighborhood, they were surrounded by neighbors who also experienced substance abuse and mental health difficulties. These neighbors, while at times supportive, promoted the involvement of family members in neighborhood conflicts and were a source of alcohol and drugs. The home itself was in poor physical condition. Samal's family had a history of conflict with the school, and the children rarely attended class. Samal was in a remedial placement, having failed two grades. School officials were dubious about Samal's ability to succeed in an academic environment due to his behavioral and emotional problems and the family's track record.

Although the family experienced complex and serious clinical and practical difficulties, the therapist was able to identify significant strengths to leverage for change. Among these was that Cal and the father were sincere and committed in their love for the children. They wanted Samal and his siblings to finish school, stay drug free, and obtain a "better life." The entire family was intent on staying together and expressed a high level of commitment to one another. They were also generally willing to allow the therapist into their home and accepted the clinical team's help.

Interventions

Samal's family worked with the MST continuum treatment team for 15 months, during which time the team provided numerous interventions.

The actions that were implemented by the family and clinical team for Samal are outlined briefly next by system.

Individual

At the individual level, Samal was treated for symptoms of depression, severe mood lability, anxiety, and substance abuse. In collaboration with the therapist and youth, the MST psychiatrist provided medication and monitored psychiatric symptoms and medication compliance. CRA interventions (described previously; Budney & Higgins, 1998) were implemented to address Samal's substance use. Thus, behavioral and cognitive behavioral approaches were used to evaluate the multiple determinants of drug use and to develop interventions to interrupt the sequence of behaviors that triggered use. Results of frequent urine drug screens were paired with rewards (for abstinence) or consequences (for use) that were implemented by the family.

Family

The clinical team worked with the caregivers to address their medical and psychiatric symptoms and to improve their ability to safely monitor and supervise the children. Interventions included psychiatric evaluations for both the father and Cal, facilitation of appropriate medical care for the father, and enrollment of the father in a detoxification and day treatment program for his substance dependence. Significant work went into teaching Cal and the father skills for monitoring the children and helping them work through problems implementing what they had learned. Family sessions focused on improving communication and interaction skills. Interventions targeting Cal's alleged criminal behavior are outlined in the safety section.

School

Extensive effort was directed toward working with the school and family to diminish truancy and improve Samal's academic performance. Assessment and intervention strategies included observing and monitoring the youth in the school; using role plays and coaching sessions to promote better school–family collaboration; and specific action plans that enabled teachers and the family to develop, implement, and maintain home follow-through of consequences for teacher-reported behaviors.

Peers

The therapist and family worked together to decrease Samal's access to deviant peers (i.e., Cal's associates, neighbors who supplied drugs) and to increase involvement with prosocial peers. This was largely accomplished through interventions intended to increase Samal's exposure to prosocial peers (e.g., school basketball team), increase the caregivers' awareness of peers, and provide significant levels of adult supervision.

In addition to system-specific interventions such as those just outlined, interventions to ensure safety at times of crisis were developed and included the use of MST continuum placement settings on two occasions.

Safety

An extensive safety evaluation of the youth, family, and home is conducted at intake and repeated periodically for every family in the MST continuum. The home and surrounding area are assessed for weapons, medications, drugs, alcohol, and other potentially harmful items. Samal's family cooperated in the safety assessment initially and worked with the team to lock up medications, remove potential weapons, and monitor processes identified in the safety plan. Although the clinical team perceived Cal's involvement in criminal activity as an ongoing safety threat, he also seemed to be the best candidate to assume the primary parent role in the family. The father's cognitive limitations, substance dependence, and medical conditions were such that he seemed to best serve the family in a secondary caregiver role. Thus, the clinical team focused substantial energies on helping Cal to step up to the role of primary parent. Leveraging his strengths (i.e., paternal feelings for siblings, parentified role in the family, skills as a mechanic), the therapist assisted Cal in developing strategies to remove criminal activity and influences from the home environment. The team was able to accomplish these goals, and Cal enrolled in an adult education program to obtain his GED and further training as a mechanic.

Placement

The team used MST therapeutic foster care twice and psychiatric hospitalization once to help Samal safely manage his symptoms of mood lability and substance use. On the first occasion, Samal was placed in an MST therapeutic foster home for 5 days after becoming intoxicated and suicidal during a time of high family conflict. On this occasion, the team was able to help the foster parent implement treatment plans in the foster home while the team made necessary changes to the family environment. Approximately 5 months into treatment, Samal became very agitated and suicidal secondary to numerous therapist, family, and individual stressors. As a result, he was placed in the psychiatric hospital by the MST team for 5 days to stabilize his psychiatric and behavioral symptoms, and then he was transferred back to the MST therapeutic foster care home. He remained at this foster home for approximately 90 days. While he was in the MST foster home, extensive MST interventions were implemented with Samal and his family of origin, with the foster parent playing a substantial clinical role in Samal's care.

Reunion

After approximately 60 days in MST foster care, Samal and his family reached many of the goals targeted for Samal's return home. The clinical team, youth, family, and foster family worked to slowly integrate Samal back into his home and school environment over a 30-day period. During this time, Samal's home visits were contingent upon family maintenance of safety standards and responsible behaviors as objectively monitored by MST team members. By the time Samal returned to the home, all ties to criminal behavior had been removed from the home, and Samal was closely monitored to ensure compliance with the goals set jointly by the clinical team, youth, and family (e.g., school attendance, medication compliance, curfew, prosocial activity). Samal's father then worked with the MST therapist to diminish his substance abuse, maintain access to appropriate medical care, and improve his parenting skills.

Prior to discharge from MST, Cal was able to demonstrate substantially improved parenting skills and worked with the MST therapist to develop behavioral and school interventions for Samal's younger brother, who was experiencing significant academic and behavior difficulties. Samal's urine drug screens indicated 3 months of abstinence, and his family was making substantial progress toward the goal of locating housing in a safer community.

SUMMARY

The development of MST to serve youth at risk of out-of-home placement due to serious psychiatric impairment is a work in progress. Although several clinical trials have supported the long-term effectiveness of MST for delinquent youth, only one study involving 156 families (half of whom received MST) supported the short-term efficacy of MST for youth and families in psychiatric crisis. Both data and clinical experience have led to the reconceptualization of MST for use with families of youth whose functional impairments are due to psychiatric illness. Modifications to MST include the incorporation of psychiatrists and crisis caseworker resources into the team. Also, training strategies have been added to supplement therapists' skills in crisis intervention, psychopharmacologic treatments, and caregiver substance abuse interventions. Finally, additional strategies have been incorporated that focus on achieving and maintaining therapists' adherence to MST. Although these changes seemed to promote short-term improvements in youth and family functioning posttreatment, they have not been shown to generalize to longer term effective management of psychiatric impairment in youth. Thus, a current project is attempting to help families sustain improved outcomes over the longer term by modifying the full array of services a youth receives in accordance with MST principles and procedures. Outcomes from this evaluation will help to determine the future viability of MST for families and youth with serious psychiatric impairments.

AUTHORS' NOTE

Preparation of this chapter was supported by National Institute of Mental Health Grants R01MH51852 and RO1MH59138, National Institute on Drug Abuse Grants 99011905 and R01 DA15844, National Institute on Alcohol Abuse and Alcoholism Grant R01 AA122202, and the Annie E. Casey Foundation.

REFERENCES

Achenbach, T. M. (1991). *Manual for the Child Behavior Checklist/4–18 and 1991 Profile.* Burlington: University of Vermont, Department of Psychiatry.

American Academy of Child and Adolescent Psychiatry. (1997). Practice standards for the assessment and treatment of children and adolescents with bipolar disorder. *Journal of the American Academy of Child and Adolescent Psychiatry, 36* (Suppl.), 157S–176S.

Barkley, R. A. (1998). *Attention-deficit hyperactivity disorder: A handbook for diagnosis and treatment* (2nd ed.). New York: Guilford Press.

Birmaher, B., Ryan, N. D., Williamson, D. E., Brent, D. A., Kaufman, J., Dahl, R. E., et al. (1996). Childhood and adolescent depression: A review of the past 10 years. Part I. *Journal of the American Academy of Child and Adolescent Psychiatry, 35*(11), 1427–1439.

Borduin, C. M., Mann, B. J., Cone, L. T., Henggeler, S. W., Fucci, B. R., Blaske, D. M., et al. (1995). Multisystemic treatment of serious juvenile offenders: Long-term prevention of criminality and violence. *Journal of Consulting and Clinical Psychology, 63,* 569–578.

Bronfenbrenner, U. (1979). *The ecology of human development.* Cambridge, MA: Harvard University Press.

Budney, A. J., & Higgins, S. T. (1998). *Therapy manuals for drug addiction. A community reinforcement plus vouchers approach: Treating cocaine addiction* (NIH Publication no. 98-4309). Rockville, MD: NIDA.

Elliott, D. S., Huizinga, D., & Ageton, S. S. (1985). *Explaining delinquency and drug use.* Beverly Hills, CA: Sage.

Ellis, D. A., Naar-King, S., Frey, M., Rowland, M. D., & Gregor, N. (2003). Case study: Feasibility of multisystemic therapy as a treatment for urban adolescents with poorly controlled type I diabetes. *Journal of Pediatric Psychology, 28,* 287–293.

Geller, B., Craney, J. L., Bolhofner, K., Nickelsburg, M. J., Williams, M., & Zimerman, B. (2002). Two-year prospective follow-up of children with prepubertal and early adolescent bipolar disorder phenotype. *American Journal of Psychiatry, 159*(6), 927–933.

Haley, J. (1976). *Problem-solving therapy.* San Francisco: Jossey-Bass.

Henggeler, S. W., & Borduin, C. M. (1990). *Family therapy and beyond: A multisystemic approach to treating the behavior problems of children and adolescents.* Pacific Grove, CA: Brooks/Cole.

Henggeler, S. W., Melton, G. B., Brondino, M. J., Scherer, D. G., & Hanley, J. H. (1997). Multisystemic therapy with violent and chronic juvenile offenders and their families: The role of treatment fidelity in successful dissemination. *Journal of Consulting and Clinical Psychology, 65*(5), 821–833.

Henggeler, S. W., Melton, G. B., & Smith, L. A. (1992). Family preservation using multisystemic therapy: An effective alternative to incarcerating serious juvenile offenders. *Journal of Consulting and Clinical Psychology, 60,* 953–961.

Henggeler, S. W., Melton, G. B., Smith, L. A., Schoenwald, S. K., & Hanley, J. H. (1993). Family preservation using multisystemic treatment: Long-term follow-up to a clinical trial with serious juvenile offenders. *Journal of Child and Family Studies, 2,* 283–293.

Henggeler, S. W., Mihalic, S. F., Rone, L., Thomas, C., & Timmons-Mitchell, J. (1998). *Blueprints for violence prevention: Multisystemic therapy.* Boulder: University of Colorado at Boulder, Center for the Study and Prevention of Violence.

Henggeler, S. W., Rodick, J. D., Borduin, C. M., Hanson, C. L., Watson, S. M., & Urey, J. R. (1986). Multisystemic treatment of juvenile offenders: Effects on adolescent behavior and family interactions. *Developmental Psychology, 22,* 132–141.

Henggeler, S. W., Rowland, M. D., Halliday-Boykins, C. A., Sheidow, A. J., Cunningham, P. B., Randall, J., et al. (2003). One-year follow-up to multisystemic therapy as an alternative to the hospitalization of youths in psychiatric crisis. *Journal of the American Academy of Child and Adolescent Psychiatry, 42*(5), 543–551.

Henggeler, S. W., Rowland, M. D., Pickrel, S. G., Miller, S. L., Cunningham, P. B., Santos, A. B., et al. (1997). Investigating family-based alternatives to institution-based mental health services for youth: Lessons learned from the pilot study of a randomized field trial. *Journal of Clinical Child Psychology, 26,* 226–233.

Henggeler, S. W., Rowland, M. D., Randall, J., Ward, D. M., Pickrel, S. G., Cunningham, P. B., et al. (1999). Home-based multisystemic therapy as an alternative to the hospitalization of youths in psychiatric crisis: Clinical outcomes. *Journal of the American Academy of Child and Adolescent Psychiatry, 38,* 1331–1339.

Henggeler, S. W., Schoenwald, S. K., Borduin, C. M., Rowland, M. D., & Cunningham, P. B. (1998). *Multisystemic treatment of antisocial behavior in children and adolescents.* New York: Guilford Press.

Henggeler, S. W., Schoenwald, S. K., Rowland, M. D., & Cunningham, P. B. (2002). *Serious emotional disturbance in children and adolescents: Multisystemic therapy.* New York: Guilford Press.

Kazdin, A. E. (1996). Problem solving and parent management in treating aggressive and antisocial behavior. In E. D. Hibbs & P. S. Jensen (Eds.), *Psychosocial treatments for child and adolescent disorders: Empirically based strategies for clinical practice* (pp. 77–408). Washington DC: American Psychological Association.

Kolko, D., & Swenson, C. C. (2002). *Assessing and treating physically abused children and their families.* Thousand Oaks, CA: Sage.

Leschied, A. W., & Cunningham, A. (2001). Intensive community-based services can influence re-offending rates of high-risk youth: Preliminary results of the multisystemic therapy clinical trials in Ontario. *Empirical and Applied Criminal Justice Research, 1,* 1–24.

Liddle, H. A. (1996). Family-based treatment for adolescent problem behaviors: Overview of contemporary developments and introduction to the special section. *Journal of Family Psychology, 10,* 3–11.

Loeber, R., & Farrington, D. P. (Eds.). (1998). *Serious and violent juvenile offenders: Risk factors and successful interventions.* Thousand Oaks, CA: Sage.

Minuchin, S. (1974). *Families and family therapy.* Cambridge, MA: Harvard University Press.

Olson, D. H., Portner, J., & Lavee, Y. (1985). *FACES–III.* St. Paul: University of Minnesota, Department of Family Social Science.

Randall, J., Henggeler, S. W., Cunningham, P. B., Rowland, M. D., & Swenson, C. C. (2001). Adapting multisystemic therapy to treat adolescent substance abuse more effectively. *Cognitive and Behavioral Practice, 8,* 359–366.

Rowland, M. D., Halliday-Boykins, C. A., Henggeler, S. W., Cunningham, P. B., Lee, T. G., Kruesi, M. J., et al. (2003). *A randomized trial of multisystemic therapy with Hawaii's Felix class youth.* Manuscript submitted for publication.

Saigh, P. A., Yasik, A. E., Sack, W. H., & Koplewicz, H. S. (1999). Child–adolescent posttraumatic stress disorder: Prevalence, risk factors, and comorbidity. In P. A. Saigh & J. D. Bremner (Eds.), *Posttraumatic stress disorder: A comprehensive text* (pp. 18–43). Needham Heights, MA: Allyn & Bacon.

Satin, R. (2000). *A test of the efficacy of multisystemic therapy for reducing recidivism and decreasing the length of residential treatment.* Paper presented at the First International MST Conference, Savannah, GA.

Schoenwald, S. K., Sheidow, A. J., & Letourneau, E. J. (2004). Toward effective quality assurance in evidence-based practice: Links between expert consultation, therapist fidelity, and child outcomes. *Journal of Clinical Child and Adolescent Psychology, 33*(1), 94–104.

Schoenwald, S. K., Sheidow, A. J., Letourneau, E. J., & Liao, J. G. (2003). Transportability of evidence-based treatments: Evidence for multi-level influences. *Mental Health Service Research, 5,* 235–239.

Schoenwald, S. K., Ward, D. M., Henggeler, S. W., Rowland, M. D., & Brondino, M. J. (2000). MST vs. hospitalization for crisis stabilization of youth: Placement outcomes 4 months post-referral. *Mental Health Service Research, 2*(1), 3–12.

Swenson, C. C., Henggeler, S. W., Schoenwald, S. K., Kaufman, K. L., & Randall, J. (1998). Changing the social ecologies of adolescent sexual offenders: Implications of the success of multisystemic therapy in treating serious antisocial behavior in adolescents. *Child Maltreatment, 3,* 30–38.

Wagner, B. M. (1997). Family risk factors for child and adolescent suicidal behavior. *Psychological Bulletin, 121*(2), 246–298.

Washington Institute for Public Policy. (1998). *Watching the bottom line: Cost-effective interventions for reducing crime in Washington* (pp. 1–6). Olympia, WA: Evergreen State College.

Effective Schoolwide Discipline

CHAPTER 18

J. Ron Nelson, Jorge Gonzalez, Ronald C. Martella, and Nancy Marchand-Martella

For approximately 180 days per year and 6 hours each day, educators strive to provide learning environments that are conducive to learning. Unfortunately, a growing number of children exhibit problem behaviors that make it difficult to achieve such environments. For example, estimates provided in the recently published Surgeon General's report on children and mental health (U.S. Department of Health and Human Services, 1999) indicate that 21% of youth within the general population have a diagnosable mental health disorder. Additionally, approximately 11% of youth meet the diagnostic criteria for a significant impairment that adversely affects relationships at home, with peers, and in the community.

What is the importance of schoolwide discipline in improving the mental health status of children? The simple, most direct answer is that schools are where the majority of mental health services are provided, and effective schoolwide discipline supports positive child functioning and provides the foundation for such services. The research base on mental health needs and services demonstrates quite clearly that many children receive mental health services outside of the traditional mental health/health sciences service sectors. Perhaps in the most dramatic study to date, the Great Smoky Mountains Study, Costello and colleagues (1996) reported on the mental health needs and service provisions of 4,500 children in western North Carolina. According to the authors,

> The data presented here show that the majority of children with recent mental health care needs were not receiving professional help for those needs … When children did receive care it was likely to be from a provider outside of the specialty mental health sector. The major player in the de facto system of care was the education sector—more than three-fourths of children receiving mental health services were seen in the education sector, and for many this was the sole source of care. The general health care system played a relatively minor role in the provision of mental health care for children. (p. 155)

It is unsurprising that many teachers report that they are unprepared to deal with problem behaviors exhibited by the increasing numbers of children with mental health disorders (Furlong & Morrison, 1994). As a result, only one-half of classroom time is used for instruction, while the majority of the other half is taken up with discipline problems (Cotton, 1990). Even special education teachers experience problems dealing with students who exhibit problem behaviors, and they feel ill prepared to deal with these behaviors. For example, only 25% of resource teachers reported feeling adequately prepared to deal with social problems, 56% reported feeling fairly or poorly prepared, and 18% indicated they had no preparation to deal with these problems (Baum, Duffelmeyer, & Geelan, 1988). Parents are also concerned about problem behaviors within schools: Thirty-six percent of general public school parents rated fighting, violence, and gangs; lack of discipline; lack of funding; and use of drugs as the top four biggest problems facing local schools; these four problems have been rated within the top four for the last 15 years (Rose & Gallup, 2001).

Problem behaviors not only confront schools and families with serious challenges, they also have an adverse impact on individual students. Research has consistently painted a bleak picture for postschool adjustment of students with emotional and behavioral disorders (EBD; Edgar & Levine, 1987; Neel, Meadow, Levine, & Edgar, 1988; Wagner, 1992; Wagner & Shaver, 1989). Data from the SRI National Longitudinal Transition Study documented that those with EBD experienced the highest unemployment, poorest work history, and highest number of social adjustment problems post–high school of any disability group (Wagner, 1992). The presence of problem behaviors is among the most common reasons students, including those with disabilities, are excluded from school, community, and work environments (Sugai, Sprague, Horner, & Walker, 2000).

In response to this growing concern, three-tiered behavior prevention programs have been recommended to help schools create more positive teaching and learning environments (e.g., Nelson, Martella, & Marchand-Martella, 2002; Sugai et al., 2000; Walker et al., 1996). Such programs are designed to help schools establish a set of progressively more comprehensive, intense, and specific intervention programs designed to address the educational and social needs of three types of children that exist in any school setting: (a) typical children not at risk for problems, (b) children at risk for developing antisocial behavior problems, and (c) children who show signs of life-course-persistent antisocial behavior patterns and involvement in delinquent acts (Moffitt, 1994; Walker et al., 1996). Members of each group are candidates for differing levels or types of intervention that represent greater specificity, comprehensiveness, expense, and intensity (Reid, 1993).

Interventions appropriate for each child group are primary, secondary, and tertiary forms of prevention. Primary prevention services focus on enhancing protective factors on a schoolwide basis so that students do not become at risk. Interventions used for primary prevention are universal—all students are exposed to the services. Secondary prevention programs provide behavioral, social, or academic support; mentoring; skill development; and assistance to at-risk students. Students who do not respond to universal interventions or demonstrate specific risk factors are candidates for secondary prevention services. Tertiary prevention services are appropriate for severely involved children who evince a life-course-persistent pattern of antisocial behavior. Successful interventions for these students are likely to be comprehensive, intensive, and long term; to involve parents, siblings, peers, and natural supports; and to be collaborative across agencies.

The focus of this chapter is on describing how to create and maintain an effective schoolwide discipline or primary-level intervention program. Effective schoolwide discipline programs not only provide a predictable environment that promotes positive behaviors and maximizes learning opportunities, they also provide the foundation from which to link and coordinate secondary- and tertiary-level interventions. Indeed, the three primary goals of an effective schoolwide discipline program are (a) to establish effective policies and procedures that create positive norms for behaviors, (b) to improve the ecological arrangements of the school to promote positive behaviors, and (c) to identify and implement evidence-based secondary- and tertiary-level intervention programs and strategies.

This chapter will describe the behavior and academic support and enhancement (BASE) model. BASE is a strategic planning model for developing, implementing, maintaining, and evaluating an effective schoolwide discipline program that supports the identification and implementation of evidence-based secondary- and tertiary-level interventions and supports. We first provide an overview of the outcome research conducted on BASE. This overview is followed by a discussion of the elements and organizational systems that are considered within BASE. This discussion is followed by a detailed description of the school evaluation rubric (SER; Nelson & Ohlund, 1999) assessment and planning tool that underlies BASE. The SER is a continuum-of-progress evaluation rubric that is integrated within a strategic planning process to guide educators through the development of a comprehensive three-tiered prevention program. Finally, the process used to administer the SER is detailed.

OUTCOME RESEARCH CONDUCTED ON BASE

The SER and its associated action planning process have been field-tested and validated in numerous schools across the country (Nelson, 1996; Nelson et al., 2002). Two U.S. Department of Education grants from the Office of Special Education Programs (OSEP) and Office of Educational Research and Innovation (OERI) supported the development and evaluation of BASE. A quasi-experimental design was used to evaluate BASE in both cases. Comparative analyses were conducted on the school (experimental schools were compared to a matched group of comparison schools) and student (pre- and posttest comparisons made between children with and without EBD) levels. The effects of BASE were assessed in two urban elementary schools over a 2-year period (Nelson, 1996). Comparisons with two matched elementary schools indicated strong positive effects on disciplinary actions (80% decrease in formal office referrals, 65% decrease in suspensions, 90% decrease in emergency removals) of the schools and on the teachers' perceptions of their ability to work with children who exhibit problem behaviors, as well as the extent to which there were shared goals among staff for working with such behaviors. Additionally, comparisons between target (i.e., those with or at risk of EBD) and criterion (i.e., those without and not at risk of EBD) students indicated positive effects on the social adjustment, academic performance, and school survival skills of the target students.

Nelson and colleagues (2002) replicated and expanded the BASE prevention model to include an academic emphasis (i.e., tertiary-level reading program). In other words, BASE focused on integrating a reading program (i.e., *Sound Partners;* Vadasy, Jenkins, Antil, Wayne, & O'Connor, 1997) within a three-tiered prevention program (i.e., schoolwide discipline program featuring conflict resolution, parenting skills development, and functional behavioral assessment–driven intervention development). Seven elementary schools were studied over a period of 2 years (Nelson, Martella, & Marchand-Martella, 2002). Comparisons with the remaining 28 elementary schools in the district indicated strong positive effects on the formal disciplinary actions (60% decrease in formal office referrals, 75% decrease in suspensions, 80% decrease in emergency removals) and academic performance of the participating schools. Comparisons between target and criterion students indicated positive effects on the social adjustment and academic performance of the target students.

KEY ELEMENTS

BASE, like other research-based schoolwide discipline models (e.g., effective behavior support; Colvin, Kameenui, & Sugai, 1993), includes a number of key elements: (a) a behaviorally based conceptual framework, (b) a consensus-based participatory approach, (c) research-validated and practical interventions, (d) attention to social validity, and (e) a systems approach (Sugai & Horner, 1999). Specifically,

1. BASE is founded on a science of human behavior that emphasizes that much of human behavior is learned, comes under the control of environmental factors, and can be changed. Additionally, the most effective interventions and programs are based on a behavioral or behavioral–cognitive framework (Gottfredson et al., 2000).

2. BASE uses a consensus-based participatory process in which staff, students, parents, and community members work together to design and implement a schoolwide discipline program that supports the identification and implementation of evidence-based secondary- and tertiary-level interventions. This process is used to diagnose and strengthen problem areas.

3. BASE emphasizes the adoption and maintained use of research-based and practical interventions. Although procedures to prevent and reduce the likelihood of occurrences of problem behaviors often are associated with behavioral interventions, BASE emphasizes academic and behavioral interventions and strategies that use assessment information (such as screening pro-

cedures and functional behavioral assessment) to build students' skills and arrange learning environments so factors that are likely to trigger or maintain problem behaviors are less likely to be present and adaptive behaviors are more likely to be taught, occasioned, and supported.

4. BASE emphasizes the social validity of the learning options available to the student and to the student's peers. Thus, a central tenet of BASE is that behavior change and the means by which behavior change is achieved need to be socially significant by being (a) comprehensive, considering all parts of a student's day (before, during, and after school) and important social contexts (home, school, neighborhood, and community); (b) durable, so that change lasts for long periods of time; and (c) relevant, enhancing both prosocial and academic behaviors that affect learning and living opportunities (academic, family, social, work).

5. BASE emphasizes a systems approach. A systems approach considers the many contexts or organizational systems in which adaptive behavior is required. In schools, six organizational systems (described next) must be considered. A systems approach also focuses on prevention-based practices, team-based problem solving, active administrative support and participation, data-based decision making, and a full continuum of behavior support to accommodate the range of intensities of problem behaviors that occur in schools.

ORGANIZATIONAL SYSTEMS

Six organizational systems are included within the BASE model: (a) leadership, (b) schoolwide, (c) nonclassrooms, (d) classrooms, (e) individual students, and (f) the academic support system. The first four systems focus on the schoolwide discipline program, whereas the remaining two systems center on the identification and implementation of evidence-based secondary- and tertiary-level interventions and supports provided to children at risk of or experiencing school failure, respectively. Each of these systems is described in this section.

Leadership Organizational System

This area examines the school's role in facilitating a leadership team that implements a continual strategic planning process to achieve a safe and disciplined school environment that maximizes student learning. This system is central to the development, implementation, maintenance, and evaluation of a schoolwide discipline program. Although this system is not necessarily distinct from other leadership activities used to direct and support the school efforts, it focuses on establishing positive teaching and learning environments within all key organizational structures of the school: schoolwide (i.e., all students, all staff, and all settings), nonclassroom (i.e., particular times or places where supervision is emphasized), classroom (i.e., instructional settings), individual student support (i.e., specific supports for students who are at risk of or engage in chronic problem behaviors), and academic support (i.e., early screening and secondary- and tertiary-level academic interventions). The goal of the leadership organizational system is to improve the school's vision and organization; stakeholder involvement and communication; allocation of resources (human, fiscal, and time); development, implementation, and maintenance of systems to support positive teaching and learning environments; and continual self-assessment and modifications based on feedback gained through this iterative process.

There are seven key attributes of the leadership organizational system: (a) administrator support and representation, (b) parent involvement, (c) behavioral capacity, (d) building-level status, (e) support and commitment of staff, (f) sustained effort, and (g) its status as integral to school improvement goals. The first key attribute of the leadership system is the support of the administrator. Support from the administrative staff is necessary because they are central to discipline policies and procedures, and they provide a vision for all aspects of the school. Additionally, the leadership team should be representative in terms of key areas addressed in BASE. However, we have found that it is important to limit the number of members. We have found that six to eight members help to ensure the representativeness of the leadership team and its efficiency.

Second, parental involvement is important for two primary reasons. First, parental involvement plays an important role in establishing community support and commitment for the schoolwide discipline program. The community can provide many valuable resources to support the schoolwide discipline program and improve its outcomes. Second, parental involvement will facilitate communication of the goals, procedures, and practices of the schoolwide discipline program with families and others.

The third key attribute of the leadership system is behavioral capacity. At least one of the members of the team should have training and experience in applied behavior analysis. Furthermore, the members of the leadership team should have broad and complementary expertise (e.g., academic, social, family, community), particularly when developing a schoolwide discipline program that supports the identification and implementation of evidence-based secondary- and tertiary-level interventions and supports. All of the members of the leadership team should be knowledgeable regarding evidence-based academic and behavioral programs. It is difficult for the team to develop an effective schoolwide discipline program if the members are not knowledgeable about basic applied behavior analysis and evidence-based programs.

Fourth, the leadership team must have building-level status. This simply means that the leadership team developing the schoolwide discipline program is a key part of the school's organizational structure. Because the schoolwide discipline program affects essentially all areas of the school (e.g., rules, curriculum), the leadership system should be coordinated with the remaining functions of the school's overall organizational system. Additionally, the team should not be seen as temporary or tangential to the organizational structure of the school.

The support and commitment of the staff is the fifth attribute of the leadership system. The leadership system should not be based on a top-down process to develop the schoolwide discipline program. Rather, the team should work to build consensus on all of the policies, procedures, and practices. Although there is not a set standard, schools generally try to achieve 80% consensus among staff prior to implementing any aspect of the schoolwide discipline program.

Sixth, sustained effort on the part of the leadership team is necessary to develop, implement, maintain, and evaluate a schoolwide discipline program. Building a schoolwide discipline program is an ongoing refinement and maintenance process that requires sustained effort and multiple iterations over time. Given the comprehensive nature of a schoolwide discipline program that supports the identification and implementation of evidence-based secondary- and tertiary-level interventions and supports, it is beyond the capacity of staff to develop and implement such a program in less than 2 to 3 years. This time frame, coupled with changes in personnel and the need to update current staff, requires sustained effort.

The final attribute of the leadership system is that developing a schoolwide discipline program should be seen as central to achieving the school improvement goals. It is our contention that achieving a school environment that maximizes the learning of all students should be a key part of the school improvement goals of all schools. The efforts of the leadership team must also be linked and coordinated to school reform efforts and activities and maintained over time. Achieving a safe and disciplined learning environment is a process of continual refinement.

Schoolwide Organizational System

The schoolwide organizational system is defined as involving all students and staff in all settings within a school. The goal of the schoolwide organizational system is to create a common language among staff, students, and families regarding the school's culture; to clarify staff roles in regard to discipline issues, problems, and crisis procedures; and to provide feedback to staff on a regular basis.

There are four key attributes of the schoolwide organizational system: (a) schoolwide guidelines for success (e.g., be safe, be accountable, be respectful); (b) strategies for teaching staff, students, and families the guidelines for success; (c) clearly defined discipline roles and responsibilities; and (d) a clearly defined crisis response plan. The first key attribute of the schoolwide organizational system is the guidelines for success. These guidelines are a limited set of general expectations that represent the overall culture the school wants to achieve. The general nature of the guidelines for success not only encompass a great deal of behavior but also provide the flexibility necessary for staff to connect more specific nonclassroom and classroom expectations to them. The guidelines for success provide a "common language" that staff can use to communicate with students and among themselves (e.g., "Were you safe, accountable, or responsible?") about behavioral issues. Using a common language improves the predictability in the day-to-day interactions between students and staff, as well as among staff. Additionally, the guidelines for success provide a common foundation with which to connect nonclassroom and classroom rules or expectations.

Strategies for teaching staff, students, and families the guidelines to success and associated nonclassroom and classroom expectations are the second key attribute of the schoolwide organizational system. Developing and implementing such teaching strategies is critical because educators often assume that students already know what appropriate school behavior is. Indeed, this is one of the most unchallenged assumptions in schools today. Related to this issue is the notion that telling students the guidelines for success and associated nonclassroom and classroom expectations is the same as teaching students what is expected. Effective schools acquaint students with the key areas of the school (e.g., gym, cafeteria, break areas) and actively teach the guidelines for success and associated nonclassroom and classroom expectations.

The third key attribute of the schoolwide organizational system is defined discipline roles and responsibilities. It is important for all staff members to understand the problem behaviors they are expected to handle and their role in doing so. For example, problem behaviors requiring an administrative response and the respective roles of the administrator and staff should be clearly defined. Clearly defined discipline roles and responsibilities reduce staff conflicts and improve communication among administrators, students, staff, and families.

A crisis response plan is the fourth key attribute of the schoolwide organizational system. When a school achieves an exemplary level of implementation in each of the six areas of the schoolwide organizational system, the occurrence of crisis is reduced. However, crises can happen anytime and anywhere. The crisis response plan should help schools to prepare for and resolve a range of crisis situations. Although the number of crisis events or situations that can be included in the response plan can vary, many schools focus on school-level events (e.g., anonymous threats to school safety, a school shooting), nonclassroom and classroom-level situations (e.g., defiance or verbal or physical aggression), and student-level events (e.g., suicide threat). The crisis response plan should (a) clearly define the roles and responsibilities for all school staff, (b) establish an effective communication system, and (c) establish an efficient process for securing support (internally and externally when needed).

Nonclassroom Organizational System

The nonclassroom organizational system is defined as particular times or places outside the classroom where supervision is emphasized (e.g., hallways, cafeteria, playground, bus). The goal of the nonclassroom organizational system is to improve the predictability of the day-to-day interactions between staff and students and among staff by ensuring that the behavioral expectations are linked to the schoolwide guidelines for success; increase the participation of all staff in creating safe and disciplined nonclassroom areas; maximize the ecological arrangements of the nonclassroom areas of the school to promote positive student behaviors; and ensure active supervision of students and effective use of discipline procedures by supervisory staff.

The key attributes of the nonclassroom organizational system are (a) behavioral expectations that are linked to the schoolwide guidelines for success, (b) strategies for teaching behavioral expectations to students, (c) ecological arrangements that maximize positive student behaviors, and (d) training staff on active supervision and discipline procedures.

The first key attribute is the linkage of the behavioral expectations of the nonclassroom areas with the schoolwide guidelines to success. This linkage is more general and flexible in nature and improves the predictability in the day-to-day interactions between students and staff, as well as among staff.

Strategies for teaching staff and students about expectations for each of the nonclassroom areas is the second key attribute of the nonclassroom organizational system. Establishing strategies for teaching students, regardless of age, is critical to creating a safe and disciplined learning environment that maximizes student learning. Again, staff who work with older students often mistakenly assume that students already know the expectations required of them. Although the teaching strategies would differ (e.g., less rehearsing with older students), all staff should commit time at the beginning of the year to teaching students the expectations associated with each of the nonclassroom areas of the school. In this process, the behavioral expectations for each of the nonclassroom areas should be linked to the guidelines to success.

The third key attribute of the nonclassroom organizational system is adjusting the ecological arrangements of the nonclassroom areas of the school to maximize positive student behavior. The basic assumption is that the proper design and effective use of the school environment reduces the incidence of problem behaviors in the nonclassroom areas of the school. Critical examination of the ecological arrangements is difficult because the human tendency is to overlook obvious solutions to problems. Clichés such as "If it had been a snake, it would have bit me!" apply to the ecological arrangements of the school. Staff need to view the ecological arrangements through a different lens and take advantage of the solutions that are inherent in the school environment itself.

Typical modifications to the ecological arrangements in the nonclassroom areas of the school include (a) eliminating or adjusting unsafe physical arrangements and (b) improving the scheduling and use of space. Eliminating or adjusting unsafe physical arrangements involves actual structural changes and adjustments in the use of the space. Although each site plan is unique, some problems are typical. First, campus and specific area borders are sometimes poorly defined. Even when fencing is used, it is sometimes obscured by foliage that shields the campus from natural surveillance. Second, undifferentiated campus areas (e.g., a hidden corner of the playground) present opportunities for informal gathering areas that are beyond adult supervision. These areas are often used for prohibited activities and also provide fertile ground for problem behaviors. Third, building layout and design often produce isolated spots (e.g., end of the hallway) where students gravitate and either commit prohibited activities or may be exposed to victimization. Finally, bus-loading areas are often in direct conflict with traffic flow or create conflict and congestion with automobile parking areas. These zones also tend to be in direct conflict with the flow of students leaving the school grounds or entering for extracurricular activities. Congestion created by traffic and student flow provides ample opportunities for problem behaviors and increases safety concerns.

One of the most effective ecological strategies for promoting positive social behaviors centers on improving the scheduling and use of space. For example, it not only takes longer to get groups through the lunch line because of congestion, but it also provides the occasion for more physical and undesirable social interactions among students. In elementary schools, reversing lunch and recess, as well as mixing grades, may eliminate many problems typically associated with the lunch and recess periods. Although there are no set rules, general guidelines can be used to improve the scheduling and use of space. These include reducing the density of students by using all entrances and exits to a given area; increasing the space between groups, lines, or classes; mixing age groups as the density of students increases; keeping wait time at a minimum; decreasing travel time and distance as much as possible; using physical signs to control movement, such as clearly marked transition zones that indicate movement from less controlled to more controlled space or behavioral expectations for the common areas of the school; and sequencing events in common areas designed to facilitate the type of behavioral momentum desired (e.g., going to recess before lunch rather than going to lunch before recess results in students being better prepared for instruction).

Training supervisory staff to supervise and use the discipline procedures is the final key attribute of the nonclassroom organizational system. Both certified and classified staff need training because the ratio of students to staff is the largest in the nonclassroom areas. The ability of staff to affect behavior in a positive fashion is greatly decreased. Teaching staff to move, observe, and engage students when they are exhibiting positive or problem behaviors is key to creating positive nonclassroom areas. Additionally, supervisory staff need to understand the disciplinary procedures in place for each of the common areas and how to challenge students who are exhibiting problem behaviors in a nonconfrontational and unemotional matter.

Classroom Organizational System

The classroom organizational system is defined as instructional settings in which teachers supervise and teach groups of students. The goal of this system is to ensure student learning outcomes; to improve the predictability of the day-to-day interactions between staff and students, as well as among staff; and to build staff knowledge of and competencies in effective teaching and behavioral interventions and supports.

There are several key attributes of the classroom organizational system. These are (a) a curriculum that focuses on promoting academic success for all students, (b) behavioral expectations that are linked to the schoolwide guidelines for success, (c) consistent discipline procedures used by teachers, (d) teachers having access to effective assistance and recommendations for student behavioral and academic concerns, and (e) teachers having access to ongoing staff development activities.

The first key attribute of the classroom organizational system is a curriculum focus on achieving positive student outcomes. This attribute focuses on establishing not only the overall curriculum but also a full continuum of academic supports (e.g., one-to-one tutoring programs) to ensure the success of all students. Focusing on achieving positive academic outcomes is critical; many empirical studies have demonstrated a strong relationship between academic competence and social functioning (e.g., Hawkins, Farrington, & Catalano, 1998; Herrenkohl et al., 1998; Huizinga & Jakob-Chien, 1998; Lipsey & Derzon, 1998; Maguin & Loeber, 1996; McEvoy & Welker, 2000). The results from more than 100 cross-sectional and longitudinal analyses revealed that (a) poor academic performance is related to the onset, frequency, persistence, and seriousness of social functioning problems in both boys and girls and (b) the relationship between academic performance and social functioning is independent of major sociological variables, such as socioeconomic status.

Second, behavioral expectations should be linked to the schoolwide guidelines for success. The linkage of each teacher's specific expectations to these guidelines, which are more general and flexible in nature, improves the predictability of day-to-day interactions between students and staff, as well as among staff. This is not to say that every teacher has to have the same expectations. Rather, the linkage of each teacher's expectations to the schoolwide guidelines for success provides a common language with which to discuss student behaviors (both appropriate and inappropriate).

The third key attribute of the classroom organizational system of the school is the use of consistent disciplinary procedures for common classroom problem behaviors (e.g., off task, noncompliance). The goal is to provide a common disciplinary response by teachers to improve the predictability in the day-to-day interactions between teachers and students. Behavioral expectations linked to the schoolwide guidelines for success, coupled with a common disciplinary response by the teachers, are crucial. Although there are numerous common disciplinary responses, effective ones tend to reduce or eliminate warnings, provide the student a chance to regain control, and plan or problem-solve alternative responses. It is important to maintain flexibility in administrative and classroom disciplinary responses for more severe problem behaviors (e.g., fighting, defiance). Such responses should be adjusted according to the context associated with the problem behavior.

Ensuring that teachers have access to effective assistance and recommendations for student behavioral and academic concerns is the fourth key attribute of the classroom organizational system. Schools must develop efficient and simple structures (e.g., common planning time once a week focused on academic and behavioral concerns) to support problem solving by teachers.

Schools must also develop the knowledge and competencies of key members of their staff to ensure that teachers have access to evidence-based practices. That is, a number of staff should have in-depth knowledge of academic and behavioral interventions and supports, as well as the collaborative skills necessary to work with staff.

Finally, staff should have access to ongoing staff development opportunities. These opportunities should be designed to sustain current practices in the school as well as to explore potential additions. Staff development activities should be targeted and strategic in nature if they are to facilitate the implementation, refinement, and maintenance of the schoolwide discipline program.

Individual Organizational System

The individual organizational system is defined as specific supports for students who are at risk of or are experiencing school failure. The goals of this system are to establish prevention intervention procedures for students who are at risk of school failure and to provide individualized interventions and supports to students who are experiencing school failure.

Key attributes of the individual organizational system include (a) evidence-based prevention and intervention procedures for students who are at risk of or are experiencing school failure, (b) a common solutions-focused language or conceptual lens used by all staff to develop effective prevention and intervention practices, (c) an established behavioral support team that is easy to access and is not seen solely as a step in the special education referral process, and (d) the use of community resources as prevention and intervention practices for students and families.

The first key attribute of the individual organizational system is the use of evidence-based prevention and intervention practices. The critical need to use evidence-based prevention and intervention practices is punctuated by the fact that the major federal agencies (e.g., National Institute of Mental Health) and professional organizations (e.g., National Association for School Psychologists) have established criteria for determining whether a particular practice is evidence based or not. These criteria were generated on the basis of observations of schools' and social service agencies' tendencies to apply ineffective practices.

Second, a common language or conceptual model with which to view problem behaviors should be established. It is difficult to assess problem behaviors and to develop behavioral intervention plans to treat the problem behaviors if staff use different conceptual models. An effective conceptual model for viewing problem behaviors should incorporate principles and concepts that are easily understood. If the concepts are too complex, the model will be difficult to use with all staff in a school setting. The conceptual model should also lead naturally to school-based interventions. A conceptual model is of little use if it does not logically connect to variables that can be manipulated in a school setting. Finally, the conceptual model should be legally defensible. Courts will look closely to see if schools have applied evidence-based processes and practices if a legal issue should arise in the treatment of a student. We believe that the only conceptual model that meets all three of these criteria is the one used as the foundation for BASE—the behavioral model. Some of the more common conceptual models, such as psychoanalytic (i.e., behaviors are the function of the constant interplay of unconscious processes within the individual), psychoeducational (i.e., similar to the psychoanalytic except the focus of treatment is on the volitional aspect [ego] of the unconscious processes), and control theories (i.e., behaviors are internally controlled and not influenced by external events or individuals), do not meet the criteria for an effective conceptual model (Gottfredson et al., 2000; Zirpoli & Melloy, 2001).

The third attribute of the individual organizational system is an established behavioral support team that is easy to access and is not seen solely as a step in the special education referral process. The team should be integrated into the organizational structure of the school to ensure easy and efficient access. Behavioral support teams are composed of teachers, administrators, and support staff who possess the knowledge and competencies necessary to address complex student problems. The team works collaboratively with teachers to analyze the problem and to design interventions and supports to improve student outcomes (academic and social). The team should use functional behavioral analysis processes and procedures. Additionally, the team should receive ongoing staff development to expand their capacity to address such behaviors.

Fourth, community resources should be used in individual organization systems. The educational focus and training in today's schools often limits their ability to respond to the most serious needs of some students. Thus, schools must establish collaborative relationships and procedures to access and collaborate with those agencies in the community charged with meeting the more complex needs of student and family systems. Procedures should be developed to improve communication and networking among social service agencies, law enforcement, the juvenile justice system, and other relevant community resources. Community resources can be used to provide a wide range of services to students and families that extend beyond the boundaries of the school, from mentoring programs to multisystemic approaches to therapy.

Academic Support System

The academic support system is defined as the integration of evidence-based academic skill support programs in three key skill areas (i.e., beginning reading, language, and mathematics) at the secondary (for students who are at risk of developing learning problems) and tertiary (for students who are experiencing learning problems) levels. The secondary and tertiary academic programs should build on the existing primary universal curriculum delivered to all students. In other words, the secondary- and tertiary-level programs should align and fit contextually within the primary universal curriculum program provided all students. Furthermore, the interventions should address key skill areas in reading, language, and mathematics, rather than the entire set of skills.

There are three key attributes of the academic support organizational system: (a) evidence-based secondary- and tertiary-level curricula and instructional procedures; (b) coordinated and integrated primary, secondary, and tertiary curriculum and instructional procedures; and (c) early identification procedures. The first attribute of the academic support organizational system is the use of evidence-based secondary- and tertiary-level curricula and instructional practices. Selecting such a curriculum and practices is critical because children with or at risk of learning problems need intensive sequenced instruction.

The second attribute of the academic support organizational system is the integration and coordination of the primary-, secondary-, and tertiary-level curricula and instructional practices. The overall goal of establishing these three levels of curricula and instruction practices is to provide an interconnected continuum of support for students with or at risk of learning problems, rather than offering distinct and unrelated approaches. In other words, the secondary- and tertiary-level curricula and instruction practices should target key skill areas necessary for students to access the primary-level curriculum.

The final attribute of the academic support organizational system is the early identification of students with or at risk of learning problems. The goal of early identification is to prevent the emergence of learning problems in the case of at-risk students and to provide immediate support to those already possessing problems. Gated assessment processes are commonly used to identify students with or at risk of learning and behavior problems. These processes consist of a series of assessments designed to systematically screen out such students (Walker & Severson, 1990). Each assessment level (or "gate") consists of a finer grained assessment. Initial gates are very broad and will include many students. Subsequent gates are finer grained and pass only those students potentially at risk. The process should be designed to be simple, efficient, and quick so as to impose as little as possible on teachers.

SCHOOL EVALUATION RUBRIC

The SER is a continuum-of-progress evaluation rubric that describes three levels of implementation (beginning, developing, and exemplary) for each of the six organizational systems. An abbreviated version (service gap analysis and strategic planning forms are removed) of the SER is given in Appendex 18.A (a complete version of the SER is available from the first author). The goal of the SER strategic planning process is to ensure that all six organizational systems are exemplary (i.e., include all of the key attributes associated with each system). A description of the key attributes of each of the organizational systems is detailed in the next sections. Studying the three levels of implementation (i.e., beginning, developing, exemplary) detailed in the abbreviated SER will help us to understand the attributes of each of the six organizational systems.

ADMINISTERING THE SER

Overcoming Barriers

The SER is designed to help schools overcome several barriers that often arise in the process of developing a comprehensive schoolwide discipline program. First, the SER is designed to overcome the tendency of schools to adopt a narrow focus when developing a three-tiered schoolwide program. The SER enables schools to systematically evaluate each of the six interrelated organizational systems that underlie a safe and disciplined school environment. Evaluating each of the six systems allows schools to create a more comprehensive schoolwide discipline program.

The second barrier that the SER is designed to overcome is the susceptibility of schools to adopt practices that have little or no empirical support or their failure to apply practices in their particular context. The SER supports data-based decision making regarding the current status and analysis of service gaps relative to key attributes of the six organizational systems identified earlier. The organizational systems are designed to support staff in the implementation of safe school practices, which are designed to maximize student learning. Additionally, the consensus-based strategic planning process embedded within the SER ensures that the adopted policies and practices are contextually fitted to the school.

Third, the SER is designed to overcome the time constraints associated with developing a schoolwide discipline program. The SER diminishes time constraints in several ways. First, the SER provides schools a clear and efficient structure for developing, implementing, maintaining, and evaluating a schoolwide discipline program. Schools do not have to spend extensive time thinking through the process they will use to develop, implement, maintain, and evaluate their program. Second, the SER is an effective staff development tool. Schools do not have to commit extensive time toward staff development activities or rely on outside expertise to develop, implement, maintain, and evaluate a schoolwide discipline program because all staff become fluent in the key attributes of effective schoolwide discipline programs as they use the SER. Finally, the SER serves to improve and maintain the schoolwide discipline program over time. The readministration process embedded within the SER not only sets the context for the continual refinement of the program but also its renewal by providing a natural context for reeducating existing staff and educating new individuals each academic year.

Finally, the SER is designed to overcome the conflicts that often arise with the development of a schoolwide discipline program. Discipline-related issues in schools are often difficult because staff have different levels of expertise, perspectives, and commitment. In addition to ensuring that all staff understand the key attributes of an effective schoolwide discipline program, which in itself reduces conflict, the SER is a truly bottom-up process that helps build a common focus and commitment among staff.

Implementing the SER

Numerous data collection procedures can be used to assess school environments. Thus, the SER and the other data collection procedures presented here are not exhaustive, and there will be times when additional procedures (e.g., observations, staff surveys, inspection of formal disciplinary referrals) should be used along with the SER.

It is important to preface our description of how to administer the SER by noting that basic management responsibilities, such as open communication, fair assignment of duties, and access to appropriate instructional materials, must be attended to prior to the deeper discussion evoked by implementing the SER. Problems with inappropriate instructional materials, learning environments, or a school culture that is unwilling to accept the diversity and individuality of the students (especially those who exhibit problem behaviors) and families all take precedence over high-level discussions about creating a safe and disciplined school environment designed to maximize student learning.

This is not to say that implementing the SER and developing an action plan to create a safe school environment requires a perfectly functioning leadership and management system to move forward. Indeed, many of the problems just identified may be detected through the administration and implementation of the SER. Nevertheless, such problems must be addressed before individuals of the school community can develop confidence that the school leadership has the ability to tackle the problems presented by students who exhibit problem behaviors.

The SER incorporates a four-stage strategic planning model to develop, implement, maintain, and evaluate a comprehensive safe school plan that encompasses the six organizational systems. Positive teaching and learning environments are maximized when a school is exemplary in all six systems. This model includes a set of concepts common to most strategic planning models. The strategic planning model features the following stages:

1. consensus-based administration of the SER (identification of problems and service gap analysis);
2. formation of leadership team (guide the development, implementation, maintenance, and evaluation of the schoolwide discipline program);
3. development and implementation of safe school action plan (practices to fill gaps in current services); and
4. monitoring effectiveness (ongoing evaluation of the effectiveness and refinement of the organizational systems).

The administration of the SER is truly a bottom-up process in which all staff have input into the development of the schoolwide discipline program from the beginning. The first stage in the strategic planning model involves the consensus-based administration of the continuum-of-progress evaluation rubric within the SER. In the second stage, a leadership team is formed to guide the development, implementation, maintenance, and effectiveness of the safe school action plan. The remaining two stages focus on the development, implementation, and maintenance of the plan, and the evaluation of it, respectively.

The SER presents each of the six organizational systems in sequence to facilitate its use (see Appendix 18.A). The continuum-of-progress rubric for each organizational system and associated service gap analysis form are presented in sequence. The rubrics and associated service gap analysis forms are used in Stage 1. The leadership team (formed in Stage 2) uses the final page of the SER to develop and implement the schoolwide discipline program in Stage 3. The SER is readministered on a regular basis in Stage 4.

Stage 1: Consensus-Based Administration of the SER

A consensus-based administration process is used to identify the current status (i.e., beginning, developing, and exemplary) of and service gaps for each of the six organizational systems. The goal of the consensus-based administration process is not only to ensure that everyone has input but also to increase staff's understanding of the key attributes associated with each of the six organizational systems.

A four-step process is used for each organizational system in Stage 1. First, a staff member presents a brief overview of the key attributes of one of the organization systems. Second, small groups study the continuum-of-progress rubric for each of the six organizational systems and achieve consensus on the current status (beginning, developing, and exemplary) of each one. Third, each group completes the associated service gap analysis form and preliminary action plan (i.e., potential solutions to fill the service gap needs) associated with each of the organizational systems. Finally, the results from each group are reported and discussed by the larger group until they achieve consensus on the current status of and service gaps for each organizational system. The potential solutions are not typically discussed at this time. Rather, the leadership team will consider potential solutions suggested by staff when developing the schoolwide discipline program.

Stage 2: Formation of High-Status Leadership Team

As mentioned, a leadership team should be formed to guide the development, implementation, maintenance, and evaluation of the schoolwide discipline program. The formation of this team and the designation of its responsibilities are important prerequisites to the success of the program. Although the committee will direct and guide the development, implementation, and evaluation process, the schoolwide discipline program is a joint venture, with staff at all levels working together. Achieving consensus on all aspects of the plan is essential to ensuring its implementation and maintenance.

The overall responsibility of the leadership team is to direct the development, implementation, maintenance, and evaluation of the schoolwide discipline program action plan. The following are the responsibilities and general activities of the committee: to attend all planning meetings; to develop, implement, maintain, and revise the schoolwide discipline program; to evaluate new or revised components of the schoolwide discipline program; to communicate with staff members regarding the activities of the committee; and to conduct staff meetings to ensure the implementation and maintenance of the schoolwide discipline program. In addition, team members must be persistent in their efforts because effecting school change may be slow, can be intense, and may result in heated exchanges. Committee members must push through these dialogues in a positive and constructive manner.

Stage 3: Development, Implementation, and Maintenance of the Schoolwide Discipline Program

The leadership team uses the results obtained during Stage 1 to develop a strategic schoolwide discipline program. The results obtained in Stage 1 provide direction and momentum that the leadership team can use to develop the plan. Planning for a safe and disciplined school environment requires priority attention above and beyond the routine planning process that is common to schools. Schools must change current practices; these are not always easy to change. The leadership team may be faced with the following three challenges in relation to the planning process.

1. Adequate time is unavailable for planning due to the demand for immediate change.
2. Staff may pressure the leadership team to designate a significant amount of time toward immediate planning for a particularly troubling group of students.
3. The school may not have adequate resource support readily available to implement all of the necessary practices.

Although the total planning, implementation, maintenance, and evaluation process may seem overwhelming, the leadership team can respond to these demands in a prudent manner by prioritizing and working toward acquiring the resources necessary to implement the safe school plan. For example, schools commonly focus on the first four organizational systems (i.e., leadership, schoolwide, nonclassroom, and classroom) in the first year. Making adjustments to achieve exemplary status in these systems, in most cases, does not require extensive resources and time and enables the leadership team to actively engage the entire staff in a proactive manner. Additionally, the leadership team should use an efficient team meeting format to reduce the time demands associated with the planning, implementation, maintenance, and evaluation process.

The leadership team uses a three-step process during Stage 3. First, the overall consensus on the current status (beginning, developing, and exemplary) of each of the organizational systems is formally recorded. This baseline information provides the team with a basis for assessing their progress toward achieving a schoolwide discipline program that is exemplary in each of the organizational systems. Second, the leadership team should record the results of the service gap analysis and prioritize those gaps that are most important. Prioritizing the service gaps will enable the leadership team to develop a long-term strategic plan that will not overwhelm the staff. Third, the leadership team develops a strategic plan to guide the development and implementation of the schoolwide discipline program. The plan of action form requires the team to identify the actions and associated strategies to achieve them. Additionally, the team identifies a target date, the resources necessary, person(s) responsible, and evaluation procedure. The plan of action form included in the SER helps by providing a framework for making all decisions, facilitating teamwork through the development and implementation of the plan, providing effective communication for sharing progress in achieving goals, providing a mechanism for analyzing and enhancing the coordination of resources, focusing efforts on specific goals and objectives, and serving as a tool for measuring and demonstrating effectiveness.

Stage 4: Monitoring Effectiveness

The leadership team readministers the SER and collects any other data (e.g., administrative contacts, academic performance, attendance) necessary to evaluate the effectiveness of and to refine the schoolwide discipline program. In addition to serving an evaluative function, the readministration of the SER serves to reeducate existing staff and to educate new staff on the elements of the schoolwide discipline program. The dialogue associated with the readministration process provides a natural context for clarifying the elements of the schoolwide discipline program and provides corrective feedback and associated changes.

The leadership team uses the same steps detailed in Stage 1 to evaluate the schoolwide discipline program. Staff's views of the current status of each of the organizational systems are compared to those obtained with the previous administration of the SER. Additionally, the readministration process will provide staff an opportunity to identify additional service gaps and potential solutions. The leadership team then uses the same process detailed under Stage 3 to refine the schoolwide discipline program. The overall goal is to achieve an exemplary status in each of the organization systems.

SUMMARY

Effective schoolwide discipline programs that support the identification and implementation of evidence-based secondary- and tertiary-level interventions represent one of the more important educational advances that have occurred in recent years. For the most part, traditional approaches to school discipline are based on punitive and exclusionary policies developed in the early

1900s, when schools were oriented toward academically inclined students. Success in school was not necessary to obtain a job. Times have changed, however. Without a high school education today, prospects for life success tend to be very poor. Although times have changed, schools have not followed suit. As a result, administrators and teachers often fail to develop a coordinated schoolwide discipline program that considers the full range of factors necessary to provide children a predictable, positive, and supportive learning environment. Failure to develop an effective schoolwide discipline program often leads to lists of prohibitive rules and a series of increasingly severe punishments for the violators of these rules, with little regard to their long-term effect on children.

BASE provides schools a systematic process with which to apply academic and behavioral interventions and supports across all of the school organizational systems. The goal of BASE is to apply a behaviorally based systems approach to enhance the capacity of schools, families, and communities to design school environments that improve the fit or link between evidence-based practices and the environments in which teaching and learning occur. The practices and processes of BASE emphasize the systematic examination of the environments in which academic problem behaviors are observed; development of proactive evidence-based interventions and supports; and the importance of the acceptability of procedures and outcomes by the school staff, families, and community members.

The SER, which incorporates the key attributes of the six organizational systems of the school, provides staff with an efficient process from which to develop, implement, maintain, and evaluate a schoolwide discipline program that supports the identification and implementation of evidence-based secondary- and tertiary-level interventions and supports. The SER serves several important functions. First, the SER enables schools to systematically evaluate each of the six interrelated organizational systems that underlie a schoolwide discipline program (i.e., leadership, schoolwide, nonclassroom, classroom, and individual). Evaluating each of the six systems naturally leads schools to create a more comprehensive program.

Second, the SER supports data-based decision making regarding the current status, analysis of service gaps, and evaluation of the implementation and maintenance of practices in each of the six organizational areas. The organizational systems are designed to support staff in the implementation of interventions and supports, which are designed to positively influence students' behaviors. Additionally, the strategic planning process embedded with the SER ensures that the policies and practices adopted are contextually fitted to the school.

Third, the SER provides schools with an efficient process from which to develop, implement, maintain, and evaluate a schoolwide discipline program. The SER also serves to promote, improve, and maintain the schoolwide discipline program over time. The readministration process embedded within the SER sets the context for the continual refinement of the program and also facilitates its renewal by providing a natural context for reeducating existing staff and educating new individuals each academic year.

Finally, the SER reduces conflicts that often arise among staff when they are developing a schoolwide discipline program. The SER reduces such conflict because it ensures that all staff understand and subscribe to the key attributes of an effective schoolwide discipline program. The SER is also a truly bottom-up process that helps build a common focus and commitment among staff.

APPENDIX 18.A

School Evaluation Rubric (SER)

Leadership Team To Guide the Strategic Planning Process

This area of the SER examines the school's role in establishing a leadership team that implements the strategic planning process. This process focuses on establishing positive teaching and learning environments within all systems in the school: schoolwide (i.e., all students, all staff, and all settings); non-classroom (i.e., particular times or places where supervision is emphasized); classroom (i.e., instructional settings), individual student support (i.e., specific supports for students who engage in chronic problem behaviors); and academic support (i.e., early identification and academic support in key skill areas). Specifically, this area involves the school's development of a leadership team that is capable of improving the school's (a) vision and organization; (b) stakeholder involvement and communication; (c) allocation of resources (human, fiscal, and time); (d) development, implementation, and maintenance of systems to support positive teaching and learning environments; and (e) continual self-assessment.

Describe how the school's leadership team support a focus on establishing positive teaching and learning environments within all systems of the school: schoolwide, nonclassroom, classroom, individual student support, and academic support.

Beginning

Leadership and decision making are in the hands of a few people and are not fully supported by the administration. Stakeholder involvement in major decisions and activities is limited or nonexistent. Data are not examined to determine the school's strengths and areas for development within the systems in the school (i.e., schoolwide, classroom, nonclassroom, and individual support systems). There is no common language used to discuss the strategic planning process.

Developing

Leadership and decision making now include representatives of some stakeholders and are supported by the administration. The system is beginning to focus on establishing positive teaching and learning environments within some of the systems in the school (e.g., classroom system is in place but others are not). Some data are examined to determine the school's strengths and areas for development within some of the systems in the school. A common language is instituted to facilitate clear discussions on the strategic planning process.

Exemplary

Leadership and decision making representing all key stakeholders are well established and are fully supported by the administration. The system works to maintain the school's focus on establishing positive teaching and learning environments within all systems of the school. The leadership team includes general and special educators, a school counselor or psychologist, an administrator, someone with in-depth knowledge of behavioral interventions and supports, and parent(s). Data are examined to determine the school's strengths and areas for development within all systems of the school. One common language is used to discuss the strategic planning process.

Schoolwide System

The schoolwide organizational system is defined as involving all students and all staff in all settings within a school. Specifically, this area involves (a) schoolwide guidelines for success, (b) strategies for teaching expectations, (c) clearly defined discipline procedures, (d) clearly defined crisis response plans (threats, actual events, classroom, and individual), and (e) continual self-assessment.

Describe the current schoolwide system in place at your school in terms of schoolwide guidelines for success, teaching, discipline, and continuous assessment.

Beginning

Schoolwide guidelines for success that provide a framework from which to create a common culture and language, as well as linkages across systems, are not clearly articulated. Teachers and staff are able to state guidelines for success, but these differ from person to person. Teachers and staff do not know what behaviors they should manage and what behaviors the office should manage. There are no procedures for emergency or dangerous situations. Teachers, staff, and students are not systematically taught the schoolwide guidelines for success and discipline procedures. Assessment of the schoolwide system does not occur. There is little or no feedback given to the school staff.

Developing

Guidelines for success are articulated. Teachers and staff are able to state the guidelines for success but do not use them or have a uniform interpretation of them. Some teachers and staff know what behaviors they should manage and what behaviors the office should manage. Options are being developed for emergency or dangerous situations. Schoolwide guidelines for success are reviewed by school staff and students but are not taught systematically. Some assessment of the schoolwide system occurs. Some feedback is given to the school staff when needed.

Exemplary

The school has a small number (e.g., 3–5) of clearly stated guidelines for success that are linked across systems. Teachers and staff are able to state and use the guidelines for success and interpret them uniformly. Teachers and staff know what behaviors they should manage and what behaviors the office should manage. Procedures are in place to address emergency or dangerous situations. Teachers, staff, and students are systematically taught the school-wide guidelines for success and discipline procedures. Booster training activities for students are conducted when needed (e.g., after holiday breaks). Continuous assessment of the schoolwide system is conducted. Feedback is given to school staff on a regular basis (monthly or quarterly).

Nonclassroom Organizational System

The nonclassroom organizational system is defined as particular times or places where supervision is emphasized (e.g., hallways, cafeteria, playground, bus). Specifically, this area involves (a) nonclassroom behavioral expectations, (b) strategies for teaching expectations, (c) clearly defined discipline procedures, (d) ecological arrangements, and (e) continual self-assessment.

Describe the current nonclassroom system in place at your school in terms of nonclassroom behavior expectations, teaching, discipline, ecological arrangements, and continuous assessment.

Beginning

There are no stated behavioral expectations for the nonclassroom settings or they are unrelated to the schoolwide ones. Only selected staff are involved in the management of student behavior in nonclassroom settings. Little or no training is provided to staff on how to actively supervise (teach students the behavioral expectations, move, scan, positively engage) students. Teachers, staff, and students are not systematically taught the behavioral expectations. Discipline procedures for nonclassroom problem behaviors may exist; however, they remain fairly ineffective. Ecological arrangements (physical arrangements and scheduling) have not been examined closely to reduce wait time, decrease the density of students, and improve safety. Assessment of the nonclassroom settings does not occur. There is little to no feedback given to the school staff.

Developing

The stated schoolwide behavioral expectations apply to nonclassroom settings. Only selected staff are involved in the management of student behavior in nonclassroom settings, but they are supported by some staff (e.g., assist in supervision when needed). Some training is provided to staff on how to actively supervise students. Behavioral expectations are reviewed by school staff and students but are not taught systematically. Some booster training is provided to school staff and students. Discipline procedures for nonclassroom problem behaviors exist; however, staff are not systematically taught how to use them. Ecological arrangements have been considered but not systematically examined. Some assessment of the nonclassroom settings occurs. Some feedback is given to the school staff when needed.

Exemplary

The stated schoolwide behavioral expectations (3–5) apply to nonclassroom settings. All staff are involved (to some degree) in the management of student behavior in nonclassroom settings. Training is provided to selected staff on how to actively supervise students. Teachers, staff, and students are systematically taught the nonclassroom behavioral expectations. Booster training is provided to school staff and students. Discipline procedures for nonclassroom problem behaviors exist, and staff are systematically taught how to use them. Ecological arrangements have been adjusted to maximize positive student behaviors. Continuous assessment of the nonclassroom settings is conducted. Feedback is given to school staff on a regular basis (monthly or quarterly).

Classroom Organizational System

The classroom organizational system is defined as instructional settings in which teachers supervise and teach groups of students. Specifically, this area involves a school's (a) focus on instruction, (b) classroom behavioral expectations and routines, (c) consistent discipline procedures used by teachers, (d) access to assistance, and (e) continual self-assessment.

Describe the current classroom system in place at your school in terms of classroom behavior expectations, teaching, discipline, and continuous assessment.

Beginning

There is not a clear curriculum focus on achieving student outcomes. There is variability across teachers in the degree to which classroom behavioral expectations and routines are established. Behavioral expectations are not linked to schoolwide ones. Little training is provided or made available to teachers on classroom management. Discipline procedures for classroom problem behaviors may exist; however, they remain fairly ineffective and there is a great deal of variability across teachers. Teachers have few, if any, opportunities for access to assistance and recommendations (observation, instruction, and coaching). Assessment of the classroom system does not occur. There is little to no feedback given to teachers.

Developing

There is a clear curriculum focus on achieving student outcomes in some areas but not others (e.g., strong focus in reading but weak in mathematics). Most teachers establish clear classroom behavioral expectations and routines; however, the behavioral expectations are not linked to the schoolwide ones. Some training is provided or made available to teachers on classroom management. Discipline procedures for classroom problem behaviors exist and are fairly effective; however, there is variability across teachers. Teachers have access to assistance and recommendations (observation, instruction, and coaching); however, it is generally ineffective or viewed as a step in the special education referral process. Some assessment of the classroom system occurs. Some feedback is given to teachers when needed.

Exemplary

There is a clear curriculum focus on achieving student outcomes in all areas. All teachers establish clear classroom behavioral expectations and routines, and the behavioral expectations are linked to the schoolwide ones. Training is provided or made available to teachers on classroom management. Discipline procedures for classroom problem behaviors exist and are effective, and there is consistency across teachers. Teachers have access to assistance and recommendations (observation, instruction, and coaching), and it is generally effective. Continuous assessment of the classroom system is conducted. Feedback is given to teachers on a regular basis (monthly or quarterly).

Individual Support System

The individual organizational system is defined as specific supports for students who are, or are at risk of, experiencing school failure. Specifically, this area involves a school's (a) data-based prevention and intervention procedures for students at risk of school failure, (b) common solutions-focused language used by all staff, (c) established behavioral support team (not seen as a step in the special education referral process), (d) procedures for providing intervention and supports to students who are experiencing school failure, and (e) continual self-assessment.

Describe the current individual system in place at your school in terms of data-based prevention and intervention procedures for students at risk of school failure, common solutions-focused language used by all staff, established behavioral support team, procedures for providing intervention and supports to students experiencing school failure, and continual self-assessment.

Beginning

The school has not developed specific prevention and intervention procedures for students at risk of school failure (e.g., one-to-one tutoring program in reading, mentor program). There is not a common solutions-oriented language (functional behavioral analysis) used by school staff to guide the development of interventions and supports for students who are experiencing school failure. The school has no or an ineffective behavior support team to assist staff in developing, implementing, and evaluating interventions and supports for students who are experiencing school failure.

Developing

The school has developed some prevention and intervention procedures for students at risk of school failure, but no data have been used to guide their development and implementation. Some staff use a common solutions-oriented language to guide the development of interventions and supports for students who are experiencing school failure. The school has a relatively effective behavior support team to assist staff in developing, implementing, and evaluating interventions and supports for students who are experiencing school failure, but it is viewed as a step in the special education referral process.

Exemplary

The school has developed prevention and intervention procedures for students at risk of school failure. A data-based decision-making process has been conducted to guide the development and implementation of the procedures to ensure that they meet the specific needs of students. All staff use a common solutions-oriented language to guide the development of interventions and supports for students who are experiencing school failure. The school has an effective behavior support team to assist staff in developing, implementing, and evaluating interventions and supports for students who are experiencing school failure. The team is not necessarily viewed as part of the special education referral process.

Academic Support System

The academic support system is defined as the integration of evidence-based academic skills support programs in key skill areas (i.e., language, reading, and mathematics) at the secondary (for students who are at risk of developing learning problems) and tertiary (for students who are experiencing academic failure) levels. Specifically, this area involves a school's (a) strategies for the early identification of learning problems in language, reading, and mathematics; (b) curriculum and instruction procedures in key skill areas (e.g., code-based instruction in reading) that enhance (not replace) the primary-level ones (curriculum provided to all students); (c) tertiary (not necessarily special education) curriculum and instruction procedures in key skill areas that enhance or replace the primary-level ones for students experiencing significant learning problems; and (d) continual self-assessment.

Describe the current academic support system in place at your school in terms of (a) specific secondary- and tertiary-level curricula and instruction procedures for students at risk of or who are experiencing learning problems, respectively, and (b) continual self-assessment.

Beginning

The school has not developed specific secondary and tertiary curricula procedures for students at risk of or who are experiencing learning problems, respectively. There are no early identification procedures in place to identify students in need of academic supports.

Developing

The school has developed some secondary- or tertiary-level curricula and instruction procedures for students at risk of or who are experiencing learning problems, respectively. The school provides secondary or tertiary curricula and instruction procedures in some areas, but they are delivered only to students formally classified as having a disability or do not fully address the need. The curricula and instruction procedures are not connected or integrated with one another. Procedures for identifying students in need of academic supports are in place, but they are part of the special education referral process.

Exemplary

The school has developed, coordinated, and integrated secondary- and tertiary-level curricula and instruction procedures for students at risk of or who are experiencing learning problems, respectively. The school provides evidence-based secondary- or tertiary-level curricula and instruction procedures in language, reading, and mathematics. The curricula and instruction procedures are connected and integrated with one another to improve their effectiveness. Procedures for identifying students in need of academic supports are in place and are not necessarily part of the special education referral process.

REFERENCES

Baum, D. D., Duffelmeyer, F. A., & Geelan, M. (1988). Resource teacher perceptions of the prevalence of social dysfunction among students with learning disabilities. *Journal of Learning Disabilities, 21,* 180–194.

Colvin, G., Kameenui, E. J., & Sugai, G. (1993). Reconceptualizing behavior management and school-wide discipline in general education. *Education and Treatment of Children, 16,* 361–381.

Costello, E. J., Angold, A., Burns, B. J., Stangl, D. K., Tweed, D. L., Erkanli, A., et al. (1996). The Great Smoky Mountains Study of youth: Goals, design, methods, and the prevalence of DSM–III–R disorders. *Archives of General Psychiatry, 53,* 1129–1136.

Cotton, K. (1990). *School improvement series, close-up #9: School wide and classroom discipline.* Portland, OR: Northwest Regional Educational Laboratory.

Edgar, E., & Levine, P. (1987). *Special education students in transition: Washington state data 1976–1986.* Seattle: University of Washington, Experimental Education Unit.

Furlong, M. J., & Morrison, R. L. (1994). School violence to school safety: Reframing the issue for school psychologists. *School Psychology Review, 23,* 236–256.

Gottfredson, G. D., Gottfredson, D. C., Czeh, E. R., Canter, D., Crosse, S. B., & Hantman, H. (2000). *Final report: National study of delinquency prevention in schools.* Ellicott City, MD: Gottfredson Associates.

Hawkins, J. E., Farrington, D. P., & Catalano, R. F. (1998). Reducing violence through the schools. In D. S. Eliot, B. A. Hamburg, & K. R. Williams (Eds.), *Violence in American schools: A new perspective* (pp. 188–216). Cambridge, England: Cambridge University Press.

Herrenkohl, T., Maguin, E., Hill, K., Hawkins, J., Abbott, R., & Catalano, R. (1998). *Childhood and adolescent predictors of youth violence.* Seattle: University of Washington, Seattle Social Development Project.

Huizinga, D., & Jakob-Chien, C. (1998). The contemporary co-occurrence of serious and violent juvenile offenders and other problem behaviors. In R. Loeber & D. Farrington (Eds.), *Serious and violent juvenile offenders: Risk factors and successful interventions* (pp. 47–67). Thousand Oaks, CA: Sage.

Lipsey, M. W., & Derzon, J. (1998). Predictors of violent or serious delinquency in adolescence and early adulthood: A synthesis of longitudinal research. In R. Loeber & D. P. Farrington (Eds.), *Serious and violent juvenile offenders: Risk factors and successful interventions* (pp. 86–105). Thousand Oaks, CA: Sage.

Maguin, E., & Loeber, R. (1996). Academic performance and delinquency. In M. Tonry (Ed.), *Crime and justice: An annual review of the research* (Vol. 20, pp. 145–264). Chicago: University of Chicago Press.

McEvoy, A., & Welker, R. (2000). Antisocial behavior, academic failure, and school climate. *Journal of Emotional and Behavioral Disorders, 8,* 130–140.

Moffitt, T. (1994). Adolescence-limited and life-course-persistent antisocial behavior: A developmental taxonomy. *Psychological Review, 100,* 674–701.

Neel, R., Meadow, N., Levine, P., & Edgar, E. (1988). What happens after special education: A statewide follow-up study of secondary students who have behavioral disorders. *Behavioral Disorders, 13,* 209–216.

Nelson, J. R. (1996). Designing schools to meet the needs of students who exhibit disruptive behavior. *Journal of Emotional and Behavioral Disorders, 4,* 147–161.

Nelson, J. R., Martella, R. C., & Marchand-Martella, N. E. (2002). Maximizing student learning: The effects of a comprehensive school-based program for preventing disruptive behaviors. *Journal of Emotional and Behavioral Disorders, 10,* 136–148.

Nelson, J. R., & Ohlund, B. J. (1999). *School Evaluation Rubric.* Tempe: Arizona State University.

Reid, J. (1993). Prevention of conduct disorder before and after school entry: Relating interventions to developmental findings. *Development and Psychopathology, 5*(1/2), 243–262.

Rose, L. C., & Gallup, A. M. (2001). Thirty-third annual Phi Delta Kappa/Gallup poll of the public's attitude toward public education. *Phi Delta Kappan, 83,* 41–48.

Sugai, G., & Horner, R. H. (1999). Discipline and behavioral support: Preferred processes and practices. *Effective School Practices, 17,* 10–22.

Sugai, G., Sprague, J. R., Horner, R. H., & Walker, H. M. (2000). Preventing school violence: The use of office discipline referrals to assess and monitor schoolwide discipline intervention. *Journal of Emotional and Behavioral Disorders, 8,* 94–112.

U.S. Department of Health and Human Services. (1999). *Mental health: A report of the Surgeon General.* Washington, DC: Author.

Vadasy, P. F., Jenkins, J. R., Antil, L. R., Wayne, S. K., & O'Connor, R. E. (1997). The effectiveness of one-to-one tutoring by community tutors for at-risk beginning readers. *Learning Disability Quarterly, 2,* 202–216.

Wagner, M. (1992). Long-term outcomes of transition. Reported in *Grants and Contracts Weekly.*

Wagner, M., & Shaver, D. (1989). *Educational programs and achievements of secondary special education students: Findings from the National Longitudinal Transition Study.* Menlo Park, CA: SRI International.

Walker, H. M., Horner, R. H., Sugai, G., Bullis, M., Sprague, J. R., Bricker, D., et al. (1996). Integrated approaches to preventing antisocial behavior patterns among school-age children and youth. *Journal of Emotional and Behavioral Disorders, 4,* 193–256.

Walker, H., & Severson, H. (1990). *Systematic Screening for Behavior Disorders* (SSBD). Longmont, CA: Sopris West.

Zirpoli, T. J., & Melloy, K. J. (2001). *Behavior management: Applications for teachers and parents* (3rd ed.) Upper Saddle River, NJ: Merrill.

Achievement and Emotional Disturbance

Academic Status and Intervention Research

Michael H. Epstein, J. Ron Nelson, Alexandra L. Trout, and Paul Mooney

In the U.S. Department of Education's definition of emotional disturbance (ED; 1997 amendments to the Individuals with Disabilities Education Act), academic problems are described as both a characteristic of the disorder (i.e., "an inability to learn that cannot be explained by intellectual, sensory, or health factors") and as a condition of the characteristic (i.e., "a condition ... which adversely affects educational performance"; 34 C.F.R. § 300.7(c)(4)). Highlighting the significant relationship between ED and academic functioning, the federal definition describes academic underachievement as a primary, significant marker of the disorder. An awareness of the occurrence of academic underachievement in students with ED is critical for policymakers, researchers, and practitioners who are responsible for making important decisions about educational and social resources, financial allocations, and teacher training programs for children and youth with ED. In addition, knowledge about specific academic interventions that have shown success with children with ED will allow for informed and effective academic programming designed to alleviate the patterns of educational underachievement that lead to lifelong academic and social deficits.

A primary focus of research and interventions for students with ED has been on managing or changing children's maladaptive social behaviors. Much less attention has been given to the significant relationship between ED and academic failure. In this chapter, we focus on the academic status and intervention research conducted with students with ED. Five general areas will be discussed. First, we briefly review the possible theoretical causal models for the linkage between ED[1] and academic underachievement. Second, we highlight child, family, school, and cultural risk factors for ED and academic

---

[1]The literature assessing the theories of possible causal pathways between academic underachievement and ED has focused on studies of students presenting only externalizing behavior problems. This literature describing these pathways (e.g., Hinshaw, 1992b) suggests that students with externalizing behaviors may exhibit different academic patterns of achievement than students with internalizing behavior disorders. However, the literature assessing the academic status and interventions for students with ED does not discriminate between students with externalizing and internalizing behavior disorders. Thus, it may be assumed that the status and intervention literature described in this chapter represents students presenting externalizing or internalizing behavior disorders.

451

underachievement. Third, we detail the prevalence, magnitude, and stability of academic deficits and variables (e.g., sampling) that may influence the estimates of underachievement. Fourth, we summarize the literature on academic interventions for students with ED. Finally, we discuss two bodies of evidence that can inform future educational research and practice related to students with ED.

POSSIBLE THEORETICAL CAUSAL MODELS

Determining the nature of the causal link between ED and academic underachievement could play a critical role in the design of intervention programs for students in this population. For example, if a clear direction were found between the failure to develop early academic skills and the ensuing development of ED, early interventions focusing on academics might prove to be more effective than those attempting to decrease or alter problem behavior. In contrast, if ED leads to academic underachievement, interventions focusing on behavior management might prove to be more effective. Olweus (1983) proposed four possible causal models for the linkage between ED and underachievement. The four models are discussed next and summarized in Figure 19.1.

According to Model 1, the poor grades–aggression hypothesis, academic underachievement is the causal factor for ED. Along with basic skills deficits (e.g., reading failure), this model suggests that other factors related to academic underachievement, such as student demoralization as a response to negative academic experiences and a heightened frustration level due to poor grades, negatively affect the student's behavior due to feelings of inadequate academic abilities. In turn, the student becomes aggressive and acts out with peers, teachers, and other school staff. Olweus (1983) described these students as the "loser in the system" (p. 354) because they cannot achieve in the schools due to the instructional demands necessary for academic success.

According to Model 2, the aggression–poor grades hypothesis, ED causes academic underachievement. In this model, children enter the educational

Model	Hypothesis	Directionality of Influence
1	Poor grades–aggression	Poor grades ----------------➤ Aggression
2	Aggression–poor grades	Aggression -------------------➤ Poor grades
3	Reciprocal causation	Academic failure ◄-------➤ ED
4	Spurious relationship	Underlying factors ---------➤ ED and academic failure

FIGURE 19.1. Possible theoretical causal models linking the co-occurrence of emotional disturbance (ED) and academic underachievement.

environment with preestablished problem behaviors that interfere with the attainment of early academic skills and school-related behaviors (e.g., ability to follow directions) necessary for academic success. Maladaptive and aggressive social behaviors are said to interfere with the student's desires or abilities to complete academic demands (e.g., homework, attention to task), and academic failure ensues. Moreover, the school personnel's response to the aggressive behaviors may result in negative feedback to the student, reflected by poor teacher ratings or grades.

According to Model 3, the reciprocal causation hypothesis, a reciprocal relationship exists between ED and academic underachievement. In this case, neither academic underachievement nor ED is assumed to be the precursor. In the reciprocal model, both pathological behaviors and academic failure occur simultaneously, with both factors directly influencing the degree of severity of the other.

According to Model 4, the spurious relationship hypothesis, underlying etiological factors cause the simultaneous occurrence of academic failure and ED. This model hypothesizes that a host of environmental and child-related characteristics (e.g., familial, socioeconomic status, intelligence, speech and language deficits) may precede the simultaneous occurrence of ED and academic underachievement. In this model, Olweus (1983) suggested that neither academic failure nor ED is present first; rather, both conditions occur as a result of previously established variables that influence the development of ED and academic underachievement.

The differences among the causal models suggest that the conditions under which the development of problem behavior and academic underachievement evolve may vary considerably. Generally, causal models are used for policy decisions, program design, and the making of decisive rulings about factors that may influence the phenomenon. However, due to the difficulty of assessing the hypothetical causes linking problem behavior and underachievement (e.g., costs of longitudinal studies, methodological issues), to date little research has been able to conclusively determine a consistent causal pathway (Hinshaw, 1992b; Lane, 1999). Thus, more accessible factors, such as risks, have been examined to determine their direct influence on the development of co-occurring underachievement and ED.

ETIOLOGICAL RISK FACTORS FOR ED AND UNDERACHIEVEMENT

Early behavioral characteristics (e.g., irritability, temperament), social interactions, and exposure to learning experiences influence the developing child and either promote or inhibit early school success. Children with ED generally contend with risk factors that limit their social and academic experiences. These risks include a host of child, family, school, and cultural variables, such as difficult temperament, harsh and coercive parenting, inadequate behavior management, and poverty (see Table 19.1; Hann & Borek, 1998; Hinshaw,

TABLE 19.1
Examples of Risk Factors Common to Students with Emotional Disturbance

Child	Family	School	Cultural
Biological factors (e.g., autism)	Maternal stress/depression	Insufficient training	Low socioeconomic status
Difficult temperament	Large families	High student–teacher ratios	High crime neighborhoods
Substance use	Divorce	Poor instruction	Negative peer relationships
Neuropsychological deficits (e.g., language impairments)	Antisocial parent/sibling	Maladaptive working conditions	Peer rejection
Antisocial	Ineffective behavior management	Poor behavior management	Cultural expectations
Academic deficits	Abuse	Inconsistent expectations	
Low intelligence	Harsh or coercive parenting	Little academic emphasis	

1992a; Huffman, Mehlinger, & Kerivan, 2000; Kauffman, 2001; Reid, Patterson, & Snyder, 2002; Wagner, 1995). For example, prenatal exposure to drugs or toxins increases the incidence of birth defects and damage to the nervous system of the child. This damage often results in delayed social, emotional, and academic development (Erickson, 1998; Osofsky & Thompson, 2000; Shonkoff & Meisels, 2000; Wicks-Nelson & Israel, 2003).

Familial influences, such as parental psychopathology (e.g., depression), inadequate communication methods, and maladaptive family functioning, have also been linked to the development of ED (Haggerty, Sherrod, Garmenzy, & Rutter, 1996; Shonkoff & Meisels, 2000). When children are raised in challenging family situations, maladaptive behaviors often become part of their repertoire and are evident in social relationships and behaviors with peers and teachers in the school. The school experiences of children also affect their academic success and social behaviors. For example, if the school curriculum fails to focus on functional academic and behavioral skills, the probability that the child will complete the task decreases, while problem behaviors increase (Kauffman, 2001). School demands that are functional, relevant, and worthwhile to the child increase the child's attention to the task and willingness to participate in classroom demands (Kauffman, 2001). Finally, cultural and socioeconomic (SES) factors have also been found to influence early experiences and later academic success. For instance, children raised in dangerous, low-SES neighborhoods often face more restrictions by their parents. These restrictions have been associated with increased levels of acting-out behavior, aggression, and low scores on measures of intelligence (Wicks-Nelson & Israel, 2003).

For decades, researchers have investigated the direct or indirect influence of these and other risk factors on children and youth with ED. Collectively, these risks have frequently been found to interfere with the development of the social behaviors and academic skills (e.g., following directions) necessary for academic success (Hinshaw, 1992a; Rock, Fessler, & Church, 1997). (For a more extensive discussion of the impact of risks on students with ED, see Erickson, 1998; Haggerty et al., 1996; Osofsky & Thompson, 2000; Shonkoff & Meisels, 2000; Wicks-Nelson & Israel, 2003.)

ACADEMIC STATUS OF CHILDREN AND YOUTH WITH ED

The academic status of children and youth with ED has been studied across a broad range of academic domains. However, very few studies have examined subjects such as oral expression (e.g., Barnes & Forness, 1982; Fessler, Rosenberg, & Rosenberg, 1991), history (e.g., Scruggs & Mastropieri, 1986), science (e.g., Scruggs & Mastropieri, 1986), and listening comprehension (e.g., Scruggs & Mastropieri, 1986). Therefore, we detail the academic underachievement of students with ED in three primary subject areas: reading, arithmetic, and written expression. The prevalence, magnitude, and stability of deficit within each of these areas will be discussed (see Table 19.2).

Reading

Prevalence
Prevalence rates of underachievement in reading for students with ED range from 31% to 81%, varying across samples, age, and dependent measures (Duchnowski, Johnson, Hall, Kutash, & Friedman, 1993; Forness, Bennett, & Tose, 1983; Glassberg, Hooper, & Mattison, 1999; Greenbaum et al., 1996; Kutash et al., 2000; Shimota, 1964; Silver et al., 1992; Stone & Rowley, 1964; Zimet & Farley, 1993). For example, Shimota studied the prevalence rates of reading deficits in 74 children with ED aged 13 to 15 placed in state hospitals. Using the California test bureau's norms to determine students' expected grade placement, Shimota described underachievement as scores falling 25% or more below normal. Of the 74 children, 31% presented some degree of

TABLE 19.2
Summary of Academic Deficits Described in the Status
Literature for Children and Youth with Emotional Disturbance

	Prevalence (%)	Magnitude (Years Behind)	Stability	
			Maintains	Increases
Reading	31–81	.53–2+	Yes	Yes
Arithmetic	42–93	1.0–2.0	Yes	Mixed
Written expression	50–54	.48–2.4	Yes	No[a]

[a] Only one study assessed the stability of deficit for written expression.

reading disability. In contrast, Duchnowski and colleagues (1993) studied 87 children aged 7 to 18 served in five community-based alternatives to residential treatment facilities across the country. The results revealed that 81% of the children's reading scores obtained from the *Wide Range Achievement Test* (WRAT; Jastak & Wilkinson, 1984) and the *Slosson Oral Reading Test* (Slosson, 1963) were below expected grade level.

Differences in sampling (e.g., age of students); criteria for underachievement (e.g., standardized reading score cutoffs, grade level, teacher identification); and sources of ratings (e.g., teacher ratings, formal diagnoses) may account for the range of deficits observed between samples of students (Forness et al., 1983; Hinshaw, 1992a). Moreover, the use of convenience sampling, which is common to the majority of studies assessing children with ED, may provide a limited overall picture of the reading skills of students with ED and may not be generalizable to the overall population.

Magnitude

Similar to prevalence, the magnitude of reading deficits for students with ED spans a wide range, from a low of .53 to a high of more than 2 grade levels behind same-age peers without disabilities (Coutinho, 1986; Cowen, Zax, Izzo, & Trost, 1965; Graubard, 1967; Greenbaum et al., 1996; Levy & Hobbes, 1989; Luebke, Epstein, & Cullinan, 1989; Motto & Lathan, 1966; Motto & Wilkins, 1968; Sullivan, 1926; Wagner, 1995; Wilson, Cone, Bradley, & Reese, 1986). For instance, in a sample of 68 students with ED, teacher reports of standardized test scores indicated that students as a whole performed 2.2 grades behind expected grade level (Wagner, 1995). In contrast, Wilson and colleagues (1986) revealed a .53 deficit between expected grade equivalent scores and actual grade level for 90 students with ED. It appears that external factors, such as sampling, may account for the differences in the magnitude of reading deficit. For instance, Wagner's sample of children with ED was nationally representative, whereas all the students in Wilson and colleagues' study were from one state.

Stability

Research on the stability of reading deficits has resulted in two major findings: (a) Reading deficits occur early in a child's academic career, and (b) deficits are persistent and are likely to increase with age. For example, Coutinho (1986) assessed the status of reading delays in students with ED to determine the trajectory of reading failure from elementary through senior high school. The *Stanford Achievement Test* (Madden & Gardner, 1972) and *Iowa Test of Basic Skills* (ITBS, 1996) reading scores of 45 secondary students (Grades 7–9 and 10–12) with ED were compared to the scores of 45 same-age peers without disabilities. Differences were revealed both between groups and across grade levels. Children with ED presented significant reading delays across all grade levels, with deficits increasing with each successive academic year. An initial difference of 1.5 to 2.0 grade-equivalency units behind at Grades 7 through 9 increased to almost 3.5 grade-equivalency units by Grades 10 through 12 (Coutinho, 1986). These differences reflect the fact that children with ED frequently fail to keep up with their same-age peers in reading as they progress throughout their education.

Arithmetic

Prevalence

Children with ED appear to evidence the most severe deficits in arithmetic (e.g., Epstein, Kinder, & Bursuck, 1989; Greenbaum et al., 1996). Prevalence estimates of arithmetic underachievement range from 42% to 93% (Duch-nowski et al., 1993; Fessler et al., 1991; Forness et al., 1983; Greenbaum et al., 1996; Silver et al., 1992; Stone & Rowley, 1964; Zimet & Farley, 1993). Zimet and Farley, for example, assessed the arithmetic performance of 131 children ages 6 to 14 enrolled in a psychoeducational day treatment facility for students with ED. Of the students presenting arithmetic deficits, 38% were considered moderately impaired, and the remaining 14% were considered to be severely deficient in arithmetic skills (Zimet & Farley, 1993). In contrast, Greenbaum and colleagues (1996) revealed much higher rates of arithmetic underachievement in children and youth diagnosed with ED who were served in either mental health or public school systems across six states. Their results revealed that 93% of the total 629 children and youth with ED presented deficits 1 year or more behind expected grade levels on scores obtained from the WRAT.

Magnitude

The magnitude of arithmetic underachievement in the ED population consistently ranges between 1 year and 2 years below grade level (Forness, Kavale, Guthrie, Scruggs, & Mastropieri, 1987; Luebke et al., 1989; Rosenblatt & Rosenblatt, 1999; Wagner, 1995). For example, in a study of 61 youth with ED, Rosenblatt and Rosenblatt found that the arithmetic skills as measured by scores on the WRAT were significantly below average, with mean scores 1.9 years below expected achievement. Similar deficits were revealed in Wagner's sample of the teacher-reported standardized achievement scores for 68 students with ED. Mean differences between expected ability and grade-level achievement revealed deficits of 1.8 years below expected ability (Wagner, 1995).

Stability

As with studies assessing the stability of reading failure, arithmetic achievement in the ED population does not appear to improve with age (Anderson, Kutash, & Duchnowski, 2001; Glassberg et al., 1999). However, mixed results have been found in studies assessing the increase in deficits over time. For example, Glassberg and colleagues studied the prevalence of arithmetic deficits in 233 students with ED across three age categories: ages 6 to 8, 9 to 11, and 12 to 16. Arithmetic deficits were apparent across all three age categories; however, children aged 6 to 8 scored significantly higher than those aged 12 to 16 (Glassberg et al., 1999). These results suggest that the arithmetic underachievement of students with ED increased with age. Anderson and colleagues (2001) found a different pattern of arithmetic underachievement. Scores obtained from standardized measures of achievement taken at two separate times (i.e., kindergarten and first grade, and fifth and sixth grades) revealed significant arithmetic deficits across both time periods. However, no age differences were revealed, suggesting that the deficits were constant and did not increase with age (Anderson et al., 2001).

Written Expression

Prevalence

Written expression (i.e., spelling, writing samples, and writing fluency) has received much less research attention than reading and arithmetic. Prevalence estimates for written expression deficits are generally around 50% (Forness et al., 1983). For example, Zimet and Farley (1993) reported that 54% of 131 school-age students with ED have at least a moderate degree of deficit on standardized measures of written expression. Forness and colleagues (1983) reported similar estimates in 92 students aged 9 to 13 with ED. Specifically, on standardized achievement tests, 6.5% of the students with ED presented moderate (.5–1 year behind) and 46.7% presented severe (more than 1 year behind) levels of written expression underachievement.

Magnitude

The magnitude of underachievement in written expression ranges from .48 to 2.4 years below expected grade level (Forness et al., 1983; Luebke et al., 1989; Rosenblatt & Rosenblatt, 1999; Wilson et al., 1986). For example, standardized scores of 92 students with ED 6 to 13 years of age enrolled in a psychiatric inpatient ward revealed written expression deficits of nearly half (.48) a year behind expected achievement (Forness et al., 1983). In contrast, Rosenblatt and Rosenblatt examined the written expression skills of 143 children and youth aged 5 to 18 served in community-based mental health programs and found that as a group, students with ED scored 2.4 years below expected achievement.

Stability

To our knowledge, only one study assessing the stability of written expression deficits over time has been conducted with students with ED. In this study, Glassberg and colleagues (1999) reported the average Woodcock–Johnson written expression scores of 233 students with ED aged 6 to 8, 9 to 11, and 12 to 16. Although deficits were present in all three age groups, no differences in written expression ability were revealed across the age categories (Glassberg et al., 1999). These results suggest that the written expression deficits of these students maintained but did not increase with age.

Academic Status Summary

The examination of causal models (e.g., poor grades–aggression hypothesis, reciprocal causation hypothesis) has revealed several possible factors that may link the co-occurrence of ED and academic underachievement. Although these possible causal models may provide researchers and practitioners with a theoretical base for the development of intervention programs, the examination of risk factors also allows for an evaluation of an individual child's propensity for developing ED and academic underachievement. Some of the risk factors discussed in this chapter are common to many students with ED and include low SES, maternal stress and depression, inconsistent school expectations, and difficult temperaments. These risks, especially when combined, have been shown to negatively influence the development of the early academic skills and social behaviors necessary for school success (Hinshaw, 1992a; Rock et al., 1997).

Research Limitations

Academically, we know that students with ED often present significant, persistent, broad-based deficits that span academic content areas and frequently increase over time. Very likely, these deficits significantly affect school functioning and ultimately may negatively affect later life events (e.g., competitive employment). Although the literature has clearly documented these deficits in children with ED, several limitations in the quality of the research must be addressed. Specifically, as the indicators of these deficits (i.e., prevalence, degree, and stability) have shown significant variability across studies, one may suspect that mitigating variables are responsible for some of this variance. Four of these variables are (a) sampling procedures, (b) measurement instruments, (c) deficit cutoff criteria, and (d) diversity within subcategories of ED populations.

First, convenience samples have most often been used to determine the academic status of students with ED. More representative sampling procedures (e.g., random sampling) might clarify both the prevalence rates and magnitude of academic deficit, allowing for greater generalization of the results across students diagnosed with ED. Second, there has been wide variability in the type and quality of the measures used to determine status. For example, although the majority of studies have used standardized measures, others have assessed status through standardized teacher ratings or teacher judgments. Differences among assessment measures may increase the variability related to judgment or assessment rather than reflecting differences between students' actual academic deficits. Third, no consistent cutoff criterion has been established for the definition of deficit. Although some studies indicate students significantly underperform across academic areas, it is often not clear what constitutes significant underachievement (e.g., 2 years behind, greater than 1 *SD* below). Finally, much of the variability within the measures of deficit may relate to the limited information on subcategories of students with ED. Mediating factors specific to some subgroups (e.g., lower IQ, low SES, gender) may relate more significantly to academic deficit than others. However, little research has been conducted on subgroups of students with ED, allowing for only general conclusions about the academic status of students with ED.

Future Research

Although the research has documented that academic deficits are prevalent in the ED population, several areas in the status literature need further exploration. For example, additional research on specific populations of students with ED should be examined. Although researchers investigating cultural and gender differences among children have found that these individual differences may affect educational achievement (e.g., Dixon-Floyd & Johnson, 1998; Meece & Kurtz-Costes, 2001), few investigators have assessed the academic status of students with ED across race/ethnicity, gender, and SES (Trout, Nordness, Pierce, & Epstein, 2003). An examination of the relationship between these student characteristics and academic achievement may prove to be critical to the development of individualized instruction for students with ED. Another area warranting future investigation is the specific skill sets of students in the ED population. Although it is clear that deficits exist in the core academic areas (i.e., reading, arithmetic, and written expression), few studies have assessed specific limitations (e.g., phonemic awareness skills, reading comprehension) within each of these domains. Moreover, more advanced academic subject areas have been overlooked (Trout, Nordness, et al., 2003). For example, the functioning of students with ED with respect to such important learning strategy skills as outlining, note taking, homework, and test taking have not been investigated. Third, few studies have followed the academic skill development of children with ED over time. The use of longitudinal studies would allow for the assessment of the possible causal pathways models, the implications of risks for students with ED, the development of specific academic skill sets over time, and the effects of mitigating variables (e.g., problem behavior, placement settings) on students' academic achievement. Moreover, longitudinal studies would increase our abilities to target and evaluate the long-term effects of curriculum programs, instructional strategies, and intervention programs. Finally, few studies have assessed children served in general education settings (Epstein et al.,1989; Trout, Nordness, et al., 2003). Although a majority of students with ED are increasingly being served in the general education setting (U.S. Department of Education, 2001), we know little about the academic functioning of these students in relation to their peers without disabilities.

To develop instructional programs designed to meet the individual academic needs of students with ED, we must be able to first define and address the specific areas of strengths and limitations common to this population. To do so, researchers must attempt to (a) systematically assess the areas of limitations by making use of sampling procedures that reflect the broad population of students with ED and (b) follow these children from school entry through graduation to determine the development of academic skills and failure over time. If we can present a more comprehensive picture of the academic functioning of students in this population, preventative programs and effective interventions can be better targeted to the special academic needs of students with ED.

ACADEMIC INTERVENTION FOR STUDENTS WITH ED

The evidence as presented clearly indicates that students with ED enter school underachieving in basic academic skills and fall further and further behind as time passes. Moreover, their postschool adjustment problems are related in part to poor academic and social adjustment. Clearly there is a need to effectively address the issue of academic underachievement in this student population. In this section, we focus on academic interventions for students with ED as well as sound instructional practices that can be implemented with this population. First, we review the evidence base on academic interventions for students with ED. Next, we discuss teaching practices that have been shown to positively affect student academic achievement. Finally, we address effective curriculum design principles, highlighting the positive impacts that evidence-based interventions have had on the academic skills of students at risk for ED. Throughout the discussion that follows, we describe strengths of the evidence and provide directions for future research to ameliorate what we believe to be deficits.

Research on Academic Interventions

A number of researchers over the years (e.g., Gunter & Denny, 1998; Lakin, 1983; Ruhl & Berlinghoff, 1992; Skiba & Casey, 1985) have summarized the evidence base with respect to academic interventions for students with ED. Overall, the effects of the academic treatments reviewed for students with ED have been shown to be promising. Recently, researchers at the Center for At-Risk Children's Services at the University of Nebraska comprehensively examined the literature on both the types and effects of academic intervention research for students with ED. For example, Mooney, Epstein, Reid, and Nelson (2003) offered a descriptive analysis of the entire body of evidence, as well as trends related to academic intervention research for students with ED, completed since the passage in 1975 of legislation designed to offer appropriate educational opportunities to students with disabilities (i.e., the Education for All Handicapped Children Act, now known as the Individuals with Disabilities Education Act). A total of 55 academic intervention studies were identified through searches of computer databases, selected journals, and ancestral reviews.

The research studies were organized into three types of interventions: (a) teacher mediated, (b) peer mediated, and (c) child mediated. Teacher-mediated interventions refer to those treatments in which the teacher maintains responsibility for treatment throughout the entire process through manipulation of antecedents (e.g., curriculum modification, choice making) or consequences (e.g., token economy, praise). Peer-mediated interventions refer to peer tutoring and cooperative learning treatments. Child-mediated interventions refer to self-regulation treatments. Mooney and colleagues (2003) found that teacher-mediated interventions were both the most prevalent and consistently implemented interventions over a 28-year time span (i.e., 1975–2002). In contrast, implementation of child- and peer-mediated interventions varied across time, with the majority of child- and peer-mediated treatment studies conducted between 1982 and 1995. Relatively few have been carried out since that time.

The effectiveness of treatment of teacher-mediated (Pierce, Reid, & Epstein, 2003), peer-mediated (Ryan, Reid, & Epstein, 2002), and child-mediated (Mooney, Ryan, Uhing, Reid, & Epstein, 2003) interventions for students with ED was examined in three separate meta-analyses. In this research, effectiveness of treatment was determined by calculating effect sizes. An effect size represents the strength of a treatment on outcome measures (Kromrey & Foster-Johnson, 1996). In group design research, effect sizes are generally determined by subtracting the value of the treatment condition from the value of the baseline or control condition and then dividing that difference in scores by a measure of statistical error. The larger the effect size value, the greater the change in the outcome measure used. Effect sizes in the range of 0 to 0.3 are considered small, 0.3 to 0.8 are considered medium, and 0.8 and above are considered large (Cohen, 1988).

Because the majority of studies involving students with ED used single-subject designs, and effect sizes from single-subject studies are inflated when compared to those of group design studies, in these three reviews statistical corrections were made to account for the correlation between baseline and treatment phases in the single-subject studies. The meta-analytic correction procedure used was identical to that used by Swanson and Sachse-Lee (see Swanson & Sachse-Lee, 2000, for a detailed description) in their meta-analysis of single-subject interventions for students with learning disabilities. Effect size calculations were completed only on single-subject studies in which three data points could be determined for both the baseline and treatment phases. To be conservative, the mean intercorrelation between the last three sessions of baseline and the last three sessions of treatment phase was set at .80. As in Swanson and Sachse-Lee, all adjusted effect sizes greater than 3.0 were considered outliers (i.e., extremely unlikely results, given the population) and removed from the respective syntheses. From the original 55 studies, researchers were able to calculate effect sizes on 9 studies overall (8 teacher mediated and 1 child mediated). Each of the treatment types is discussed in the next section.

Teacher-Mediated Intervention

Teacher-mediated interventions are those in which the teacher maintains responsibility for treatment through manipulation of antecedents or consequences. How the teacher arranges the classroom, designs the curriculum, and delivers the material contributes to successful or unsuccessful academic experiences for students with ED. Mooney and colleagues (2003) determined that the largest proportion of academic intervention studies for students with ED (44%; $n = 24$) were teacher mediated. Table 19.3 reports results of eight academic teacher-mediated intervention studies for which effect sizes could be calculated. Mean effect sizes ranged from 0.32 to 2.61, indicating that all eight studies produced at least moderately strong findings. Effect sizes could not be calculated for the other 16 teacher-mediated studies because (a) there were not three data points determinable in both the control and experimental conditions for single-subject studies, (b) means and standard deviations for group studies were not included, or (c) effect sizes for any dependent variables in the single-subject studies exceeded 3.0.

One example of a teacher-mediated intervention study that reported positive findings was a reading comprehension intervention by Babyak, Koorland, and Mathes (2000). Babyak et al. taught 4 boys (ages 10-10 to 11-8) in a

TABLE 19.3

Academic Interventions, Citations, and Effect Sizes
for Students with Emotional Disturbance

Intervention (Citation)	Design	Mean Effect Size (Range)
Teacher mediated[a]		
Teacher delivery adjustments (West & Sloan, 1986)	SS	0.52 (0.0–1.62)
Teaching test-taking skills (Scruggs & Marsing, 1987)	G	1.03
Mnemonics instruction (Mastropieri et al., 1988)	G	1.30
Personalized instruction (McLaughlin, 1991)	G	0.92
Structured teaching (Foley & Epstein, 1993)	G	0.32
Incorporating student interest (Clarke et al., 1995)	SS	1.47
Story mapping (Babyak et al., 2000)	SS	2.61 (2.54–2.68)
Individual curricular modifications (Kern et al., 2001)	SS	1.62 (0.69–2.54)
Peer mediated[b]		
None		—
Child mediated[c]		
Cover, copy, and compare (Skinner et al., 1991)	SS	1.0 (0.09–2.31)

Note. (SS) = single subject design; (G) = group design.

[a] Interventions in which the teacher maintains responsibility for treatment through manipulation of antecedents (e.g., curriculum modification, choice making) or consequences (e.g., token economy, praise).

[b] Interventions in which peers were actively involved in the instruction of a person of similar status or standing in academic skills. Examples include peer tutoring and cooperative learning.

[c] Interventions in which the ultimate responsibility for implementation of the intervention rested with the student. Examples include self-management strategies.

summer school program for students with ED how to use an empirically validated strategy for organizing stories designed to improve comprehension of text. Students were instructed on the importance of story mapping and understanding the elements of stories prior to receiving guided and independent practice in story-mapping procedures. Results of the instruction indicated that the median percentage of comprehension questions answered correctly increased from 50 to 60 during baseline to 80 to 100 during treatment for the 3 boys who completed the intervention. Moreover, all 4 students improved the accuracy of their oral retell statements (Babyak et al., 2000). A mean effect size of 2.61 (range 2.54–2.68) was calculated for the 2 students for whom effect sizes could be calculated (Pierce et al., 2003). There were not enough data points provided to calculate effect sizes for the other 2 students.

Peer-Mediated Intervention

A peer is a matched companion, a person of relatively equal standing, age, or rank (Topping & Ehly, 1998). Peer-mediated instruction is the process of actively teaching a person of similar status or standing in academic skills. Examples of peer-mediated interventions include same-age and cross-age tutoring. Same-age peer tutoring refers to tutoring efforts between peers of a same age or grade; cross-age peer tutoring refers to tutoring between students of different ages or grade levels. In both types of tutoring, students can take the role of tutor (i.e., providing instruction), tutee (i.e., receiving instruction), or both. Peer-assisted instruction has a well-established record of promoting academic gains across learner types, settings, and subject areas (Maheady, 2001; Mastropieri, Spencer, Scruggs, & Talbott, 2000; Mathes, Torgesen, & Allor, 2001). Twenty percent ($n = 11$) of the academic intervention studies for students with ED involved peer-mediated interventions (Mooney et al., 2003).

Peer tutoring designed to improve the academic functioning of students with ED has primarily been applied to the area of reading. For example, three cross-age peer-tutoring studies were identified in a recent review of the research on teaching reading to students with ED (Coleman & Vaughn, 2000). All three studies examined cross-age peer tutoring's influence on reading and social outcomes for elementary-age students with ED (Cochran, Feng, Cartledge, & Hamilton, 1993; Resnick, 1987; Shisler, Top, & Osguthorpe, 1986). The three interventions lasted from 8 weeks to 5 months and resulted in improvements on several measures of reading skills (e.g., sight word inventories, standardized tests). Effect sizes could not be calculated for any of the three studies because they did not meet inclusionary criteria (i.e., Resnick, 1987), did not report sufficient data to calculate effect sizes (i.e., Cochran et al., 1993), or reported effect sizes that were considered outliers (i.e., Shisler et al., 1986).

More recently Falk and Wehby (2001) demonstrated the value of peer tutoring for improving the reading skills of students with ED. They examined the effectiveness of the kindergarten version of *Peer-Assisted Learning Strategies* (K–PALS; Fuchs, Fuchs, Mathes, & Simmons, 1997), an evidence-based instructional reading program that has been shown to successfully teach reading skills to students with learning disabilities. Six kindergarten boys with disabilities, served in a self-contained classroom for students with ED, were administered the K–PALS peer-tutoring component three times a week for 11 weeks. Results indicated that the peer-tutoring component of K–PALS was effective in increasing student performance on measures of letter–sound identification and blending but was not successful in improving segmenting skills. Effect sizes were not reported for the Falk and Wehby study, however, because at least one effect size was considered an outlier.

Child-Mediated Intervention

Child-mediated interventions generally refer to self-regulation interventions and are those in which the ultimate responsibility for implementation of the intervention rests with the student. Much like peer-mediated treatments, child-mediated interventions have a long history of demonstrated effectiveness for students with disabilities. Mooney and colleagues (2003) found that 33% of the academic intervention studies reviewed ($n = 18$) focused on child-mediated interventions.

The child-mediated interventions reviewed generally involved use of self-regulation procedures. According to Zimmerman (2001), self-regulation refers to a "self-directive process through which learners transform their mental abilities into task-related academic skills" (p. 1). Self-regulation procedures, then, are those in which students learn to change or monitor their own behavior, in a sense taking charge of their own learning. A number of the most common self-regulation procedures include goal setting, self-instruction, self-monitoring (also called self-assessment or self-recording), self-evaluation (also called self-management), and self-reinforcement (Harris, Reid, & Graham, in press).

One self-regulation technique that has been demonstrated as effective for students with ED is self-monitoring. Self-monitoring occurs when a student assesses whether or not a behavior has occurred and then self-records the results (R. O. Nelson & Hayes, 1981). Levendoski and Cartledge (2000) taught 4 boys with ED who ranged in age from 9 years 10 months to 11 years 6 months to monitor their academic productivity (i.e., the number of arithmetic problems completed correctly during the daily arithmetic period). Students were instructed to place a check-mark in the appropriate box (i.e., completing work or not) when they heard a timer bell chime about once every 10 minutes. Results demonstrated that students overall were more productive during the self-monitoring phases than during baseline. Effect sizes for all students were excluded from the meta-analysis, however, because at least one was considered an outlier (effect size >3.0).

Intervention Summary

Table 19.3 presents a description of the treatment types we have described in this chapter (i.e., teacher mediated, peer mediated, child mediated), along with names of individual academic intervention studies included in the meta-analytic reviews (i.e., Mooney et al., 2003; Pierce et al., 2003; Ryan et al., 2002), their citations, design, and a magnitude of effects indicator. The majority of research studies for which effect sizes could be calculated (78%; 7 of 9) yielded mean effect sizes at or above Cohen's (1988) threshold for a substantial finding (i.e., .80). Of the three intervention types, teacher-mediated interventions accounted for the greatest proportion of studies with substantial findings (89%; 8 of 9).

Although these findings support the notion that targeted intervention can positively affect the academic performance of students with ED, there are two major caveats that must be considered. First, the studies summarized in Table 19.3 represent a small minority of the published academic intervention studies (see Mooney et al., 2003). The overwhelming majority of studies (84%; 46 of 55) either did not report data sufficient enough to calculate effect sizes or reported effect sizes considered outliers and thereby removed from analysis. The proportion of studies excluded from the meta-analyses of studies involving students with ED (i.e., 72%, $n = 23$ of 32) far exceeded the proportion of studies excluded from the summary of intervention research on students with learning disabilities (i.e., 19%, $n = 20$ of 105; Swanson & Sachse-Lee, 2000). Second, findings from Mooney et al. (2003) and those of other reviewers (e.g., Gunter & Denny, 1998; Ruhl & Berlinghoff, 1992) have indicated that the results of research on academic interventions for students with ED are difficult to generalize because of the limited number of students studied ($N = 358$), poor descriptions of participants, problematic experimental designs, and inadequate attention to treatment integrity and generalization and maintenance of results. In sum, anyone attempting to describe the evidence base with respect to academic interventions for students with ED should do so cautiously. Although it appears there is a case to be made for optimism in terms of the positive impact academic interventions can have on the academic skills of students with ED, there certainly is a need for more scientifically rigorous replication of previous findings and expansion of the research.

TEACHER EFFECTS AND CURRICULUM DESIGN

Any expansion of the literature base on academic interventions for students with ED must be theoretically and empirically sound. Such a message is not only logical; it is timely, given passage of legislation (i.e., No Child Left Behind Act of 2001, 2002) that is based on principles demanding accountability for outcomes and use of evidence-based teaching practices. There are two sound bodies of research that can inform researchers and practitioners who aim to improve the academic performance of students with ED: teacher effects and curriculum design. Curriculum design refers to a body of research identifying characteristics of quality educational tools for students with learning difficulties (Carnine, 1994).

Teacher Effects

The teacher effects literature refers to a cumulative line of research that was designed to identify teacher behaviors related to student achievement gain (Rosenshine, 1997). These teacher behaviors are particularly appropriate for curriculum material that is well structured. Rosenshine (1997) and Rosenshine and Stevens (1986) summarized the available research base on effective teacher practices involving well-structured academic content and skills. They concluded that effective teachers

- began a lesson with a short review of previous, prerequisite learning;
- began a lesson with a short statement of goals;
- presented new material in small steps, with student practice following each step;
- gave clear and detailed instructions and explanations;
- provided a high level of active practice for all students;
- asked a large number of questions, checked for student understanding, and obtained responses from all students;
- guided students during initial practice;
- provided systematic feedback and corrections; and
- provided explicit instruction and practice for seatwork exercises and, where necessary, monitored students during seatwork.

There is research in the academic intervention literature base for students with ED that has incorporated the principles summarized by the teacher effects research. For example, Scruggs and Marsing (1987) taught 34 students with ED to use four strategies when taking content-area tests. The four strategies were designed to improve test performance by helping students focus on the most logical choices to multiple-choice questions. One example of a strategy was the removal of "absurd" options, thereby increasing the odds of selecting the correct response. Students in the experimental condition were taught these strategies in small groups and by using principles of effective instruction, including review, presentation of a general rule for each strategy being taught, questioning and feedback, guided and independent practice, and daily formative evaluation through a practice test. Results indicated statistically significant differences in scores for the experimental and control conditions following intervention. A large mean effect size of 1.03 was calculated for the test-taking intervention (Pierce et al., 2003).

There is also evidence that the use of effective instructional principles positively affects school-related academic and social behaviors. For example, J. R. Nelson, Johnson, and Marchand-Martella (1996) compared the effects of instructional practices incorporating teacher presentation of new material with modeling, guided practice, and student independent practice (i.e., direct instruction) to two other types of instruction (i.e., cooperative learning and independent learning) with 4 boys with ED (ages 8 years 4 months to 9 years 10 months) enrolled in a self-contained public-school classroom. The two target variables measured were the percentages of on-task behavior and disruptive behavior. On-task behavior was noted when students were observed to be either engaging in an academic task (e.g., marking academic task materials) or acting appropriately under the circumstances (e.g., asking the teacher a question). Disruptive behavior was noted, for example, when students were observed to hit another person or engage in a nonacademic task without the permission of the teacher. Results indicated that students displayed higher rates of on-task behavior and lower rates of disruptive behavior during the direct instruction condition compared to the cooperative learning and independent learning conditions. Findings from these studies and others (e.g., Mastropieri, Emerick, & Scruggs, 1988) indicate that teacher behaviors can positively affect the academic performance of students with ED.

Curriculum Design

Effective curriculum design principles have been culled from research that has identified characteristics of quality educational tools for students with diverse learning needs, including students with disabilities (Carnine, 1994; Coyne, Kame'enui, & Simmons, 2001). Developed by researchers at the National Center to Improve the Tools of Educators (NCITE) at the University of Oregon, this framework incorporates the following six organizing principles:

- big ideas, which are the fundamental concepts and principles that facilitate efficient acquisition of knowledge in a content area;
- mediated scaffolding, which refers to the personal guidance, assistance, and support that teachers, materials, or tasks provide a learner early in the content-learning process;
- conspicuous strategies, which are a series of steps that proficient learners purposely follow in solving a problem or achieving an outcome;
- strategic integration, which is the combining of essential information in meaningful ways that results in new and more complex learner understanding of a topic;
- primed background knowledge, which involves providing learners with a brief reminder that acts as a memory trigger and allows them to remember what they need to do to solve a task or retrieve pertinent information;
- judicious review, which involves enough practice of previously learned information that the learner performs the task or recalls the information without hesitation, over time, cumulatively, and in such a way that the knowledge can be applied to a wide variety of situations and settings. (Carnine, 1994; Coyne et al., 2001; Kame'enui & Carnine, 1998)

Coyne and colleagues (2001) recently applied these organizing principles to the process of beginning reading instruction for students with disabilities. The big ideas that educators and researchers must attend to in designing instruction include (a) phonological awareness (i.e., knowledge of the sound structure of the language), (b) alphabetic principle (i.e., the notion that letters are linked to sounds), and (c) fluency (i.e., translating letters to sounds and sounds to words quickly). Teachers then design mediated scaffolding, conspicuous strategies, strategic integration, primed background knowledge, and judicious review around these big ideas. Mediated scaffolding, for example, can be instituted through individualized instruction, such as tutoring. Use of conspicuous strategies can be systematically built into individualized instruction and, again, around the big ideas essential to effective beginning reading instruction. Conspicuous strategies related to phonological awareness, for example, might include teachers or tutors overtly modeling sounds in words and students practicing those sounds.

Effective implementation of these organizing principles, which builds on the knowledge of the teacher effects literature, has been shown to affect the reading performance of students at risk of ED. Trout, Epstein, Mickelson, Nelson, and Lewis (2003) examined the effects of a supplemental reading curriculum that incorporates such design principles as mediated scaffolding and judicious review. In this study, 12 kindergarten students at risk of ED were randomly assigned to either a treatment ($n = 6$) or control ($n = 6$) condition. Their scores were also compared to those of 6 kindergartners not at risk of ED. Students in the treatment group received daily 30-minute one-on-one tutoring sessions by four trained graduate students over a 7-month period as a supplement to their regular classroom instruction. The supplemental reading curriculum consisted of two reading programs based on direct instruction principles: *Reading Mastery I* (Engelmann & Bruner, 1988) and *Great Leaps* (Mercer & Campbell, 1998). *Reading Mastery I* is a structured phonics program; *Great Leaps* is a fluency-building program. After 7 months, students in the treatment condition outperformed both comparison groups (i.e., at-risk control, normal control) on measures of individual letter sounds (e.g., /a/) and sound blends (e.g., /fl/). Further, students in the treatment condition outperformed students in the at-risk condition on measures of high-frequency words. These findings indicate that intensive implementation of curricula firmly grounded in direct instruction principles can enable students at risk of ED and reading difficulties to catch up to their typically achieving peers. With respect to the organizing principles, researchers have also applied these curriculum design principles to the areas of writing (Stein, Dixon, & Issacson, 1994), mathematics (Carnine, Jones, & Dixon, 1994), social studies (Carnine, Miller, Bean, & Zigmond, 1994), and science (Grossen, Romance, & Vitale, 1994).

Teacher Effects and Curriculum Design Summary

Individuals interested in positively affecting the academic functioning of students with ED have rich and developing literature bases in teacher effects and curriculum design from which to build effective instructional programs.

Rosenshine (1997) described the teacher effects literature as "an impressive run of cumulative research" (p. 201) and indicated that more than 100 experimental and correlational studies were conducted using a common design and in such a way that researchers "cited and built on the instructional findings of others" (p. 201). The work of researchers at NCITE is also impressive. The six organizing principles that compose the framework of sound curriculum design were derived from "numerous studies and investigations that have identified the characteristics or features of high-quality educational tools for students with diverse learning needs" (Coyne et al., 2001, p. 63). Researchers have demonstrated that instructional practices based on effective instructional practices and a well-designed curriculum have the ability to positively affect the academic lives of students with ED (e.g., J. R. Nelson et al., 1996; Scruggs & Marsing, 1987), as well as those at risk of developing ED (e.g., Trout, Epstein, et al., 2003).

There is much to be gained from synthesizing research on teacher effects and curriculum design with academic research on students with ED. At times, it seems these two bodies of literature have been unnecessarily separated from each other. Three considerations lead us to comment on this divide. First, consider Rosenshine's (1997) comments with respect to the cumulative nature of the teacher effects evidence base. Researchers in that era of science built upon the findings of others. In the field of ED, it seems as though we have not used the results we have accumulated to build a science to inform the teaching of students with ED. There is yet to be a cumulative knowledge base documenting academic interventions for students with ED. Second, consider what happened to the "evidence" when a quantitative technique (i.e., meta-analysis for single-subject research) was applied to the research base. From a quantitative standpoint, much of it was deemed uninterpretable. Granted, positive findings remain in many of the studies, even if effect sizes cannot be calculated. However, determination of "positive findings" relies on visual inspection that unfortunately has repeatedly been shown to be unreliable. Third, much has already been made of the difficulty in generalizing results from the evidence in the academic intervention literature base. Specifically, researchers have noted problems with the research designs (Skiba & Casey, 1985), dependent measures (Gunter & Denny, 1998), sketchy participant description (Mooney et al., 2003), and lack of evidence of treatment integrity (Mooney et al., 2003).

Although these limitations are significant, opportunities remain for researchers to contribute with respect to academic interventions for students with ED. To paraphrase Rosenshine (1997), there is a great deal we can do to build a cumulative knowledge base. We suggest the following as starting points:

- Delineate a theoretical and conceptual framework for future research on academic interventions for students with ED that is based on the evidence-based principles set forth in the teacher effects and curriculum design literatures. Next, build a cumulative body of evidence around teacher-, peer-, and child-mediated interventions.

- Place more emphasis on randomized clinical trials. Consider the effects of conducting large-scale studies that compare intervention types (e.g., teacher mediated) to controls, each other, and combinations of types (e.g., teacher and child mediated). Clinical trials may offer researchers opportunities to more effectively answer the question, "What works for whom?"
- Finally, attend to deficits in the current academic intervention literature with respect to participant information, settings, content, and use of scientific procedures. More specifically, consider the following: (a) Increase the numbers of studies and sample sizes; (b) provide detailed descriptions of participants, including age, gender, race/ethnicity, SES, identification procedures, and IQ; (c) conduct studies with female and minority students with ED; (d) conduct research in settings other than the special education classroom; (e) ensure that treatments are being implemented as intended and that consumer opinions are being taken into account; (f) increase the use of dependent variables with benchmarks (e.g., opportunities to respond); (g) broaden the focus of academic studies to include content areas such as social studies, science, learning strategies, and vocational skills; and (h) incorporate the features of progress monitoring (e.g., *Dynamic Indicators of Basic Early Literacy Skills* probes; Good & Kaminski, 2002) into research designs.

CONCLUSION

Professionals have a number of child, family, and societal variables to consider when designing mental health interventions for children and youth with emotional and behavioral disorders and their families. Treatments developed for these children and youth and their families often focus on reducing antisocial behavior patterns. Although it is important to reduce inappropriate behaviors, it also seems proper that mental health professionals address the academic deficiencies that appear to be so prevalent in this population. Much can be done to improve the academic functioning of students with, as well as those at risk of, ED. Research supports the notion that children and youth benefit from academic intervention. Moreover, there is a substantial literature base from which we can draw in designing effective academic intervention programs for students with ED. It is imperative that all of us who aim to improve the lives of students with ED and their families incorporate academic intervention into multifaceted treatment plans.

AUTHORS' NOTE

This research was supported by Grants H325D990035 and H324X010010 from the U.S. Department of Education, Office of Special Education Programs. The statements in this chapter do not necessarily represent the views of the U.S. Department of Education.

REFERENCES

Anderson, J. A., Kutash, K., & Duchnowski, A. J. (2001). A comparison of the academic progress of students with EBD and students with LD. *Journal of Emotional and Behavioral Disorders, 9,* 106–115.

Babyak, A. E., Koorland, M., & Mathes, P. G. (2000). The effects of story mapping instruction on the reading comprehension of students with behavioral disorders. *Behavioral Disorders, 25,* 239–258.

Barnes, T. R., & Forness, S. R. (1982). Learning characteristics of children and adolescents with various psychiatric diagnoses. *Behavioral Disorders, 8,* 32–41.

Carnine, D. (1994). Introduction to the mini-series: Educational tools for diverse learners. *School Psychology Review, 23,* 341–350.

Carnine, D., Jones, E. D., & Dixon, R. C. (1994). Mathematics: Educational tools for diverse learners. *School Psychology Review, 23,* 406–427.

Carnine, D., Miller, S., Bean, R., & Zigmond, N. (1994). Social studies: Educational tools for diverse learners. *School Psychology Review, 23,* 428–441.

Clarke, S., Dunlap, G., Foster-Johnson, L., Childs, K. E., Wilson, D., White R., et al. (1995). Improving the conduct of students with behavioral disorders by incorporating student interests into curricular areas. *Behavioral Disorders, 20,* 221–237.

Cochran, L., Feng, H., Cartledge, G., & Hamilton, S. (1993). The effects of cross-age tutoring on the academic achievement, social behaviors, and self-perceptions of low-achieving African-American males with behavioral disorders, *Behavioral Disorders, 18,* 292–302.

Cohen, J. (1988). *Statistical power analysis for the behavioral sciences* (2nd ed.). Mahwah, NJ: Erlbaum.

Coleman, M. C., & Vaughn, S. (2000). Reading interventions for students with E/BD. *Behavioral Disorders, 25,* 93–104.

Coutinho, M. J. (1986). Reading achievement of students identified as behaviorally disordered at the secondary level. *Behavioral Disorders, 11,* 200–207.

Cowen, E. L., Zax, M., Izzo, L. D., & Trost, M. A. (1965). Prevention of emotional disorders in the school setting: A further investigation. *Journal of Consulting Psychology, 30,* 381–387.

Coyne, M. D., Kame'enui, E. J., & Simmons, D. C. (2001). Prevention and intervention in beginning reading: Two complex systems. *Learning Disabilities Research and Practice, 16,* 62–73.

Dixon-Floyd, I., & Johnson, S. W. (1998). Variables associated with assigning students to behavioral classrooms. *Journal of Educational Research, 91,* 123–127.

Duchnowski, A. J., Johnson, M. K., Hall, K. S., Kutash, K., & Friedman, R. M. (1993). The alternatives to residential treatment study: Initial findings. *Journal of Emotional and Behavioral Disorders, 1,* 17–26.

Engelmann, S., & Bruner, E. C. (1988). *Reading mastery I.* Chicago: Science Research Associates.

Epstein, M. H., Kinder, D., & Bursuck, B. (1989). The academic status of adolescents with behavioral disorders. *Behavioral Disorders, 14,* 157–165.

Erickson, M. T. (1998). *Behavior disorders of children and adolescents: Assessment, etiology, and intervention* (3rd ed.). Upper Saddle River, NJ: Prentice Hall.

Falk, K. B., & Wehby, J. H. (2001). The effects of Peer-Assisted Learning Strategies on the beginning reading skills of young children with emotional or behavioral disorders. *Behavioral Disorders, 26,* 344–359.

Fessler, M. A., Rosenberg, M. S., & Rosenberg, L. A. (1991). Concomitant learning disabilities and learning problems among students with behavioral/emotional disorders. *Behavioral Disorders, 16,* 97–106.

Foley, R. M., & Epstein, M. H. (1993). A structured instructional system for developing the school survival skills of adolescents with behavioral disorders. *Behavioral Disorders, 18,* 139–147.

Forness, S. R., Bennett, L., & Tose, J. (1983). Academic deficits in emotionally disturbed children revisited. *Journal of the American Academy of Child Psychiatry, 22,* 140–144.

Forness, S. R., Kavale, K. A., Guthrie, D., Scruggs, T. E., & Mastropieri, M. A. (1987). Academic levels and achievement gains of children hospitalized for psychiatric disorders. *Child Psychiatry and Human Development, 18,* 71–81.

Fuchs, D., Fuchs, L. S., Mathes, P. G., & Simmons, D. C. (1997). Peer-assisted learning strategies: Making classrooms more responsive to diversity. *American Educational Research Journal, 34,* 174–206.

Glassberg, L. A., Hooper, S. R., & Mattison, R. E. (1999). Prevalence of learning disabilities at enrollment in special education students with behavior disorders. *Behavioral Disorders, 25,* 9–21.

Good, R. H., & Kaminski, R. A. (2002). *Dynamic indicators of basic early literacy skills* (6th ed.). Eugene, OR: Institute for the Development of Educational Achievement. Retrieved April 3, 2003, from http://dibels.uoregon.edu/

Graubard, P. S. (1967). Psycholinguistic correlates of reading disability in disturbed delinquent children. *The Journal of Special Education, 1,* 363–368.

Greenbaum, P. E., Dedrick, R. F., Friedman, R. M., Kutash, K., Brown, E. C., Lardieri, S. P., et al. (1996). National Adolescent and Child Treatment Study (NACTS): Outcomes for children with serious emotional and behavioral disturbance. *Journal of Emotional and Behavioral Disorders, 3,* 130–146.

Grossen, B., Romance, N. K., & Vitale, M. R. (1994). Science: Educational tools for diverse learners. *School Psychology Review, 23,* 442–463.

Gunter, P. L., & Denny, R. K. (1998). Trends and issues in research regarding academic instruction of students with emotional and behavioral disorders. *Behavioral Disorders, 24,* 44–50.

Haggerty, R. J., Sherrod, L. R., Garmezy, N., & Rutter, M. (1996). *Stress, risk, and resilience in children and adolescents: Processes, mechanisms, and interventions.* Cambridge, England: Cambridge University Press.

Hann, D. M., & Borek, N. B. (1998). *Taking stock of risk factors for child/youth externalizing behavior problems.* Retrieved March 1, 2003, from http://www.nimh.nih.gov/childhp/takingstock.pdf

Harris, K. R., Reid, R., & Graham, S. (in press). Self-regulation in children with learning disabilities. In B. Wong (Ed.), *Learning about learning disabilities.* San Diego, CA: Elsevier.

Hinshaw, S. P. (1992a). Academic underachievement, attention deficits, and aggression: Comorbidity and implications for intervention. *Journal of Consulting and Clinical Psychology, 60,* 893–903.

Hinshaw, S. P. (1992b). Externalizing behavior problems and academic underachievement in childhood and adolescence: Causal relationships and underlying mechanisms. *Psychological Bulletin, 111,* 127–155.

Huffman, L. C., Mehlinger, S. L., & Kerivan, A. S. (2000). *Risk factors for academic and behavioral problems at the beginning of school.* Retrieved March 8, 2000, from http://www.nimh.nih.gov/childhp/huffman.pdf

Individuals with Disabilities Education Act Amendments of 1997, 20 U.S.C. § 1401 (26).

Iowa Tests of Basic Skills. (1996). Itasca, IL: Riverside.

Jastak, S., & Wilkinson, G. S. (1984). *The Wide Range Achievement Test–Revised Administration Manual.* Wilmington, De: Jastak Associates.

Kame'enui, E. J., & Carnine, D. W. (1998). *Effective teaching strategies that accommodate diverse learners.* Columbus, OH: Merrill, Prentice Hall.

Kauffman, J. M. (2001). *Characteristics of emotional and behavioral disorders of children and youth* (6th ed.). Upper Saddle River, NJ: Merrill, Prentice Hall.

Kern, L., Delaney, B., Clarke, S., Dunlap, G., & Childs, K. (2001). Improving the classroom behavior of students with emotional and behavioral disorders using individualized curricular modifications. *Journal of Emotional and Behavioral Disorders, 9,* 239–247.

Kromrey, J. D., & Foster-Johnson, L. (1996). Determining the efficacy of intervention: The use of effect sizes for data analysis in single-subject research. *Journal of Experimental Education, 65,* 73–93.

Kutash, K., Duchnowski, A. J., Robbins, V., Calvanese, P. K., Oliveria, B., Black, M., et al. (2000). The school and community study: Characteristics of students who have emotional and behavioral disabilities in restructuring public schools. *Journal of Child and Family Studies, 9,* 175–190.

Lakin, K. C. (1983). Research-based knowledge and professional practice in special education for emotionally disturbed students. *Behavioral Disorders, 8,* 128–137.

Lane, K. L. (1999). Young students at risk for antisocial behavior: The utility of academic and social skills interventions. *Journal of Emotional and Behavioral Disorders, 7,* 211–223.

Levendoski, L. S., & Cartledge, G. (2000). Self-monitoring for elementary school children with serious emotional disturbances: Classroom applications for increased academic responding. *Behavioral Disorders, 25,* 211–224.

Levy, F., & Hobbes, G. (1989). Reading, spelling, and vigilance in attention deficit and conduct disorder. *Journal of Abnormal Child Psychology, 17,* 291–298.

Luebke, J., Epstein, M. H., & Cullinan, D. (1989). Comparison of teacher-rated achievement levels of behaviorally disordered, learning disabled, and nonhandicapped adolescents. *Behavioral Disorders, 15,* 1–8.

Madden, R., & Gardner, E. F. (1972). *Stanford Achievement Test.* New York: Harcourt Brace Jovanovich.

Maheady, L. (2001). Peer-mediated instruction and interventions and students with mild disabilities. *Remedial and Special Education, 22,* 4–14.

Mastropieri, M. A., Emerick, K., & Scruggs, T. E. (1988). Mnemonic instruction of science concepts. *Behavioral Disorders, 14,* 48–56.

Mastropieri, M. A., Spencer, V., Scruggs, T. E., & Talbott, E. (2000). Students with disabilities as tutors: An updated research synthesis. *Advances in Learning and Behavioral Disabilities, 14,* 247–279.

Mathes, P. G., Torgesen, J. K., & Allor, J. H. (2001). The effects of peer-assisted literacy strategies for first-grade readers with and without additional computer-assisted instruction in phonological awareness. *American Educational Research Journal, 38,* 371–410.

McLaughlin, T. F. (1991). Use of a personalized system of instruction with and without a same-day retake contingency on spelling performance of behaviorally disordered children. *Behavioral Disorders, 16,* 127–132.

Meece, J. L., & Kurtz-Costes, B. (2001). Introduction: The schooling of ethnic minority children and youth. *Educational Psychologist, 36,* 1–7.

Mercer, C. D., & Campbell, K.U. (1998). *Great leaps reading program.* Gainesville, FL: Diarmuid, Inc.

Mooney, P., Epstein, M. H., Reid, R., & Nelson, J. R. (2003). Status and trends of academic intervention research for students with emotional disturbance. *Remedial and Special Education, 24,* 273–287.

Mooney, P., Ryan, J. B., Uhing, B. M., Reid, R., & Epstein, M. H. (2003). *A review of treatment outcomes of self-regulated learning interventions for students with emotional and behavioral disorders.* Lincoln, NE: Center for At-Risk Children's Services.

Motto, J. J., & Lathan, L. (1966). An analysis of children's educational achievement and related variables in a state psychiatric hospital. *Exceptional Children, 32,* 619–623.

Motto, J. J., & Wilkins, G. S. (1968). Educational achievement of institutionalized emotionally disturbed children. *Journal of Educational Research, 61,* 218–221.

Nelson, J. R., Johnson, A., & Marchand-Martella, N. (1996). Effects of direct instruction, cooperative learning, and independent learning practices on the classroom behavior of students with behavioral disorders: A comparative analysis. *Journal of Emotional and Behavioral Disorders, 4,* 53–62.

Nelson, R. O., & Hayes, S. C. (1981). Theoretical explanations for reactivity in self-monitoring. *Behavior Modification, 5,* 3–14.

No Child Left Behind Act of 2001. (2002). Retrieved November 20, 2002, from http://www.ed.gov/offices/OESE/esea/

Olweus, D. (1983). Low school achievement and aggressive behavior in adolescent boys. In D. Magnusson (Ed.), *Human development: An interactional perspective* (pp. 353–365). San Diego, CA: Academic Press.

Osofsky, J. D., & Thompson, M. D. (2000). Adaptive and maladaptive parenting. In J. P. Shonkoff & S. J. Meisels (Eds.), *Handbook of early childhood intervention* (pp. 54–75). New York: Cambridge University Press.

Pierce, C. D., Reid, R., & Epstein, M. H. (2003). *Teacher-mediated interventions for children with emotional disturbance and their academic outcomes: A review.* Lincoln, NE: Center for At-Risk Children's Services.

Reid, J. B., Patterson, G. R., & Snyder, J. (2002). *Antisocial behavior in children and adolescents: A developmental analysis and model for intervention.* Washington, DC: American Psychological Association.

Resnick, M. J. (1987). The use of seriously emotionally disturbed students as peer tutors: Effects of oral reading rates and tutor behaviors. (Doctoral dissertation) *Dissertation Abstracts International, 49,* 5B. (Abstract no. 1989-53011-001)

Rock, E. E., Fessler, M. A., & Church, R. P. (1997). The concomitance of learning disabilities and emotional/behavioral disorders: A conceptual model. *Journal of Learning Disabilities, 30,* 245–264.

Rosenblatt, J. A., & Rosenblatt, A. (1999). Youth functional status and academic achievement in collaborative mental health and education programs: Two California care systems. *Journal of Emotional and Behavioral Disorders, 7,* 21–30.

Rosenshine, B. (1997). Advances in research on instruction. In J. W. Lloyd, E. J. Kame'enui, & D. Chard (Eds.), *Issues in educating students with disabilities* (pp. 197–220). Mahwah, NJ: Erlbaum.

Rosenshine, B., & Stevens, R. (1986). Teaching functions. In M. C. Wittrock (Ed.), *AERA handbook of research on teaching* (3rd ed., pp. 376–391). New York: Macmillan.

Ruhl, K. L., & Berlinghoff, D. H. (1992). Research on improving behaviorally disordered students' academic performance: A review of the literature. *Behavioral Disorders, 17,* 178–190.

Ryan, J. B., Reid, R., & Epstein, M. H. (2002). *A review of peer-mediated intervention studies on academic achievement for students with emotional and behavioral disorders.* Lincoln, NE: Center for At-Risk Children's Services.

Scruggs, T. E., & Marsing, L. (1987). Teaching test-taking skills to behaviorally disordered students. *Behavioral Disorders, 13,* 240–244.

Scruggs, T. E., & Mastropieri, M. A. (1986). Academic characteristics of behaviorally disordered and learning disabled students. *Behavioral Disorders, 11,* 184–190.

Shimota, H. E. (1964). Reading skills in emotionally disturbed, institutionalized adolescents. *Journal of Educational Research, 58,* 106–111.

Shisler, L., Top, B. L., & Osguthorpe, R. T. (1986). *British Columbia Journal of Special Education, 10,* 101–117.

Shonkoff, J. P., & Meisels, S. J. (2000). Early childhood intervention: A continuing evolution. *Handbook of early childhood intervention* (2nd ed.). New York: Cambridge University Press.

Silver, S. E., Duchnowski, A. J., Kutash, K., Friedman, R. M., Eisen, M., Prange, M. E., et al. (1992). A comparison of children with serious emotional disturbance served in residential and school settings. *Journal of Child and Family Studies, 1,* 43–59.

Skiba, R., & Casey, A. (1985). Interventions for behaviorally disordered students: A quantitative review and methodological critique. *Behavioral Disorders, 10,* 239–252.

Skinner, C. H., Ford, J. M., & Yunker, B. D. (1991). A comparison of instructional response requirements on the multiplication performance of behaviorally disordered students. *Behavioral Disorders, 17,* 56–65.

Slosson, R. L. (1963). *Slosson Oral Reading Test* (SORT). East Aurora, NY: Slosson Educational Publications.

Stein, M., Dixon, R. C., & Isaacson, S. (1994). Effective writing instruction for diverse learners. *School Psychology Review, 23,* 392–405.

Stone, F. B., & Rowley, V. N. (1964). Educational disability in emotionally disturbed children. *Exceptional Children, 30,* 423–426.

Sullivan, E. B. (1926). Age, intelligence, and educational achievement of boys entering Whittier State School. *Journal of Delinquency, 11,* 23–38.

Swanson, H. L., & Sachse-Lee, C. (2000). A meta-analysis of single-subject intervention research for students with LD. *Journal of Learning Disabilities, 33,* 114–136.

Topping, K., & Ehly, S. (1998). Introduction to peer-assisted learning. In K. Topping & S. Ehly (Eds.), *Peer-assisted learning* (pp. 1–23). Mahwah, NJ: Erlbaum.

Trout, A. L., Epstein, M. H., Mickelson, W. T., Nelson, J. R., & Lewis, L. M. (2003). Effects of a reading intervention for kindergarten students at-risk of emotional disturbance and reading deficits. *Behavioral Disorders, 28,* 313–326.

Trout, A. L., Nordness, P. D., Pierce, C. D., & Epstein, M. H. (2003). Research on the academic status of children with emotional and behavioral disorders: A review of the literature from 1961 to 2000. *Journal of Emotional and Behavioral Disorders, 11,* 198–210.

U.S. Department of Education. (2001). *Twenty-third annual report to Congress on the implementation of the Individuals with Disabilities Act.* Washington, DC: Author.

Wagner, M. M. (1995). Outcomes for youths with serious emotional disturbance in secondary school and early adulthood. *The Future of Children: Critical Issues for Children and Youths, 5,* 90–112.

West, R. P., & Sloane, H. N. (1986). Teacher presentation rate and point delivery rate: Effects on classroom disruption, performance, accuracy, and response rate. *Behavior Modification, 10,* 267–286.

Wicks-Nelson, R., & Israel, A. C. (2003). *Behavior disorders of childhood* (5th ed.). Upper Saddle-River, NJ: Prentice Hall.

Wilson, L., Cone, T., Bradley, C., & Reese, J. (1986). The characteristics of learning disabled and other handicapped students referred for evaluation in the state of Iowa. *Journal of Learning Disabilities, 19,* 553–557.

Zimet, S. G., & Farley, G. K. (1993). Academic achievement of children with emotional disorders treated in a day hospital program: An outcome study. *Child Psychiatry and Human Development, 23,* 183–202.

Zimmerman, B. J. (2001). Theories of self-regulated learning and academic achievement: An overview and analysis. In B. J. Zimmerman & D. H. Schunk (Eds.), *Self-regulated learning and academic achievement: Theoretical perspectives* (2nd ed., pp. 1–37). Mahwah, NJ: Erlbaum.

The Linking the Interests of Families and Teachers (LIFT) Prevention Program for Youth Antisocial Behavior

CHAPTER 20

Description, Outcomes, and Feasibility in the Community

J. Mark Eddy, John B. Reid, Rebecca Ann Fetrow, Margaret Lathrop, and Celeste Dickey

Despite falling rates of crime in the United States (e.g., Rennison, 2002), both youth delinquency and adult crime remain serious public health problems. The United States has a property crime rate that is similar to that of most other industrialized nations but a homicide rate that far exceeds that of any other industrialized nation (Zimring & Hawkins, 1997). Of particular concern is violent crime among juveniles and young adults. The age group with the highest risk of nonfatal assault is 12- to 24-year-olds (U.S. Department of Justice, 1992), and homicide is one of the leading causes of death for youth and young adults. Youths and young adults are disproportionately involved in the commission of these violent crimes (Potter & Mercy, 1997).

For the past three decades, the primary public policy response to delinquency, crime, and violence throughout the country has been punishment in the form of "just desserts" incarceration, where more severe offenses garner more lengthy periods "under lock and key." This has led to a significant increase in the numbers of incarcerated Americans (e.g., from 100 per 100,000 in 1975 to more than 400 per 100,000 in 1995; U.S. Bureau of Justice Statistics, 1997), but it has not led to an overall decrease in crime (Mauer, 1999). However, the increase has resulted in corrections departments subsuming an increasingly larger and mandated proportion of state budgets, which in turn has led to a decrease in the amount of money available for other traditional government services, such as public education, child welfare, and other social services (e.g., Rubin, 1997). Increased incarceration has also had far-reaching social consequences for children and families, particularly within impoverished minority communities (Mauer & Chesney-Lind, 2002). Given these outcomes, it seems unlikely that over the long run, incarceration will continue to serve as *the* public policy "solution" for delinquency and crime in American society.

A potential alternative to the status quo is to employ a range of complementary strategies on a wide scale, including programs designed to prevent the development of delinquent and criminal behavior in the first place (commonly referred to as "prevention"), programs designed to prevent the continuation of such behaviors once they have begun (commonly referred to as "intervention"), and incarceration. Over the past 20 years, there have been increasing efforts expended within the scientific community toward the creation of effective prevention and intervention programs targeting a variety of social and psychological problems, including delinquency and crime (Reid & Eddy, 1997). Of particular interest has been the impact of such programs on the subgroup of children who first begin to display high rates of antisocial behaviors (i.e., oppositional and defiant behavior toward adults, verbal and physical fighting with peers, lying and stealing) during preschool or elementary school. Such "early starter" youth (Patterson, Capaldi, & Bank, 1991) compose only 5% of the population of their cohort but during adolescence and adulthood account for at least 50% of reported crimes (Blumstein, Cohen, Roth, & Visher, 1986). Further, these children are the most likely to go on to commit violent acts during late adolescence and young adulthood (e.g., Capaldi & Patterson, 1996; Lipsey & Derzon, 1998).

At present, there is a strong consensus among scientists that prevention and intervention programs for youth antisocial behavior are most likely to be effective if they are grounded in scientifically based and tested developmental models (Mrazek & Haggerty, 1994). Developmental models summarize the risk and protective factors that are particularly salient to antisocial behavior at various points across the life span and specify how factors and problems at one age are related to factors and antisocial behavior at later ages. Most developmental models highlight two key points: (a) Multiple risk and protective factors in the home, school, peer, and community domains are important in the genesis and maintenance of persistent and serious antisocial behavior; and (b) persistent and serious antisocial behaviors often co-occur with other youth problem behaviors of public health significance (e.g., heavy substance use, early sexual behavior). Thus, researchers guided by developmental models favor prevention and intervention programs that target multiple-risk and protective factors (Conduct Problems Prevention Research Group, 2002; Hawkins et al., 1992). Most such programs comprise several components or modes (and thus are called multimodal programs), with each mode targeting certain risk and protective factors within a specific setting (e.g., the home, the classroom, the peer group, the community).

One of the best known multimodal prevention programs created to interrupt the development of delinquency and related behaviors is the Social Development Project (SDP; Hawkins et al., 1992). The SDP includes teacher training in classroom management and teaching skills, child problem-solving skills training, and parent behavior management skills training. Improvements in these skills are hypothesized to increase protection and decrease risk for delinquency in the school, peer, and home settings. In a nonrandomized comparison study, the program began in first grade, and some type of teacher, child, and parent skills training continued throughout the elementary school years (Hawkins et al., 1992). In that study, compared to youth in a control group, a variety of positive outcomes were found for SDP youth, including significantly lower self-reported rates of cigarette use and a trend for lower rates of marijuana and alcohol use for low-income girls by age 11 (O'Donnell, Hawkins, Catalano, Abbott, & Day, 1995), a trend for lower self-reported delinquency initiation for low-income boys by age 11 (O'Donnell et al., 1995), and lower rates of self-reported violent delinquency and heavy drinking for boys and girls by age 18 (Hawkins, Catalano, Kosterman, Abbott, & Hill, 1999).

Multimodal *intervention* programs most frequently have targeted risk and protective factors in the individual child and the family, but they have also attempted to change some factors in school and community settings. Two examples are the outpatient program Multisystemic Treatment (MST; Henggeler, Schoenwald, Borduin, Rowland, & Cunningham, 1998) and the residential program Multidimensional Treatment Foster Care (MTFC; Chamberlain, 1994). In MST, a clinician/case manager works intensely with a delinquent youth and his or her family. Clinicians are available on a continuous basis (24 hours a day, 7 days a week) during the intervention period and attempt to address both the physical and psychological needs and problems faced by the youth and his or her family. Depending on the case, multiple intervention strategies may be used, including parent skills training, youth cognitive behavioral therapy, and family strategic and structural therapies. In MTFC, delinquent youth live in a foster home managed by parents with a high level of training in behavior management techniques. During the program, foster parents receive intensive support (through a weekly support group and as needed 24 hours a day, 7 days a week); youth receive individual therapy and behavioral skills training; and natural parents receive behavioral parent training. A case manager coordinates all services. In several randomized controlled studies, youth in MST and MTFC have been found to have better outcomes in terms of lower rates of general delinquency, as well as lower rates of violent behavior, for up to several years after the end of intervention (e.g., Borduin et al., 1995; Chamberlain & Reid, 1998; Eddy, Whaley, & Chamberlain, 2004; Henggeler, Clingempeel, Brondino, & Pickrel, 2002).

In this chapter, we describe an elementary school–based multimodal prevention program, the Linking the Interests of Families and Teachers program (LIFT; Reid, Eddy, Fetrow, & Stoolmiller, 1999). The components of the LIFT were created by members of our workgroup in cooperation with many of our colleagues at the Oregon Social Learning Center (OSLC). The primary intent of LIFT is to reduce the proportion of youth who display serious and chronic delinquency, violence, and related problem behaviors during adolescence.

BACKGROUND

LIFT is based on a model of the development of life-course-persistent antisocial behavior proposed by Gerald R. Patterson, John B. Reid, and colleagues at the OSLC (see Patterson, 1982; Patterson, Reid, & Dishion, 1992; Reid, Patterson, & Snyder, 2002). The key aspects of the OSLC model were conceptualized during clinical case studies conducted at the University of Oregon in the early 1960s and then refined through the findings from group comparison studies during the 1970s (see Patterson, Reid, & Eddy, 2002). Most recently, the model was expanded on the basis of findings from a series of long-term and large-scale investigations of child development conducted at OSLC and elsewhere during the 1980s and 1990s. At various points during its tenure, the social learning research group has been supported by competitive grants from the federal government to three independent entities: the University of Oregon, the Oregon Research Institute, and the OSLC. The research projects funded by these grants have included more than 5,000 children and families from the Willamette Valley in Oregon.

OSLC Developmental Model

The OSLC developmental model (see Eddy, Reid, & Curry, 2002; Reid & Eddy, 1997) summarizes risk and protective factors that have been identified as significant in the development of youth antisocial behavior, delinquency, violence, and other problem behaviors. In our view, the most significant risk and protective factors reside in the daily social relationships a child has with his or her parents, teachers, and peers (Snyder, 2002; Snyder & Stoolmiller, 2002), and thus the driving force in the model is daily social interaction. Figure 20.1 illustrates prominent risk factors across the youth life course that have been shown to be highly predictive of behavior problems. The arrow on the top of the figure illustrates that within the model, contextual factors, such as family income, parent depression, and neighborhood environment, are assumed to have their biggest impact on the child through their impact on parenting and the parent–child relationship. We summarize the key aspects of the OSLC model in the following paragraphs.

Within the home setting, irritable, unskilled, and inconsistent parenting and aversive child behavior have been jointly implicated as key factors in the development of acting-out behavior problems. Despite how much parents care for and love their child, some parents and children get locked in ongoing and intense verbal and sometimes physical battles in the home. These battles may be initiated over seemingly inconsequential affairs, but when they are repeated over and over, they intensify. This is because such battles are usually "won" when the child or the parent finally gives in following a highly aversive behavior or a string of such behaviors by the other person (e.g., yelling, spanking, hitting). The victor learns that aversion works, and he or she becomes likely to repeat it under similar circumstances in the future. We refer to this pattern of conflict as "coercive family interaction." Unfortunately, coercion experiences provide a child with early training in "effective" but ultimately unproductive ways for terminating interpersonal conflicts. They also provide no training in how to resolve and productively move beyond conflict.

When children enter the school setting, the uncooperative and aggressive behaviors they have learned and practiced during conflicts at home may lead to aggressive relationships with peers that not only accelerate the development of child antisocial behaviors but also decrease opportunities for positive peer experiences. Most peers ultimately do not like aggressive children

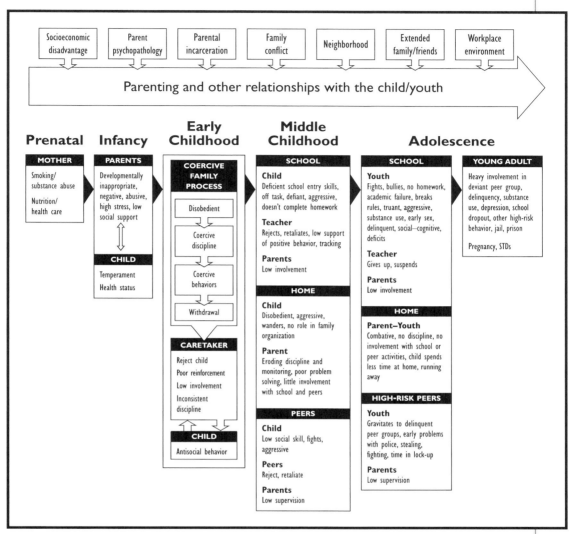

FIGURE 20.1. Oregon Social Learning Center developmental model. *Note.* From "The Prevention of Anti-social Behavior: Considerations in the Search for Effective Interventions," by J. M. Reid and J. B. Eddy, in *Handbook of Antisocial Behavior,* by D. M. Stott, J. Breiling, and J. D. Maser (Eds.), 1997, New York: Wiley. Copyright 1997 by John Wiley and Sons. Adapted with permission. Also adapted from "The Adolescent Children of Incarcerated Parents," by J. B. Eddy and J. M. Reid, in *Prisoners Once Removed: The Impact of Incarceration and Reentry on Children, Families and Communities,* by Travis and Wauls (Eds.), 2004, Washington, DC: The Urban Institute.

and stay away from them as much as possible. Aggressive children also have trouble in their relationships with teachers and other adults and are likely to end up being rejected, labeled, and tracked into an increasingly limited set of options.

With few other options, rejected children may end up spending much of their time hanging out with children from similar social–interactional cir-cumstances. Children who spend a significant amount of time in the presence of such deviant peers are at high risk for committing a host of other problem behaviors, particularly if their time together is unsupervised (see Reid & Eddy, 1997). Thus, what began as a lack of cooperation with parents and teachers eventually can lead to fighting on the playground and then later stealing, vandalism, early substance use, and early sexual behavior. As children continue to engage in problem behaviors during adolescence, their deviant peer network enlarges. Once established, the relationships within such networks tend to actively encourage further deviant and antisocial behaviors and may lead to more serious and organized groups, such as formal gangs. Throughout these myriad difficult experiences, youth miss the opportunities that other children have to develop the cognitive and behavioral skills needed to succeed as an adult in conventional society.

A child may enter this developmental course at any point in time: The model does not specify one particular cause of the initiation of patterns of child antisocial behavior. Some children from the start are more irritable, impulsive, hyperactive, or aggressive than their peers, and some of these children have parents who, for a myriad of reasons, have difficulty parenting them. Other children are members of families that live in highly stressful circumstances, such as intense poverty or severe marital conflict, and these factors may lead to a significant breakdown in parenting, which in turn fosters the development of child behavior problems, which leads to further difficulties in parenting, and so on. Alternatively, a child may seem to be doing quite well until mid-adolescence and then for some reason become involved in a deviant peer group and delinquency (so called late starters; see Patterson & Yoerger, 2002). In short, there are many possible entry points into the developmental process: No single family stressor or circumstance necessarily leads to youth delinquency. In fact, many families find ways to thrive in the presence of one or many stressors. What is key, however, is that no matter what the age of a child, once parenting is seriously disrupted and discipline and supervision break down, a child is at high risk for entering the antisocial developmental pathway. This risk is exponentially compounded when a child links up with a deviant peer group and begins to spend a significant amount of time in settings unsupervised by adults.

THE LIFT PROGRAM

When we originally conceptualized the LIFT program, our goal was to create a program that would have a reasonable chance at maximally affecting the prevalence of delinquency at the lowest possible cost. This led to several key decisions about the content and implementation of LIFT (see also Reid et al., 1999). First, on the basis of our developmental model and our previous clinical work with delinquent youth, we decided that LIFT should be conducted as early as possible in the life of the child. Once begun, persistent child antisocial behavior leads to a variety of failure experiences that can cascade into a series of very serious, highly stressful, and ultimately dangerous situations for everyone involved. We hypothesized that the less exposure a child and his or her close relations have to these failures, the more likely that the child could stop behaving in antisocial ways. Second, we decided that LIFT should target antecedents of later antisocial behavior problems that were not only theoretically important but that were also possible to change within the context of the program. Thus, we targeted aspects of social interaction within the settings that we could access in some way.

Third, and on a more practical note, we decided that LIFT should be delivered through and utilize available resources within an existing service system with widespread access to the general population. In this regard, we did not want to create a program that "worked" but that was most likely impossible to deliver on an ongoing basis outside of a research context. Programs must be relatively easy to set up and maintain within service structures that already exist (Spoth & Redmond, 2002). Further, we preferred a system with population access because predicting exactly which young children will go on to display high rates of antisocial behavior as teenagers and adults is difficult (Derzon, 2001), and thus, a universal intervention available to everyone in the population seemed to make more sense to us than a pull-out intervention for high-risk individuals. Prior to LIFT, we had research experience with pull-out interventions and found that one of our programs actually led to increases in youth problem behaviors, perhaps because it offered participating youth a chance to enlarge their deviant peer networks (Dishion & Andrews, 1995; Dishion, McCord, & Poulin, 1999).

The only system with population access to children in communities throughout the United States is the public school system. LIFT was thus designed for elementary school–aged children and their families. However, in keeping with our goal to keep costs down, we realized that a universal intervention could probably not be delivered in every school in a region, and thus we chose to target children and families living in neighborhoods where it was most likely for a child and his or her peers to be arrested by the police as a juvenile. On the basis of this reasoning, and informed by our developmental model, we created a low-cost, easy-to-implement prevention package that simultaneously targets key risk and protective factors of later antisocial behavior within the home, the school, and the peer group settings. The three interventions that compose the LIFT target factors in the home, school, and peer group are reviewed in the following sections. Key aspects of the interventions are summarized in Table 20.1.

Home Intervention

The LIFT home intervention is an adaptation of the OSLC parent management training (PMT) program (Eddy, 2001; Forgatch & Martinez, 1999). In a review of 82 studies of the psychosocial treatment of children with persistent antisocial behavior problems (Brestan & Eyberg, 1998), OSLC PMT was one of only two interventions that met stringent scientific criteria for a well-established intervention (the other was Carolyn Webster-Stratton's parenting program, e.g., Webster-Stratton, 1989, which is based on the same social

TABLE 20.1

Key Concepts in the LIFT Home, School, and Peer Group Interventions

Home

Discipline fundamentals
    Paying attention sooner rather than later
    Appearing calm; disengagement
    Using small positive and negative consequences
    Consistency

Family management skills
    Creating daily routines
    Creating behavior change contracts
    Listening and tracking
    Making effective requests
    Defining cooperation
    Giving encouragement along the way
    Giving consequences: time-out, work chores, privilege removal
    Solving problems: definition, brainstorming, evaluating, and trying solutions
    Monitoring: networking with teachers and parents

School

Relationship fundamentals
    Listening
    Giving and receiving compliments
    Understanding and following rules
    Identifying feelings
    Responding appropriately to others
    Dealing with anger
    Asking appropriate questions
    Being flexible

Peer group skills
    Joining a group
    Cooperating within groups
    Following the four steps of problem solving: Clearly state the problem; brainstorm solutions;
        if I do this, *then* what will happen; try out a solution
    Including new people in a group
    Responding to closed groups

Peer Group

Recess monitor role
    Keep moving all over the playground; don't get stuck in one spot for very long
    Keep alert for the desirable behaviors that students are doing
    Pass out armbands to students who are displaying desirable behaviors
    Explain rationale for armbands when passing them out
    Pass out many armbands

Teacher role
    Post playground rules in the classroom
    Remind students of the good behavior game
    Comment on the effort of students each day as they work to fill the armband jar
    Brainstorm possible class rewards
    Reward the class when the armband jar is full

learning principles as the OSLC program). The primary goal of the home intervention is to teach and support the use of consistent, proactive, and non-aversive discipline and supervision techniques (see Reid et al., 1999). This goal is met primarily through a six-session group-based (i.e., 10–15 families per group) parent training course offered during a 6-week period at the participating public school. To accommodate changing schedules, the session of the week is offered multiple times during the week, and free childcare is provided. Even with such conveniences, however, we have long been aware that getting parents to attend a series of parent training classes is difficult (e.g., Forehand, Middlebrook, Rogers, & Steffe, 1983). To address this problem, we offer home visits to families who are unable to attend any of the group sessions in a given week. During a home visit, the session of the week is taught just as it would be in the group setting. If a home visit is not convenient, we offer to send all class materials, including videotapes, via the mail. During each LIFT parent session, interventionists utilize a variety of formats to teach and reinforce positive parenting behaviors, including brief lectures, illustrative videos, role-plays, and homework review. In this last regard, homework is assigned at the end of each session and usually includes some reading and home practice activities. An additional key aspect of the program is a weekly check-in phone call between the parent trainer and participating families. During these calls, trainers inquire about the progress of the home practice for the week and answer any questions that arose in the family concerning the content for the week.

School Intervention

The LIFT school intervention is an adaptation and expansion of the cognitive–behavioral social and problem-solving skills programs that have been popular in the United States since the 1970s (e.g., Meichenbaum, 1977). Although the evidence is mixed on the efficacy of these programs in terms of treating or preventing youth antisocial behavior when delivered in isolation (see Taylor, Eddy, & Biglan, 1999), multimodal programs that include such interventions have demonstrated some promising (albeit modest) findings (Hawkins et al., 1999; O'Donnell et al., 1995; Tremblay, Pagani-Kurtz, Masse, Vitaro, & Pihl, 1995). For the purposes of the LIFT package, the 20-session classroom-based social and problem-solving skills program we developed served not only as an opportunity to introduce all youth to positive ways for relating with peers but also as a coordinating center for the other LIFT intervention components. The 10-week (i.e., twice a week sessions) classroom program provides a platform to set up and modify the context for the ongoing peer group intervention as well as a place to reward and recognize successes in the peer group setting. The content in the classroom program is linked to the content in the parent program, and weekly newsletters pointing out the parallels are sent home from the classroom. Also included in the newsletters are suggestions for family activities that complement the school activities for the week. The classroom is the location for the "LIFT Line," which is a phone and answering machine located within each LIFT classroom. Teachers are encouraged to leave brief messages on the LIFT Line about class activities and assignments, and to update these daily. Parents are encouraged to call in to hear the messages and to leave messages for teachers, if desired. This provides a low-key and relatively nonthreatening way for parents and teachers to communicate more frequently. As in the home intervention sessions, during each classroom session, interventionists use didactic instruction and role playing to teach and reinforce skills for prosocial peer interaction as well as for coping with aggression and rejection from peers. Problem solving with peers is divided into four steps: clearly stating the problem, brainstorming solutions, evaluating solutions, and trying solutions.

Peer Group Intervention

The LIFT peer group intervention is embedded in the school intervention but can be used independently of the other components. This intervention is an adaptation of the Good Behavior Game (GBG), a behavioral intervention originally developed by Barrish, Saunders, and Wolf (1969) and adapted for use more recently by a number of prevention research and intervention groups (e.g., Dolan et al., 1993; Kellam, Ling, Merisca, Brown, & Ialongo, 1998). As used in prior studies, the GBG is a classroom, team-based behavior management intervention. Teams are rewarded if individuals on the team do not commit specific aggressive or disruptive behaviors during a specific period of the school day. During each new period of the day, a team is eligible to win regardless of the behaviors of the individuals in the group during the prior period. As used in the LIFT, the peer group intervention is intended to provide immediate consequences for specific positive and negative peer behaviors during school recess. These same peer behaviors are highlighted and either encouraged or discouraged during the classroom social and problem-solving skills sessions. The key to the success of the peer group intervention is increasing the usual number of adult playground monitors, training them and continually encouraging them to move about the playground rather than to stand and talk with other adults, and providing them something very concrete to do that has high visibility: passing out colorful nylon armbands to children who are observed displaying good problem-solving and otherwise socially skilled behaviors during recess. The monitors are taught to log individual negative child behaviors and respond appropriately but to keep such responses short and to the point. Lecturing and lengthy on-the-spot write-ups of playground infractions are discouraged because they decrease the opportunities monitors have to reward positive child behaviors. LIFT classrooms are divided into small groups of approximately five children each, and individual students can earn rewards for both their small groups and their classrooms by earning armbands (which count toward classroom rewards, such as an extra recess or a pizza) and not violating playground rules (which counts against small-group rewards, such as small prizes from a class grab bag). In the LIFT evaluation discussed next, the peer group intervention occurred concurrently with the school intervention (i.e., 20 sessions across a 10-week period). However, this is the type of intervention that could continue on an ongoing basis and provides an ideal opportunity for a school to continually encourage and recognize prosocial child behaviors.

OUTCOME EVALUATION RESEARCH

The LIFT is currently being evaluated in a scientifically rigorous, randomized trial that involves 671 families from 12 original schools (see Reid et al., 1999, and Eddy, Reid, Stoolmiller, & Fetrow, 2003, for full details on the trial). The schools were randomly chosen from at-risk neighborhoods in the Eugene–Springfield, Oregon, metropolitan area. These neighborhoods were chosen on the basis of one characteristic: They were higher than the local average in terms of the number of households in the neighborhood that had at least one police contact due to juvenile misbehavior. Participating schools had an average juvenile police arrest rate of 13% of the households in their neighborhood area, an average yearly student turnover rate of 43%, and an average free-lunch rate of 47%. Participating parents tended to be European American (90%), in the lower to middle socioeconomic classes, and to have completed high school and some college. Approximately 50% of the target children in the study were girls.

During each of the 3 intervention years of the study (1991–1994), four schools were randomly chosen to participate, and then two schools were randomly chosen as LIFT program schools and two as control schools (i.e., no LIFT prevention program provided, but $2,000 in unrestricted funds awarded to the school). In each year, within the intervention and control conditions, one school was randomly assigned to participate as a "first-grade" school (i.e., only students in first- or first/second-grade classrooms participated in the study) or as a "fifth-grade" school (i.e., only students in fifth- or fourth/fifth-grade classrooms participated in the study). In the fall before the intervention and the spring following the intervention, children, parents, and teachers were interviewed and completed a variety of questionnaires; school and juvenile court records were collected; children were observed interacting with their peers on the playground and during their regular classroom time; and families were observed during family problem sessions in our clinic. In subsequent years, children, parents, and teachers were assessed on a yearly basis, and school and court records were collected.

To date, three types of outcome data have been examined: intervention fidelity and consumer satisfaction (Reid et al., 1999), immediate impacts (Reid et al., 1999; Stoolmiller, Eddy, & Reid, 2000), and 3-year impacts (Eddy, Reid, & Fetrow, 2000; Eddy, Reid, et al., 2003; Reid & Eddy, 2002). In terms of the first issue, more than 90% of the planned intervention content was delivered in the home and the school interventions to approximately 90% of children and families. However, this was achieved only through the use of home visits and mail-outs to families when they were unable to attend parenting sessions. Notably, only 28% of families actually received all parenting materials through the group sessions alone. Consumer satisfaction in terms of parent and teacher reports was quite high. For example, 94% of parents said they would recommend the LIFT to other parents, and 75% of teachers said they would recommend the LIFT to other teachers.

In terms of immediate impacts, the LIFT significantly decreased child physical aggression on the playground and parent aversive behavior during family problem-solving interactions and significantly increased teacher ratings of child positive behaviors toward classmates (Reid et al., 1999). These effects held for both first- and fifth-grade children and families, as well as for boys and girls. The positive effects on the playground were particularly pronounced for children with the highest levels of physical aggression on the playground prior to the intervention (Stoolmiller et al., 2000).

Finally, in terms of 3-year impacts, the LIFT significantly limited growth in attention-deficit behaviors in the first-grade sample (Reid & Eddy, 2002) and significantly reduced the likelihood of the first appearance of a variety of problem behaviors in the fifth-grade sample (Eddy, Reid, et al., 2003). The effects in the fifth-grade sample are of particular public health significance. Relative to intervention participants, control participants were about 1.5 times more likely to be arrested by the police and 1.5 times more likely to report patterned alcohol use during middle school. LIFT did not affect reports of marijuana or tobacco use initiation during middle school, however. Arrest during middle school has been identified as a marker of later and more severe youth behavior problems (see Reid et al., 2002), including chronic delinquency and violent behavior. It remains to be seen what impact LIFT has on these longer term outcomes. The follow-up of LIFT participants continues, and answers to such questions are forthcoming.

FEASIBILITY STUDIES

The findings from the initial LIFT randomized trial have been promising enough that we have begun to explore the feasibility of exporting the LIFT to a variety of other settings. In this work, we have been interested in how consumers adapted the program for their setting, how satisfied they were with the program, and whether the program continued after our research staff members were no longer involved. However, we have not yet investigated program effects on parent or child behavior. The first two major exports of LIFT were to a summer day camp and to a public elementary school.

Wyoming LIFT Program

In 1997, UPLIFT, a parent advocacy group in Wyoming, decided to provide a summer day camp program for children diagnosed with attention-deficit/ hyperactivity disorder. These children often have difficulty in regular summer camp settings, where most staff members do not have experience or training in how to handle the behavior management challenges that inevitably arise.

Summer camps have long been thought to have therapeutic benefit (e.g., McCord, 1992), and in the past several decades, researchers (e.g., Pelham & Hoza, 1996) have pioneered camps as a treatment modality for children with attention-deficit problems (see also Wells et al., 2000). UPLIFT worked with staff from OSLC and the mental health clinic at the local U.S. Air Force base to adapt the LIFT package into a 10-day, 2-week-long summer day treatment program for elementary and middle school–aged children (Eddy, Winebarger, Fisher, Sonnek, & Nikkel, 2003). Funding for the camp, christened the Wyoming Attention Camp Program (WACP), was provided by the Wyoming Children's Trust Fund and the Governor's Council on Disabilities.

The original version of the WACP maintained each of the interventions of the LIFT. The school intervention was delivered during the course of the 5-hour summer camp day (12:00 P.M. to 5:00 P.M.), with social and problem-solving skill instruction alternating with academic, sports, and craft experiences. So that the various activities throughout the day could be tailored to child age, children were assigned to groups of five to eight children of similar age, and two counselors were assigned to guide each group. The peer group intervention was delivered during the various recesses throughout the day. The home intervention was delivered each evening following the summer camp day. Free meals were provided (donated by local restaurants) for all family members, and free childcare was provided during parent class time. A key addition over and above the original LIFT program was the use of "star charts" (Patterson & Gullion, 1968) throughout the camp day that were identical to the type of charts that parents were encouraged to start at home with their children to encourage positive child behaviors.

Consumer satisfaction for the first WACP was high for parents and staff (Eddy, Winebarger, Fisher, & Nikkel, 1997). Ratings were quite similar to those obtained in the initial LIFT research study. Further, the program was well liked by the UPLIFT administrator and board of directors. The next year, funding was obtained to expand the program to two communities and three camps, including an overnight camp with a focus on older children and adolescents. Consumer satisfaction ratings for children, parents, and staff were high again during the second summer (Eddy, Winebarger, Fisher, & Nikkel, 1998). In the first 2 years, OSLC staff members were heavily involved in delivering the program. In subsequent years, involvement has been minimal to nonexistent. UPLIFT continues to operate the day camp version of the WACP each summer at several sites in Wyoming, and consumer satisfaction continues to be high (e.g., Sonnek, 2001).

Clear Lake LIFT Program

Moving interventions from researcher-driven efficacy trials to community settings is notoriously difficult, and relatively little is known about how to increase the chances that this type of technology transfer will be effective. When it was clear to us that the LIFT was having some positive long-term impacts on youth outcomes, we decided to investigate how the LIFT would operate without the benefits of a research environment (i.e., relatively abundant staff, regular staff supervision, ongoing measurement of intervention processes and outcomes). With this in mind, we approached the local public school district with the highest percentage of high-risk students in our county (based on measures of factors such as academic failure, youth antisocial behavior, child abuse, and poverty), and asked administrators if, for 2 years, we could support a half-time school counselor position that was dedicated to LIFT activities in one school. In addition, we offered to supply a half-time OSLC staff member well versed in the LIFT package to train the school counselor in the various interventions and to assist in intervention delivery.

The district was interested in our proposal. Cuts in school funding during the 1990s had reduced the number of counselors in the district, and most schools had only half-time counselors. With the approval of the school principal and staff, the district ultimately decided to use our funds to increase the counselor position at Clear Lake Elementary School to full time. Clear Lake serves a population of 400 students and families, including some Spanish-speaking-only Mexican immigrant families. During the next 2 years, the counselor and the OSLC staff member worked as a team with the school staff, students, and families to determine what about LIFT was most desirable, useful, and possible within the context of the day-to-day life of a public elementary school. The adaptations they made were revealing.

In terms of the school intervention, the team decided to make the four problem-solving steps the centerpiece of the program. At the beginning of the year, all school staff, including noninstructional staff, received training in use of the problem-solving steps, and posters listing the steps were put up around the school. Students in the first and fifth grades received the 20-session social and problem-solving skills program each year, but students in the other grades received a revised 8-session program that included some problem-solving instruction and a class meeting. All LIFT sessions were taught by the counselor, the OSLC staff member, or undergraduate interns. Because of already heavy responsibility loads, teachers were not interested in taking on LIFT teaching responsibilities. The LIFT Line was not tried due to lack of resources.

In terms of the home intervention, group parent training sessions were offered in the fall, winter, and spring to first- and fifth-grade families only. Although interest was often high, attendance was usually light (from 4 to 20 families). Attendance was best when free dinner, free childcare, and a Spanish translator were provided. In the second year, all families in the school were invited to attend, but attendance levels were similar. However, there was not sufficient staff time to conduct home visits for parent training or to make frequent phone calls home to families. Further, funds were not available to copy and mail home intervention materials.

In terms of the peer group intervention, which the staff renamed the Recess Intervention Program (RIP), the principal provided several paraprofessionals (PPs) to pass out armbands on the playground. Each day, the OSLC staff member served not only as an example to the PPs on what to do on the playground but also as a coach, providing encouragement for PPs' efforts on a daily basis, as well as during monthly staff meetings. The counselor also passed out armbands on the playground. With all staff present on the playground, the ratio of staff to students was approximately 1 to 45, which did pose challenges to staff in terms of being able to have regular contact with all students and deal with the inevitable behavior problems that pull one or more staff members away to focus on a small group of students for a period of time. With staff missing, the staff to student ratio could become quite unmanageable. RIP was initially used with only the fifth- and first-grade classes but eventually was expanded to all classes in the school.

The Clear Lake LIFT program worked well when all staff members were present but suffered when they were not. This was most noticeable for the RIP. During part of the winter of the first year, the OSLC staff member went on a short-term leave. This increased the workload on the counselor in terms of the school and home interventions and decreased her availability to be on the playground. Without the presence and coaching of these two key individuals on the playground, the RIP was not practiced as intended, and few armbands were passed out by the remaining staff. During the second year, the counselor left to take another position, and the OSLC staff member was so well liked by the school that she was offered a job as the new counselor. She accepted the position, taking on a half-time position as counselor and a half-time position as LIFT interventionist. Once prevention and intervention service delivery was centered within one individual rather than two, the tension between these activities increased. The biggest impact of this was again felt on the playground, where PPs were often on their own to pass out armbands without supervision and coaching. To cope with this situation, OSLC hired a part-time person to assist on the playground. However, rather than solely have this person pass out armbands, the staff decided to encourage students who tended to get in more trouble on the playground to engage in sports activities that were supervised by this new staff person as well as by the school counselor, when possible. The PPs passed out armbands to the remaining students but were again left in a relatively unsupervised situation with a large number of students.

As with the WACP, consumer satisfaction ratings for the Clear Lake LIFT were high for both parents and staff (Eddy, Lathrop, Dickey, Reid, & Fetrow, 2003). Students also liked LIFT and were particularly fond of the RIP. Before armbands were passed out to all students, they were becoming a coveted item among the first- and fifth-grade students and highly desired by students in other grades. This passion for armbands lessened when the program went schoolwide, but it remained nonetheless. The program was also well liked by the principal and the district, and it also brought the school and the district positive attention from a variety of media sources, including newspapers and television. Probably the most telling practical outcome for the program was that when OSLC stopped paying for the half-time school counselor position dedicated to LIFT activities, the school staff voted to continue the position, using funds that could have been used to hire a classroom teacher. The principal supported this decision, and thus LIFT continued after OSLC pulled out.

RECOMMENDATIONS FOR FUTURE WORK

LIFT shows promise as a primary prevention strategy for serious and chronic delinquency, violence, and related problem behaviors. LIFT is well liked by participants, fits well within the regular activities of a typical elementary school, and, within the context of a randomized study, has shown significant and meaningful impacts on a variety of important precursors to more serious behavior problems. Adaptations of LIFT appear feasible for use in community settings and have shown remarkable staying power over the years in such settings. Once started, LIFT activities have continued, at least in some fashion. However, whether these activities affect youth behavior as the LIFT program did in the original research study is not yet known.

Probably the biggest challenge to LIFT as an intervention is how to support some of the key aspects of the original trial. The peer group intervention clearly needs more staff members on the playground than schools usually provide. Further, the peer group intervention needs a "point person" on the playground who knows how to do the intervention well, models appropriate behavior to other staff, and provides other staff with encouragement to keep moving around the playground and passing out armbands. The home intervention will clearly not help many families if offered only through groups. The additional activities engaged in during the original LIFT trial, such as visiting at home to families who do not attend groups, sending materials home, and calling to check in with families, cannot be accomplished without additional staff time and funds. Our experiences at Clear Lake suggest that (a) if a person were hired on a full-time basis to do LIFT activities only, (b) if enough PPs were hired to reduce the staff to student ratio to 1 to 30 on the playground, (c) if a variety of volunteers were utilized well, and (d) if a sufficient budget was available for the reproduction of curriculum materials for home mail-outs, an approximation of the original LIFT intervention could occur in a moderately sized elementary school (i.e., 400 students). Volunteers would need to shoulder a large burden, however, and would need sufficient training and supervision. Even with this scenario, it is likely that only limited home visiting could be done. The addition of an additional full-time interventionist would enable further home visits.

The biggest advantage of the LIFT to a school is that the LIFT simply puts together two programs that already exist in many schools (i.e., parent education and social skills training), adds a recess program, and provides some coordination among the three programs. Adopting the LIFT may not require major changes in what schools typically do with children and families. A variety of quality parenting and child social skills training programs that are based on behavioral principles similar to those of the LIFT are already available (see Eddy, Lathrop, et al., 2003), and many schools already own these. However, the LIFT requires the coordination of these programs (i.e., delivering them at about the same time and working to make links between them for parents and children), as well as financial investments to increase the numbers of lower-paid positions present on the playground (e.g., our PPs were hourly, noninstructional workers) and to increase school counselor or parent educator time. From our experience, the LIFT also requires the presence of a person or persons (ideally, the principal and the LIFT interventionist) who have a strong passion for prevention; who can get along well with students, staff, and families; and who can build and sustain enthusiasm for the program over the long run.

Multimodal prevention programs like LIFT have promise, but much is yet to be learned about how well they operate in practice. The formal documentation and dissemination of information about how programs like LIFT succeed or fail in the real world would be of great benefit to both researchers and other practitioners. We strongly encourage school personnel who attempt to implement best practices types of programs to partner with researchers and graduate students in their area and to write up their experiences for publication. The best practices movement needs this type of formal dialogue, from research to practitioner and from practitioner to researcher, to move forward and to find the best possible best practice for children and for families.

AUTHORS' NOTES

Support for this project was provided by Grant R01 MH 54248 from the Prevention and Behavioral Medicine Research, Division of Epidemiology and Services Research, National Institute of Mental Health (NIMH), U.S. Public Health Service (PHS); by Grant P30 MH 46690 from Prevention and Behavioral Medicine Research Branch, Division of Epidemiology and Services Research, NIMH and ORMH, U.S. PHS; and by a center infrastructure development grant from the McConnell Clark Foundation. Special thanks to the children, families and school, nonprofit, and OSLC staff who participated in each of the LIFT projects, including executive director Peggy Nikkel and clinical directors Allen Winebarger and Scott Sonnek of UPLIFT and principal Betsy Fernandez of Clear Lake Elementary School.

REFERENCES

Barrish, H. H., Saunders, M., & Wolf, M. M. (1969). Good behavior game: Effects of individual contingencies for group consequences on disruptive behavior in a classroom. *Journal of Applied Behavior Analysis, 2,* 119–124.

Blumstein, A., Cohen, J., Roth, J. A., & Visher, C. A. (Eds.). (1986). *Criminal careers and "career criminals."* Washington, DC: National Academy Press.

Borduin, C. M., Mann, B. J., Cone, L. T., Henggeler, S. W., Fucci, B. R., Blaske, D. M., et al. (1995). Multisystemic treatment of serious juvenile offenders: Long-term prevention of criminality and violence. *Journal of Consulting and Clinical Psychology, 63*(4), 569–578.

Brestan, E. V., & Eyberg, S. M. (1998). Effective psychosocial treatments of conduct-disordered children and adolescents: Twenty-nine years, 82 studies, and 5,272 kids. *Journal of Clinical Child Psychology, 27,* 180–189.

Capaldi, D. M., & Patterson, G. R. (1996). Can violent offenders be distinguished from frequent offenders: Prediction from childhood to adolescence. *Journal of Research in Crime and Delinquency, 33*(2), 206–231.

Chamberlain, P. (1994). *Family connections: Treatment foster care for adolescents with delinquency.* Eugene, OR: Northwest Media.

Chamberlain, P., & Reid, J. (1998). Comparison of two community alternatives to incarceration for chronic juvenile offenders. *Journal of Consulting and Clinical Psychology, 66,* 624–633.

Conduct Problems Prevention Research Group. (2002). Evaluation of the first 3 years of the Fast Track prevention trial with children at high risk for adolescent conduct problems. *Journal of Abnormal and Child Psychology, 30*(1), 19–35.

Derzon, J. H. (2001). Antisocial behavior and the prediction of violence: A meta-analysis. *Psychology in the Schools, 38*(2), 93–106.

Dishion, T. J., & Andrews, D. W. (1995). Preventing escalation in problem behaviors with high-risk young adolescents: Immediate and 1-year outcomes. *Journal of Consulting and Clinical Psychology, 63*(4), 538–548.

Dishion, T. J., McCord, J., & Poulin, F. (1999). When interventions harm: Peer groups and problem behavior. *American Psychologist, 54*(9), 755–764.

Dolan, L. J., Kellam, S. G., Brown, C. H., Werthamer-Larsson, L., Rebok, G. W., Mayer, L. S., et al. (1993). The short-term impact of two classroom-based preventive interventions on aggressive and shy behaviors and poor achievement. *Journal of Applied Developmental Psychology, 14,* 317–345.

Eddy, J. M. (2001). *Aggressive and defiant behavior: The latest assessment and treatment strategies for the conduct disorders.* Kansas City, MO: Compact Clinicals.

Eddy, J. M., Lathrop, M., Dickey, C., Reid, J. B., & Fetrow, R. A. (2003). *Moving science to practice: Adapting the LIFT program to a non-experimental public school setting.* Manuscript in preparation.

Eddy, J. M., & Reid, J. B. (2004). The adolescent children of incarcerated parents. In J. Travis & M. Waul (Eds.), *Prisoners once removed: The impact of incarceration and reentry on children, families and communities* (pp. 233–258). Washington, DC: The Urban Institute.

Eddy, J. M., Reid, J. B., & Curry, V. (2002). The etiology of youth antisocial behavior, delinquency, and violence and a public health approach to prevention. In M. R. Shinn, H. M. Walker, & G. Stoner (Eds.), *Interventions for academic and behavior problems II: Preventive and remedial approaches* (pp. 27–51). Bethesda, MD: National Association of School Psychologists.

Eddy, J. M., Reid, J. B., & Fetrow, R. A. (2000). An elementary school–based prevention program targeting modifiable antecedents of youth delinquency and violence: Linking the interests of families and teachers (LIFT). *Journal of Emotional and Behavioral Disorders, 8*(3), 165–176.

Eddy, J. M., Reid, J. B., Stoolmiller, M., & Fetrow, R. A. (2003). *Outcomes during middle school for an elementary school-based preventive intervention for conduct problems: Follow-up of a randomized trial.* Manuscript submitted for publication.

Eddy, J. M., Whaley, R. B., & Chamberlain, P. (2004). The prevention of violent behavior by chronic and serious male juvenile offenders: A randomized clinical trial. *Journal of Emotional and Behavioral Disorders, 12*(1), 2–8.

Eddy, J. M., Winebarger, A., Fisher, P., & Nikkel, P. (1997). *Final report of the 1997 Cheyenne Attention Camp Program.* Cheyenne, WY: UPLIFT.

Eddy, J. M., Winebarger, A., Fisher, P., & Nikkel, P. (1998). *Wyoming Attention Camp Program, Phase I: Development and refinement, 1997–1998.* Cheyenne: UPLIFT.

Eddy, J. M., Winebarger, A., Fisher, P., Sonnek, S., & Nikkel, P. (2003). *An adaptation of the LIFT prevention program for a summer camp setting: The Wyoming Attention Camp Program.* Manuscript submitted for publication.

Forehand, R., Middlebrook, J., Rogers, T., & Steffe, M. (1983). Dropping out of parent training. *Behaviour Research and Therapy, 21*(6), 663–668.

Forgatch, M. S., & Martinez, C. R., Jr. (1999). Parent management training: A program linking basic research and practical application. *Tidsskrift for Norsk Psykologforening, 36,* 923–937.

Hawkins, J. D., Catalano, R. F., Kosterman, R., Abbott, R., & Hill, K. G. (1999). Preventing adolescent health-risk behaviors by strengthening protection during childhood. *Archives of Pediatrics and Adolescent Medicine, 153,* 226–234.

Hawkins, J. D., Catalano, R. F., Morrison, D. M., O'Donnell, J., Abbott, R. D., & Day, L. E. (1992). The Seattle social development project: Effects of the first four years on protective factors and problem behaviors. In J. McCord & R. E. Tremblay (Eds.), *Preventing antisocial behavior: Interventions from birth through adolescence* (pp. 139–161). New York: Guilford Press.

Henggeler, S. W., Clingempeel, W. G., Brondino, M. J., & Pickrel, S. G. (2002). Four-year follow-up of multisystemic therapy with substance-abusing and substance-dependent juvenile offenders. *Journal of the American Academy of Child and Adolescent Psychiatry, 41*(7), 868–874.

Henggeler, S. W., Schoenwald, S. K., Borduin, C. M., Rowland, M. D., & Cunningham, P. B. (1998). *Multisystemic treatment of antisocial behavior in children and adolescents.* New York: Guilford Press.

Kellam, S. G., Ling, X., Merisca, R., Brown, C. H., & Ialongo, N. (1998). The effect of the level of aggression in the first grade classroom on the course and malleability of aggressive behavior into middle school. *Development and Psychopathology, 10*(3), 165–186.

Lipsey, M. W., & Derzon, J. H. (1998). Predictors of violent or serious delinquency in adolescence and early adulthood: A synthesis of longitudinal research. In R. Loeber & D. P. Farrington (Eds.), *Serious and violent juvenile offenders: Risk factors and successful interventions* (pp. 86–105). Thousand Oaks, CA: Sage.

Mauer, M. (1999). *Race to incarcerate.* New York: The New Press.

Mauer, M., & Chesney-Lind, M. (2002). *Invisible punishment: The collateral consequences of mass imprisonment.* New York: The New Press.

McCord, J. (1992). The Cambridge–Somerville Study: A pioneering longitudinal experimental study of delinquency prevention. In J. McCord & R. E. Tremblay (Eds.), *Preventing antisocial behavior: Interventions from birth through adolescence* (pp. 196–206). New York: Guilford Press.

Meichenbaum, D. (1977). *Cognitive-behavior modification: An integrative approach.* New York: Plenum Press.

Mrazek, P. G., & Haggerty, R. J. (Eds.). (1994). *Reducing risks for mental disorders: Frontiers for preventive intervention research.* Washington, DC: National Academy Press.

O'Donnell, J., Hawkins, D., Catalano, R. F., Abbott, R. D., & Day, L. E. (1995). Preventing school failure, drug use, and delinquency among low-income children: Long-term intervention in elementary schools. *American Journal of Orthopsychiatry, 65*(1), 87–100.

Patterson, G. R. (1982). *Coercive family process.* Eugene, OR: Castalia.

Patterson, G. R., Capaldi, D., & Bank, L. (1991). An early starter model for predicting delinquency. In D. J. Pepler & K. H. Rubin (Eds.), *The development and treatment of childhood aggression* (pp. 139–168). Hillsdale, NJ: Erlbaum.

Patterson, G. R., & Gullion, M. E. (1968). *Living with children: New methods for parents and teachers.* Champaign, IL: Research Press.

Patterson, G. R., Reid, J. B., & Dishion, T. J. (1992). *A social interactional approach: Antisocial boys* (Vol. 4). Eugene, OR: Castalia.

Patterson, G. R., Reid, J. B., & Eddy, J. M. (2002). A brief history of the Oregon Model. In J. B. Reid, G. R. Patterson, & J. Snyder (Eds.), *Antisocial behavior in children and adolescents: A developmental analysis and model for intervention* (pp. 3–21). Washington, DC: American Psychological Association.

Patterson, G. R., & Yoerger, K. (2002). A developmental model for early- and late-onset antisocial behavior. In J. B. Reid, J. Snyder, & G. R. Patterson (Eds.), *Antisocial behavior in children and adolescents: A developmental analysis and model for intervention* (pp. 147–172). Washington, DC: American Psychological Association.

Pelham, W. E. Jr., & Hoza, B. (1996). Intensive treatment: A summer treatment program for children with ADHD. In E. D. Hibbs & P. S. Jensen (Eds.), *Psychosocial treatments for child and adolescent disorders: Empirically based strategies for clinical practice* (pp. 311–340). Washington, DC: American Psychological Association.

Potter, L. B., & Mercy, J. A. (1997). Public health perspective on interpersonal violence among youths in the United States. In D. M. Stoff, J. Breiling, & J. D. Maser (Eds.), *Handbook of antisocial behavior* (pp. 3–11). New York: Wiley.

Reid, J. B., & Eddy, J. M. (1997). The prevention of antisocial behavior: Some considerations in the search for effective interventions. In D. M. Stoff, J. Breiling, & J. D. Maser (Eds.), *Handbook of antisocial behavior* (pp. 343–356). New York: Wiley.

Reid, J. B., & Eddy, J. M. (2002). Preventive efforts during the elementary school years: The Linking the Interests of Families and Teachers Project. In J. B. Reid, G. R. Patterson, & J. Snyder (Eds.), *Antisocial behavior in children and adolescents: A developmental analysis and model for intervention* (pp. 219–233). Washington, DC: American Psychological Association.

Reid, J. B., Eddy, J. M., Fetrow, R. A., & Stoolmiller, M. (1999). Description and immediate impacts of a preventive intervention for conduct problems. *American Journal of Community Psychology, 27*(4), 483–517.

Reid, J. B., Patterson, G. R., & Snyder, J. (2002). *Antisocial behavior in children and adolescents: A developmental analysis and model for intervention.* Washington, DC: American Psychological Association.

Rennison, C. (2002). *Criminal victimization 2001* (Bureau of Justice Statistics report). Retrieved September 23, 2002, from http://www.ojp.usdoj.gov/bjs/pub/pdf/cv01.pdf

Rubin, E. L. (Ed.). (1997). *Minimizing harm as a goal for crime policy in California* (Policy Research Program Report), policy seminar, University of California, Berkeley.

Snyder, J. (2002). Reinforcement and coercion mechanisms in the development of antisocial behavior: Peer relationships. In J. B. Reid, J. Snyder, & G. R. Patterson (Eds.), *Antisocial behavior in children and adolescents: A developmental analysis and model for intervention* (pp. 147–172). Washington, DC: American Psychological Association.

Snyder, J., & Stoolmiller, M. (2002). Reinforcement and coercion mechanisms in the development of antisocial behavior: The family. In J. B. Reid, G. R. Patterson, & J. Snyder (Eds.), *Antisocial behavior in children and adolescents: A developmen-*

tal analysis and model for intervention (pp. 65–100). Washington, DC: American Psychological Association.

Sonnek, S. (2001). *Wyoming's Attention Camp Program: Final report, 2001.* Cheyenne: UPLIFT.

Spoth, R. L., & Redmond, C. (2002). Project Family prevention trials based in community–university partnerships: Toward scaled-up preventive interventions. *Prevention Science, 3*(3), 203–221.

Stoolmiller, M., Eddy, J. M., & Reid, J. B. (2000). Detecting and describing preventive intervention effects in a universal school-based randomized trial targeting delinquent and violent behavior. *Journal of Consulting and Clinical Psychology, 68*(2), 296–306.

Taylor, T. K., Eddy, J. M., & Biglan, A. (1999). Interpersonal skills training to reduce aggressive and delinquent behavior: Limited evidence and the need for an evidence-based system of care. *Clinical Child and Family Psychology Review, 2*(3), 169–182.

Tremblay, R. E., Pagani-Kurtz, L., Masse, L. C., Vitaro, F., & Pihl, R. O. (1995). A bimodal preventive intervention for disruptive kindergarten boys: Its impact through mid-adolescence. *Journal of Consulting and Clinical Psychology, 63*(4), 560–568.

U.S. Bureau of Justice Statistics. (1997). *Sourcebook of criminal justice statistics.* Washington, DC: U.S. Department of Justice.

U.S. Department of Justice. (1992). *Recidivism of felons on probation, 1986–1989.* Washington, DC: U.S. Bureau of Justice Statistics.

Webster-Stratton, C. (1989). Systematic comparison of consumer satisfaction of three cost-effective parent training programs for conduct problem children. *Behavior Therapy, 20,* 103–115.

Wells, K. C., Pelham, W. E. Jr., Kotkin, R. A., Hoza, B., Abikoff, H. B., Abramowitz, A., et al. (2000). Psychosocial treatment strategies in the MTA study: Rationale, methods, and critical issues in design and implementation. *Journal of Abnormal Child Psychology, 28*(6), 483–505.

Zimring, F. E., & Hawkins, G. (1997). *Crime is not the problem: Lethal violence in America.* New York: Oxford University Press.

The First Step to Success Program

Achieving Secondary Prevention Outcomes for Behaviorally At-Risk Children Through Early Intervention

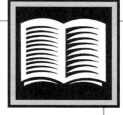

Hill M. Walker, Jeffrey R. Sprague, Kindle Anne Perkins-Rowe, Kelli Y. Beard Jordan, Bonita M. Seibert, Annemieke M. Golly, Herbert H. Severson, and Edward G. Feil

In our view, there are two primary developmental periods in which intervention efforts can be mounted effectively to prevent or reduce the destructive outcomes that so many behaviorally at-risk children experience later in their lives. These are the prenatal to age 5 developmental period and the elementary school years (i.e., ages 6 to 10). In the prenatal to age 5 period, some of the generic risks for later destructive outcomes (e.g., weak parenting practices, families experiencing severe levels of stress, parental drug use) can be addressed and sometimes reduced or eliminated via comprehensive, community-based interventions (see Olds, Hill, & Rumsey, 1998). Once a child begins the schooling experience, however, educators are faced with the responsibility of developing and enhancing protective factors that can buffer and offset the damaging effects of prior risk exposure because they typically can do little to affect such nonschool risks as parental neglect or abuse, which can powerfully affect school performance (see Hawkins, Catalano, Kosterman, Abbott, & Hill, 1999).

THE ROLE OF RISK AND PROTECTIVE FACTORS IN PROBLEMATIC CHILD BEHAVIOR

The recently released report by the U.S. Surgeon General on youth violence (see Satcher, 2001) calls for the continuing development and broad-based application of systematic, comprehensive approaches to address the growing and very serious threats to the well-being of our children, youth, and the larger society. This report provides substantive information about the roles of risk and protective factors associated with poor mental health outcomes for children and youth. The more risks and the fewer offsetting protective factors there are in a child's life, the more likely it is that vulnerable children and youth will experience destructive outcomes at some time in their lives. Further, the earlier such risk exposure begins, the longer it lasts, and the more severe it is, the greater the odds that the impact will be extensive (Loeber & Farrington, 2001; Patterson, Reid, & Dishion, 1992; Reid, 1993). The social conditions of our society over the past three decades seem to have accelerated the numbers of such children who manifest the palpable effects of pervasive prior risk exposure as they begin their school careers.

Many of the conditions of risk that set up vulnerable children for school failure and other negative outcomes exert their influence in the prenatal and early developmental periods (e.g. prenatal drug use during pregnancy, poverty, chaotic family situations). As noted previously, it is usually beyond the reach of schools and educators to prevent, eliminate, or reduce the impact of these "out-of-school" risks that have so much to do with how children respond to the ordinary demands of schooling. However, the Olds Nurse Home Visitation Program, which provides advocacy, support services, and direct training by public health nurses to young, first-time mothers who meet a characteristic risk profile, is an example of a very early intervention (prenatal to age 2) that can effectively address some of these risk factors. Further, early Head Start and regular Head Start have the potential to produce a similar but generally less powerful or enduring impact.

SCHOOLING AS A PROTECTIVE FACTOR

Research and meta-analyses have converged in documenting the protective influences of schooling in preventing and attenuating numerous destructive outcomes that occur in adolescence and young adulthood (see Hawkins et al., 1999; Malecki & Elliott, 2002; Najaka, Gottfredson, & Wilson, 2001). For example, in a meta-analysis of the dimensions that predict problem behavior in school, Najaka et al. (2001) found that school bonding emerged as a significant positive influence. Similarly, Malecki and Elliott (2002) reported an experimental study of a universal school intervention in which school bonding and attachment were identified as key factors in the favorable outcomes achieved. Finally, Hawkins and his colleagues reported a 12-year longitudinal intervention study that was designed to enhance the protective influences of school success and bonding/attachment to schooling. They also examined the role of early (Grades 1–3) versus later (Grades 5–6) intervention with at-risk students in reducing long-term destructive outcomes. Their intervention involved direct child skills training in social and academic domains, teacher training, support and coaching, and instruction of parents in proven techniques of effective parenting.

These researchers located and followed up on 598 of the 643 original study participants at age 18 and assessed them on a number of outcomes. Results showed no differences between the later intervention group and the control group. However, there were highly significant differences favoring the early intervention participants over the untreated control group on the following outcomes at age 18: violent, delinquent acts; heavy drinking; academic underachievement; teenage pregnancy; multiple sex partners; sexually transmitted diseases; behavioral episodes at school; and school failure. These authors concluded that (a) bonding and attachment to schooling served as a powerful protective factor against some very serious health risk behaviors in adolescence and (b) early intervention, delivered at the point of school entry, was highly effective in fostering such bonding and attachment.

FACILITATING SCHOOL BONDING AND ATTACHMENT

We believe that one of the very best ways to develop bonding and attachment to the schooling process is to try and ensure that all children, especially those who are behaviorally at risk, get off to the best possible start in school and receive the monitoring, supports, attention, and services necessary to achieve continuing school success within the elementary school years. To achieve this important goal, it is essential that schools have the capacity to intervene effectively with those students who enter the schoolhouse door not ready to learn and who manifest maladaptive behavior patterns that prove to be disruptive of the teaching/learning process. Children from chaotic family environments who experience significant risk exposure are especially vulnerable and in need of such supports.

High-level child aggression and oppositional-defiant behavior can be very problematic in this regard because they severely disrupt the two most important social–behavioral adjustments a student is required to make in school: teacher related and peer related (Leff, Power, Manz, Costigan, & Nabors, 2001; Walker, Colvin, & Ramsey, 1995; Walker, Irvin, Noell, & Singer, 1992). Failure in either of these critically important social–behavioral adjustments is very significant; failure in both can put the student's school success and life chances at risk. The behavioral correlates of successful and unsuccessful forms of these two types of adjustment are known and should be used as a road map by educators and mental health professionals alike in either designing or selecting interventions to enhance the school success of behaviorally at risk-students.

THE DEMAND FOR EVIDENCE-BASED INTERVENTIONS

From parent advocates, to school professional consumers, to legislators and policymakers alike, uniform demand has accelerated in recent years for (a) access to evidence-based interventions that are reasonable in their costs and (b) the efforts necessary for their effective implementation. Further, there is a critical need for proven and promising interventions that can be scaled up and applied on a broad scale while preserving their effectiveness (see Elias et al., 1997).

The reasons underlying this change are not completely clear. However, it is likely that the plethora of school shooting tragedies during the mid- to late-1990s helped fuel an intense demand and search by school officials for effective interventions to ensure the safety of schools. Further, educators now seem much more open to preventive approaches that were rejected in the past as excessive in their fiscal costs or in the effort required for their implementation. In particular, school personnel have been more open to schoolwide interventions that have the potential to reduce discipline problems and to create a positive school climate (see Horner, Sugai, Lewis-Palmer, & Todd, 2001). These outcomes are broadly viewed by educators as enhancing the school's relative safety.

The important work of Hoagwood and Erwin (1997) in evaluating school systems' accommodation of behaviorally at-risk youth may be a contributing factor in this regard as well. They conducted a 10-year review of school-based mental health services for children and found that (a) approximately 75% of child mental health services are typically delivered within school settings, (b) the mental health needs of school-age children and youth are severely underserved in the context of schooling, and (c) the school-based services that *are* delivered tend to be ineffective due to the common practice of applying interventions that have not been empirically tested or proven. The work of Hoagwood and her colleagues has received broad attention in the professional literature and has positively influenced the funding decisions of federal agencies providing support to schools for coping with at-risk students. For example, both the U.S. Department of Education's Office of Safe and Drug Free Schools and the U.S. Office of Juvenile Justice and Delinquency Prevention have invested substantially in funding the adoption and implementation of the *Blue Print Series* of proven interventions that have been validated by the Center for the Study and Prevention of Violence at the University of Colorado (Elliott, 1994). Hoagwood (2000, 2001) and her colleagues continue to be a powerful voice in promoting evidence-based interventions by schools and mental health systems and in identifying the barriers to implementing what we know to be effective. Burns and Hoagwood (2002) have recently profiled effective, evidence-based interventions for use in child mental health and school contexts that represent a seminal contribution to the professional literature on this critical issue.

Jensen (2001) has recently contributed an important commentary on the critical features of such evidence-based interventions and has identified specific criteria for evaluating them. Jensen's work has been especially noteworthy in influencing the movement toward adoption of evidence-based practices. He is the founding editor of the *Report on Emotional and Behavioral Disorders in Youth,* which is dedicated to the promotion of evidence-based assessments and interventions for at-risk children and youth. This report is receiving increasingly strong support among child mental health and school professionals.

This chapter is focused on the First Step to Success early intervention program, which is designed to assist behaviorally at-risk students in getting off to the best start possible in their school careers (see Walker et al., 1998; Walker et al., 1997). This program has three modular components (screening, school intervention, parent training) and is applied to one behaviorally at-risk child at a time in K–2 classroom settings. First Step is an early intervention program designed to achieve secondary prevention goals and outcomes for students with behavior problems who show clear effects of risk exposure prior to beginning their school careers. Two of the most important features of this program are that it is a school-based intervention that addresses child mental health problems and it uses parents, teachers, and peers as natural helpers/ therapists in the intervention process.

The remainder of this chapter focuses on the following topics: (a) overview and description of the First Step program, (b) development and trial testing of the intervention, (c) replication and extension of First Step program applications, (d) the Oregon First Step Replication Initiative, (e) cultural appropriateness of First Step, and (f) ongoing research. The chapter concludes with some observations about the school and preschool contexts in which the First Step program is applied.

OVERVIEW AND DESCRIPTION OF THE FIRST STEP PROGRAM

The First Step program has been described previously in several venues (see Epstein & Walker, 2002; Golly, Stiller, & Walker, 1998; Walker et al., 1998). As noted previously, First Step to Success contains three interrelated modular components. These are (a) a screening and early detection procedure that provides four different options for use by adopters in identifying target participants, (b) a school intervention component that teaches an adaptive behavior pattern for fostering school success and satisfactory adjustment to the normal demands of schooling, and (c) a parent component, called homeBase, that teaches parents how to develop and strengthen their child's school success skills (e.g., cooperating, accepting limits, sharing, doing one's work). First Step is a carefully manualized intervention program that comes in a kit containing both consumable (forms, stickers) and nonconsumable (behavioral coach's guidebook, parent handbook) materials. Resupply kits of consumable materials are available from the publisher for a nominal cost.

Screening

The First Step screening procedures are universal in nature and are designed to ensure that every child is given an equal chance to be identified for the intervention. Classrooms of students in Grades K–2 are screened for the presence of emerging patterns of antisocial behavior. Four screening options are provided, ranging from less expensive (teacher nominations) to more expensive (a three-stage, multiple-gating process). Option 1, for example, requires the general education classroom teacher to nominate and rank-order students who show the behavioral indicators of aggressive or disruptive behavior. Option 4, in contrast, uses the Early Screening Project (ESP) measures and three-stage, multiple-gating procedures (Walker, Severson, & Feil, 1995) to accomplish the universal screening of all children in the classroom. We consider the ESP screening procedures to be more robust, comprehensive, and accurate; however, they are also more expensive in terms of the time and effort required for their administration.

School Intervention

The school intervention component of the First Step program is designed to teach target participants an adaptive pattern of behavior that will facilitate academic success and improved peer relations. A group-dependent contingency procedure is used in the school intervention to enlist peer support for the target child's attempts at changing his or her behavior. In this procedure, the target of the intervention earns points and praise for such things as following classroom rules; responding to teacher requests, instructions, and commands; cooperating with others; and doing appropriate work. If 80% or more of the available points are earned for appropriate behavior, the target child earns a group activity reinforcement or privilege (e.g., extra recess time, classroom games) for the entire class. If the reinforcement criterion is met in both daily sessions, the target child also earns a home reward or privilege prearranged with parents and caregivers. This procedure has been highly effective in assisting First Step target children to change their behavior in desired directions.

Home Intervention

The home intervention component of the First Step program, called home-Base, is designed to enlist parents and caregivers as natural therapists in the intervention process. Their major role is to support the school intervention and to teach their children school success skills at home. We find that approximately 60% of First Step parents actively participate in this portion of the intervention while the remaining 40% agree to it but do not follow through. In all cases, the school intervention component of the program is implemented, regardless of whether parents choose to participate in homeBase.

Over approximately a 6-week period, parents are taught how to teach their children key school success skills at home using a variety of techniques, including modeling and demonstration, role play, shaping, and home-based activities and games. These skills include the following: communication and sharing, cooperation, limits setting, problem solving, friendship making, and self-confidence. Parents are provided with a homeBase program manual and a box of games and activities targeted to each of the six homeBase skills. Parents teach the homeBase skills, the target child displays the skill(s), and teachers monitor, support, and praise the child's use of the skills at school.

The First Step program is set up and operated initially in regular K–2 classrooms by a behavioral coach (school psychologist, counselor, early interventionist, behavioral specialist) who invests 50 to 60 hours of professional time during the approximately 3-month implementation period. After Program Day 10, the general education teacher assumes full control of the program and operates it on a daily basis until Program Day 30 is completed and the program is terminated. The behavioral coach contacts the target child's parents after Program Day 10 to enlist their participation and support in learning how to teach their child school success skills at home. During this program phase, the behavioral coach conducts six home visits, one per week, in which parents are instructed in how to teach the homeBase school success skills at home. One skill is covered per visit, with reviews of previously taught skills provided as needed.

Although not a formal part of the program procedures, it is strongly recommended that behavioral coaches continue to monitor the child's progress after program termination and to stay in contact with the parents and participating teacher(s), as appropriate. In some cases, it may be necessary to reinstitute part of the First Step program in the form of "booster shots" to sustain previously achieved behavior changes.

The First Step program has been evaluated primarily through the use of teacher report measures, by direct observations recorded in classroom settings, and via less formal social validity measures (questionnaires, focus groups). Typically, the program produces an effect size of approximately .80 and above across the teacher report and observational measures in pre/post assessments of behavioral changes (see Walker et al., 1998, for details). Longer term follow-up assessments in the primary and intermediate grades have indicated moderate to good durability of treatment effects in most cases (see Epstein & Walker, 2002; Walker et al., 1998). Consumer satisfaction results from caregivers, teachers, and coaches also tend to be generally positive (see Golly et al., 1998); however, some teachers see the program as too demanding, and school personnel have reported from time to time that it is too expensive in terms of the materials required and the behavioral coach's time investment. Thus far, the specific contributions of the homeBase component of First Step to overall program outcomes have not been assessed.

First Step is considered to be a promising, evidence-based early intervention for diverting behaviorally at-risk children from a destructive pathway at the point of school entry. To date, the program has been listed in a number of reviews of recommended early intervention programs for achieving prevention outcomes. Appendix 21.A contains a listing of these reviews and contact information for accessing them.

DEVELOPMENT AND TRIAL TESTING OF THE FIRST STEP INTERVENTION

The First Step program was developed through a 4-year grant to the senior author from the U.S. Office of Special Education Programs. This grant supported a collaborative development effort between the Institute on Violence and Destructive Behavior (IVDB) at the University of Oregon, the Oregon Social Learning Center, the Eugene 4J School District, and the Oregon Research Institute. Each of these affiliating agencies made unique contributions to the First Step program's development and final form. Year 1 of the project was focused on planning, program design, creating a context for implementing the intervention, and recruitment; Years 2 and 3 involved implementation and trial testing of the intervention; Year 4 activities were concentrated on packaging, dissemination, and staff training efforts associated with adoption of the First Step program by school districts.

In the original trial testing of the First Step program reported in Walker et al. (1998), two cohorts of 24 and 22 kindergartners and their families, teachers, and peers were recruited from the Eugene 4J School District across 2 school years. These kindergartners were assigned to the First Step intervention using a wait-list control group design; that is, half of Cohort 1 participants were assigned to receive the First Step program and half served as wait-list controls who, in turn, received the intervention following program completion by those who received it first. This procedure was implemented successfully for Cohort 1 participants in Year 2 and was repeated exactly for Cohort 2 participants during Year 3.

A trainer-of-trainers model was used to implement the intervention. A cadre of eight program consultants or behavioral coaches was recruited and trained by project coordinators. They included school counselors, psychologists, behavioral specialists, and graduate students. The coaches were trained and supervised by IVDB personnel (i.e., the project coordinators), who also were developers and authors of the First Step program. First Step coaches were assigned two to three target participants each, which they then ran in succession. The project coordinators also ran First Step cases in addition to their other supervisory and coordinating duties (see Walker et al., 1998, for complete details of these staff training and monitoring/supervision procedures).

Five measures were used to assess program outcomes in the Walker et al. (1998) study. They included four teacher report measures and one behavioral observation measure. The teacher report measures consisted of the adaptive and maladaptive teacher rating scales from the ESP, the Aggression and Social Withdrawal subscales of the *Child Behavior Checklist* (CBCL; Achenbach, 1991), and in vivo recordings of academic engaged time (AET) within the classroom settings where the First Step Program was implemented. The teacher report measures are validated and nationally normed Likert rating scales of child behavior that provide frequency estimates of occurrence. The AET measure uses a stopwatch duration recording procedure. These five measures were completed on a pre/post basis for each target child included in Cohorts 1 and 2 who participated in the intervention.

Table 21.1 presents outcome data for Cohorts 1 and 2. Analyses of covariance were conducted in which baseline scores on these measures were used as covariates. Mean differences were statistically significant for four of the five dependent measures. The social withdrawal measure was not sensitive to the First Step intervention.

Cohort 1 participants were followed up annually through Grade 4 and Cohort 2 participants through Grade 3. The same measures used in the initial program evaluation were readministered during each of the follow-up years. Maintenance outcome data showed that a substantial portion of the original program gain was sustained across the follow-up assessments, with the AET observational measure showing greater durability than the teacher report measures. The long-term follow-up data referenced here are reported in Walker et al. (1998) and in Epstein and Walker (2002). Although these results were encouraging, they represent a relatively small number of participants and call for confirmation through replication with larger and more diverse samples by the developers and other investigators. A series of replication and extension studies of the First Step program are briefly described next.

REPLICATION AND EXTENSION OF FIRST STEP PROGRAM APPLICATIONS

This section briefly describes some of the program replications and extensions of First Step that have been conducted by the program's developers and other investigators (see Beard, 1998; Golly, Sprague, Walker, Beard, & Gorham, 2000; Golly et al., 1998; Overton, McKenzie, King, & Osborne, 2002; Perkins-Rowe, 2001; Zolna, Kimmich, & Hawkinson, 2001). The reader is referred to primary sources for details on these efforts.

In the first of several intersubject replications of the First Step program and its effects, Golly and colleagues (1998) reported an investigation involving two studies. Study 1 was a replication of the First Step program in which 20 kindergartners participated; a total of 16 to 18 children (depending upon the dependent measure) for whom useable data could be obtained were included in the analyses. Participant selection procedures and dependent measures in this study were identical to those used by Walker et al. (1998) in the initial trial testing of First Step. The data from this study closely replicated the results obtained by Walker et al. (1998) in terms of the magnitude and direction of behavior change(s) achieved for the target participants. Also, four of the five dependent measures registered statistically significant effects, as in the Walker et al. (1998) study. The Social Withdrawal subscale of the CBCL again was not sensitive to the First Step intervention.

Beard (1998) conducted a study of 6 kindergartners (4 boys and 2 girls) in a rural school district in southern Oregon using single-case methodology

TABLE 21.1
Raw Score Intervention and Follow-up Results: Means and Standard Deviations by Cohort (1993–1994 and 1994–1995)

Cohort 1 (1993–1994)

Measures	Normal Range	Kindergarten		Grade 1 (n = 21)	Grade 2 (n = 18)	Grade 3 (n = 17)	Grade 4 (n = 10)
		Pre- (n = 24)	Post- (n = 23)				
Teacher Ratings							
ESP Adaptive[a]	(35.9)	21.96 (4.57)	28.83 (6.25)	25.43 (4.70)	26.72 (5.66)	30.60 (5.60)	29.43 (8.36)
ESP Maladaptive[b]	(13.5)	32.58 (7.61)	22.26 (8.86)	23.48 (6.50)	23.83 (9.37)	19.40 (5.58)	18.14 (12.50)
CBC Aggression[c]	(7.0)	20.33 (11.10)	11.04 (8.31)	14.19 (10.06)	14.55 (11.79)	8.60 (7.22)	7.00 (11.25)
CBC Withdrawn[d]	(0–1)	7.04 (4.87)	4.50 (4.41)	4.62 (4.05)	6.11 (4.08)	4.90 (3.07)	5.29 (4.89)
AET observations[e]	(75.19%)	(n = 24) 62.54% (16.35)	(n = 24) 79.83% (22.16)	(n = 20) 90.65% (10.62)	(n = 17) 83.67% (14.02)	(n = 17) 78.68% (12.90)	(n = 10) 90.40% (5.52)

Cohort 2 (1994–1995)

Measures	Normal Range	Kindergarten		Grade 1 (n = 15)	Grade 2 (n = 12)	Grade 3 (n = 8)	Grade 4
		Pre- (n = 22)	Post- (n = 22)				
Teacher Ratings							
ESP Adaptive[a]	(35.9)	21.73 (5.26)	26.68 (4.86)	26.47 (5.78)	28.33 (3.05)	29.63 (9.12)	—
ESP Maladaptive[b]	(13.5)	31.45 (6.97)	26.27 (8.04)	23.67 (6.95)	21.33 (7.50)	23.00 (10.11)	—
CBC Aggression[c]	(7.0)	24.82 (10.41)	16.77 (10.56)	17.27 (9.17)	16.00 (7.00)	16.88 (12.33)	—
CBC Withdrawn[d]	(0–1)	4.00 (3.49)	2.64 (3.40)	1.20 (1.90)	0.33 (.58)	2.88 (4.73)	—
AET observations[e]	(75.19%)	(n = 22) 59.64% (14.41)	(n = 22) 90.77% (6.71)	(n = 13) 81.85% (10.31)	(n = 12) 89.85% (9.63)	(n = 8) 75.00% (20.25)	—

Note. From *Community Treatment for Youth: Evidence-Based Interventions for Severe Emotional and Behavioral Disorders,* by B. Burns and K. Hoagwood (Eds.), 2002, New York: Oxford University Press. Copyright 2002 by Oxford University Press, Inc. Reprinted with permission.
[a]ESP Adaptive = Early Screening Project, *Adaptive Behavior Rating Scale.* [b]ESP Maladaptive = Early Screening Project, *Maladaptive Behavior Rating Scale.* [c]CBC Aggression = *CBC Aggression subscale.* [d]CBC Withdrawn = *Child Behavior Checklist,* Aggression subscale. [e]CBC Withdrawn = *Child Behavior Checklist,* Withdrawn subscale. [e]AET observations = academic engaged time.

to assess behavior changes over time. Two observational measures were used to record baseline, intervention, and maintenance outcomes. The first was a composite measure of maladaptive classroom behaviors that included talking out, out-of-seat, touching others, off-task actions, and noncompliance with teacher instructions and commands. The second observational measure was a duration measure of AET in which students were evaluated as to the level of their engagement with academic tasks and activities. Results indicated substantial changes on both dependent measures for each of the 6 participants in this study. That is, the proportion of academic engaged time displayed during allocated instructional periods showed approximately a 20% gain from a baseline average of approximately 75% across the 6 participants, as indicated by behavioral observations recorded during the intervention period. The frequency of problem behavior showed a decrease during intervention to zero levels for 2 of the participants and to near-zero levels for the remaining 4.

More recently, this investigator (Beard) has successfully applied the First Step program to a number of African American K–2 boys ($n = 15$) in urban areas in southern California. Figure 21.1 presents single-case observational data for 6 of Beard's target participants. Three of her participants received the school-only component of the First Step program (i.e., Class) and the remaining 3 received the home and school components (Class and homeBase). Figure 21.1 shows the participants' percentage of AET and the frequency of instances of disruptive, inappropriate classroom behavior (e.g., noisy, out-of-seat, disturbing others).

These results are very similar to those obtained with a rural, non–African American sample reported by Beard (1998). In addition, all 6 participants responded well to the intervention, regardless of whether school-only or school and home components were in effect. It is encouraging to see such responsiveness from young African American male students within urban settings to a high-quality implementation of the First Step program.

In a similar replication effort using single-case methodology, Golly et al. (2000) reported results that closely replicated those of Beard's (1998) work with rural students in Oregon. Target participants were two sets of identical twins enrolled in kindergarten settings in a rural, southern Oregon school district. A multiple baseline design was used in this study across each set of twins to establish a causal relationship between the First Step program's implementation and documented changes in the observational measures used. The results of this study were quite similar in direction and magnitude of achieved effects to those reported by Beard (1998).

Using a case study approach and direct observational measures, Overton and her associates at the University of Oklahoma (Overton et al., 2002) conducted a 3-year replication study of the First Step to Success program supported by an outreach grant from the U.S. Office of Special Education Programs. These investigators also conducted extensive analyses of the social validity and implementation fidelity of First Step as part of their study, which involved more than 20 students who were behaviorally at risk and their families within school districts across Oklahoma. The results of Overton et al.

(*text continues on p. 515*)

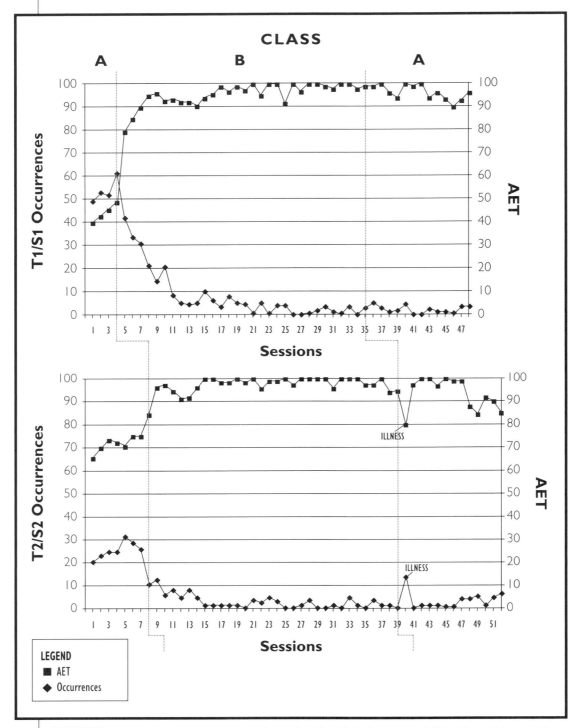

FIGURE 21.1. Percentage of academic engaged time (AET) and the frequency of disruptive or inappropriate classroom behavior for 6 African American boys in the First Step program.

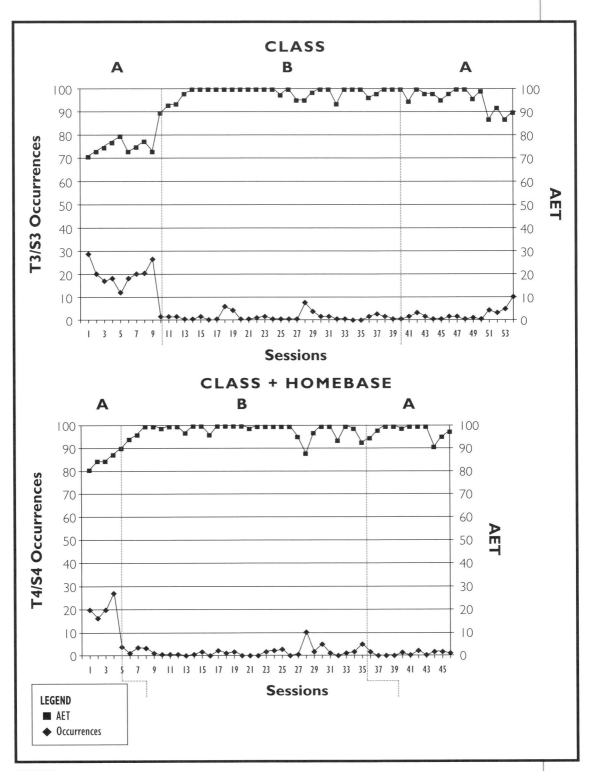

FIGURE 21.1. *Continued.*

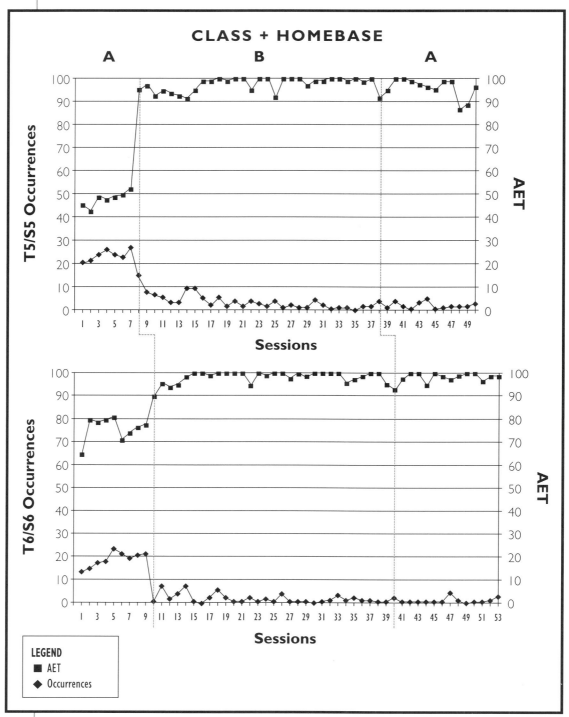

FIGURE 21.1. *Continued.*

paralleled those of Walker and his colleagues (see Walker et al., 1998) in some respects but not in others. For example, the magnitude of effect of the First Step intervention upon child behavior from pre- to postintervention assessments was very similar across the two investigations. However, the maintenance effects reported by Overton et al. were much more variable and generally of a lower level than those of Walker et al. following termination of intervention. In addition, Overton and her colleagues experienced more implementation barriers (i.e., lack of administrative support, uncooperative teachers, program cost) and more diverse consumer satisfaction outcomes. The First Step program applications in the Overton study involved primarily rural and suburban school settings.

Perkins-Rowe (2001) conducted an extension of the First Step program while examining both direct and collateral effects of the intervention. Using a multiple baseline design across 4 target participants and general education classrooms, she investigated the magnitude of the intervention's effect on the target participants, with observational procedures as the primary dependent measure. In addition, she examined the collateral impact of the intervention on the behavior of teachers and peers and on the overall classroom environment. Results indicated that target student problem behaviors decreased while rates of academic engagement increased substantially. Further, there was a moderately positive effect on these measures for "problem behavior" peers, while "average" or typical peers in each classroom maintained appropriate levels of behavior. In addition, teacher rates of positive interactions with students increased. Classwide AET, assessed on four separate occasions per classroom, increased substantially from pre- to postintervention (i.e., from approximately 50% to 85%). Teachers rated the intervention as effective and as moderately easy to use. This study was impressive in demonstrating clear collateral positive effects of a targeted intervention on nontargeted participants (i.e., teacher, peers, and the entire class of students). Replication of these effects will be important to demonstrate, and a study to do so is currently being conducted.

THE OREGON FIRST STEP REPLICATION INITIATIVE

The First Step program was the focus of an independent, state-funded evaluation conducted by the Oregon Human Services Research Institute (HSRI) and reported in the spring of 2001. During the 1999–2001 biennium, the Oregon state legislature appropriated approximately $500,000 to begin making the First Step program available statewide for all schools and districts interested in adopting it. These funds supported the cost of program materials, staff training in the implementation of First Step, provision of technical assistance, and independent evaluation of the program's effects and outcomes. This initiative, known as the Oregon First Step Replication Initiative, is the first example of an application of the the program on a widespread basis in the real-world conditions of classroom settings and schools without the careful supervision and monitoring of the implementation process by the program's developers.

Between January 2000 and April 2001, a total of 31 First Step training sessions were conducted in Oregon school district sites involving 22 of the state's 36 counties. These training sessions were conducted by the First Step program's developers and involved 244 behavioral coaches selected by their respective school districts to implement the program. The HSRI evaluation of the program's implementation examined (a) the impact of the First Step intervention on the participating children and its broader impact on peers, schools, and families and (b) the impact of implementing the program in the absence of close monitoring by program developers. The HSRI evaluators worked closely with the First Step developers during the implementation process and used the same dependent measures as Walker et al. (1998) in evaluating the program's effects. These measures included direct observations of AET, teacher ratings of adaptive and maladaptive behavior, and the Aggression subscale of the CBCL. In addition, the HSRI evaluators also developed an implementation fidelity tool for use during classroom observation sessions to assess how well the First Step program had been implemented.

HSRI evaluators also developed surveys to assess teacher and parent perceptions of the First Step program to supplement the child behavior change data. The teacher and parent surveys were relatively brief and asked a series of questions that required both quantitative and open-ended, qualitative responses. The survey questions included queries about parents' and teachers' expectations for the program prior to its implementation, as well as their assessment of its impact and their satisfaction with it.

HSRI evaluators developed evaluation packets for each behavioral coach and distributed them during staff training sessions in First Step implementation procedures prior to the beginning of the evaluation study. The staff training sessions were conducted by IVDB experts in the First Step intervention who, along with the HSRI evaluators, reviewed and discussed their contents and study measures with coach trainees. Behavioral coaches were instructed in guidelines for administering and recording each of the study measures. In addition, participating coaches were trained in how to accurately record AET using a stopwatch recording procedure. Coaches were trained to an 80% interrater agreement criterion prior to recording behavioral observations. Following the staff training sessions, HSRI sent a follow-up letter reviewing the data collection requirements and the importance of meeting posted timelines to each coach.

Each evaluation packet contained the following items: (a) a letter and checklist of tasks for coaches, (b) three teacher report behavior rating scales (ESP Adaptive, ESP Maladaptive, CBCL Aggression), (c) an observation recording form for use by coaches in recording AET during pre- and postintervention time periods, (d) a student profile sheet on which coaches entered the rating scale scores, (e) teacher and parent surveys, (f) letters introducing First Step to teachers and parents, and (g) a one-page summary of the evaluation. Participating classroom teachers completed the three teacher rating scales at pre- and postintervention time points; the behavioral coaches recorded AET observations on these same occasions.

HSRI received First Step data from 30 behavioral coach participants representing 11 of Oregon's 36 counties by the May 2001 deadline for inclusion in the evaluation report. A total of 24 coaches returned useable data that were included in the final evaluation report. Coaches were asked to distribute and collect the teacher and parent surveys. Only 19 teachers completed the pre- and postintervention surveys; 17 sets of parents completed and returned the parent surveys.

Pre- and postintervention change scores for target participants for whom useable data were received by the HSRI evaluators in time for inclusion in its evaluation report are displayed in Table 21.2.

The results in Table 21.2 show substantial changes in the desired directions for each of the four dependent measures. All of the pre/post changes for the target participants were statistically significant at $p < .001$ and closely replicated those obtained by Walker et al. (1998).

HSRI evaluators conducted an additional analysis to assess responses to the intervention of students with more severe behavior problems versus those who had less serious involvements. A subgroup of 30 children were identified who were rated as "most severe" by their teachers on a least one of the three teacher rating scales (Adaptive, Maladaptive, and Aggression) at the beginning of the evaluation study. The mean score changes were statistically significant in favor of the most severe group on all three teacher rating measures but not for the AET observational measure. The average gain scores on these three measures for the severe group were nearly twice the magnitude of those for all other target children in the HSRI evaluation sample. It is important to note that the more severe participants had greater room for improvement on the study measures due to lower baseline scores.

The teacher survey asked only one question specifically about the target child, with the remaining questions focused on the class as a whole. The child-specific question asked how positively or negatively other children in the class viewed the target child on a scale of 1 to 4 (1 = *very positively;* 4 = *very negatively*). The baseline survey average for this question across the 19 teachers

TABLE 21.2

Mean Scores Across Four Measures for Participants in the Oregon Human Services Research Institute Evaluation

Measure and Group	Preintervention		Postintervention		
	M	SD	M	SD	n
Adaptive—Experimental	21.38	4.42	27.90	5.50	181
Aggression—Experimental	25.41	9.27	16.04	9.62	123
Maladaptive—Experimental	32.33	6.57	23.10	7.38	123
AET—Experimental	64.05	20.90	86.66	12.80	128

Note. AET = academic engaged time.

was 2.68 and the postintervention average was 2.05—a change that was in the right direction but that was not statistically significant. The remaining questions asked the teacher to estimate the First Step program's impact on the classroom as a whole. Overall, participating teachers saw the First Step program as valuable and especially liked the classwide impact of the program—a finding that replicates that of the Perkins-Rowe (2001) investigation.

For parents, the strongest positive changes occurred in the following areas: (a) their concerns about the child's behavior at home, (b) their concerns about the child's school behavior, (c) negative school reports from the child's teacher(s), and (d) the child's ability to get along with others. Parents cited family gains resulting from First Step as their favorite part of the program.

The overall results of this program evaluation were positive and encouraging. The findings of the HSRI evaluators closely replicated the level and direction of the First Step program's impact, as indicated by the close correspondence between results for the HSRI sample ($N = 181$) and the Walker et al. (1998) cohorts (n's $= 24$ and 22). Achieving intervention effects of this magnitude when the program is scaled up and applied under far less than controlled experimental conditions is a positive sign. Two other positive outcomes of this study were that (a) both parents and teachers saw collateral positive effects on the classroom and the family resulting from their participation and (b) evidence emerged that the First Step program is particularly effective with more intensely involved children.

These positive outcomes are, however, buffered and offset to some extent by several limitations resulting from logistical problems, data collection difficulties, and use of behavioral coaches as both evaluators and interventionists. Due to the nature of the HSRI study's design and execution, it was not possible to randomly assign children to experimental and control groups for comparative purposes. Thus, the effects noted cannot be attributed to a causal relationship between the First Step program and the observed changes in ratings and behavioral observations. Further, having coaches perform the dual roles of data collectors and interventionists introduces the very real possibility of bias in the data that favors the possibility of finding positive program effects. However, it was encouraging to see the close correspondence to and replication of the HSRI and Walker et al. (1998) investigations, in which these potentially biasing conditions were controlled. Finally, usable evaluation data were available from only 24 of the 244 behavioral coaches trained in First Step implementation, which represents only 11 of Oregon's 36 counties. Thus, it is unlikely that the sample adequately represented the population and geographic diversity of Oregon.

Many of these problems were due to inadequate funding of the evaluation study and delays in its onset, which resulted in a limited number of coaches participating from the available pool of trained personnel across the state who were capable of such participation. Although the evaluation data for the HSRI sample closely matched that for Cohorts 1 and 2 of the Walker et al. (1998) study, which were collected under much more rigorous conditions, the fact remains that their data may not adequately reflect the true impact of the First Step program's implementation.

HSRI evaluators' observations of the First Step program's implementation fidelity indicated that the integrity or quality of implementation varied substantially. They found that in some cases, all the key steps in the model's implementation were followed closely and rigorously adhered to, but in other cases there was significant deviation from intervention protocols and instructions contained in the First Step program materials. HSRI evaluators concluded that the First Step program produces reliable changes in child behavior even when there is relatively poor implementation fidelity.

It is hoped that a more thorough and scientifically rigorous program evaluation of the First Step intervention can be accomplished in subsequent years as a part of continuing State of Oregon funding of the program's implementation in Oregon schools. At a minimum, such an evaluation would need to have the following features: (a) random assignment to treatment and control conditions, or at least to wait-list control groups; (b) recording of pre- and postintervention measures by trained individuals who have nothing to do with the intervention and are blind to the treatment or control status of participating children, and (c) long-term follow-up monitoring and assessments to measure the durability of intervention-based behavioral gains.

THE CULTURAL APPROPRIATENESS OF FIRST STEP

The First Step program has been demonstrated to work effectively in rural, suburban, and urban settings and with a diverse array of students representing different cultural backgrounds (Caucasian, African American, Latino, Asian, and Native American). In addition, the First Step program has been translated into Spanish and is currently being translated into French and Japanese. To date, the program has been implemented in Australia and New Zealand, both English- and French-speaking Canadian provinces, and approximately 20 U.S. states. Plans are also under way to replicate the First Step program within Japanese schools. These program applications have proved successful and effective. They expand the range of populations, contexts, and cultural conditions under which the First Step program can produce reliable improvements in the behavior patterns of at-risk children.

ONGOING RESEARCH

The First Step program is currently the focus of several federally funded initiatives to intervene effectively with young children experiencing problem behavior primarily of an externalizing nature. Researchers at the University of Nebraska, Lincoln, and the University of Oregon are current recipients of large 5-year programmatic grants to demonstrate the effective integration of intervention approaches to achieve primary, secondary, and tertiary prevention goals and outcomes. In both these initiatives, the First Step program has been incorporated as an intervention to address secondary prevention goals. Results of these investigations will significantly expand the research base on First Step and should demonstrate its effects as implemented within the context of a schoolwide, universal intervention. The Washington County Mental Health Department in Oregon recently received a 4-year prevention grant from the Substance Abuse and Mental Health Services Administration (SAMHSA) to study the comparative efficacy of First Step. This ongoing study compares the results from an intervention using the standard version of First Step with data from an untreated control group and also with results from an enhanced version of the program in which participating families receive mental health support services in addition to the homeBase component of the program. Finally, the senior author, along with Severson, Feil, and Golly, recently received a 5-year grant award from the U.S. Agency for Children, Youth and Families (ACYF) to adapt the First Step program for effective use with Head Start children, teachers, and families. The results of this research will include a program version of First Step for exclusive use by Head Start programs. We are hopeful that these research initiatives involving First Step will increase its effectiveness and expand the range of applications in which the program will be considered for adoption and implementation. We look forward to seeing the results of these research efforts over the next 5 years.

CONCLUDING REMARKS

First Step appears to be an effective intervention with acceptable social validity, as indicated by feedback from consumers, although some teachers see it as too demanding of their time and effort. Additional research is need to establish its impact within urban school and community settings, where powerful risk factors operate at child, family, school, and community levels. Examination is also needed of the school contexts in which the program can and will likely be applied, including schoolwide or universal interventions, specialized alternative settings for at-risk students within school districts, and day treatment or residential treatment centers that include schooling components. The relative contributions of the home and school components of First Step to an overall treatment effect is a question that also needs further investigation. It is possible that a substantial treatment effect can be achieved from the school-only part of the program, and the recent results of Beard, reported earlier herein, suggest that this may indeed be the case. If so, this would be an important finding to document. Finally, it is important to research the relative contributions of these program components to long-term maintenance outcomes as indicated by longitudinal follow-up assessments.

APPENDIX 21.A

Reviews of Effective Early Intervention Programs

The First Step to Success program has been included or featured in the following compilations of effective interventions to address at-risk children and youth and to identify approaches for making schools safer and violence free.

1. *Preventing Mental Disorders in School-Age Children: A Review of the Effectiveness of Prevention Programs.* Mark T. Greenberg, PhD, Director, Prevention Research Center for the Promotion of Human Development, College of Health and Human Development, Pennsylvania State University, University Park, PA 16802; phone: 814/863-0112; fax: 814/865-2530; Web site: http://www.psu/edu/dept/prevention

2. *Effective Interventions for Children Having Conduct Disorders in the 0 to 8 Age Range.* Carolyn H. Webster-Stratton, PhD, Professor and Director, Parenting Research Clinic; Professor, Family and Child Nursing; Box 354801, 305 University District Building, School of Nursing, University of Washington, Seattle, WA 98195; phone: 206/543-6010; fax: 206/543-6040; e-mail: cws@u.washington.edu

3. *Effective Programs and Strategies to Create Safe Schools.* Paul Kingery, PhD, Director, Hamilton Fish National Institute on School and Community Violence—National Office, 2121 K Street NW, Suite 200, Washington, DC 20037-1830; phone: 202/496-2201; fax: 202/496-6244; e-mail: kingery@gwu.edu; Web site: www.hamfish.org

4. *Compilation of Early Violence Prevention Programs and Resources.* Julia M. Silva, PhD, APA Public Interest Directorate, American Psychological Association, 750 First Street NE, Washington, DC 20002-4242; phone: 202/336-5817; fax: 202/336-5723; e-mail: publicinterest@apa.org; Web site: www.apa.org/pi

5. *Programs and Interventions to Make Schools Safer.* Video Series on Safe Schools, National Education Association, 1201 16th Street NW, Washington, DC 20036; phone: 202/833-4000.

6. *Preventing Delinquency Through Early Interventions: Prenatal to Age 10.* Ray Mathis, Children's Delinquency Reduction Committee; Executive Director, Citizens Crime Commission, Affiliate of the Portland Metropolitan Chamber of Commerce, 221 NW Second Avenue, Portland, OR 97209-3999; phone: 503/228-9736; fax: 503/228-5126; e-mail: ccc@pdxchamber.org

REFERENCES

Achenbach, T. (1991). *The Child Behavior Checklist: Manual for the teacher's report form.* Burlington: University of Vermont, Department of Psychiatry.

Beard, K. (1998). The effects of a teacher and parent directed, proactive early intervention on the behaviors of elementary school children at-risk for antisocial behavior (Doctoral dissertation, University of Oregon, 1998). *Dissertation Abstracts International, 59,* 157.

Burns, B. J., & Hoagwood, K. (Eds.). (2002). *Community treatment for youth: Evidence-based interventions for severe emotional and behavioral disorders.* New York: Oxford University Press.

Elias, M., Zins, J., Weissberg, R., Frey, K., Greenberg, M., Haynes, N., et al. (1997). *Promoting social and emotional learning: Guidelines for educators.* Alexandria, VA: Association for Supervision and Curriculum Development.

Elliott, D. S. (1994). Serious violent offenders: Onset, developmental course, and termination (American Society of Criminology 1993 Presidential Address). *Criminology, 32,* 1–21.

Epstein, M. H., & Walker, H. M. (2002). Special education: Best practices and First Step to Success. In B. J. Burns & K. Hoagwood (Eds.), *Community treatment for youth: Evidence-based interventions for severe emotional and behavioral disorders* (pp. 179–197). New York: Oxford University Press.

Golly, A., Sprague, J., Walker, H. M., Beard, K., & Gorham, G. (2000). The First Step to Success program: An analysis of outcomes with identical twins across multiple baselines. *Behavioral Disorders, 25*(3), 170–182.

Golly, A., Stiller, B., & Walker, H. M. (1998). First Step to Success: Replication and social validation of an early intervention program for achieving secondary prevention goals. *Journal of Emotional and Behavioral Disorders, 6*(4), 243–250.

Hawkins, J. D., Catalano, R. F., Kosterman, R., Abbott, R., & Hill, K. G. (1999). Preventing adolescent health-risk behaviors by strengthening protection during childhood. *Archives of Pediatrics and Adolescent Medicine, 153,* 226–234.

Hoagwood, K. (2000). Research on youth violence: Progress by replacement, not addition. In H. Walker & M. Epstein (Eds.), *Making schools safer and violence free: Critical issues, solutions, and recommended practices* (pp. 1–4). Austin, TX: PRO-ED.

Hoagwood, K. (2001). Evidence-based practice in children's mental health services: What do we know? Why aren't we putting it to use? *Report on Emotional and Behavioral Disorders in Youth, 1*(4), 84–87.

Hoagwood, K., & Erwin, H. D. (1997). Effectiveness of school-based mental health services for children: A 10-year research review. *Journal of Child and Family Studies, 6,* 435–451.

Horner, R., Sugai, G., Lewis-Palmer, T., & Todd, A. (2001). Teaching school-wide behavioral expectations. *Report on Emotional and Behavioral Disorders of Youth, 1*(4), 77–80.

Jensen, P. S. (2001). The search for evidence-based approaches to children's mental health. *Emotional and Behavioral Disorders in Youth, 1*(3), 49, 50, 65.

Leff, S. S., Power, T. J., Manz, P. H., Costigan, T. E., & Nabors, L. A. (2001). School-based aggression prevention programs for young children: Current status and implications for violence prevention. *School Psychology Review, 30*(3), 344–362.

Loeber, R., & Farrington, D. (2001). *Child delinquents: Development, intervention, and service needs.* London: Sage.

Malecki, C., & Elliott, S. (2002). Children's social behaviors as predictors of academic achievement: A longitudinal analysis. *School Psychology Quarterly, 17*(1), 1–23.

Najaka, S., Gottfredson, D., & Wilson, D. (2001). A meta-analytic inquiry into the relationship between selected risk factors and problem behavior. *Prevention Science, 2*(4), 257–271.

Olds, D., Hill, P., & Rumsey, E. (1998). *Prenatal and early childhood nurse home visitation* (Juvenile Justice Bulletin NCJ172875). Washington, DC: U.S. Department of Justice, Office of Juvenile Justice and Delinquency Prevention.

Overton, S., McKenzie, L., King, K., & Osborne, J. (2002). Replication of the First Step to Success model: A multiple-case study of implementation effectiveness. *Behavioral Disorders, 28*(1), 40–56.

Patterson, G. R., Reid, J. B., & Dishion, T. J. (1992). *Antisocial boys.* Eugene, OR: Castalia.

Perkins-Rowe, K. (2001). Direct and collateral effects of the First Step to Success program: Replication and extension of findings (Doctoral dissertation, University of Oregon, 2001). *Dissertation Abstracts International, 62*(12A), 4058.

Reid, J. B. (1993). Prevention of conduct disorder before and after school entry: Relating interventions to developmental findings. *Development and Psychopathology, 5,* 311–319.

Satcher, D. (2001). *Youth violence: A report of the Surgeon General.* Washington, DC: U.S. Public Health Service, U.S. Department of Health and Human Services.

Walker, H. M., Colvin, G., & Ramsey, E. (1995). *Antisocial behavior in schools: Strategies and best practices.* Pacific Grove, CA: Brooks/Cole.

Walker, H. M., Irvin, L. K., Noell, J., & Singer, G. H. S. (1992). A construct score approach to the assessment of social competence: Rationale, technological considerations, and anticipated outcomes. *Behavior Modification, 16,* 448–474.

Walker, H. M., Kavanagh, K., Stiller, B., Golly, A., Severson, H. H., & Feil, E. G. (1998). First Step to Success: An early intervention approach for preventing school antisocial behavior. *Journal of Emotional and Behavioral Disorders, 6*(2), 66–80.

Walker, H. M., Severson, H. H., & Feil, E. G. (1995). *The Early Screening Project: A proven child-find process.* Longmont, CO: Sopris West.

Walker, H. M., Stiller, B., Golly, A., Kavanagh, K., Severson, H. H., & Feil, E. (1997). *First Step to Success: Helping young children overcome antisocial behavior.* Longmont, CO: Sopris West.

Zolna, J., Kimmich, M., & Hawkinson, L. (2001). *Final report: Evaluation of First Step to Success replication.* Salem: Oregon Commission on Children and Families.

The Longitudinal Comparison Study of the National Evaluation of the Comprehensive Community Mental Health Services for Children and Their Families Program

CHAPTER 22

*Robert L. Stephens, Tim Connor, Hoang Nguyen, E. Wayne Holden,
Paul Greenbaum, and E. Michael Foster*

The longitudinal comparison study of the national evaluation of the Comprehensive Community Mental Health Services for Children and Their Families Program was first implemented in 1997 among the grant communities funded initially in 1993 and 1994. The study contributes to nearly a decade of research designed to determine the efficacy of systems of care for improving child and family outcomes. Although the literature has consistently demonstrated the positive effects of system reform, it is less clear whether these system-level changes translate into greater symptom improvement for children served in systems of care than for those served in more traditional service delivery systems (Farmer, 2000; U.S. Department of Health and Human Services, 1999).

The 1999 *Mental Health: A Report of the Surgeon General* concluded that although results of studies on the effectiveness of systems of care seem promising, more research is necessary to determine conclusively whether changes at the system level will result in improved clinical outcomes for children served in systems of care (U.S. Department of Health and Human Services, 1999). An obvious need exists to develop evidence of the mechanisms through which system changes affect changes in outcomes for individual children and families. Farmer (2000) recently observed that there has been a shift in focus as system-building initiatives have grown from their historical roots in the Child and Adolescent Service System Program (CASSP). Although the principles of a system of care, as outlined by CASSP (Stroul & Friedman, 1986), have continued to drive these initiatives, an emphasis on individual-level outcomes as measures of effectiveness has replaced the initial focus on macrolevel changes and system performance. However, the heterogeneity of the populations that are served, the complexity of the interventions that are implemented, the lack of clarity in defining how effectiveness should be determined, and the lack of well-defined theories of change as the basis for intervention development have all contributed to the difficulties encountered in evaluations of the effectiveness of a system of care at the individual level (Duchnowski, Kutash, & Friedman, 2002; Farmer, 2000).

The primary research question addressed by the longitudinal comparison study was the extent to which observed changes in child and family outcomes can be attributed to differences in service delivery approaches. Secondary research questions were as follows: (a) Do outcomes change over time? (b) If outcomes do change over time, is there a differential rate or magnitude of change as a function of treatment delivery approach? and (c) Are there subgroups of children and families for whom a system of care is more effective? The study addressed these questions by comparing the outcomes of children and families served by systems of care funded by Community Mental Health Services (CMHS) with the outcomes of those served in communities without CMHS funding, within the context of a quasi-experimental matched-groups design.

DESIGN AND COMPONENTS OF THE LONGITUDINAL COMPARISON STUDY

A multimethod approach was used to evaluate system characteristics, child clinical and functional outcomes, services delivered and their associated costs, and family service experiences. The clinical outcome measures included the *Child and Adolescent Functional Assessment Scale* (CAFAS; Hodges, 1990) and the *Child Behavior Checklist* (CBCL; Achenbach, 1991). Functional indicators included measures of school placements, school attendance, contacts with law enforcement, social support, and living arrangements. In addition, a measure of family functioning, the *Caregiver Strain Questionnaire* (CGSQ), was included; it measures the degree of strain experienced by a caregiver as a result of his or her responsibilities related to caring for a child with behavioral problems (Brannan, Heflinger, & Bickman, 1998).

Children and families were interviewed at intake into services. Follow-up interviews occurred at 6-month intervals for up to 2 years. Field staff in each community interviewed families in their homes or at a convenient location in the community. In addition, a system-of-care assessment was conducted in each community to assess the system's infrastructure and service delivery practices relative to the system-of-care principles. Furthermore, a select sample of children and families participated in a system-of-care practice review (Hernandez et al., 2001) that assessed the extent to which their service experience conformed with system-of-care principles. These components of the study were included to evaluate implementation fidelity (i.e., the degree to which system-of-care principles were implemented in each of the communities and the consistency with which services experiences embodied system-of-care principles). Finally, management information system data were obtained from mental health agencies to examine service use and costs over time.

COMMUNITY SELECTION AND CHARACTERISTICS

Selection of three grant communities from among the 22 communities funded in 1993 and 1994 was initiated in the summer of 1997. All comparison study communities were selected based on the following criteria:

- *Service delivery approach.* Grant-funded communities were selected based on the extent of their progress in developing a system of care. "Mature" systems were identified based on system-of-care assessment data and information from state and local experts familiar with the communities. Eligible comparison communities were identified that did not have federal funding to support the development of a system of care.
- *Geographic, demographic, and economic characteristics.* Data from the 1990 Census were used in selecting matching comparison communities. Characteristics that communities were matched on included population size, child age distributions, racial and ethnic composition, income, size of catchment area, the percentage of people living below the poverty level, and the percentage of adults with high school educations. When possible, geographical proximity was also considered in selecting comparison communities to ensure they would be subject to the same state mental health structure and health-care changes (e.g., managed care). Statewide adoption of the system-of-care service delivery approach made this infeasible for one grant community.
- *Rate of child enrollment.* Communities had to be able to enroll the number of children needed to meet the required sample size during the proposed study period.
- *Child referral patterns.* To facilitate the selection of children with similar degrees and types of emotional and behavioral problems, similarity in referral patterns was examined in the selection of matching communities.

The final selection criterion was willingness to participate. Based on these criteria, the following matched pairs were selected: (a) the Stark County, Ohio, system of care matched to the Mahoning County, Ohio, comparison system; (b) the Santa Cruz County, California, system of care matched to the Travis County, Texas, comparison system; and (c) the East Baltimore, Maryland, system of care matched to the West Baltimore, Maryland, comparison system.

CHILD AND FAMILY SELECTION CRITERIA

Children were eligible for the study if they were between the ages of 6 and 17.5 years and presented with serious emotional or behavioral problems. In addition, at least one of the following four criteria had to be met: (a) a *Diagnostic and Statistical Manual of Mental Health Disorders* (*DSM–IV;* American Psychiatric Association, 1994) diagnosis of a mental health disorder and a clinical or functional assessment score above the clinical range on either the CAFAS or the CBCL; (b) a history of services received from multiple child-serving agencies (e.g., juvenile justice, education, child welfare, substance abuse); (c) currently at risk of, or past history of, out-of-home placement; or (d) participation in a special education program for children with serious emotional disturbance. Children and families recruited for the study were asked to participate for up to 2 years after entering the study.

RECRUITMENT, RETENTION, AND DATA COMPLETION

Overall, 1,042 children and their families were enrolled across the six sites. The retention rates were generally acceptable. Through the end of data collection in December 2000, 84% of families had been retained. Total data completion rates across communities ranged from 73% to 84%. The overall data completion rate of 80% across the four follow-up waves of data collection compared favorably to those of other longitudinal studies. For example, in the Fort Bragg evaluation, completion rates at 18 months ranged from 65% to 81% for key outcome measures (Hamner, Lambert, & Bickman, 1997), and in their Stark County study (Bickman, Summerfelt, & Noser, 1997), a data completion rate of 76% at the 6-month follow-up interview was reported. Angold, Costello, Burns, Erkanli, and Farmer (2000) reported a 70% completion rate across four data collection waves in the Great Smoky Mountains Study.

SYSTEM-LEVEL AND SERVICES EXPERIENCES DIFFERENCES

The system-of-care theoretical model posits that implementation of a system of care within a community will produce system-level changes (e.g., increased interagency collaboration, a wider array of traditional and innovative services, flexible funding arrangements, increased involvement of consumers, culturally competent services) that will alter the care that is provided directly to children and families and result in positive outcomes. This major tenet of the model required the development of a measurement approach for evaluating system-of-care implementation and development that did not previously exist in the children's mental health arena. To address this methodological challenge, the system-of-care assessment protocol was developed (Brannan, Baughman, Reed, & Katz-Leavy, 2002; Vinson, Brannan, Baughman, Wilce, & Gawron, 2001). This protocol consisted of a mixed quantitative and qualitative methodology with data collected via semistructured interviews conducted with multiple stakeholders during regular site visits to grant-funded communities. The data obtained were scored within a conceptual framework to evaluate the operationalization of the major system-of-care principles across the infrastructure and service delivery dimensions of children's mental health services. To complement this system-level measure, an individual case study protocol was developed to assess the experiences of services at the interface between providers and families (Hernandez et al., 2001).

To evaluate fidelity of implementation, system-level assessment site visits were conducted at each of the six study sites during the spring of 1999. Site visitors, who had been trained to an interrater agreement criterion of 85%, conducted the visits at each of the six study sites. In addition to evaluating interrater agreement as part of their training, agreement was evaluated in the field during the six site visits. During each of these visits, both site visitors simultaneously participated in an interview and independently rated the responses. Agreement in the field across these six site visits averaged 89% and ranged from 84% to 92%.

Comparisons of system scores across paired sites suggested that the federal program that funded the systems of care helped those sites come closer than the comparison sites to the ideals articulated in the principles. There was also less variability in scores across the funded systems of care, with greater variability found across the comparison sites' scores. Some movement toward the system-of-care approach was demonstrated in the comparison sites, however, despite their lack of federal funding. The systems of care performed especially well in the principles of interagency involvement and community-based service delivery. Although they generally performed better than the comparison sites, the system-of-care sites continued to struggle in their system-level quality improvement efforts and in culturally competent service delivery. A more detailed discussion of the differences between grantee communities on the system-of-care assessment can be found in Brannan et al. (2002).

The system-of-care practice review (SOCPR) provided an assessment of service experiences at the practice level. It was included in the comparison study for a subsample of children and families in each community (total $N = 96$ across all six communities) to determine whether system-of-care principles were being expressed directly in practice-level interactions between them and their service delivery personnel (Hernandez et al., 2001). Results of initial analyses of SOCPR data indicated that the service experiences of families were more consistent with system-of-care principles in the CMHS-funded systems than in the matched communities. Another set of analyses was conducted to explore the relationship of the experience of care that embodies the principles of a system of care to subsequent clinical outcomes for children being served in CMHS-funded systems of care and matched comparison communities (Stephens, Holden, & Hernandez, 2002). Results of those analyses indicated that children and families in systems of care reported experiencing services that embodied system-of-care principles at high levels. Their service experiences were more consistent, and their symptom severity did not vary as a function of intensity of their experiences (i.e., those with higher symptom scores had similar services experiences to those with lower symptom scores). In contrast, children and families in matched comparison communities reported more variability in their experiences of services that embodied system-of-care principles, and their symptom severity varied inversely as a function of their experiences. These findings mirror those of the system-of-care assessment described earlier regarding the operationalization of the system-of-care principles. System scores across the systems of care were less variable than those across the traditional service delivery systems, yet there was some movement toward the system-of-care approach in the traditional service delivery systems (Brannan et al., 2002).

CHARACTERISTICS OF SAMPLES AT INTAKE

Data quality control procedures began with interviewers reviewing each interview for completeness, clarity of recording, proper use of skip patterns, and proper use of missing values. Interviewers were also asked to describe any issues affecting the reliability of the data with the local field coordinator (e.g., a respondent who said "yes" to every question would be discarded). Field coordinators then conducted a second review for the same issues. A third abbreviated editing review was conducted at the central office. All interviews were entered into an aggregate electronic data file using double data entry procedures. The electronic data file was then cleaned using SPSS software. Verification of the data records included a search for duplicate records and a test of out-of-range or incorrect child identifiers, community identifiers, and interview wave identifiers. A review of individual variables was then conducted to verify the structure of the data file. In addition, individual variables were tested for out-of-range values and appropriate missing values. In addition, comments from the field staff were used to identify any unreliable interview data, which were then removed from the aggregate data file. Crucial demographic characteristics, including the child's gender, age, and race, were then reviewed across data collection waves for consistency and accuracy, and the appropriate use of skip patterns was also tested.

Following the application of data quality control procedures, the resulting analysis sample contained 1,033 children and their families. The demographic and behavioral characteristics of children and families in the comparison study communities were examined to assist in addressing baseline differences between samples in data analyses. Results are presented for each comparison pair separately (see Table 22.1).

TABLE 22.1

Demographic Characteristics of Children in the Comparison Study

Characteristic	Pair 1		Pair 2		Pair 3	
	Stark County[a]	Mahoning County[b]	Santa Cruz County[a]	Travis County (Austin)[b]	East Baltimore[a]	West Baltimore[b]
Gender	(n = 232)	(n = 216)	(n = 130)	(n = 214)	(n = 137)	(n = 100)
Male	64.7%	69.0%	60.0%	65.0%	63.5%	73.0%
Female	35.3%	31.0%	40.0%	35.0%	36.5%	27.0%
Age[c]	(n = 232)	(n = 216)	(n = 130)	(n = 214)	(n = 137)	(n = 100)
6–8 years	25.4%	22.7%	8.5%	28.0%	16.1%	16.0%
9–11 years	27.2%	25.9%	15.4%	29.0%	29.2%	27.0%
12–14 years	34.1%	28.7%	26.2%	32.2%	31.4%	23.0%
15–17 years	13.4%	22.7%	50.0%	10.7%	23.4%	34.0%
Mean (SD)	11.1 (3.1)	11.5 (3.3)	13.6 (2.9)	10.8 (3.0)	11.7 (3.1)	12.4 (3.3)
Race/Ethnicity[d]	(n = 232)	(n = 216)	(n = 126)	(n = 211)	(n = 136)	(n = 100)
African American	19.4%	46.8%	0.8%	28.4%	95.6%	96.0%
White	69.4%	38.4%	49.2%	31.8%	2.2%	2.0%
Hispanic/Latino	0.9%	5.1%	29.3%	27.0%	1.5%	1.0%
Mixed race	7.8%	9.3%	15.9%	12.3%	0%	1.0%
Other	2.5%	0.5%	4.8%	0.5%	0.7%	0%
Stability of living situation[e]	(n = 231)	(n = 216)	(n = 130)	(n = 213)	(n = 137)	(n = 100)
1 placement	67.1%	64.8%	39.2%	62.4%	75.2%	80.0%
2 placements	21.2%	21.4%	31.5%	26.3%	15.3%	18.0%
3 placements	8.2%	6.9%	20.0%	7.0%	7.3%	2.0%
4+ placements	3.5%	6.9%	9.2%	4.2%	2.2%	0%

[a]Community Mental Health Services (CMHS)–funded system-of-care community. [b]Non–CMHS-funded, non–system-of-care community. [c]Pair 2: χ^2 (3, N = 344) = 70.99, $p < .001$; $t(342) = -8.51, p < .001$. [d]Pair 1: χ^2 (4, N = 448) = 55.82, $p < .001$; Pair 2: χ^2 (4, N = 337) = 47.45, $p < .001$. [e]Pair 2: χ^2 (3, N = 333) = 23.54, $p < .001$.

Demographic Characteristics

Of the 1,033 children in the analyses, about two-thirds were boys. Gender was not significantly different among any of the three pairs. The ages of children in the Stark and Mahoning Counties pair were not significantly different, nor were there significant differences in the East Baltimore–West Baltimore pair. However, children in Santa Cruz County were significantly older than children in Travis County. Half of the children in Santa Cruz County were 15 to 17 years old when enrolled, whereas only 11% of children in Travis County were in that age range, $\chi^2(3, N = 344) = 70.99, p < .001$. This difference in ages reflects, in part, the difference in referral sources between the two communities. Santa Cruz County placed special emphasis on serving children referred from juvenile justice. Travis County had no special emphasis on a particular referral source and served children referred from a variety of sources.

Forty-two percent of children enrolled were African American, 37% were White, 11% were Hispanic or Latino, and another 8% had a mixed racial and ethnic background. Although the samples of children enrolled from the East and West Baltimore communities were almost all African American, samples of children enrolled from the Stark–Mahoning Counties, $\chi^2(4, N = 448) = 55.82, p < .001$, and the Santa Cruz–Travis Counties, $\chi^2(4, N = 337) = 47.45, p < .001$, had significantly different racial and ethnic distributions. Children in the Mahoning County and Travis County communities were more likely to be African American, whereas children in the Stark County and Santa Cruz County communities were more likely to be White. However, similar proportions of children with Hispanic backgrounds were enrolled in Santa Cruz and Travis Counties.

The demographic characteristics of the caregivers and families participating in the comparison study were also examined at intake. Caregivers who had spent the most time with the child in the past 6 months were sought as interview respondents. Biological mothers were the most frequent respondents, and 92% of all caregiver respondents across the six communities were women. Between 5% and 12% of respondents in each community were the children's biological fathers. Within all three pairs, the relationship of caregiver respondents to children was fairly similar. Caregiver respondents in West Baltimore and Santa Cruz County were more likely to have completed their high school education than the respondents in their paired communities: East–West Baltimore, $\chi^2(1, N = 237) = 10.88, p < .001$; Santa Cruz–Travis Counties, $\chi^2(1, N = 342) = 4.87, p < .05$. Caregivers in Stark County, West Baltimore, and Santa Cruz County were more likely to have a higher family income than caregivers in their paired communities: Stark–Mahoning Counties, $\chi^2(1, N = 444) = 10.84, p < .001$; East–West Baltimore, $\chi^2(1, N = 233) = 7.53, p < .01$; Santa Cruz–Travis Counties, $\chi^2(1, N = 340) = 23.10, p < .001$. Overall, 59% of all families participating in the study made less than $15,000 per year.

Child Behavior and Functioning at Intake

As noted previously, the primary behavioral and functional measures for the comparison study were the CAFAS and the CBCL. Samples of children in five of the six communities had mean CAFAS scores in the marked or severe range (see Table 22.2). The mean score for children from West Baltimore was slightly below the marked/severe range at 65.7, but their mean score was not significantly different from the mean score of children in the East Baltimore community. Children from Santa Cruz County and Travis County were also comparable on the CAFAS. However, children enrolled from Mahoning County had significantly more serious levels of functional impairment than the children from Stark County, $t(440) = 3.08$, $p < .005$. Generally, at entry into the study, caregivers of children in each of the six communities rated their children in the clinical range on the CBCL Total Problems scale. Although mean scores indicated similar levels of behavioral and emotional problems in two of the three pairs, children served in Travis County had significantly higher CBCL Total Problems scores than children in Santa Cruz County, $t(341) = 2.67$, $p < .01$.

TABLE 22.2

Children's Mean Scores on Clinical and Family Outcomes at Intake in the Comparison Study[a]

	Pair 1		Pair 2		Pair 3	
	Stark County[b]	Mahoning County[c]	Santa Cruz County[b]	Travis County (Austin)[c]	East Baltimore[b]	West Baltimore[c]
CAFAS Total Score[d]	($n = 227$)	($n = 215$)	($n = 125$)	($n = 205$)	($n = 135$)	($n = 95$)
M	70.7	78.1	79.2	74.9	70.9	65.7
SD	25.4	24.6	25.6	30.3	26.5	25.9
CBCL Total Problems[e]	($n = 232$)	($n = 215$)	($n = 129$)	($n = 214$)	($n = 137$)	($n = 100$)
M	68.9	70.2	65.6	68.7	65.2	65.0
SD	9.5	9.7	10.4	10.6	10.8	10.9
CGSQ Global Strain[f]	($n = 223$)	($n = 213$)	($n = 111$)	($n = 208$)	($n = 134$)	($n = 99$)
M	7.5	7.3	8.4	7.5	7.2	6.6
SD	2.6	2.3	2.4	2.5	2.6	2.4

Note. CAFAS = *Child and Adolescent Functional Assessment Scale* (Hodges, 1990); CBCL = *Child Behavior Checklist* (Achenbach, 1991); CGSQ = *Caregiver Strain Questionnaire* (Brannan et al., 1998).

[a] CAFAS total scores greater than or equal to 70 indicate children in the marked or severe ranges; CBCL and *Youth Self-Report* Total Problems scores greater than or equal to 63 are considered to be in the clinical range.

[b] Community Mental Health Services (CMHS)–funded system-of-care community.

[c] Non-CMHS-funded, non–system-of-care community.

[d] Pair 1: $t(440) = 3.08$, $p < .005$.

[e] Pair 2: $t(341) = 2.67$, $p < .01$.

[f] Pair 2: $t(317) = 23.22$, $p < .005$.

Family Functioning at Intake

Overall, caregivers of children in the Stark County and the East Baltimore systems of care did not experience significantly more strain in their lives than caregivers of children in the respective comparison communities of Mahoning County and West Baltimore (see Table 22.2). However, caregivers in the Santa Cruz County community reported more overall strain on average than caregivers in Travis County, $t(317) = -3.22, p < .005$.

In summary, populations across all six communities were very diverse. Although children and caregivers in paired communities generally were well matched on gender, marital status, and caregiver education, some samples did not match on age, racial identity, family employment, and family income. Although communities were fairly well matched during the community selection process, the local children's mental health agencies' enrollment processes did not always mirror predictions or census information used to match communities. As a result, some significant differences were also reported in functional and behavioral measures across matched pairs.

LONGITUDINAL ANALYSIS STRATEGY

Longitudinal analyses of child and family outcomes involved the use of a two-level hierarchical linear model (Bryk & Raudenbush, 1992). Hierarchical linear modeling (HLM) provides the ability to model data with a nested structure by allowing submodels at each level of the data structure. In Level 1 of the model, individual change trajectories were generated for each child in the sample to model change in symptomatology over time, with intercept, linear slope, and quadratic slope parameters included in the model (if appropriate based on significance tests of variance in each of the parameters in an unconditional model). In Level 2 of the model, the intercepts and slopes from the Level 1 model were treated as outcome variables. Variability in Level 1 intercepts, linear slopes, and quadratic slopes was predicted using individual demographic characteristics and site as covariates, as well as interactions between site and the other covariates. Both discrete continuous and dichotomous measures were included as covariates. The following continuous covariates were included: age and number of missing waves of outcome data. The dichotomous covariates were coded as follows: site (1 = *system of care*; 0 = *non–system of care*), gender (1 = *male*; 0 = *female*), annual family income (1 = *less than $15,000*; 0 = *$15,000 or more*). Race was coded differently for the Stark–Mahoning Counties pair and the Santa Cruz–Travis Counties pair (1 = *White*; 0 = *non-White* and 1 = *Hispanic*, 0 = *non-Hispanic*, respectively). Race was not entered in the East–West Baltimore models because the samples for analyses contained only African American children.

The modeling process began with the calculation of unconditional models to determine the appropriateness of including the linear and quadratic time slope components in the Level 1 model. If there was no significant variability in linear or quadratic time slopes in the unconditional model with both components free to vary, an unconditional model was calculated, with the variability of the quadratic term fixed at 0. If the variability in linear time slopes was significant in this model, the covariate models were calculated, with the quadratic time slope fixed. If the linear time slope variability was still not significant, an unconditional model was calculated, with the quadratic time slope component removed. In all cases where this step was required, the resulting unconditional model indicated significant variability in the linear time slope component, and models including the covariates were calculated with only the linear time slope component in the model.

CLINICAL OUTCOMES

To assess the relative effectiveness of systems of care to effect change in emotional and behavioral symptoms and functioning for children with serious emotional disturbance, CAFAS Total scores and CBCL Total Problems, Internalizing Problems, and Externalizing Problems scores were analyzed across data collection waves.

Stark–Mahoning Counties Pair

Analysis of change in functional impairment, as measured by CAFAS Total scores, from baseline to 24 months for children in Stark and Mahoning counties revealed a Site $\times$ Race $\times$ Gender interaction, $t(436) = 2.27, p < .05$. At intake, boys in both communities were more functionally impaired than girls, regardless of race. In the Stark County system of care, White boys improved at a greater rate than non-White boys, and non-White girls improved at a greater rate than White girls. In the Mahoning County non–system of care, the reverse pattern was obtained. Non-White boys improved at a greater rate than White boys, and White girls improved at a greater rate than non-White girls.

Analysis of change in CBCL Total Problems raw scores indicated no significant differences in rates of improvement between children in the Stark County system of care and the Mahoning County non–system of care. On average, children in both communities improved over time from intake to 24 months. However, analysis of change in CBCL Externalizing Problems raw scores revealed significant differences between children in the Stark County system of care and the Mahoning County non–system of care. At intake, caregivers in Stark County reported slightly fewer externalizing behavioral problems for their children than did caregivers in Mahoning County. Rates of improvement were initially greater in Stark County than in Mahoning County, $t(438) = -2.72, p < .01$. This trend continued from intake to 12 months. Beyond 12 months, deceleration of improvement was greater for Stark County than Mahoning County, $t(440) = 2.90, p < .005$, resulting in equivalent levels of improvement for children in both communities by 24 months.

Santa Cruz–Travis Counties Pair

Analysis of change in functional impairment from baseline to 24 months, as measured by CAFAS Total scores, for children in the Santa Cruz County system of care and the Travis County matched comparison site revealed a significant Site $\times$ Age interaction for the quadratic time parameter, $t(323) = -2.53, p < .05$. For both younger and older children served in Santa Cruz County, the rate of improvement increased over time. In contrast, the rate of improvement for both older and younger children served in Travis County slowed over time. The difference between the two communities in the rate at which improvement changed over time was more pronounced for older children than for younger children. This suggests that the Santa Cruz County system of care had a greater impact than the Travis County comparison system on reducing the functional impairment of older children.

Analysis of change in behavioral and emotional symptoms from baseline to 24 months, as measured by CBCL Total Problems raw scores, revealed a Site $\times$ Age interaction on the intercept parameter $t(330) = -5.04, p < .001$. For children served in the Santa Cruz County system of care, younger children had higher symptom scores at entry than older children, whereas for children served in the Travis County matched comparison site, older children had higher symptom scores at entry than younger children. Only the amount of missing data affected the rate of change in symptom scores over time, and this effect was the same for children in both communities, $t(330) = 2.17, p < .05$. The slowing of the rate of improvement was greater for those children with more missing data, possibly because families of children with more chronic behavior and emotional problems were more likely to have difficulty keeping scheduled appointments with data collectors.

The findings for CBCL Externalizing Problems scores mirrored those for CBCL Total Problems scores at entry into services, with level of symptoms at entry into services being predicted by a Site $\times$ Age interaction, $t(330) = -2.42, p < .025$. In addition, the linear time parameter for Externalizing Problems scores also revealed a Site $\times$ Age interaction, $t(1,099) = -1.96, p < .05$. Older children served in Santa Cruz County and younger children served in Travis County showed steeper slopes for change over time and less slowing of the rate of improvement than their counterparts. For CBCL Internalizing Problems scores, the Site $\times$ Age interaction was also predictive of the level of symptoms at entry into services, $t(327) = -4.19, p < .001$. However, the linear and quadratic time parameters were not related significantly to site.

East–West Baltimore Pair

Analysis of change in CAFAS Total scores from baseline to 24 months for children in the East Baltimore system of care and the West Baltimore comparison system revealed a significant Site $\times$ Missingness interaction on the quadratic time parameter, $t(680) = -2.64, p < .01$, that indicated children served in East Baltimore had greater deceleration of improvement compared to children served in West Baltimore, and the difference was greatest for those children with more missing data. This potentially could reflect a greater likelihood of children with more severe functional impairment remaining in services longer in East Baltimore than in West Baltimore.

Analysis of change in behavioral and emotional symptoms from baseline to 24 months, as measured by the CBCL, indicated that the Total Problems raw scores of children served in the West Baltimore comparison system improved at a greater rate than those of children served in the East Baltimore system of care, $t(220) = 2.54, p < .05$. Although the effect was statistically significant, the magnitude of the difference was minimal prior to 24 months.

This effect was not observed in analyses of Externalizing Problems or Internalizing Problems raw scores. However, there were significant Site $\times$ Missingness interactions on the linear time parameter for both Externalizing Problems, $t(716) = -2.05, p < .05$, and Internalizing Problems, $t(715) = -3.38, p = .001$, scores. These interactions reflect the relatively greater decrease in the rate of improvement at 24 months for children with missing data who were served in the East Baltimore system of care compared to children served in the West Baltimore comparison system, for whom missing data were associated with an increase in the rate of improvement. Again, this may reflect a tendency for children with more severe behavioral and emotional symptoms to remain in services longer in the East Baltimore system of care.

FUNCTIONAL INDICATORS

Stark–Mahoning Counties Pair

Equally as important as improvements in clinical outcomes for children are improvements in indicators of functioning in school and in the community. Involvement with the juvenile justice system is an important community indicator of functional impairment and behavioral problems.

To evaluate variations in juvenile delinquent behavior for children in the study, data were collected from the management information systems (MIS) of both Stark and Mahoning counties' juvenile court departments from 1997 to 2000. The juvenile courts maintain current and historical information on all juvenile offenses in each county, including offense type, degree of offense, date of court referral, adjudication decision, and disposition decision. Offenses recorded in each MIS included violent crimes, property crimes, criminal trespassing, disorderly conduct, alcohol- and drug-related offenses, weapons-related offenses, truancy and curfew violations, and probation violations.

Of the 232 children in the Stark County sample, 91 children (39%) had been charged with an offense at least once during the 1997–2000 period. Of the 217 children in the Mahoning County sample, 103 children (47%) had been charged with an offense. Although more children from Mahoning County were involved with the juvenile justice system during the study period, similar percentages of children in Stark County (37%) and Mahoning County (38%) committed offenses before entry into the study. Survival analysis (i.e., a hazard or Cox regression model) was used to compare juvenile delinquency between the two communities, controlling for important child characteristics that influence juvenile delinquent behavior, such as the child's age, gender, race, family structure, family socioeconomic status, school performance, baseline symptomatology (i.e., CBCL Total Problems score), and baseline functional impairment (i.e., CAFAS Total score). The survival analysis technique was applied to determine how long children "survive" without committing an offense in the system of care relative to children served in the non–system of care. The technique measures the time between intake and an ensuing offense. Based on the number of offenses committed by children in the sample, the survival analysis technique also generates the relative risk of delinquency. The relative risk of delinquency for this analysis is the risk of committing an offense after study entry relative to the risk of committing an offense prior to study entry.

Results indicated the relative risk of committing an offense after study entry for children in the Stark County system of care was slightly lower than that for children in Mahoning County. More specifically, the risk of committing an offense in Stark County after study entry was 43% of the risk prior to study entry. In Mahoning County, the risk of committing an offense after study entry was 67% of the risk prior to study entry. The risk of delinquency declined after study entry in both communities. Although it declined slightly more in Stark County, the difference in the risk of delinquency between the communities was only marginally significant, $t = -1.68, p < .10$.

In a second analysis of serious offenses only, the offense data were reduced to include only violent crimes, property crimes, alcohol and drug offenses, weapons offenses, criminal damaging and trespassing, and sexual offenses. Probation violations, disorderly conduct offenses, truancy, runaway, and curfew offenses were not included. When only serious offenses were analyzed, the risk of delinquency after study entry for children in Stark County was 67% of the risk prior to study entry. The risk of delinquency after study entry for children in Mahoning County was actually 44% *higher* than the risk prior to study entry. The risk of committing a serious offense after study entry for children in Stark County was significantly lower than the risk for children in Mahoning County, $t = -2.11, p < .05$.

Santa Cruz–Travis Counties Pair

Data were collected from the county juvenile court departments in Santa Cruz and Travis counties from July 1997 to December 2000. The quantity of offenses and dates on which they occurred were available from both counties, but data on the specific types of offenses were not consistently available across counties and could not be analyzed.

A comparison of the percentage of study children who committed offenses between Santa Cruz and Travis counties revealed that rates of juvenile delinquency were not dramatically different. Of the 130 children in the Santa Cruz County sample, 40% were charged with an offense at least once during the July 1997–December 2000 period, compared to 31% of children in Travis County. In the first year after study entry a similar pattern existed, with 31.5% of the children in Santa Cruz County committing an offense, compared with 22.8% of children in Travis County. A comparison of children based on the number of offenses each child committed in the first year after study entry revealed that 6.2% and 7.9% of children committed exactly one offense in Santa Cruz and Travis counties, respectively. Slightly more children committed two or more offenses in Santa Cruz County (25.4%) than did children in Travis County 14.9%).

To examine potential changes in delinquency in Santa Cruz and Travis counties, survival analysis was again used, controlling for the child's gender, age, race, and family income. Despite the focus on serving children with juvenile delinquent behaviors in Santa Cruz County, the relative risk of committing an offense after study entry was exactly the same (17% of the risk prior to study entry) for children in the two communities. Thus, both the Santa Cruz County and Travis County mental health systems significantly reduced the risk of juvenile delinquency in their communities. Although slightly more children from Santa Cruz County committed offenses overall, this difference was eliminated when age was entered as a covariate in the model. It is important to note that the Santa Cruz County system of care was able to reduce the relative risk of juvenile delinquency after study entry to 17% of its prestudy level while targeting children with delinquent behavior problems.

FAMILY FUNCTIONING

Given the family focus of the system-of-care program, the examination of how the system affects family life is important in determining the effectiveness of the program. Families can play an important role in their children's use of services and continuation in treatment.

Stark–Mahoning Counties Pair

Results of analysis of global strain scores for caregivers in Stark and Mahoning counties indicated that caregivers in both communities reported similar levels of strain at entry into services. Further, their global strain scores were reduced similarly over time ($p > .05$).

Santa Cruz–Travis Counties Pair

For caregivers in the Santa Cruz–Travis counties pair, change in global strain was predicted by a Site $\times$ Age interaction on the quadratic time parameter, $t(1,022) = -3.08$, $p < .005$. Although there was initial reduction in global strain for caregivers of both younger and older children in both communities, by 24 months there was a tendency for global strain to increase to levels similar to those at entry into services. This increase was most pronounced for caregivers of younger children in Santa Cruz County and for caregivers of older children in Travis County.

East–West Baltimore Pair

Results of analysis of change of global strain in the East–West Baltimore pair indicated that caregivers in East Baltimore reported higher levels of global strain at entry into services than those in West Baltimore, $t(219) = 2.11, p < .05$. Further, the rate of reduction in strain was predicted by a Site $\times$ Age interaction on the linear time parameter, $t(219) = 2.10, p < .05$. Caregivers of older children in West Baltimore reported a greater reduction in strain than caregivers of younger children in West Baltimore. In contrast, caregivers of both younger and older children in the East Baltimore system of care reported less reduction in strain than caregivers in West Baltimore. Further, in East Baltimore, caregivers of younger children reported a slightly greater reduction than caregivers of older children. Overall, reported levels of strain were fairly low in both communities.

SERVICES EXPERIENCES

A major component of the comparison study involved the collection and analysis of mental health services and costs data to help explain differences in the success of serving children with emotional and behavioral disorders in the two systems. Primary mental health services data were collected from the community mental health centers (CMHCs) through which children were enrolled into the study in both the Stark–Mahoning counties pair and in the Santa Cruz–Travis counties pair. Each CMHC has a computerized MIS used for internal management and billing purposes.

Stark–Mahoning Counties Pair

Results in this section will focus primarily on the Stark–Mahoning counties pair because the comparison study methodology in Ohio incorporated an aggressive community-wide services and costs data collection effort for the purposes of describing services received outside the CMHCs, and replication of the effort in the remaining pairs was cost-prohibitive. In the Ohio pair, data were collected from inpatient mental health providers, child welfare departments, juvenile detention centers, and school special education programs.

For the Stark–Mahoning counties pair, the primary mental health services data were collected for the entire study period, from January 1997 through December 2000. Because the last child was enrolled in October 1999, at least 15 months of services data were available for all children. The analyses of services and costs data include only services received in the first 18 months following enrollment into the study. Ninety-five percent of children in Mahoning County and 84% of children in Stark County had a full 18 months of available services data for analysis. (In Stark County, 32% of all children received services more than 18 months after study entry, and 36% did so in Mahoning County.) Of the 232 children in the Stark County sample, the participating CMHC was able to provide services data for 229. The 3 remaining children were missing data in CMHC records. Services data for 214 of the 232 children in the Stark County sample and 206 of the 217 children from Mahoning County were included in the final services and costs data analyses.

Types of Services Delivered in Stark and Mahoning Counties

The primary types of mental health services that the Stark County and Mahoning County CMHCs recorded in their MISs were similar, including intake and assessment services, individual counseling, family or group counseling, medication monitoring, and case management. The percentage of children who received a specific type of service provided an indication of its prominence in the program's service array. All children received intake and assessment services in both communities. The percentages of children in each community who received case management services were similar (59% in Stark County vs. 57% in Mahoning County), as they were for behavioral medication monitoring (44% in Stark County vs. 45% in Mahoning County). The Stark County and Mahoning County CMHCs differed in their use of the various types of counseling. The Mahoning County CMHC relied more heavily on individual counseling, while the Stark County CMHC provided a broader mix of individual, family, and group counseling. Ninety-five percent of children received individual counseling from the Mahoning County CMHC, compared to 75% from the Stark County CMHC, $\chi^2(1, N = 420) = 30.67$, $p < .001$. However, the Stark County CMHC provided family or group counseling to 82% of children, compared to 11% of children at the Mahoning County CMHC, $\chi^2(1, N = 420) = 210.02$, $p < .001$.

Service Mix in Stark and Mahoning Counties

An agency's service mix was defined as the amount of each service delivered as a percentage of the total amount of all services delivered. Of all services delivered to children by the Mahoning County CMHC, the core of the service use pattern was individual counseling (44%) and case management (36%), with group and family counseling making up a smaller percentage of services (6%). The Stark County CMHC provided a more balanced mix of individual counseling (20%), group and family counseling (22%), and case management (46%). Medication monitoring played a much greater role in the service mix in the Mahoning County CMHC (12%) than in the Stark County CMHC (3%). In addition, although similar percentages of children in the two communities received medication monitoring and case management, the Stark County CMHC actually delivered a greater proportion of case management,

$\chi^2(1, N = 420) = 200.14, p < .001$, and a smaller proportion of medication monitoring, $\chi^2(1, N = 420) = 588.36, p < .001$, than the Mahoning County CMHC delivered in relation to other services.

Amount of Services in Stark and Mahoning Counties

A dramatic difference existed between the communities in terms of the number of services received per child. The Stark County CMHC delivered more than twice as many services ($M = 65.8$ per child) in the first 18 months after study entry as the Mahoning County CMHC ($M = 29.5$ per child), $t(418) = -5.99, p < .001$. In terms of hours of services, the Stark County CMHC and Mahoning County CMHC diverge even more. Children served by the Stark County CMHC received an average of almost three times as many hours of services (74 hours) than children served by the Mahoning County CMHC (26 hours) in the first 18 months of service delivery.

When individual services were examined, the most pronounced difference was found in the average hours of case management received per child. Although a similar percentage of children served by the Stark County and Mahoning County CMHCs received case management in the 18 months following study entry, the children served by the Stark County CMHC averaged 38 hours, compared with 11 hours for children served by the Mahoning County CMHC, $t(243) = -6.13, p < .001$. The system-of-care approach emphasizes the importance of case management activities, such as coordinating services, advocating for and supporting families, and monitoring quality. Thus, the relatively large amount of time spent on case management is a confirmation of the strength of the implementation of the system of care for families served by Stark County. In addition, the children who received assessment, $t(168) = -4.61, p < .001$; individual counseling, $t(354) = -2.82, p < .01$; and medication monitoring services, $t(185) = -4.62, p < .001$, at the Stark County CMHC received significantly more hours of each respective service compared to children served by the Mahoning County CMHC. The only service category for which the Stark County and Mahoning County CMHCs provided similar hours of service per child was group or family counseling, but the Stark County CMHC provided the service to 71% more children ($n = 175$ in Stark County [175/214 = 82%] vs. $n = 23$ in Mahoning County [23/206 = 11%]).

Duration and Intensity of Services in Stark and Mahoning Counties

The duration of service use was measured by the number of months between the child's first and last service. Examination of only the first 18 months after study entry indicated that children served by the two CMHCs did not differ significantly; both groups received services for an average of 9.5 months. Service intensity was defined as the average hours of services received per month between the first and last dates of service. The intensity of services delivered to children by the Stark County CMHC (7.5 hours per month) was significantly higher than the intensity of services delivered to children by the Mahoning County CMHC (3.9 hours per month), $t(418) = -4.25, p < .001$. This difference is related to the number of days children received service encounters in the two communities. During the 18-month period, children served by the Stark County CMHC had service encounters for an average of 49 days, compared to 23 days for children served by the Mahoning County CMHC.

Continuity of Services in Stark and Mahoning Counties

Previous analyses have suggested that continuous services can have a positive impact on children's outcomes (Center for Mental Health Services, 1998). Because the intensity of services delivered by the Stark County CMHC within the system of care was greater, continuity of services might also be greater. At the Stark County CMHC, the average break between services in the first 3 months was 3.82 days, and it increased slightly over the entire 18-month period to 5.45 days during the last 3 months of the 18-month period. At the Mahoning County CMHC, the average break between services was not only greater, but also increased dramatically over time, from 6.59 days in the first 3 months to 18.11 days during the last 3 months of the 18-month period. This was more than three times longer than the average break for children served in the Stark County system of care during the last 3 months of services, $t(1,919) = 7.81, p < .001$.

The Costs of Services in Stark and Mahoning Counties

The previous description of children's service use patterns documents how the Stark County CMHC within the system of care delivered services to children in greater amounts and with greater intensity than the Mahoning County CMHC. As would be expected, the costs of providing these more intensive services were also significantly greater. Overall, $4,690 was spent on the average child served by the Stark County CMHC, whereas $2,256 was spent on the average child served by the Mahoning County CMHC, $t(418) = -5.35, p < .001$. As was the case with the amount of services delivered, much of the difference in costs was due to the difference in case management. For children who received case management, the Stark County CMHC spent an average of $2,773 per child for these services and the Mahoning County CMHC spent an average of $946 per child. As described earlier, both CMHCs provided case management to a similar number of children, but the Stark County CMHC dedicated many more service hours to case management per child. The more frequent use of group and family counseling at the Stark County CMHC also contributed to higher total costs. For the children who received group or family counseling at the Mahoning County CMHC, an average of $1,037 per child was spent on group or family counseling. At the Stark County CMHC, an average of $1,465 per child was spent on group or family counseling, and 65% more children received this service.

One possible effect of the more intensive mental health services delivered at the Stark County CMHC could be the reduction of costs for other children's services used within the community, potentially resulting in costs savings.

Costs data collected from other child-serving agencies in each community were analyzed to compare the dollars spent outside of the CMHC on outpatient mental health services, inpatient mental health services, and community placements with child-serving agencies in the Stark–Mahoning counties pair. In Chapter 10 of this volume, Foster and Connor present a thorough discussion of an examination of cost shifting and cost offset in the Stark–Mahoning counties pair. Their findings suggest that there are potential costs savings in other child-serving sectors when comparisons are properly adjusted.

Santa Cruz–Travis Counties Pair

As with the Stark County and Mahoning County pair, services data in the Santa Cruz–Travis Counties pair were collected from the CMHCs through which children had been enrolled into the study in each county. Both CMHCs were operated by the county-based public mental health system and served as the primary source of mental health services in each community. Each CMHC has a computerized MIS for internal management and billing purposes.

Of the 130 children in the Santa Cruz County sample, the participating CMHC was able to provide services data for 129. Services data were available for 213 of the 215 children in the Travis County sample. Excluded from the data were canceled appointments with the child and family, and services received prior to study entry. Although the design of some service MISs includes only billable services, the Santa Cruz County and Travis County MISs included both billable and nonbillable services. To provide the most comprehensive analysis of service utilization, both of these types of services were included. Both the Santa Cruz County and Travis County systems contracted with other providers for day treatment and residential treatment services, which they did not record in their MISs. Santa Cruz County also directly provided some day treatment and residential services that they recorded in their MIS, but these data were excluded from the analyses to provide a more equitable comparison between the two counties.

The mental health services data were collected for the period of time beginning January 1998 and ending December 2000. To provide an appropriate comparison between communities, the analyses of service utilization data in these communities included only services received in the first 12 months following study enrollment for each child. Thus, 122 children from Santa Cruz County and 210 children from Travis County were included in the current analyses.

Types of Services Delivered and Service Mix in Santa Cruz and Travis Counties

Findings for the Santa Cruz–Travis counties pair were similar to those for the Stark–Mahoning counties pair. The primary types of mental health services included intake and assessment services, individual counseling, family counseling, group counseling, medication monitoring, and case management. As in the Stark County–Mahoning County comparison, the CMHCs in both Santa Cruz and Travis counties provided case management to essentially equivalent numbers of children (99% and 98%, respectively). However, unlike the Stark County–Mahoning County pair, the Travis County CMHC provided individual counseling to significantly fewer children (64%) than the Santa Cruz County CMHC (94%), $\chi^2(1, N = 332) = 38.17, p < .001$. Santa Cruz County also provided more family (33% vs. 16%) and group (45% vs. 0%) counseling than Travis County. In addition, a greater percentage of children served in Santa Cruz County received crisis services compared to children served in Travis County (24% vs. 4%, respectively), $\chi^2(1, N = 332) = 28.91, p < .001$. However, a greater percentage of children in Travis County received medication monitoring, compared to children in Santa Cruz County (59% vs. 44%, respectively), $\chi^2(1, N = 332) = 6.35, p < .05$. Of all services delivered to children in each community, the core of the service use pattern was individual counseling (26% of all services in Santa Cruz County vs. 24% of all services in Travis County) and case management (57% of all services in Santa Cruz County vs. 60% of all services in Travis County). However, the Santa Cruz County service mix was somewhat more balanced because of the inclusion of group counseling for children (11% of all services in Santa Cruz County vs. 0% of all services in Travis County) and the less frequent use of medication monitoring (3% of all services in Santa Cruz County vs. 5% of all services in Travis County). Although Santa Cruz County provided many more services overall, the mix of services provided by the two county CMHCs was not dramatically different, with the exception of the absence of group counseling in Travis County.

Amount of Services in Santa Cruz and Travis Counties

As in the Stark–Mahoning counties pair, a dramatic difference existed between Santa Cruz and Travis counties in terms of the number of services received per child in the first 12 months after study entry. The Santa Cruz County CMHC delivered more than twice as many services ($M = 110$ per child) as the Travis County CMHC ($M = 46$ per child), $t(330) = -10.05$, $p < .001$. When hours of services were examined, the Santa Cruz County CMHC and Travis County CMHC diverged even more. Children served by the Santa Cruz County CMHC received an average of three times as many hours of service (119 hours) than children served by the Travis County CMHC (37 hours) in the first 12 months of service delivery, $t(330) = -12.18$, $p < .001$. When individual services were examined, the most pronounced difference was found in the average hours of case management received per child. Although a similar percentage of children served by the Santa Cruz County and Travis County CMHCs received case management in the 12 months following study entry, the children served by the Santa Cruz County CMHC averaged 55.3 hours, compared to 12.5 hours for children served by the Travis County CMHC, $t(325) = -12.30, p < .001$.

Duration, Intensity, and Continuity of Services in Santa Cruz and Travis Counties

The children served at the Santa Cruz County CMHC received more overall services in the first 12 months because of the longer duration and greater intensity of their services. Children served by the Santa Cruz CMHC averaged 9.3 months in service, compared to 7.4 months for children at the Travis County CMHC,[1] $t(330) = -4.30$, $p < .001$. Although children in Travis County received 7.4 hours of service per month, children in Santa Cruz County received 13.1 hours of service per month, $t(330) = -4.07$, $p < .001$. At the Santa Cruz County CMHC, the average break between services in the first 3 months was about 2 days, and it gradually increased over the first 12 months to 3.43 days in the last 3 months (9–12 months after entry). At the Travis County CMHC, the average break between services was not only greater but also increased at a greater rate over time. At the Santa Cruz County CMHC, the average break between services in the first quarter was approximately 2 days, and it gradually increased over the first 12 months to 3.43 days in the last quarter. Thus, service contacts with children in Santa Cruz County were consistently an average of 2 to 3 days apart during the first 12 months. The average break in services at the Travis County CMHC during the first quarter was similar to Santa Cruz County at 3.52 days. However, the average break between services during the second quarter was twice as long at the Travis County CMHC, $t(6,552) = 12.34$, $p < .001$, and was more than twice as long during the last quarter of services, $t(3,156) = 8.73$, $p < .001$.

The Cost of Services in Santa Cruz and Travis Counties

As was the case with the Stark and Mahoning counties comparison, the system of care delivered more services to children, resulting in greater expenditures for the system of care. In the first 12 months after study entry, an average of $8,518 of billable services per child was recorded in the Santa Cruz County MIS, compared to $1,200 per child in the Travis County MIS, $t(330) = -15.83$, $p < .0001$. In Travis County, $1,000 or less was spent on 63.8% of children, compared to 5.7% of children in Santa Cruz County. A portion of the difference in expenditures can be directly attributed to the greater quantity and intensity of services offered by the Santa Cruz County system of care. The use of behavioral medications as the primary therapeutic intervention in Travis County also contributes to the dramatic difference in expenditures. One out of five children (19.5%) served by the Travis County CMHC received behavioral medications without any individual, family, or group therapy in the first 12 months after entry, compared to less than 1% of children served by the Santa Cruz County CMHC. When compared to the average expenditures per child served at the Stark and Mahoning counties CMHCs, the Travis County

---

[1] These figures do not represent the average overall duration for children but rather the average duration during the first 12 months after study entry. Several children received services for longer than 12 months, but not all of these data are included in the analyses in this report.

expenditures per child were similar to the Mahoning County expenditures per child, whereas the expenditures per child in Santa Cruz County were nearly double the expenditures per child in Stark County. The amount of nonbillable services for which costs are not available also affects the comparison of expenditures collected from MISs. Most agencies do not record an expenditure amount for any service for which they cannot bill, although these services are paid for by other public sources (e.g., state and county subsidies). In the data collected from Travis County, 59.4% of all services were nonbillable, compared to just 1.2% of services collected from Santa Cruz County. Thus, the gap in expenditures between the communities would close if the costs of these services were included.

CONCLUSIONS

The longitudinal comparison study conducted as part of the National Evaluation of the Comprehensive Community Mental Health Services for Children and Their Families Program was implemented to address the question of the effectiveness of systems of care, which has received support in uncontrolled outcome studies (Duchnowski et al., 2002) but has been questioned by the results of investigations using comparison groups (Bickman et al., 1995; Bickman, Noser, & Summerfelt, 1999; Bickman et al., 1997). This chapter has presented a number of findings from the initial analyses of data from the comparison study. Portions of the study conducted to evaluate implementation fidelity indicated that federal funding had a discernible impact on the development and operationalization of system-of-care principles within both the infrastructure and service delivery components of funded programs relative to their matched comparison communities. In addition, experiences at the level of service delivery for select subsamples were more consistent with system-of-care principles in the communities with federal funding. It should be noted, however, that despite the absence of CMHS funding, comparison communities displayed some operationalization of system-of-care principles and penetration of these principles to the level of service delivery experiences. This finding underscores the difficulties inherent in conducting quasi-experimental comparison studies on a service delivery approach that has widespread clinical appeal and has incompletely penetrated across community service delivery settings (Friedman & Hernandez, 2002).

Analyses of differential clinical and functional outcomes revealed a more mixed picture. Improvement across time was observed for each of the six communities on major symptom and functional indicators. Ratings of externalizing behavior problems from caregivers showed a significantly greater rate of improvement during the first 18 months of services, which was accompanied by an overall decreased risk for juvenile justice involvement for Stark County relative to the Mahoning County comparison site. Functional impairment improved at a significantly greater rate in Santa Cruz relative to the Travis County comparison site, and the risk for continued juvenile justice involvement was greatly reduced in both communities. In East and West

Baltimore, however, overall levels of caregiver-rated behavioral problems appeared to improve at a faster rate in the comparison community than the CMHS-funded community, especially during the latter 6 months of the study. Although there were no significant differences in family functioning found in the Stark–Mahoning counties pair, caregivers did report a differential reduction of strain in the Santa Cruz–Travis counties and East–West Baltimore pairs that varied across communities as a function of the child's age. The results of analyses of clinical and functional outcomes suggest that for those children with greater functional impairment, high delinquency scores, and contact with law enforcement for serious offenses, a federally funded system of care may be more beneficial than services delivered as usual in a matched comparison community.

Although the services data available from the MIS databases in the CMHCs in the Stark–Mahoning counties and Santa Cruz–Travis counties pairs did not provide complete detail on the entire array of services offered to children, a distinct and significant difference still existed among the mental health services delivered through the two CMHCs in the systems of care compared to the two CMHCs in the comparison systems. The more intensive use of case management, in particular, highlights the strength of a system of care and reflects the implementation of multiagency collaboration and service coordination. The cost analyses presented here are more extensive than previous such analyses and suggest that increased mental health expenditures occur in communities with a federally funded system of care. Increased expenditures within the Stark County system of care may have been offset by lowered expenditures in other child-serving agencies within the community.

A complex set of issues was involved in conducting and analyzing the results of these studies. The advantages of the design were that it allowed for studying the effects of services delivery within a naturalistic context and it was consistent with the overall structure and direction of the grant program. Differential outcomes using symptom-based and functional impairment measures continue to be difficult to detect clearly within these large quasi-experimental designs. Lack of assessment of the specific types of treatments delivered within outpatient settings and interactions at the service provider–family level have limited the ability to determine who benefits most from what treatment. This is compounded by the heterogeneity of presenting problems for the samples that are being treated within community settings.

The Surgeon General's report on mental health (U.S. Department of Health and Human Services, 1999) and the evidence-based treatment movement within children's mental health (Burns & Hoagwood, 2002) are recent events that have affected the evolution of research questions regarding systems of care. Systems of care are an area in need of further study, especially with respect to the integration of evidence-based interventions within these community-based programs. More recent special studies within the national evaluation employing randomized clinical trial designs are beginning to address these concerns. These studies not only will assess the effectiveness of evidence-based interventions within systems of care on clinical outcomes but also will collect both quantitative and qualitative information to identify facilitators and barriers to the faithful implementation of evidence-based interventions within community settings.

Although many questions continue about the effectiveness of systems of care at the clinical outcome level (Burns & Hoagwood, 2002; U.S. Department of Health and Human Services, 1999), data exist to support continued work on implementation of the approach within community settings. Strong consumer advocacy for alterations in traditional mental health services approaches for children with serious emotional disturbance and their families is an important driving factor in sustaining federal- and state-level efforts. The most important question for the field is how to integrate effectively evidence-based interventions within the system-of-care philosophy, with the underlying hypothesis being that the effects of these interventions will maintain and generalize more effectively within the context of coordinated, community-based service systems.

REFERENCES

Achenbach, T. M. (1991). *Manual for the Child Behavior Checklist/4–18 and 1991 Profile.* Burlington: University of Vermont, Department of Psychiatry.

American Psychiatric Association. (1994). *Diagnostic and statistical manual of mental disorders* (4th ed.). Washington, DC: Author.

Angold, A., Costello, E. J., Burns, B. J., Erkanli, A., & Farmer, E. M. Z. (2000). Effectiveness of nonresidential specialty mental health services for children and adolescents in the "real world." *Journal of the American Academy of Child and Adolescent Psychiatry, 39*(2), 154–160.

Bickman, L., Guthrie, P. R., Foster, E. M., Lambert, W., Summerfelt, W. T., Breda, C. S., et al. (1995). *Evaluating managed mental health services: The Fort Bragg experiment.* New York: Plenum Press.

Bickman, L., Noser, K., & Summerfelt, W. M. (1999). Long-term effects of a system of care on children and adolescents. *Journal of Behavioral Health Services and Research, 26*(2), 185–202.

Bickman, L., Summerfelt, W., & Noser, K. (1997). Comparative outcomes of emotionally disturbed children and adolescents in a system of services and usual care. *Psychiatric Services, 48,* 1543–1548.

Brannan, A. M., Baughman, L. N., Reed, E. D., & Katz-Leavy, J. (2002). System-of-care assessment: Cross-site comparison of findings. *Children's Services: Social Policy, Research, and Practice, 5,* 37–56.

Brannan, A. M., Heflinger, C. A., & Bickman, L. (1998). The Caregiver Strain Questionnaire: Measuring the impact on the family of living with a child with serious emotional disturbance. *Journal of Emotional and Behavioral Disorders, 5,* 212–222.

Bryk, A. S., & Raudenbush, S. (1992). *Hierarchical linear models.* Newbury Park, CA: Sage.

Burns, B. J., & Hoagwood, K. (Eds.). (2002). *Community treatment for youth: Evidence-based interventions for severe emotional and behavioral disorders.* New York: Oxford University Press.

Center for Mental Health Services. (1998). *Annual report to Congress on the evaluation of the Comprehensive Community Mental Health Services for Children and Their Families Program, 1998.* Atlanta, GA: Macro International.

Duchnowski, A. J., Kutash, K., & Friedman, R. M. (2002). Community-based interventions in a system of care and outcomes framework. In B. J. Burns & K. Hoagwood (Eds.), *Community treatment for youth: Evidence-based interventions for severe emotional and behavioral disorders* (pp. 16–37). New York: Oxford University Press.

Farmer, E. M. Z. (2000). Issues confronting effective services in systems of care. *Children and Youth Services Review, 22,* 627–650.

Friedman, R. M., & Hernandez, M. (2002). The national evaluation of the Comprehensive Community Mental Health Services for Children and Their Families Program: A commentary. *Children's Services: Social Policy, Research, and Practice, 5,* 67–74.

Hamner, K. M., Lambert, E. W., & Bickman, L. (1997). Children's mental health in a continuum of care: Clinical outcomes at 18 months for the Fort Bragg Demonstration. *Journal of Mental Health Administration, 24*(4), 465–471.

Hernandez, M., Gomez, A., Lipien, L., Greenbaum, P. E., Armstrong, K., & Gonzalez, P. (2001). Use of the system-of-care practice review in the national evaluation: Evaluating the fidelity of practice to system-of-care principles. *Journal of Emotional and Behavioral Disorders, 9,* 43–52.

Hodges, K. (1990). *Child and Adolescent Functional Assessment Scale* (CAFAS). Ypsilanti: Eastern Michigan University, Department of Psychology.

Stephens, R. L., Holden, E. W., & Hernandez, M. (2002). *System-of-care practice review scores as predictors of behavioral symptomatology and functional impairment.* Manuscript submitted for publication.

Stroul, B. A., & Friedman, R. M. (1986). *A system of care for children and youth with severe emotional disturbances* (Rev. ed.). Washington, DC: Georgetown University Child Development Center, CASSP Technical Assistance Center.

U.S. Department of Health and Human Services. (1999). *Mental health: A report of the Surgeon General.* Rockville, MD: U.S. Department of Health and Human Services, Substance Abuse and Mental Health Services Administration, Center for Mental Health Services, National Institutes of Health, National Institute of Mental Health.

Vinson, N., Brannan, A. M., Baughman, L., Wilce, M., & Gawron, T. (2001). The system-of-care model: Implementation in 27 communities. *Journal of Emotional and Behavioral Disorders, 9,* 30–42.

The Oregon Multidimensional Treatment Foster Care Model

CHAPTER 23

Research, Community Applications, and Future Directions

Stephanie A. Shepard and Patricia Chamberlain

he Oregon Multidimensional Treatment Foster Care Program (MTFC; Chamberlain, 1994) was designed to provide treatment to emotionally and behaviorally troubled youth in need of out-of-home placements. In this model, treatment is provided in a nonrestrictive community setting (i.e., family setting) as an alternative to traditional institutional, residential, and group care placements. Several randomized clinical trials of MTFC have been completed that demonstrate that MTFC is a feasible, cost-effective, community-based alternative for a variety of youth and their families. In this chapter we describe the theoretical basis for the MTFC model and provide detail about the various treatment components and staff roles. Next, we review the evidence demonstrating that MTFC is an effective approach for working with youth with severe, chronic delinquent behavior who are involved in the juvenile justice system, as well as young children through adolescents who have been referred by the mental health and child welfare systems. Implications of research on MTFC for work in these broader systems will then be discussed, and we will provide a brief description of recent efforts to disseminate MTFC within a state-supported foster care setting. In conclusion, we will explore further the issues involved in disseminating MTFC for use in different contexts with diverse samples.

THEORETICAL BASIS OF THE MTFC MODEL

The MTFC model is based on a social-learning treatment approach. The underlying assumption of the model is that the contingencies that exist within the contexts in which individuals interact reinforce their behaviors, attitudes, and emotions. As such, the model dictates that interventions be implemented across multiple settings (i.e., home, school, peer group, community) through moment-to-moment feedback (i.e., positive reinforcement for appropriate behavior and clear, well-specified consequences for rule transgressions) provided within a consistent, reinforcing environment such as a family setting. It is designed to address antecedents of adolescent antisocial behavior and delinquency, including poor parental supervision and monitoring, lack of consistent discipline, low parental involvement, associations with deviant peers, and school failure (Chamberlain, 1994, 1996; DeBaryshe, Patterson, & Capaldi, 1993; Reid, 1993; Reid & Eddy, 1997).

The intervention work conducted at the Oregon Social Learning Center (OSLC) over the last 40 years served as a basis for developing the treatment. It was developed as an extension of OSLC's parent training and behavioral family therapy treatments in particular. Research on parent training treatments (e.g., Bank, Marlowe, Reid, Patterson, & Weinrott, 1991) has supported placing youth in family settings in MTFC, demonstrating that systematic interventions applied by parents within the home have positive effects on children's behavior. Placing the youth in need of out-of-home placements in an alternative family setting is expected to have a positive socializing influence, and learning skills within a setting similar to his or her aftercare setting (i.e., a family setting vs. a group home or residential setting) is likely to increase the likelihood that skills will generalize to posttreatment contexts. Visits between the youth and his or her family of origin (or other aftercare resource, including long-term foster care with MTFC parents or other family) that take place while the youth lives in a MTFC home allow the youth and biological parents opportunities for skill development and practice in a supportive context outside the everyday pressure of family conflict and chaos.

Available research on the important contributions parents and peers can make to either exacerbate or ameliorate problem behaviors also informed program development. Extant research conducted at OSLC and elsewhere (e.g., Prinz & Miller, 1994; Webster-Stratton & Hammond, 1997) elucidated processes within the family context that shape prosocial behavior and discourage antisocial behavior. These include (a) the extent to which adults provide clear structure and limits in addition to well-specified consequences for behavior, (b) the extent to which they monitor or supervise the youth's whereabouts, and (c) the extent to which adults provide a consistent, reinforcing environment in which the youth is mentored and encouraged. These processes are targeted in parent management training (PMT), provided to both MTFC parents and the youth's biological parents. In addition, Dishion and colleagues (Dishion, McCord, & Poulin, 1999) reviewed evidence suggesting that delinquent peer associations also serve as a powerful context for exacerbating adolescent antisocial behavior. Dishion and colleagues (Dishion, Capaldi, Spracklen, & Li, 1995; Dishion, Spracklen, Andrews & Patterson, 1996) found that deviant peers engage in "deviancy training," providing positive reinforcement for engaging in deviant behavior and limiting youths' access to socializing processes that encourage the development of appropriate social skills. While in MTFC, the youth's access to deviant peers is limited and skills necessary to maintain relationships with prosocial peers are fostered. It is assumed that improving social adjustment with family members and within the peer group through MTFC will alter the negative trajectory of antisocial behavior.

The goals of MTFC and the roles of the treatment team staff members follow from its theoretical assumptions. The first goal is to facilitate the youth in living successfully within the community by providing him or her with intensive supervision, support, and skill development. Skills that have been shown to decrease parent–child conflict and disruptive child behaviors and to improve children's relationships with adults are targeted. Accomplishing this goal is the responsibility of the program supervisor,[1] who coordinates the efforts of the foster family with whom the youth is placed. The program supervisor is assisted by the youth's individual therapist and behavioral skills trainer. Daily monitoring of the youth's behavior in the foster home and school, and with peers in the community, as well as moment-to-moment feedback and direct coaching, are used to accomplish this goal. The second goal of MTFC is to prepare the youth's parents, extended family, or other adult aftercare resource to provide an environment that will maintain treatment gains once the youth is returned to their care. Under the supervision of the program supervisor, a family therapist works with the youth's family or other aftercare resource (e.g., long-term foster care) to teach the same family management strategies used in the foster home. Home visits are organized so parents or other aftercare resources can practice skills in preparation for the youth's eventual reunification to this context. Treatment team roles and program components will be reviewed in further detail later.

Finally, the MTFC model specifically addresses serious limitations in traditional modes of treatment for this population (i.e., group homes, residential treatment centers, and state training schools). First, placing individual youth (i.e., usually one youth per home) in foster homes avoids aggregating youth experiencing similar difficulties and decreases exposure to peer deviancy training, which maintains and exacerbates delinquent behavior (Chamberlain & Moore, 1998). MTFC instead takes advantage of the potential of families to provide a positive socializing influence. Next, family involvement and aftercare services are central to MTFC because they maximize the likelihood that treatment gains will be maintained within the youth's posttreatment environment. Although significant treatment effects have been demonstrated in traditional residential institutions, these gains typically fade when the youth leaves the treatment context (Jones, Weinrott, & Howard, 1981; Leichtman & Leichtman, 2001). Providing treatment within a family context, involving the youth's family of origin or other aftercare resource in treatment to establish a posttreatment environment that provides similar socialization experienced in the foster home, and providing the youth and his or her family aftercare services all increase the likelihood that treatment effects

[1] Until recently, program supervisors were referred to as "case managers." However, in most other treatment models, case managers are less experienced or trained than therapists. In the MTFC model, this individual supervises all of the team members. The title "program supervisor" more accurately depicts their training, responsibilities, and status on the treatment team.

will generalize to the youth's natural ecology and maximize the likelihood of maintaining treatment gains long term.

POPULATIONS SERVED BY MTFC

The MTFC model is an out-of-home intervention approach and therefore targets youth with emotional and behavioral disturbances who are unable to be maintained in the family home. Within this broad category, results of several randomized clinical trials have demonstrated that MTFC is a viable approach for intervening with several different hard-to-treat populations. MTFC serves boys and girls ages 12 to 17 who are referred from the juvenile justice system because of severe, chronic delinquent behavior (Chamberlain & Reid, 1994, 1998). On average, the boys served in MTFC receive their first criminal referral by 12 to 13 years of age and have 14 previous criminal referrals, including more than 4 previous felonies. Girls have 11 previous criminal offenses, and 82% are characterized as heavy drug and alcohol users (vs. 9% of the boys). All youth have had a number of previous placement disruptions. The utility of MTFC with this population has been well established for boys (see Chamberlain & Reid, 1998), and we currently are conducting a large-scale longitudinal study adapting MTFC for use with adolescent girls referred by the juvenile justice system.

The MTFC model also has the flexibility to address the needs of other populations of troubled youth. The program has been validated for addressing the needs of children and adolescents with serious mental health issues coming from the state mental hospital (Chamberlain & Reid, 1991). In addition, research has demonstrated positive outcomes of MTFC for both preschoolers (Fisher, Ellis, & Chamberlain, 1999; Fisher, Gunnar, Chamberlain, & Reid, 2000) and older children and adolescents who are placed in foster care by state child protective services (Chamberlain, Moreland, & Reid, 1992; Chamberlain & Price, in press; Smith, Stormshak, Chamberlain, & Bridges-Whaley, 2001). These are children involved in the child welfare system who have severe emotional needs or challenging aggressive and oppositional behavior. They have been removed from multiple previous foster home placements (on average, 4.75 previous placements) and have received multiple psychiatric diagnoses (see Smith et al., 2001). Finally, MTFC currently is being applied to and evaluated for youth with delayed development and borderline intellectual functioning (i.e., IQ testing results between 70 and 85). These are youth referred through the state child welfare office who have had multiple placement failures and have had problems with inappropriate sexual behaviors.

Reflecting the demographics of the community served, a vast majority of the youth and families (approximately 85%) served through the Oregon MTFC to date are of European American descent and come from a small urban area. However, efforts to explore the effectiveness of MTFC with more diverse samples currently are under way. For example, a version of MTFC is being implemented in a large, urban, ethnically diverse population in San Diego County, California.

DESCRIPTION OF SERVICES

Treatment in MTFC was designed to be flexible and is individualized to address the specific needs of each youth and his or her family (Chamberlain, 1994). Typical placements range from 6 to 9 months, and treatment also includes several months of aftercare services. During placement and aftercare, the youth is mentored and encouraged to perform specific behaviors that will increase his or her skill base. This mentoring and encouragement is provided within a structured environment in which expectations and limits are clear, well-specified consequences are consistently delivered, and in which the youth's whereabouts are closely supervised. An additional key element of treatment is providing support and assistance in building a prosocial peer network and preventing access to deviant peers. At the same time, treatment is provided to the youth's parents or other aftercare resource to prepare for and facilitate the transition home.

MTFC Treatment Components

Treatment teams consist of the MTFC foster parent(s), an individual therapist, a skills trainer, a family therapist, and a consulting psychiatrist. This team is coordinated by a program supervisor, who develops and monitors daily each youth's individualized treatment plan. The program supervisor also serves as a liaison to others in the community who play key roles in each case (e.g., juvenile court judge, parole/probation officers, teachers). The roles of each team member are well defined so that minimal overlap exists in services provided. Program components and the role of each member of the treatment team in implementing the components are described next.

Program Supervisor

MTFC program supervisors coordinate and supervise all aspects of the treatment program. Due to the high levels of contact, support, and intervention required to implement the program, program supervisors carry small caseloads (i.e., approximately 10 youth and families). Initially, the program supervisor works with the youth's foster parents to develop his or her individualized treatment program. Each program is based on a point/level system originally adapted from the Achievement Place Program (Phillips, Phillips, Fixsen, & Wolff, 1972). Program supervisors monitor each child's progress throughout placement and adjust the individualized program to fit the youth's changing needs to target new problems as they develop and to reflect progress made.

Program supervisors also monitor the youth's performance in the home and at school through daily telephone communication with foster parents. The *Parent Daily Report Checklist* (PDR; Chamberlain, 2003; Chamberlain & Reid, 1987) is used to structure these calls to collect information about the youth's behavior during the past 24 hours. PDR callers enter data directly into a PDR software program on a Web site that then can be accessed by members of the treatment team. During PDR calls, potential problems are identified and discussed, and plans for the subsequent day are reviewed. Program supervisors review the Web-based PDR data daily and use the information provided to monitor implementation of the model in the foster home, to track case progress, and to coordinate each youth's treatment team. Daily collection of PDR data helps program supervisors catch and address problems early, before serious problems develop. The PDR data also provide a way for program supervisors to track foster parent stress levels so they are aware of when foster families require extra support or respite care for the youth. Program supervisors conduct a weekly mandatory group meeting for all foster families during which they review PDR, provide support and encouragement, and supervise the implementation of the point/level system. Program supervisors are on call to provide consultation and crisis intervention to the foster parents 24 hours a day.

Program supervisors work with foster parents to ensure a successful school placement. The program supervisor often serves as a liaison between the school staff and the foster parent, including frequent phone contact and meetings with the youth's teachers, school counselor, and other school officials. Program supervisors and other MTFC staff are available on call to intervene at school if the youth becomes disruptive, and they also are available to conduct school-based interventions, when needed.

Coordinating all additional services (i.e., individual therapy, behavioral skills training, family therapy) is the program supervisor's responsibility. Program supervisors hold weekly clinical supervision meetings during which family and individual therapists present the progress and problems that arose in the past week for each case, and program supervisors provide direction and feedback. Formal and informal systems of communication among team members and foster parents that is well coordinated by a central individual (i.e., the program supervisor) is crucial to the success of the cases. The roles for these members of the treatment team will each be reviewed in turn.

Treatment Foster Care Families

MTFC values recruiting foster families from diverse social, ethnic, and economic backgrounds to implement the treatment program. Both one- and two-parent traditional and nontraditional families have successfully served as MTFC parents. MTFC parents are recruited, screened, trained, and supervised to provide treatment to the youth placed in their home. They are the primary agent in implementing the intervention process. That is, MTFC parents provide thorough monitoring and supervision and implement the point/level system to provide clear expectations and moment-to-moment feedback on behavior within a predictable, reinforcing environment.

Treatment foster parents first participate in 20 hours of preservice training. The content and methods used in training foster parents were adapted from clinical parent training programs and methods developed at OSLC, making foster parent training consistent with a social-learning parent-training approach. During training, the MTFC model is presented and policies and procedures are reviewed. Social learning principles also are taught. For example, MTFC parents are trained to observe and identify specific target behaviors, to effectively use praise and positive consequences to encourage positive behavior, to deliver clear and consistent limit setting, and to preteach strategies to coach desired behaviors. They learn how to turn problem situations into "teachable moments" and practice responding to rule violations and aggressive behavior in nonreactive ways. The individual daily program (i.e., the point/level system) also is presented and practiced. Finally, ways to promote engagement in prosocial, enriching activities and to prevent association with antisocial peers are emphasized in training and reviewed throughout treatment.

The point/level system is used to systematize treatment in MTFC homes. The program specifies the youth's daily schedule of activities and clearly spells out behavioral expectations (e.g., getting up on time, attending school and completing homework, doing chores, following adults' instructions, maintaining positive attitudes and behavior). MTFC parents monitor the youth's performance throughout the day and assign points (or other contingencies) based on his or her performance on each activity. They also take away points for minor misbehavior and rule violations. MTFC parents hold daily meetings with the youth to review points earned and to provide feedback that informs the youth about what he or she did well and where improvement is needed. The point/level system also defines three levels of supervision and privileges (e.g., bedtime, permission to make phone calls, opportunities for free time in the community). Progression through the levels is dictated by performance and compliance with program rules as reflected in the number of points earned daily.

Assigning points to the youth's performance and taking away points for unsatisfactory performance throughout the day is a vehicle through which MTFC parents can provide frequent positive reinforcement for normative and prosocial behavior and consequences for rule-breaking behavior. This system allows for ways to "catch" and deal with minor problems early rather than waiting to address the problems when they become more serious. Taking away points for transgressions discourages foster parents from engaging in lengthy conversations about problem behaviors that may inadvertently reinforce those behaviors. Using the point/level system also helps avoid power struggles between the youth and the foster parents. It provides a way to deliver consistent, nonpunitive consequences for behavior and allows for a concrete way for the youth to track his or her success. For more serious rule violations or persistent or intense problems, MTFC parents deliver consequences, such as work chores, time-outs, or privilege removals. In the most serious cases, MTFC parents may solicit the support of the program supervisor to facilitate community service or a temporary removal from school or the home (e.g., short visits to the juvenile detention center).

Treatment foster parents closely monitor all activities in the home, at school, and in the community. For example, MTFC parents drive the youth to and from school while he or she is on the most restrictive level of the program. They also must preapprove and then verify the youth's whereabouts and peer associations during free time. The program requires that all participating youth carry a school card to monitor school attendance, homework completion, and classroom behavior in each class daily. Cards are collected daily, and MTFC parents incorporate the feedback provided by teachers into the point system (i.e., points are earned or lost for school attendance and behavior) on the daily program. Both MTFC parents and program supervisors have frequent contact with school officials and teachers.

Youth Therapist

The purpose of individual therapy with youth in the MTFC program is to augment the main treatment provided through the foster home by implementing interventions to target especially problematic behaviors and providing support and advocacy. Throughout treatment, individual therapists provide support and encourage the development of skills necessary to relate successfully with adults and peers. They advocate for the youth as he or she adjusts to the program and life in the foster home. Eventually they move the youth toward developing problem-solving skills and communication strategies that will allow him or her to successfully advocate for him- or herself. Typically, individual therapy involves (a) teaching negotiation and problem-solving skills, (b) developing skills required to live successfully in a family setting, (c) practicing modulation of anger expression and coping skills, (d) establishing educational and occupational goals and plans, and (e) identifying problems with associating with deviant peers and developing skills for relating to "normal" peers engaging in prosocial activities. The individual therapist also participates in therapy sessions with the youth and his or her biological parents, advocating for the youth and shaping or coaching social skills necessary for the youth to respond appropriately to parent management strategies. Role plays, preteaching and spontaneous coaching, and developing incentive programs are among the strategies individual therapists use with the youth to develop and practice skills used in the foster home and community, and during sessions with his or her biological family.

In some circumstances, therapists also may address issues of maltreatment or abuse during individual therapy. However, this is done only after a stable, predictable environment has been established for the youth and he or she has the emotional support necessary to effectively process these experiences. The individual therapist will begin to address these issues only when the youth initiates such processing, and only when his or her behavior has been stabilized. The youth also must have developed adaptive and effective coping and problem-solving skills. The individual therapist then tailors therapy to the cognitive level of the youth (considering his or her available coping strategies and emotional support systems). The youth's emotional and behavioral responses are carefully monitored to improve functioning and avoid retraumatizing or exacerbating the troubles previously experienced. The individual therapist is available to the youth 24 hours a day by phone for support in solving problems that arise and for crisis management.

Behavioral Skills Trainer

The skills trainer works with the youth to develop the social skills necessary to interact appropriately in the community. Skills trainers take youth out into the community (e.g., to restaurants and stores, to attend art classes or participate on sports teams) for 2 to 6 hours per week. They use intensive one-on-one interaction, role play, and modeling to teach prosocial behavior and problem-solving skills that will allow youth to interact with others in a positive manner. They also are trained to use applied behavioral analysis to examine the antecedents to and reinforcers for problem behaviors for the youth in a particular setting. Establishing behavioral contracts with the youth also is common, where the skills trainer contracts with the youth to provide a reward when the youth engages in a prosocial behavior (or fails to engage in a targeted problem behavior) a specified number of days.

Family Therapist

Family involvement in MTFC is based on research demonstrating that biological parents' implementation of the family management strategies used in MTFC (e.g., thorough supervision, reinforcement for positive behaviors, fair and consistent discipline, limiting association with delinquent peers) is central to maintaining treatment gains (e.g., Eddy & Chamberlain, 2000). The family therapist therefore teaches the biological family (85% of MTFC youth return to his or her family or a relative's home) or other aftercare resource to implement the same individualized program used in MTFC in an effort to establish an aftercare environment consistent with the youth's MTFC placement. Important components of the PMT provided by the family therapist include working with parents to help them understand the necessity of close supervision and fair, consistent discipline, along with emphasizing the need to limit association with delinquent peers. The PMT provided through the family therapy component of MTFC has been shown to have positive effects on child and family outcomes (Patterson, Chamberlain & Reid, 1982; Prinz & Miller, 1994; Webster-Stratton & Hammond, 1997).

Through PMT, the family therapist works with parents to implement the same or similar supervision, encouragement, support, and discipline procedures delivered during the youth's placement in MTFC. The family therapist teaches the daily behavior management system (i.e., the point/level system) and, as in most PMT models, encourages in-home practice implementing the daily program. Home visits are scheduled to give parents opportunities to practice skills taught in family therapy with the youth in the family's natural ecology. Visits progress in length as parents improve their ability to implement the program. They typically begin as supervised visits at the center, progress to day visits in the community, and then move to overnight visits at home. Implementing the daily program during visits also allows the youth and parent opportunities to practice new ways of relating to each other such that the balance of power shifts and the youth becomes more accepting of parental guidance and support. The family therapist provides parents with extensive support before and during visits. He or she also is available to families

24 hours a day for crisis intervention and consultation. After each visit, the family therapist reviews and reinforces parents' implementation of the program and makes modifications to better fit the family's circumstances.

Building a positive relationship or "alliance" with family members and gaining their perspective on effective strategies for working with their child in MTFC are helpful for "joining" with families. This is important groundwork for working with parents to develop successful parenting practices. Family therapists also work with the family to address the barriers that prevented effective parenting in the past. This includes focusing on managing general family struggles, such as management of siblings' behavior in the home, financial demands, and employment concerns. Typically this involves developing problem-solving and communication skills, establishing methods for de-escalating family conflict, and learning ways to advocate for services for the adolescent and the family (e.g., school services, financial services).

Aftercare Services

Each program youth and his or her family is offered aftercare support services to help facilitate the transition to the youth's next placement and to sustain treatment gains made while placed in MTFC. Services offered include 24-hour on-call crisis intervention, individual consultation and support, school consultation and intervention, and individual and family therapy. The MTFC treatment team (i.e., the program supervisor, individual therapist, behavioral support specialist, and family therapist) all are available to provide aftercare support services to the youth and his or her family as needed. MTFC staff also may serve as a backup for delivering consequences for serious rule violations (e.g., time-outs at the center, supervised work chores such as community service, talking with probation officers) and may provide funds for youth and family incentives that will sustain progress.

Treatment Fidelity

Several fidelity checks are built in to the treatment to ensure that the multiple treatment components adhere to the MTFC model and remain a coordinated effort. For example, the weekly foster parent support groups and clinical supervision groups provide a vehicle through which the program supervisor can monitor treatment provided in the foster homes and by the individual therapists, behavioral support specialists, and the family therapists. In addition, data collected through PDR are used to ensure foster parents' implementation of the structured daily behavior management plan. The daily phone call used to collect PDR data also allows program staff opportunities to identify and track foster parents' responses to problem behaviors and to provide coaching and feedback on alternative ways to handle problems in ways consistent with the treatment model.

OUTCOME EVALUATION RESEARCH

Several randomized clinical trials have been conducted that compare the efficacy of MTFC to commonly used treatment alternatives. These studies demonstrate that MTFC is a feasible, effective approach to addressing the needs of youth with severe behavior and complex emotional problems who are difficult to support in community settings. According to these studies, placing youth in treatment foster homes in the community is a safe, feasible, and cost-effective alternative to more restrictive treatment settings (Aos, Phipps, Barnoski, & Lieb, 1999; Chamberlain et al., 1992; Chamberlain & Reid, 1998). MTFC leads to reductions in subsequent delinquent activity and arrests among youth referred by the juvenile justice system (Chamberlain & Reid, 1998) and can be used to successfully transition youth with serious emotional and behavioral difficulties from state mental hospitals back into the community (Chamberlain & Reid, 1991). In addition, results suggest that elements of MTFC can be successfully implemented within a state-supported foster care setting (Chamberlain et al., 1992).

MTFC with Youth Referred from the Juvenile Justice System

Two large-scale, randomized clinical trials have been conducted to examine whether chronic delinquents could be maintained in community placements through MTFC and whether MTFC, when compared to traditional treatment alternatives, led to reductions in crime and arrest rates. The first of these studies examined the utility of MTFC for early to late adolescent boys referred from the juvenile justice system. The second was conducted to understand the ways in which MTFC needed to be modified to meet the unique needs of young adjudicated girls. Results of these studies and their application for future directions in adapting MTFC for youth referred from the juvenile justice system will be reviewed.

MTFC with Boys Referred from Juvenile Justice

The largest randomized clinical trial to date (Chamberlain & Reid, 1998; Eddy & Chamberlain, 2000) involved 79 boys (85% Euro-American), ages 12 to 17 ($M = 14.9$ years, $SD = 1.3$), who were mandated to out-of-home care by the juvenile justice system. Prior to their placement in MTFC or group care (GC), all of the boys had been placed in a locked detention facility for an average of 76 days. These boys were then randomly assigned to MTFC or "treatment as usual" community placements (i.e., parole/probation officers determined placement in 1 of 11 group care facilities). Participants had an average of 14 previous criminal referrals and an average of more than four felonies prior to referral; the mean age at their first arrest was 12.6 years. All of the boys had previously been placed out of the home at least once in addition to detention, and more than three-quarters had run away from at least one previous placement.

Chamberlain and Reid (1998) demonstrated that compared to GC, fewer boys in MTFC ran away from their placement (30.5% of MTFC vs. 57.8% of GC; $\chi^2(1, N = 79) = 5.59, p < .05$) and a greater proportion completed their programs (73% of MTFC vs. 36% of GC; $\chi^2(1, N = 79) = 10.96, p < .001$). In addition, boys in MTFC spent 60% fewer days incarcerated ($M = 53$ for MTFC and $M = 129$ for GC) during the year after their original referral. A 2×2 mixed analysis of variance (ANOVA; Group $\times$ Time) revealed a significant interaction, $F(1, 77) = 3.93, p < .01$, with MTFC boys showing larger drops in official criminal referral rates from the year prior to enrollment in the study ($M = 8.5, SD = 6.6$ for MTFC; $M = 6.7, SD = 4.2$ for GC) to 1 year postdischarge or expulsion from treatment ($M = 2.6, SD = 3.3$ for MTFC; $M = 5.4, SD = 4.4$ for GC). A hierarchical multiple regression analysis (see Chamberlain & Reid, 1998, for details) revealed that these results held, regardless of age of first offense, age at program entrance, or number of prior referrals. Using generalized estimating equations (GEE) and data collected every 6 months for 2 years postdischarge, Eddy, Whaley, and Chamberlain (2004) demonstrated that, compared to boys treated in GC, boys who participated in MTFC were significantly less likely to report committing violent offenses ($b = -1.11, p < .001$) and to be arrested for a violent offense ($b = -.81, p < .05$). Together, these data suggest that compared to GC, MTFC provides the community protection from the criminal activities of chronically delinquent boys by effectively maintaining community placements and reducing general and violent offending behaviors. Importantly, the program led to treatment gains even among the oldest, hardest-to-treat groups of boys (Chamberlain & Reid, 1998; Eddy et al., 2004).

In addition to examining the immediate and long-term outcomes of participating in MTFC, an experimental test of the underlying theoretical model of change was conducted. Eddy and Chamberlain (2000) examined two sets of factors guiding the theory that underlies the design of MTFC. The factors are those believed to lead to the differences in intervention effects for MTFC and GC boys. The key factors targeted in the MTFC model, but left free to vary in the GC condition, were family management (i.e., supervision, discipline, and positive reinforcement) and deviant peer associations. The results are presented in Figure 23.1. Boys in MTFC received higher levels of parent management and associated with delinquent peers less frequently than GC boys (i.e., treatment condition was significantly related to scores on the mediators), and scores on the mediators at midtreatment were associated with levels of antisocial behavior at follow-up. For example, high levels of supervision in the foster home were associated with less frequent antisocial behavior at follow-up. Finally, as can be seen in Figure 23.1, supervision, discipline, positive reinforcement, and frequency of peer associations all mediated the impact of treatment on antisocial behavior 1 year posttreatment. These results demonstrate that MTFC's influence on reductions in antisocial behavior is through the level and type of family management support provided in the foster homes (i.e., fair, consistent, nonphysical forms of discipline, effective supervision, a positive relationship with a mentoring adult) and through the program's ability to affect reductions in associations with delinquent peers.

Applying MTFC to Girls Referred from Juvenile Justice

The treatment effects of MTFC for girls and boys (ages 12–18) involved in the juvenile justice system also have been compared in a pilot study (Chamberlain & Reid, 1994). Chamberlain and Reid (1994) reported that girls ($N = 37$) in MTFC were equally likely as MTFC boys ($N = 51$) to complete the program (73% of girls vs. 71% of boys). Both boys and girls demonstrated

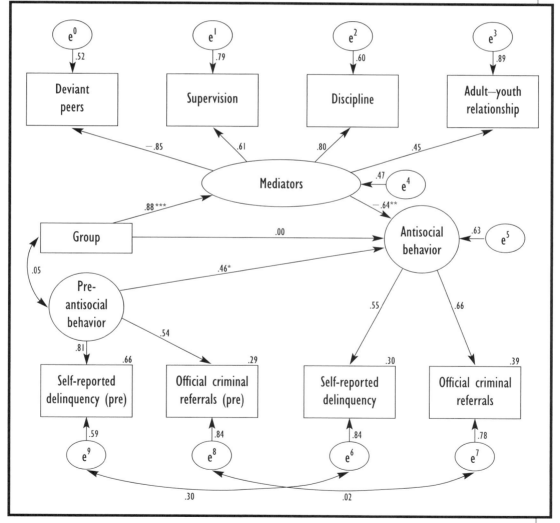

FIGURE 23.1. Mediational model, $\chi^2(22, N = 53) = 21.802$, $p = .472$, goodness-of-fit index = .920, adjusted goodness-of-fit index = .837.

$^*p < .05.$ $^{**}p < .01.$ $^{***}p < .001.$

reductions in status offenses, $F(1, 73) = 23.05, p < .001$, and arrests for person-to-person crimes, $F(1, 73) = 12.69, p < .001$, 1 year posttreatment (see Table 23.1 for pre- and posttreatment means and standard deviations). In addition, reductions in property crimes were demonstrated for both boys and girls, $F(1, 78) = 34.47, p < .001$, and a marginally significant Time $\times$ Gender interaction, $F(1, 78) = 3.65, p = .06$, suggests a trend toward boys demonstrating greater improvement than girls.

Despite the similarities in outcomes for boys and girls, differences in their responses to treatment were noted. Specifically, there was a significant Gender $\times$ Time interaction, $F(1, 47) = 8.7, p < .01$, in daily rates of problem behavior as reported by foster parents. Whereas slight reductions in boys' daily rates of conduct problems from the 1st ($M = 2.17, SD = 1.69$) to the 6th month in placement ($M = 1.73, SD = 1.33$) were demonstrated, girls' rates of conduct problems increased from the 1st ($M = 1.29, SD = .74$) to the 6th month in placement ($M = 2.17, SD = 1.26$). This pattern for girls may place them at risk of placement failure because both the foster parents and the girls may perceive such increases as deterioration or failures relative to their positive beginnings (Chamberlain & Reid, 1994). The results of this pilot study suggested that girls have unique needs that necessitate specialized treatment approaches within the MTFC model.

A 5-year randomized trial of MTFC for girls involved in the juvenile justice system was conducted based on what had been learned in this pilot study. Similar to the study described previously, girls (ages 12–17) who were referred for out-of-home placement by the juvenile justice system were ran-

TABLE 23.1
Pre- and Posttreatment Offense Rates by Gender

	Status	Person	Property
1-Year Preplacement			
Girls			
M	2.2	.45	1.50
SD	2.1	.62	1.40
Boys			
M	1.3	.52	2.80
SD	1.8	.75	2.40
1-Year Postdischarge			
Girls			
M	.84	.18	.45
SD	1.60	.47	.87
Boys			
M	.25	.13	.75
SD	.55	.49	1.30

Note. From "Differences in Risk Factors and Adjustment for Male and Female Delinquents in Foster Care," by P. Chamberlain and J. B. Reid, 1994, *Journal of Child and Family Studies, 3*(1), p. 34. Copyright 1994 by Kluwer Academic/Plenum Publishers. Reprinted with permission.

domly assigned to MTFC or "treatment as usual" settings (i.e., residential treatment, group home, hospital, inpatient drug and alcohol program). Leve and Chamberlain (in press) reviewed these girls' preplacement risk factors, and their findings confirmed previous research showing that antisocial girls come from especially adverse and dysfunctional backgrounds (e.g., Henry, Moffitt, Robins, & Silva, 1993; Rosenbaum, 1989). The girls had higher rates of parents convicted of crimes, had experienced higher rates of documented physical and sexual abuse, and had more frequent out-of-home placements than boys. In addition, the girls had run away significantly more often than the boys, had significantly more suicide attempts, and reported higher rates of symptoms of mental health disorders (i.e., anxiety, depression, paranoid/psychotic, somatization, hostility, general psychopathology). Significantly more girls than boys have been characterized as heavy drug or alcohol users (i.e., 82% of girls vs. 9.3% of boys).

To address the specific needs of girls, traditional MTFC developed for boys was supplemented in several ways. For example, MTFC foster parents were specifically trained in dealing with relational, indirect forms of aggression that is more typical of girls than boys (Björkqvist, Lagerspetz, & Kaukiainen, 1992; Underwood, 1998). Behaviors that may jeopardize girls' placements by eroding their relationship with foster parents—spreading rumors, being bossy, or presenting with a negative attitude (e.g., rolling eyes or whining in response to foster parent directives)—were often targeted on girls' individualized daily point programs.

Preliminary follow-up data are available for approximately 60% of the sample (i.e., 61 girls). These findings suggest that, consistent with results found for boys in previous studies (e.g., Chamberlain & Reid, 1998), girls' participation in MTFC (relative to GC) is associated with spending more days in treatment and fewer days in incarceration, and to greater decreases in arrests and time spent in the hospital for mental health–related problems. Despite these encouraging findings, girls in this study continue to report engaging in high-risk sexual activities, selecting antisocial partners, and using alcohol and drugs at high rates. The MTFC model currently is being revised to specifically address the prevention of these high-risk behaviors and to foster healthy adult lifestyles.

MTFC with Youth Referred from Child Welfare

Several studies have demonstrated that MTFC also is effective for troubled youth involved in the child welfare system (e.g., Chamberlain et al., 1992; Fisher et al., 2000). For example, Fisher and colleagues conducted a clinical trial examining early intervention foster care (EIFC), which is MTFC adapted to the specific needs of preschoolers involved in the child welfare system. In their pilot study, preschoolers were assigned to placement in EIFC ($N = 10$) by the state welfare system because of a history of placement disruptions or severe aggressive and oppositional behavior. Their outcomes were compared to those of equal numbers of same-age youth placed in "regular" foster care and to a community comparison group of nonmaltreated preschoolers living with their biological parent(s).

Results showed that the EIFC preschoolers' behavioral adjustment improved over time and became more similar to that of the community sample, whereas the regular foster care preschoolers exhibited increased behavioral maladjustment over the course of the study. At the same time, changes in physiological markers of distress (i.e., salivary cortisol levels) collected throughout the course of the study suggest that relative to regular foster care, the EIFC intervention may reduce stress and physiological arousal. Over time, the circadian release patterns of EIFC preschoolers came to reflect those of typically developing children. Finally, results demonstrated that systematic training and support provided to the foster parents leads them to adopt effective parenting strategies (i.e., appropriate monitoring, consistent discipline, and positive reinforcement) and to create home environments similar to those of typical families. Such training leads them to exhibit significantly more effective parenting and to experience parenting as less stressful than is typical in regular foster parents (Fisher et al., 2000). However, the nonrandomized assignment of participants to treatment conditions requires that these results be interpreted with caution. A 5-year randomized clinical trial of EIFC currently is under way.

Cost-Effectiveness

MTFC is a cost-effective intervention. The Washington State Institute for Public Policy conducted a cost–benefit analysis to compare the cost-effectiveness of MTFC to that of 31 violence prevention programs and other treatment approaches for youth involved in the juvenile justice system. They determined that MTFC saves taxpayers approximately $43,000 per participant in criminal justice and victim costs (Aos et al., 1999). Aos and colleagues estimated $22.58 of taxpayer benefits for every dollar spent on MTFC. MTFC also was found to be a cost-effective alternative to mental hospital placements, saving an average of $10,280 per child in hospital costs (Chamberlain & Reid, 1991).

IMPLICATIONS OF THE RESEARCH ON MTFC FOR WORK IN BROADER SYSTEMS

The research studies that have been conducted on the efficacy of MTFC to this point have highlighted the potential of this service type for providing alternatives to group and residential care for children and adolescents with extremely challenging behavioral and emotional problems and severe delinquency. The MTFC model has several advantages over more commonly used closed residential and group care models: It is less restrictive in that youth live in their communities and attend local schools, it is less expensive, and the gains that youth make while in placement can be directly generalized to their aftercare placement. But the question remains of whether and how the positive results observed in research-based clinical trials can be realized in implementations of MTFC models in programs in typical community agencies.

Currently the MTFC model is being implemented in a number of communities throughout the United States. The first agency to implement MTFC on a wide scale has been Youth Villages in Tennessee, which is a private, nonprofit community mental health agency that partners with the Tennessee Department of Children's Services to provide services to children with serious emotional and behavioral problem. Youth Villages currently serves more than 400 children and adolescents a day in MTFC (Mendel, 2000), making it the largest site implementing MTFC that we know of. To our knowledge, Youth Villages has not conducted a formal outcome study, but they report that they are able to serve many more youth in less restrictive placements than they did before using MTFC. Their youth are reported to be more successful at remaining at home postplacement than were youth placed before implementation of the MTFC model. In addition to getting better outcomes than they had previously using residential care beds, Youth Villages reports that MTFC costs substantially less. We are now helping agencies in several other communities implement MTFC. Future evaluations will document if our model can be effectively disseminated on a wide scale and if the inclusion of this approach into the continuum of child welfare and juvenile justice service options constitutes an improvement in choice and outcomes for youth and families.

USING ELEMENTS OF MTFC IN A STATE-SUPPORTED FOSTER CARE SETTING

Research has been conducted to examine the feasibility and utility of incorporating selected parts of MTFC into state-supported foster care. A pilot study was conducted to examine whether enhancing state-supported foster care in three Oregon counties would impact key child welfare outcomes, including placement disruption rates, foster parent retention, and child behavior problems (see Chamberlain et al., 1992). This study involved 72 children with emotional and behavioral problems (ages 4–7 years) who were involved in the child welfare system most often because of parental neglect and physical and sexual abuse. Youth were placed with 1 of 72 foster families by the state's Children's Services Division (CSD). Foster families were randomly assigned to participate in (a) foster care as usual through CSD ($N = 27$), (b) an increase of $70 in monthly stipends ($N = 14$), or (c) increased stipends plus enhanced support and training ($N = 31$, henceforth referred to as MTFC Lite). The enhanced support and training in MTFC Lite included weekly foster parent meetings during which support and training to manage day-to-day behavioral and emotional problems was provided. Foster parents in the MTFC Lite condition also received PDR calls three times per week.

The results of this study indicated that over and above the effect of providing additional financial support to foster parents, providing increased support and training in the form of weekly meetings and PDR calls increased foster parents' retention rate significantly (i.e., it resulted in a dropout rate [9.6%] that was nearly two-thirds lower than in the regular foster care group [25.9%]). There also were notable differences in child outcomes in the three groups. Children in the MTFC Lite group had the fewest disruptions in their placements (i.e., 29% vs. 53% in the other two groups). These children also demonstrated the largest reductions in the number of behavior problems reported over time on the PDR ($M = 7.50$ behaviors at baseline and $M = 3.85$ behaviors after 3 months for the MTFC Lite group; $M = 5.71$ and $M = 3.94$ for the increased payment group; $M = 3.71$ and $M = 4.56$ for the regular foster care group). Importantly, the costs associated with maintaining the level of support in the MTFC Lite condition were offset by the benefits of increasing foster parent retention rates and decreasing placement disruptions.

Based on the results of this pilot study, a large-scale clinical trial within six regions of Health and Human Services in San Diego County currently is being conducted in which the effectiveness of regular foster care and MTFC Lite are being compared. This is examining whether elements of MTFC can successfully be incorporated into preexisting state-supported foster care in a large, ethnically diverse urban area. Examining whether treatment effects generalize beyond the primarily Euro-American samples in Oregon, where MTFC was developed, to a large, ethnically diverse urban community is of particular interest in this study.

We also are especially interested in understanding the steps to implementing the MTFC model outside the original research program in which it was developed. One of the clear challenges to disseminating MTFC is in training staff and paraprofessionals to implement the model. A "cascading dissemination" design is being used in which (a) staff are directly trained and supervised by the Oregon MTFC staff who developed and have been implementing the model for several years, and (b) local San Diego staff will provide training and supervision to the subsequent staff. This design will allow us to compare the treatment effect sizes of first and second generations of dissemination. This will be an important first step toward bridging the gap between interventions run through large-scale, federally funded research programs and real-world practice.

CONCLUSION

Now that evidence exists demonstrating that MTFC is an empirically supported treatment model, we are exploring whether MTFC can be a viable treatment for a variety of populations of youth and families and are turning some of our focus toward understanding issues related to dissemination. We are continuing to adapt the MTFC model for use with other populations of troubled youth, such as children with borderline intellectual functioning. A large focus of our current work involves exploring the feasibility of disseminating the MTFC model outside the research context in which it originally was developed. The San Diego project is but one example of our efforts to bring MTFC to different contexts. To date, MTFC has been successfully implemented in Tennessee, Pennsylvania, Arizona, Virginia, and Lund, Sweden. We currently are collaborating with community organizations in several additional areas around the country to bring the MTFC model to community-based mental health agencies and social service organizations. We will continue to explore the complex issues involved in disseminating MTFC for a wide range of youth and families and to evaluate its use in large social service systems.

AUTHORS' NOTE

Support for this research was provided by grants from the National Institute for Mental Health (MH54257, MH60195, P30MH46690).

REFERENCES

Aos, S., Phipps, P., Barnoski, R., & Lieb, R. (1999). *The comparative costs and benefits of programs to reduce crime: A review of national research findings with implications for Washington state.* Olympia: Washington State Institute for Public Policy.

Bank, L., Marlowe, J. H., Reid, J. B., Patterson, G. R., & Weinrott, M. R. (1991). A comparative evaluation of parent training for families of chronic delinquents. *Journal of Abnormal Child Psychology, 19,* 15–33.

Björkqvist, K., Lagerspetz, K. M. J., & Kaukiainen, A. (1992). Do girls manipulate and boys fight? *Aggressive Behavior, 18,* 117–127.

Chamberlain, P. (1994). *Family connections: Treatment foster care for adolescents.* Eugene, OR: Northwest Media.

Chamberlain, P. (1996). Community-based residential treatment for adolescents with conduct disorder. In T. H. Ollendick & R. J. Prinz (Eds.), *Advances in clinical child psychology* (Vol. 18, pp. 63–90). New York: Plenum Press.

Chamberlain, P. (2003). *Treating chronic juvenile offenders: Advances made through the Oregon multidimensional treatment foster care model.* Washington, DC: American Psychological Association.

Chamberlain, P., & Moore, K. J. (1998). A clinical model of parenting juvenile offenders: A comparison of group versus family care. *Clinical Child Psychology and Psychiatry, 3,* 375–386.

Chamberlain, P., Moreland, S., & Reid, K. (1992). Enhanced services and stipends for foster parents: Effects on retention rates and outcomes for children. *Child Welfare, 71,* 387–401.

Chamberlain, P., & Price, J. M. (in press). *Cascading dissemination of a foster parent intervention.* Manuscript in preparation.

Chamberlain, P., & Reid, J. B. (1987). Parent observation and report of child symptoms. *Behavioral Assessment, 9,* 97–109.

Chamberlain, P., & Reid, J. B. (1991). Using a specialized foster care treatment model for children and adolescents leaving the state mental hospital. *Journal of Community Psychology, 19,* 266–276.

Chamberlain, P., & Reid, J. B. (1994). Differences in risk factors and adjustment for male and female delinquents in treatment foster care. *Journal of Child and Family Studies, 3,* 23–39.

Chamberlain, P., & Reid, J. (1998). Comparison of two community alternatives to incarceration for chronic juvenile offenders. *Journal of Consulting and Clinical Psychology, 6,* 624–633.

DeBaryshe, B. D., Patterson, G. R., & Capaldi, D. (1993). A performance model for academic achievement in early adolescent boys. *Developmental Psychology, 29,* 795–804.

Dishion, T. J., Capaldi, D., Spracklen, K. M., & Li, F. (1995). Peer ecology of male adolescent drug use. *Development and Psychopathology, 7,* 803–824.

Dishion, T. J., McCord, J., & Poulin, F. (1999). When interventions harm: Peer groups and problem behavior. *American Psychologist, 54,* 755–764.

Dishion, T. J., Spracklen, K. M., Andrews, D. W., & Patterson, G. R. (1996). Deviancy training in male adolescent friendships. *Behavior Therapy, 27,* 373–390.

Eddy, J. M., & Chamberlain, P. (2000). Family management and deviant peer association as mediators of the impact of treatment condition on youth antisocial behavior. *Journal of Consulting and Clinical Psychology, 5,* 857–863.

Eddy, J. M., Whaley, R. B., & Chamberlain, P. (2004). The prevention of violent behavior by chronic and serious male juvenile offenders: A randomized clinical trial. *Journal of Emotional and Behavioral Disorders, 12*(1), 2–8.

Fisher, P., Ellis, H., & Chamberlain, P. (1999). Early intervention foster care: A model for preventing risk in young children who have been maltreated. *Children's Services: Social Policy, Research, and Practice, 2,* 159–182.

Fisher, P. A., Gunnar, M. R., Chamberlain, P., & Reid, J. B. (2000). Preventive intervention for maltreated preschool children: Impact on children's behavior, neuroendocrine activity, and foster parent functioning. *Journal of the American Academy of Child and Adolescent Psychiatry, 39,* 1356–1364.

Henry, B., Moffitt, T., Robins, L., & Silva, P. (1993). Early family predictors of child and adolescent antisocial behaviour: Who are the mothers of delinquents? *Criminal Behaviour and Mental Health, 3,* 97–118.

Jones, R. R., Weinrott, M. R., & Howard, J. R. (1981). The national evaluation of the teaching family model. *Final Report to the Center for Studies of Antisocial and Violent Behavior.* Bethesda, MD: National Institute of Mental Health.

Leichtman, M., & Leichtman, M. L. (2001). Facilitating the transition from residential treatment into the community: I. The problem. *Residential Treatment for Children and Youth, 19,* 21–27.

Leve, L. D., & Chamberlain, P. (in press). Girls in the juvenile justice system: Risk factors and clinical implications. In D. Pepler, K. Madsen, C. Webster, & K. Levine (Eds.), *Development and treatment of girlhood aggression.* Mahwah, NJ: Erlbaum.

Mendel, R. A. (2000). *Less hype, more help: Reducing juvenile crime, what works—and what doesn't.* Washington, DC: American Youth Policy Forum.

Patterson, G. R., Chamberlain, P., & Reid, J. B. (1982). A comparative evaluation of parent training procedures. *Behavior Therapy, 13,* 638–650.

Phillips, E. L., Phillips, E. A., Fixsen, D. L., & Wolff, M. M. (1972). *The teaching-family handbook.* Lawrence: University of Kansas, Bureau of Child Research.

Prinz, R. J., & Miller, G. E. (1994). Family-based treatment for childhood antisocial behavior: Experimental influences on dropout and engagement. *Journal of Consulting and Clinical Psychology, 62,* 645–650.

Reid, J. B. (1993). Prevention of conduct disorder before and after school entry: Relating interventions to developmental findings. *Journal of Development and Psychopathology, 5,* 243–262.

Reid, J. B., & Eddy, J. M. (1997). The prevention of antisocial behavior: Some considerations in the search for effective interventions. In D. M. Stoff, J. Breiling, & J. D. Maser (Eds.), *Handbook of antisocial behavior* (pp. 205–221). New York: Wiley.

Rosenbaum, J. L. (1989). Family dysfunction and female delinquency. *Crime and Delinquency, 35,* 31–44.

Smith, D. K., Stormshak, E., Chamberlain, P., & Bridges-Whaley, R. (2001). Placement disruption in treatment foster care. *Journal of Emotional and Behavioral Disorders, 9,* 200–205.

Underwood, M. K. (1998). Competence in sexual decision-making by African-American female adolescents: The role of peer relations and future plans. In A. Colby, J. James, & D. Hart (Eds.), *Competence and character through life* (pp. 57–87). Chicago: University of Chicago Press.

Webster-Stratton, C., & Hammond, M. (1997). Treating children with early-onset conduct problems: A comparison of child and parent training interventions. *Journal of Consulting and Clinical Psychology, 65,* 93–109.

Medicaid-Managed Behavioral Health Care for Children with Severe Emotional Disturbance

CHAPTER 24

Judith A. Cook, Craig Anne Heflinger, Christina Hoven, Kelly Kelleher, Robert Paulson, Al Stein-Seroussi, Genevieve Fitzgibbon, Jane Burke, and Melissa Williams

Since the 1970s, managed care (MC) approaches have been used to control spiraling costs of Medicaid-funded health-care services to low-income women and children (Hurley, Freund, & Paul, 1993). These early efforts focused on outcomes such as reducing the use of emergency room settings for primary care among poor families (Shapiro, 1994) and ensuring adequate pre- and postnatal care for women and their children (U.S. General Accounting Office, 1994). More recently, attention has turned toward the use of MC arrangements to reduce the costs of treatment for mental health problems among low-income women and children. The purpose of the current analysis was to determine whether children and youth with severe emotional disturbance (SED) covered by Medicaid-funded MC behavioral health plans differed significantly from those covered under fee-for-service (FFS) plans in either mental health status or utilization of different types of mental health services.

BEHAVIORAL HEALTH-CARE ISSUES FOR LOW-INCOME WOMEN AND CHILDREN

Minimal attention has been paid to evaluating the effects of managed behavioral health care for Medicaid-eligible women and their families. This is true despite the fact that the costs of mental health care account for approximately 10% of overall health-care expenditures (American Managed Behavioral Health Care Association [AMBHA], 1995). Although women of childbearing age and their children represent the largest proportion of Medicaid recipients, they account for only 15% of all health expenditures (U.S. Department of Health and Human Services, 1996). Thus, the Congressional Budget Office has estimated that only a one-time 5% to 15% savings would result from the introduction of MC for nonelderly, nondisabled adults and children (White House, 1995). Because of this, policy analysts have commented on the fact that the foci of cost-containment efforts have been directed toward a group of citizens who account for a relatively small proportion of Medicaid spending: nondisabled women and children (Panda, Shapiro, & Schaps, 1995). Some have questioned the wisdom of asking such a vulnerable population of women and children to bear the brunt of cost-containment strategies when they are such a relatively inexpensive group to serve (Deal & Shiono, 1998).

Throughout the 1980s there was increasing recognition of the underfunded, overly restrictive, and fragmented system of behavioral health care for children and adolescents (Knitzer, 1982; Stroul & Friedman, 1986). Mental health services for this age group were characterized by overreliance on costly and unnecessary inpatient treatment (Weithorn, 1988), lack of system coordination in creating a continuum of care (Saxe & Dougherty, 1986), and failure to involve and support families of youths with SED (Collins & Collins, 1990). There was a general recognition that the children's mental health service system required reform along certain principles: individualized service planning, wraparound services, interagency coordination, family involvement, use of less restrictive environments, minimization of out-of-home care, and cultural sensitivity (Schlenger, Ethridge, Hansen, Fairbank, & Onken, 1992). A parallel set of principles related to financing systems of care was proposed, including strategies such as pooling of funds, use of Medicaid funds to promote community-based care, use of state resources and incentives, and wraparound funding (Kutash, Rivera, Hall, & Friedman, 1994).

Yet despite knowledge about what works, many states' Medicaid plans do not emphasize community-based services, nor do they include the innovative supports identified with the wraparound concept (Rosenblatt, 1996). For example, a 1989 state survey of Medicaid coverage for children and adolescents found that case management, school clinics, and rehabilitation services were seldom covered (Fox, Wicks, McManus, & Kelly, 1991). Moreover, treatment by clinical social workers, psychologists, and substance abuse counselors also was excluded from coverage by many state plans. Today, advocates and policymakers are concerned that the cost-saving environment applied to an already service-poor area will erode the reforms accomplished in children's services (Stroul, 1996).

A multivariate study of child mental health services in a well-insured population (the Blue Cross/Blue Shield plan for federal employees) by Padgett, Patrick, Burns, Schlesinger, and Cohen (1993) found that ethnic minority children were less likely than Caucasian children to use services. Moreover, both the rate and mean number of visits were higher in the "high option" plan, which required a higher co-payment and allowed for twice as many outpatient visits as the "low option" plan. This study also raised the issue of the critical role of parents regarding service access, given that children of high-income parents received more mental health services while those in the low-benefit plan received fewer services. This suggests that if parents cannot afford to provide outpatient care to their children—through either their insurance plan or their own economic means—those children are less likely to be treated. Moreover, the presence of a disorder and need for treatment among children typically are not perceived by parents or physicians (Hoberman, 1992). Thus, parents appear to play a major role in access to and utilization of children and youth services.

Some have argued that mental health services for youth are necessarily more complex and thus expensive. Estimates are that 50% more staff time is required to treat a youth as compared to an adult due to collateral contacts with parents, teachers, court personnel, and other professionals. Several studies have indicated that only about a third of youth with psychiatric disorders seek help (e.g., Hoberman, 1992). This underserving of the nation's children and adolescents with behavioral health problems has implications for MC, given the absence of adequate provider networks and sound formulas for capitation (Zhang, Lancaster, Clardy, & Smith, 1999).

RESEARCH ON CHILDREN'S MANAGED BEHAVIORAL HEALTH CARE

Few researchers have addressed the effects of introducing managed behavioral health-care arrangements on the outcomes and service utilization of children with mental health problems. Attkisson, Dresser, and Rosenblatt (1995) studied three California counties using managed behavioral health care along with systems of care for children's mental health disorders and found positive outcomes, such as reductions in all types of out-of-home placements and lower per capita expenditures for group home placements. In Massachusetts, with a wraparound integrated system-of-care approach for children, MC savings have been estimated at $47 million, the largest share of the savings coming from the substance abuse treatment system by shifting from high-cost hospital-based detoxification care to a lower cost public detoxification system (Gillis-Ojemann, 1995, cited in Stroul, 1996). An evaluation of a Medicaid-managed behavioral health-care carve-out for a youth demonstration program in North Carolina found that the capitated system resulted in reductions in inpatient care, increased outpatient services, and slowed growth in costs, compared to the existing Medicaid FFS system (Burns, Teagle, Schwartz, Angold, & Holtzman, 1999). In research on a recently introduced utilization management program on patterns of medical care among children and youth (Wickizer, Lessler, & Boyd-Wickizer, 1999), adolescents with depression or alcohol/drug dependence accounted for a disproportionate share of reductions in inpatient utilization. However, those admitted for mental health care and whose stay was restricted by concurrent review were significantly more likely to be readmitted within 60 days after discharge. Thus, Wickizer and colleagues questioned the effects of cost-containment strategies on the quality of care received by children and youth, especially in the mental health area.

Other recent research studies have revealed mixed findings about the effects of Medicaid MC arrangements on children's mental health and substance abuse outcomes. For example, one survey of stakeholders in 10 states (Stroul, Pires, Armstrong, & Meyers, 1998) found that although penetration rates increased under MC (i.e., an increased number of children received behavioral health services), it was more difficult for youth with SED to obtain necessary services. Given that children with SED are high service utilizers involved with multiple agencies, MC systems often have difficulties with service coordination. This survey also found that MC arrangements made it more difficult to obtain access to inpatient care in all the states surveyed. Also noted was a discernible trend toward briefer, more problem-focused treatment for behavioral health difficulties and the fact that introduction of MC had done little to increase the availability of culturally diverse providers or more culturally appropriate services.

In another study of Medicaid MC on decision making during emergency mental health screening (Nicholson, Young, Simon, Bateman, & Fisher, 1996), the total volume of screening episodes increased significantly during the year after MC implementation, as compared to the year before. However, inpatient admissions following Medicaid-funded screenings decreased significantly after implementation, compared to the prior year, and no corresponding reduction in admissions was observed among episodes not covered by Medicaid. At the same time, significant changes were noted in the pattern of dispositions following emergency screening. After MC implementation, the proportion of dispositions to the child's home decreased significantly, whereas the proportion of dispositions to crisis stabilization settings increased significantly. These findings could be indicative of interventions that result in an increased number of children being maintained in professional settings rather than their own homes in the community.

Another study compared a clinically managed continuum-of-care approach to a capitated managed mental health-care model (Heflinger & Northrup, 1998) by surveying service providers and administrators. This study found decreased coordination following the introduction of capitation. In addition, fragmentation of the service system increased following MC implementation, with provider agencies more likely to interact solely with other agencies within their immediate service cluster and less likely to coordinate with agencies outside of that cluster. The authors speculated that such fragmentation leads to more barriers in finding services appropriate to meet the diverse needs of children with SED. In addition, key informants' ratings of service coordination for children with SED decreased significantly following the introduction of capitation.

Given the lack of research on MC and the often-contradictory findings, the present study explored the effects of managed behavioral health-care arrangements on Medicaid-funded children with mental health and substance abuse difficulties. Two major research questions guided the analysis. First, do children with SED who receive services in MC versus FFS settings differ in regard to their mental health and functional impairment statuses? Second, does utilization of behavioral health services vary according to whether the child receives services in an MC versus an FFS setting?

METHOD

Background

Data were taken from the Children and Adolescents with SED Substudy, one of the four major substudies of the Managed Behavioral Health Care in the Public Sector (MBHCPS) study funded by the Substance Abuse and Mental Health Services Administration (SAMHSA). Principal investigators (PIs) from five sites (Pennsylvania, New York, Ohio, Oregon, and Tennessee/Mississippi), a PI from the University of Illinois at Chicago (UIC) multisite study coordinating center, and a consumer representative composed the steering committee for the study. The steering committee was charged with developing, administering, and overseeing the analysis of a common protocol (CP) of research instruments. At each site, Medicaid-eligible children with SED were enrolled in MC or FFS behavioral health plans. Interviews with the children's caregivers elicited information about services used by these children in the 6 months prior to study enrollment and during the period between enrollment (baseline) and 6-month follow-up, as well as the caregivers' ratings of the child's mental health status at baseline and follow-up. Interviews with children with SED age 11 years and older elicited information regarding substance use, perceptions of their own mental health, and their opinions about their behavioral health-care plan. Sites varied according to the specifics of the MC and FFS arrangements at each location, the types of children with SED who were studied, the nature of the caregivers who were interviewed, the ways services were funded, and the political and social climate at each location. More information is available at the Web site (http://www.psych.uic.edu/mhsrp/managedcarecc.htm).

Inclusion and Exclusion Criteria

Children and youth with SED were defined as those meeting the following criteria: being age 4 through 17 years at the time of study enrollment; being eligible for Medicaid; having a *Diagnostic and Statistical Manual of Mental Disorders–Fourth Edition* (*DSM–IV;* American Psychiatric Association, 1994) diagnosis of mental disorder; and using in the past year at least one type of intensive mental health service, including inpatient, residential, or day treatment; partial hospitalization; in-home support; rehabilitation; therapeutic foster care; special school; crisis services; intensive outpatient (3 days per week) treatment; or intensive case management. Exclusion criteria for the SED sample were having a *DSM–IV* mental disorder diagnosis consisting solely of the category of adjustment disorder, having a diagnosis of mental retardation or developmental disorder, and being served primarily through the mental retardation or developmental disability system. Additional inclusion criteria for the adult interviews were the presence of a knowledgeable caregiver willing and able to give informed consent. If a family member was not available to answer questions about the children, respondents were professional caregivers. For the youth interviews, additional inclusion criteria were as follows: being 11 years of age or older, being willing and able to give informed consent, and having caregiver consent to participate. Each site used a different method of recruitment, depending on its state's way of recording who was Medicaid eligible and who was enrolled in MC versus FFS plans. In addition, unique human subjects protection requirements imposed by the various sites' institutional review boards led to somewhat different recruitment strategies (see study Web site for details).

Features Associated with Study Attrition

Characteristics of the children with follow-up interviews ($N = 1,517$) were compared to those of children who had a baseline interview only ($N = 207$) to identify potential biases resulting from differential attrition rates. No differences were found between the follow-up group and those not followed in terms of child age, gender, functional impairment, health status, symptomatology, and adult caregiver burden. The only statistically significant differences between the follow-up group and those not followed were in the proportions of ethnicity/race groupings among the respondents. Caucasian children's caregivers were more likely to complete a follow-up interview (54.2% of those successfully followed up were Caucasian, whereas 44.4% of those who were not followed up were Caucasian), but caregivers of Hispanic children were less likely (8.5% of those followed vs. 13.2% of those not followed). This difference was entirely attributable to ethnicity/race differences in response rates in the FFS group, where Caucasian children were significantly more likely to be in the follow-up group than in the baseline-only group (53.7% of those followed vs. 34.8% not followed), and African American children were less likely to be followed (33.9% of those followed vs. 46.4% of those not followed). In the MC group, the only significant difference between the follow-up and baseline-only groups was a somewhat higher mean monthly household income for those who were successfully followed ($1,872.40 among those followed vs. $1,608.43 among those not followed). These variables are controlled for in all of the multivariate analyses that follow.

Interviewer Training

Interviewers at all sites attended the "train-the-trainer" CP interviewer training conducted by the UIC coordinating center at the initiation of the study in the spring of 1997. Project managers and interviewer trainers participated in this full-day seminar to ensure that identical interviewing techniques and research protocols were used across the sites. Participants were trained in general research interviewing procedures as well as techniques specific to research interviews conducted with children. Human subjects protection and confidentiality issues for both children and adults were specifically addressed. The group was then trained on the administration of the study's CP as well as how to handle typical procedural issues that might arise. Sections of the CP were simulated with role plays, and audience feedback was elicited throughout. Sites also conducted additional trainings for their interviewers based on the training seminar.

Research Instruments

Six preexisting research instruments were selected for use in the CP and constitute the major dependent and independent variables used in this analysis. The first was the *Child Behavior Checklist* (CBCL; Achenbach & Edelbrock, 1983), a 118-item scale designed to measure the behavioral problems and mental health symptoms of children and adolescents as reported by an adult who knows the child well. In addition to a Total score, two subscales of the CBCL were computed: the Internalizing subscale, designed to measure inhibited, overcontrolled behavior, and the Externalizing subscale, designed to measure aggressive, antisocial, undercontrolled behavior. In studies of referred and nonreferred boys and girls aged 4 to 18 years, the CBCL achieved good internal reliability ($\alpha = .96$) and test–retest reliability ($r = .89$). The second research instrument was the adult-response version of the *Columbia Impairment Scale* (CIS; Bird et al., 1993), a 13-item scale designed to provide a global measure of children's functional impairment. Specifically, it measures a child's interpersonal (peer) relations and functioning in school and at home. The internal consistency reliability for the CIS is excellent ($\alpha = .88$). The third research instrument was the *Child Health Questionnaire Parent Form* (CHQ; Landgraf, Abetz, & Ware, 1996), a 50-item scale designed to measure the physical and psychosocial functioning and well-being of children. In studies of a U.S. population sample, the CHQ achieved excellent internal reliability ($\alpha = .93$). For the purpose of the present analysis, the six-item General Health Perceptions subscale was used to assess the caregiver's perception of the child's health. The fourth research instrument was the *Caregiver Strain Questionnaire* (CSQ; Brannan, Heflinger, & Bickman, 1997), a 21-item scale designed to measure the strain experienced by parents and other caregivers who have primary responsibility for the needs of children younger than 18 years with SED. In studies of caregivers for a clinical population, the CSQ achieved excellent internal reliability ($\alpha = .93$). The 12-item *Short-Form Health Survey* (SF-12; Ware, Kosinski, & Keller, 1996) was used to measure an adult's physical and mental health. In studies of a general outpatient population with a longer version of the SF-12 called the SF-36, good internal reliability was reported, with alphas ranging from .76 to .86. In a study of the SF-12, test–retest reliability was excellent ($r = .89$). Finally, the *Services Utilization Instrument* (SUI) was adapted by the project steering committee from two preexisting measures: the *Service Assessment for Children and Adolescents* (SACA; Stiffman et al., 2000) and the *Child and Adolescent Services Assessment* (CASA; Burns, Angold, Magruder-Habib, Costello, & Patrick, 1996). The resulting measure was designed specifically to measure a child's receipt of health, mental health, and substance abuse services as reported by a parent or primary caregiver. This 186-item instrument is composed of sections regarding residential, nonresidential, general medical, mental retardation/developmental disabilities, child welfare, school-based, medication, general, and prevention services.

Types of Managed Care Plans Studied

The types of MC plans operating at the five sites varied widely, drawing from different funding streams, using different utilization review procedures, operating under different contract structures and provisions, using different risk-sharing mechanisms, and focused on somewhat different types of populations of children with SED. Further information regarding variations in these plans is available from a survey of their MC contracts conducted by Human Services Research Institute in Cambridge, Massachusetts (Mulkern, 1998). However, one major difference among sites was that MC at the Ohio (OH) site was not county- or statewide. At the OH site, children in the MC condition were served at a single agency and included only those defined as the "most expensive" to serve across the entire county. The MC entity was a private, not-for-profit agency that was established by county officials for the purpose of providing managed, wraparound behavioral health services to youth who were being served by multiple human service agencies or the juvenile justice system. The youth were recognized as being extremely difficult and costly to treat. Funds from five county agencies, including the Medicaid agency, were pooled to serve the youth on a case-rate basis. Over the course of the study, the MC entity began sharing fiscal risk with some of its providers. Perhaps because of this, as well as other factors, analysis results indicated that unusually high proportions of children in OH's MC condition received services relative to children in MC conditions at the other sites. It became evident through subsequent analyses that MC in Ohio operated much differently than at other sites, where MC had been introduced to a much wider range of children over a larger geographical area and delivered by a more diverse provider constituency. In cross-site analyses, the uniqueness of the OH site masked consistencies among the remaining sites that were evident once data from the OH children were excluded. Because of this, the steering committee decided to restrict the cross-site analysis to four sites, excluding OH. Single-site analyses using the same predictive models and including the OH site are presented elsewhere (Cook et al., in press).

Child Mental Health, Functional Impairment, and Service Utilization Variables

Four child mental health and functional impairment variables were selected for analysis: (a) the level of the child's functional impairment at follow-up as measured by the CIS, (b) overall psychiatric symptomatology at follow-up as measured by the CBCL, (c) internalizing symptomatology (e.g., depression, withdrawal) at follow-up from the CBCL Internalizing subscale, and (d) externalizing symptomatology (e.g., acting out, aggressive behavior) at follow-up from the CBCL Externalizing subscale. It is important to note that these variables cannot be considered outcomes of managed care per se. This is because children had been receiving services within these conditions for varying amounts of time prior to enrolling in the study and, thus, any differences that existed at follow-up might have existed prior to entry into MC or FFS settings. However, our ability to control for MC versus FFS differences at both the time of entry into the study and again at the follow-up 6 months later provided an opportunity to see whether there was differential improvement or deterioration in children's status during the 6-month study period. If such differences emerged during those 6 months, the effect might be attributable to the study condition or the MC versus FFS setting in which services were received.

Four child service utilization variables were selected for analysis: (a) any inpatient or residential service use between baseline and 6-month follow-up, (b) any traditional outpatient service use (i.e., treatment in the office of a psychiatrist, psychologist or counselor, or at a community mental health center), (c) any prescription psychotropic medication use, and (d) any nontraditional service use (i.e., day treatment, partial hospitalization, in-home treatment, school-based services, case management, or group home care).

Model Tested in the Analysis

To predict child mental health status at Time 2 (6-month follow-up), control and explanatory variables were entered into an ordinary least squares (OLS) multiple regression analysis hierarchically in six blocks: (a) Block 1 included the Time 1 (baseline) score for each model's Time 2 dependent mental health status variable (e.g., functional impairment, psychiatric symptomatology); (b) Block 2 included five child characteristics (age, gender, minority status, contact with the juvenile justice system, physical health); (c) Block 3 included seven adult caregiver characteristics (age, gender, education, physical health, mental health, caregiver strain, and satisfaction with child's behavioral health care plan); (d) Block 4 included four household characteristics (income, number of co-residents, urban neighborhood, rural neighborhood [with "mixed" neighborhood used as the reference category]); (e) Block 5 included a single variable representing study condition (MC vs. FFS); and (f) Block 6 included three of the four sites included in the analysis to control for site variation (Tennessee, Oregon, and Pennsylvania, with New York as the reference site).

To predict the child's service utilization between baseline and follow-up interviews, a model was tested that entered variables in the same blocks as described previously, except that some of the interval-level variables were dichotomized or grouped into increments to ease the interpretability of the odds ratios. Another difference is that in the logistic regression models, the child mental health status baseline measure in Block 1 was replaced by a group of three "need" variables. Need for services was defined by children's mental health status scores at baseline, including high versus low functional impairment; high versus low total psychiatric symptomatology; and use versus non-use ever of alcohol, drugs, or tobacco.

Analysis

The initial analysis involved examination of frequency distributions regarding the child and caregiver characteristics and the study's eight dependent variables at baseline. Next, cross-site OLS multiple regression analyses were conducted to predict the mental health status of children and youth regarding the child's level of functional impairment and severity of psychiatric symptomatology at the time of the 6-month follow-up interview. Finally cross-site multiple logistic regression models were run to predict the likelihood of utilization of four types of services: (a) any inpatient or residential service use between baseline and 6-month follow-up, (b) any traditional outpatient service use, (c) any medication use, and (d) any nontraditional service use.

RESULTS

Child, Caregiver, and Household Characteristics

Table 24.1 provides information about the background characteristics of the 1,206 children, their caregivers, and households. Two-thirds of the children (66%) were boys, with a mean age of 12 years, and 42% were members of racial and ethnic minority groups (27% African American, 10% Hispanic/ Latino, 5% mixed or other, <1% Asian). Around a fifth (18.5%) had prior involvement with the juvenile justice system. The majority of children scored at or above the clinical cutoff for psychiatric symptoms and functional impairment, and a third had used drugs, alcohol, or tobacco prior to entry into the study.

Most of the caregivers were women (95%) and high school graduates (72%), and their average age was 39 years. On the CSQ, half scored above the mean of 2.48 reported by caregivers of a clinical population of children (Brannan et al., 1997). Caregivers' average SF-12 physical and mental health scores fell below those of a nonclinical population of adults, indicating poorer health than the general population (Ware et al., 1996). Families reported a median household income of $1,469 per month (averaging under $18,000 per year), and 40% lived in households of 5 or more individuals.

Children's Mental Health Status at Follow-Up

At follow-up, children's CIS scores ranged from 0 to 52, with a mean of 24.2 and a median of 24. More than half of all children scored above the CIS

TABLE 24.1
Child, Caregiver, and Household Characteristic (N = 1,206 Children)

Child Characteristics

Age (M)	11.5 years
Gender	
Female	33.8%
Male	66.2%
Race/ethnicity	
Caucasian (not Hispanic)	58.3%
African American (not Hispanic)	26.7%
Hispanic	10%
Asian/Pacific Islander	<1%
Other/mixed (not Hispanic)	5%
Prior contact with juvenile justice system	
Yes	18.5%
No	81.5%
Functional impairment at Time 1 (*Columbia Impairment Scale*[a] ≥16)	79.3%
Severe psychiatric symptoms at Time 1 (*Child Behavior Checklist*[b] ≥67)	57.5%
Prior drug/alcohol/tobacco use at Time 1	
Yes	32.8%
No	67.2%
Study site	
Tennessee/Mississippi	25.6%
Oregon	20.6%
Pennsylvania	29.4%
New York	24.4%
Study condition	
Managed care	45.4%
Fee-for-service	54.6%

Caregiver Characteristics

Age (M)	39.4 years
Gender	
Male	5.0%
Female	95.0%
Education	
High school/GED or above	72.1%
Less than high school	27.9%
Caregiver Strain Scale[c] (Range 1–5, Higher = *more strain*)	2.51
SF-12[d] Physical Health subscale score (Range 0–100, Higher = *better physical health*)	43.29
SF-12 Mental Health subscale score (Range 0–100, Higher = *better mental health*)	41.33
Satisfaction with health plan score (Range 1–10, Higher = *more satisfied*)	7.5

(continues)

TABLE 24.1 *Continued.*
Child, Caregiver, and Household Characteristic (*N* = 1,206 Children)

Household Characteristics	
Monthly household income (Mdn)	$1,469
Household size, in addition to child	
2 people	10.3%
3 people	23.1%
4 people	26.8%
5 or more	39.9%
Community type	
Urban	35.8%
Mixed rural–urban	52.1%
Rural	12.1%

[a]Bird et al. (1993). [b]Achenbach & Edelbrock (1983). [c]Brannan et al. (1997). [d]*Short-Form Health Survey* (Ware et al., 1996).

clinical cutoff of 16, indicating significant impairment in their level of psychosocial functioning. Children's CBCL scores ranged from 0 to 100, averaging 66.8 (Mdn = 68). Again, more than half of all children scored above the clinical cutoff score for children in a mental health clinical population, indicating the presence of psychiatric symptomatology characteristics. The average scores on the CBCL for internalizing behavior (*M* = 62.1, Mdn = 63) indicated that just under half were at or above the clinical range, and the mean score for CBCL externalizing behavior was 66.2 (Mdn = 68), indicating that more than half of these children were at or above the clinical range.

The results of the four cross-site hierarchical linear regressions are presented in Table 24.2. Each of the models predicted a different child mental health status measure at follow-up (Time 2): functional impairment (CIS Total score), psychopathology and symptoms (CBCL Total score), externalizing problems (Externalizing score), and internalizing problems (Internalizing score). The six blocks of explanatory variables are shown in the first column on the left of Table 24.2. Across the top of the table, each of the four mental health status outcomes are listed, and repeated as each block is entered into the model. Each successive group of columns shows the regression coefficients for each of the predictor variables, repeated as blocks are entered into the models. Thus, the first four columns of the table show the models' coefficient when Block 1 is entered, the next four columns show the models' coefficients when Blocks 1 and 2 are entered, and so on up to the last four columns of the table, which show the results of the four models when all six blocks are entered. Coefficients are provided in the table for each step of the regression, indicating how the addition of each of the six blocks of independent variables altered the impact and significance of variables already entered, as well as those newly entered. Each of the models will be discussed separately.

TABLE 24.2
Cross-site Hierarchical OLS Regressions Predicting Child Mental Health Status at T2

T2 Mental Health Status	CIS[a]	CBCL[b]	EXT[c]	INT[d]	CIS[a]	CBCL[b]	EXT[c]	INT[d]	CIS[a]	CBCL[b]	EXT[c]	INT[d]	CIS[a]	CBCL[b]	EXT[c]	INT[d]	CIS[a]	CBCL[b]	EXT[c]	INT[d]	CIS[a]	CBCL[b]	EXT[c]	INT[d]
Block 1																								
Child Mental Health T1	.61**	.70***	.70***	.69***	.59***	.70***	.70***	.68***	.57***	.68***	.69***	.66***	.56***	.68***	.69***	.64***	.56***	.67***	.69***	.64***	.56***	.66***	.69***	.63***
Block 2																								
Child age					−.03	−.01	−.03	.00	−.03	−.02	−.03	−.00	−.02	−.03	−.01	−.00	−.03	−.03	−.01	−.00	−.02	−.03	−.01	−.04
Female child					−.01	−.00	.00	.00	−.02	−.02	−.00	−.02	−.00	−.00	−.00	−.02	−.00	−.00	−.00	−.02	−.02	−.01	−.00	−.02
Minority child					−.02	.04	.04	.04	−.02	−.01	.04	.02	−.02	.02	.03	.02	.02	.04	.02	.02	.02	.03	.03	.02
Juvenile justice involvement					.00	−.01	.00	−.02	−.00	−.02	−.00	−.00	−.00	−.01	−.02	−.02	.00	−.00	−.01	−.02	.00	−.01	.01	−.00
Child health					−.05*	−.04	−.03	−.06*	−.04	−.03	−.03	−.05*	−.04	−.03	−.03	−.05*	−.04	−.03	−.03	−.04*	−.03	−.02	−.02	−.04*
Block 3																								
Adult high school ed									.05*	.01	.01	.03	−.04	.02	.01	.03	.04	.02	.01	.03	.04	.02	.01	.02
Female adult									.02	−.01	.01	−.01	−.02	−.02	−.01	−.01	.02	−.02	−.01	−.01	.02	−.02	−.02	−.01
Adult age									.00	.01	−.02	−.01	−.00	.02	.01	.00	−.00	.01	−.00	.01	.02	−.02	−.02	−.01
Caregiver strain									.00	.01	.04	.01	−.00	−.00	.01	.01	−.00	.02	−.00	.00	.01	.01	.01	.01
Adult health									−.01	−.04	−.02	−.06**	−.01	−.04	−.02	−.06*	−.01	−.04	−.02	−.06*	−.01	−.03	−.02	−.06*
Adult mental health									−.08**	−.07**	−.06*	−.11***	−.09**	−.06**	−.05*	−.10***	−.09**	−.06**	−.05*	−.10***	−.08**	−.07**	−.06*	−.10***
Adult plan satisfaction									−.01	−.01	−.01	.02	−.00	−.01	−.02	.02	−.00	−.01	−.02	.02	.00	−.01	−.02	.02
Block 4																								
Household income/mo.													−.04	−.03	−.01	−.04	.04	−.03	−.01	−.04	.03	−.03	−.01	−.04
Household size													.01	.01	.01	.00	.01	.01	.00	.00	.01	.01	−.00	−.00
Urban													−.01	−.01	.02	−.01	.01	−.00	.02	−.01	.06	−.00	.03	−.00
Rural													−.01	.02	.02	.00	−.01	.02	.02	.00	.00	.01	.03	.00
Block 5																								
Managed care																	−.01	−.03	−.03	−.02	−.02	−.04	−.04	−.03
Block 6																								
Tennessee/Mississippi site																					.00	.07*	.05	.06
Oregon site																					.10*	.05	.02	.08
Pennsylvania* site																					.06	.01	−.01	.03

Note. Results of −.00 and +.00 were due to rounding.

[a] CIS = functional impairment. [b] CBCL = psychiatric symptom severity. [c] EXT = externalizing psychiatric symptom severity. [d] INT = internalizing psychiatric symptom severity.

* $p < .05$. ** $p < .01$. *** $p < .001$.

Functional Impairment

In the initial step of the model predicting functional impairment at follow-up (entry of Block 1), the baseline CIS level was significantly and positively associated with functional impairment status at Time 2 (T2). In the next step, only one child characteristic from Block 2 was significant: functional impairment at T2 was greater among those children in poorer physical health at Time 1 (T1). In the third step, addition of the caregiver's characteristics (Block 3) led the child physical health variable to become nonsignificant. In addition, child's functional impairment was greater for those caregivers at higher levels of education and those caregivers self-reporting poorer mental health at T1. In Step 4, addition of the household/neighborhood characteristics (Block 4) caused the adult education variable to become nonsignificant. In Step 5, addition of study condition (Block 5) caused no changes in the significance of variables from previous steps of the model. Finally, the addition of controls for site (Block 6) did not change the model from the previous step, but functional impairment was significantly greater among children at the Oregon site as compared with the index site (New York). Thus, in the final model of functional impairment (shown on the right of Table 24.2), children with greater functional impairment were those with greater initial functional impairment, those whose caregivers reported poorer mental health themselves, and those at the Oregon site.

Total Psychiatric Symptoms

In the model predicting the children's total psychiatric symptom severity (CBCL Total score), the baseline CBCL Total score (Block 1) was significantly and positively associated with mental health symptomatology at T2. None of the child variables (Block 2) added in Step 2 were significant. At Step 3, total symptomatology was greater for children whose caregivers reported worse mental health themselves. These results did not change with the addition of Block 4 (household characteristics), Block 5 (study condition), and Block 6 (study site), as shown in the final model of total psychiatric symptoms on the right side of Table 24.2.

Externalizing Symptoms

The child's baseline CBCL Externalizing score (Block 1) was significantly associated with greater externalizing symptomatology at follow-up. None of the child variables (Block 2) added in Step 2 was significant. At Step 3, total externalizing symptomatology was greater for children whose caregivers reported worse mental health themselves. These results did not change with the addition of Block 4 (household characteristics), Block 5 (study condition), and Block 6 (study site).

Internalizing Symptoms

Children's baseline internalizing symptomatology scores (Block 1) were positively associated with follow-up levels of internalizing symptomatology. Only one child characteristic from Block 2 was significant at Step 2, with the CBCL Internalizing score being greater for children in poorer physical health. At Step 3, internalizing symptom scores were greater for children whose caregivers reported worse mental health and worse physical health themselves. These three variables were significant throughout the remaining steps of the model, with no other significant results emerging, as shown in the final column of Table 24.2.

Overall, MC study condition was not significant at any step in any of the models. The strongest predictors of children's symptoms and functional impairment at follow-up were their symptoms and functional impairment at baseline, as might be expected. In addition, adult caregivers who rated their own mental health as poorer tended to be caring for children with higher levels of symptomatology and greater impairment.

Likelihood of Mental Health Service Utilization Between Baseline and Follow-Up

Analysis of frequencies for the service use variables indicated that 10.8% of the children received inpatient or residential services between baseline and follow-up, 64.8% received traditional outpatient services, 56.2% received psychotropic medications, and 67.4% received nontraditional services.

The results of the four cross-site hierarchical logistic regressions are presented in Table 24.3. Each of the models predicted a different type of service utilization at follow-up (Time 2): inpatient (residential), outpatient (traditional outpatient services), psychotropic medications, and nontraditional psychiatric services. As in the previous table, the six blocks of explanatory variables are shown in the first column. Across the top of the table, each of the four types of service utilization is listed and repeated as each block is entered into the model. Odds ratios are provided in the table for each step of the logistic regression, indicating how the addition of each of the six blocks of independent variables altered the impact and significance of variables already entered, as well as those newly entered. Each of the models will be discussed separately.

Use of Inpatient/Residential Services

In the multiple logistic regression model predicting likelihood of use of inpatient/residential services at follow-up, results of Step 1 (entry of Block 1 only) indicated that utilization was more likely for children with greater mental health symptomatology at baseline and for those with any history of substance use at baseline (see Table 24.3). These remained significant, although with slightly lower odds ratios, with the addition of child characteristics (Block 2) at Step 2, whereas utilization of inpatient services was more likely for children ever involved in the juvenile justice system and those in poorer physical health (as rated by their caregivers). The addition of Block 3, caregiver characteristics, caused the Block 1 need variables (baseline mental health symptoms and history of substance use) and child physical health to become nonsignificant,

TABLE 24.3

Cross-Site Hierarchical Logistic Regression Predicting Receipt of Services Between Time 1 (T1) and Time 2 (T2)

Service Receipt T1–T2	Inpt[a]	Outpt[b]	Meds[c]	NT[d]	Inpt[a]	Outpt[b]	Meds[c]	NT[d]	Inpt[a]	Outpt[b]	Meds[c]	NT[d]	Inpt[a]	Outpt[b]	Meds[c]	NT[d]	Inpt[a]	Outpt[b]	Meds[c]	NT[d]	Inpt[a]	Outpt[b]	Meds[c]	NT[d]
Block 1																								
CIS T1[e]	1.84**	2.00***	2.08***	1.48*	1.72	1.98***	1.76**	1.47*	1.16	1.87***	1.56*	1.40	1.25	1.87***	1.53*	1.37	1.27	1.87***	1.55***	1.39	1.28	1.84***	1.52*	1.36
CBCL T1[f]	2.19**	1.45**	2.37***	1.53**	1.95*	1.28	2.34***	1.50**	1.18	1.16	2.09***	1.45*	1.16	1.17	2.07***	1.46*	1.13	1.17	2.05***	1.43*	1.14	1.17	2.05***	1.57**
Substance use	2.30***	0.67**	0.81	0.91	1.70	0.92	0.85	0.92	1.51	0.90	0.80	0.90	1.62	0.90	0.80	0.89	1.67	0.90	0.82	0.93	1.70	0.87	0.88	0.87
Block 2																								
Child age					1.04	0.69***	0.92	0.90	1.07	0.67***	0.91	0.90	1.05	0.67***	0.90	0.89	1.04	0.67***	0.89	0.88	1.02	0.67***	0.80**	0.88
Female child					0.75	1.06	0.53***	0.80	0.78	1.07	0.51***	0.79	0.78	1.06	0.51***	0.79	0.80	1.06	0.52***	0.81	0.80	1.06	0.56***	0.80
Minority child					0.97	0.52***	0.39***	1.17	1.06	0.55***	0.40***	1.20	0.85	0.52***	0.46***	1.28	0.79	0.52***	0.44***	1.18	0.76	0.61*	0.53***	1.37
JD child[g]					2.16**	1.37	0.79	1.69*	1.90*	1.34	0.76	1.68*	1.89*	1.33	0.76	1.66*	1.97*	1.33	0.80	1.79*	2.02*	1.28	0.87	1.63*
Child health					0.63*	0.70	0.83	1.06	0.67	0.68**	0.81	1.03	0.65	0.68**	0.82	1.04	0.65	0.68**	0.83	1.06	0.65	0.67**	0.84	1.05
Block 3																								
Adult high school ed									1.22	1.02	1.34	1.07	1.40	0.99	1.31	1.02	1.42	0.99	1.31	1.02	1.46	0.95	1.30	1.03
Female adult									0.57	0.94	0.89	0.83	0.51	0.96	0.89	0.86	0.48	0.96	0.91	0.88	0.48	0.99	0.93	0.91
Adult age									1.14	1.17*	1.13	1.11	1.24	1.15	1.14	1.08	1.24	1.15	1.13	1.08	1.25	1.16	1.15	1.11
Caregiver strain									2.17***	1.18	1.32**	1.11	2.15***	1.18	1.33**	1.11	2.18***	1.18	1.34**	1.13	2.21***	1.17	1.32*	1.19
Adult health									1.11	0.94	0.85	1.09	1.10	0.92	0.87	1.08	1.10	0.92	0.87	1.08	1.10	0.91	0.89	1.03
Adult mental health									0.97	1.19	1.36	1.08	0.98	1.17	1.36	1.07	0.96	1.17	1.37	1.09	0.95	1.18	1.33	1.10
Adult plan satisfaction									1.41	0.79	1.20	1.09	1.34	0.80	1.20	1.12	1.35	0.80	1.18	1.09	1.34	0.82	1.21	1.14
Block 4																								
Household income/mo.													0.74*	1.09	0.98	1.10	0.75*	1.09	0.98	1.11	0.75*	1.08	1.03	1.10
Household size													1.40***	0.94	1.02	0.96	1.39**	0.93	1.01	0.95	1.39**	0.93	0.99	0.96
Urban													1.65	1.12	0.71*	0.86	1.82**	1.12	0.76	0.95	1.51	1.67*	1.15	1.11
Rural													1.78	0.99	0.95	0.83	1.66	0.99	0.90	0.76	1.60	1.06	0.83	0.86
Block 5																								
Managed care																	0.57*	0.98	0.69***	0.58***	0.59*	0.97	0.77	0.64**
Block 6																								
TN/MS[h] site																					0.79	1.34	2.61***	0.48**
Oregon site																					0.64	2.11	1.85	0.86
Pennsylvania site																					0.80	1.94*	3.58***	1.20

[a]Inpt = inpatient. [b]Outpt = outpatient. [c]Meds = psychiatric medication. [d]NT = nontraditional psychiatric services. [e]CIS = functional impairment. [f]CBCL = psychiatric symptom severity. [g]JD = juvenile justice involvement. [h]TN/MS = Tennessee/Mississippi.

* p < .05. ** p < .01. *** p < .001.

while caregiver strain was significant, with higher strain associated with greater likelihood of inpatient/residential treatment of the child. Caregiver strain and involvement with the juvenile justice system remained associated with greater likelihood of inpatient use at Step 4, with the following significant household characteristics (Block 4): Children more likely to receive inpatient/residential services were those from families with lower household incomes and those with more co-residents. None of these relationships changed with the addition of study condition (Block 5), except that urban setting became significant, with children from urban areas more likely (than those in mixed areas) to receive this kind of service. Study condition was also significant, with children in the MC condition less likely than those in the FFS condition to be hospitalized or to receive residential treatment. This did not change with the addition of site variables (Block 6), although urban setting became nonsignificant. Thus, at the model's final step, children more likely to receive inpatient or residential treatment were those ever involved in the juvenile justice system, those whose caregivers reported greater caregiving strain, those with lower household incomes, those with more household co-residents, and those children enrolled in FFS (vs. MC) behavioral health plans.

Use of Traditional Outpatient Services
Table 24.3 also presents the results of the model predicting likelihood of use of traditional outpatient services at follow-up. Here, all three baseline need variables (Block 1) were significantly associated with greater likelihood of outpatient service use. With the addition of Block 2 child characteristics in Step 2, only high baseline functional impairment remained significant, along with child age, minority status, and physical health. Throughout the remaining steps, outpatient service likelihood was greater for younger children, children in poorer physical health, Caucasian children, and those with high functional impairment. The addition of Block 3, caregiver characteristics, did not change these relationships. At this step, older caregiver age was associated with significantly greater likelihood of outpatient services to the child, although this relationship disappeared with the addition of household characteristics and study condition (Blocks 4 and 5). With the addition of site (Block 6) at the final step, urban setting was significantly associated with greater likelihood of outpatient service use, as were being in the Oregon or Pennsylvania sites (compared to the New York site). MC condition was not significant in this model.

Use of Psychotropic Medications
In the model predicting likelihood of use of psychotropic medications, two of the Block 1 baseline need variables, high functional impairment and high mental health symptoms, were significantly associated with greater likelihood of utilization of psychotropic medications throughout all of the steps of the model. Two child characteristics entered in Step 2 also were significant throughout the remainder of the model: Utilization of medications was more likely for boys and Caucasian children. One caregiver characteristic (Block 3)

was significant from Step 3 throughout the remaining steps: Higher caregiver strain was associated with greater likelihood of the child's use of medications. Addition of household/neighborhood characteristics in Step 4 did not influence variables found to be significant in prior steps; in addition, the urban variable was significant, indicating that children from urban areas were less likely (compared to mixed areas) to receive medications. This relationship became nonsignificant with the addition of Block 5, study condition, and adult mental health became significant, with better adult mental health associated with greater likelihood of the children's use of medications. Study condition was also significant at this step; here, children in the MC condition were only two-thirds as likely as those in the FFS condition to have taken psychotropic medications between baseline and follow-up. With the addition of the site control variables (Block 6), this effect of MC condition diminished to being three-quarters as likely and only approached statistical significance ($p < .08$). Additionally, adult mental health was not significant in the final step of the model, but child age was, with younger children more likely to use psychiatric medications. Children at the Tennessee and Pennsylvania sites were also more likely to use medications than those at the New York site.

Use of Nontraditional Mental Health Services

Table 24.3 also presents the results of the model predicting likelihood of use of nontraditional services at 6-month follow-up. At Step 1, utilization was more likely for children with high baseline functional impairment and high baseline mental health symptoms. At Step 2, children ever involved in the juvenile justice system also were more likely to use nontraditional services. The baseline functional impairment variable became nonsignificant with the addition of Block 3, caregiver characteristics, but no other changes were evident. Mental health symptoms and involvement with the juvenile justice system remained associated with greater likelihood of nontraditional services use throughout the rest of the model steps. Addition of Block 4 (household/neighborhood characteristics) did not change the model. At Step 5, study condition also was significant, with children in MC less than two-thirds as likely as those in FFS to receive nontraditional services. These relationships did not change with the addition of site in the final step, although children in Tennessee/Mississippi were less likely to use nontraditional services than those in New York.

Overall, MC study condition was significantly associated with reduced utilization of inpatient and nontraditional services, with a trend toward significance in lower utilization of psychotropic medications. MC condition was not a significant predictor of outpatient services use between baseline and follow-up.

SUMMARY AND CONCLUSION

This study was designed to address two primary research questions. First, do children with SED who receive services in MC versus FFS settings differ in regard to their mental health and functional impairment status? Second, does utilization of behavioral health services vary according to whether the child receives services in an MC versus an FFS setting?

Mental Health and Functional Impairment

Study findings suggest that children with SED enrolled in Medicaid-financed MC versus FFS behavioral health care plans do not differ significantly in levels of functional impairment or psychiatric symptomatology at the time of follow-up. Instead, it appears that the child's initial mental health and functional status at Time 1 had a much stronger effect on the child's psychiatric and functional status at follow-up than did any other variable.

Also noteworthy in these results was the consistent association of poorer mental and physical health among children's caregivers and greater psychiatric symptomatology and functional impairment among the children for whom they were caring. This link between the health of caregivers and their children points to the vulnerability of low-income families in which multiple members experience poor mental and physical health. It suggests that (a) treatment for behavioral health problems must be readily accessible for the entire family, and (b) a holistic approach that addresses the family as a unit is called for in benefit plan design.

Service Utilization

In the models predicting children's mental health service utilization, the likelihood of service use at follow-up was greater for children in FFS (vs. MC) plans when the service studied was inpatient/residential treatment, psychiatric medications, and nontraditional services. These study condition effects were significant even when controlling for need variables, such as baseline levels of functional impairment, total mental health symptoms, and use of drugs and alcohol. In addition, study condition effects were not influenced by controlling for study site, except that the statistical significance of the lower likelihood of psychiatric medication use diminished slightly. Thus, study condition was a noteworthy predictor of all but outpatient services utilization, with the children in the MC condition being less likely to have used most types of services examined.

An exception to these findings was the likelihood of use of traditional outpatient services, defined as visiting a mental health professional in a community mental health center or other office setting. This service was equally likely to be used by children enrolled in MC and FFS plans, suggesting that this comparatively lower cost service may be more equitably available to children who need it, regardless of type of behavioral health plan membership.

The study also found that individual characteristics of the child also were associated with the likelihood of mental health service use. For example, children with high levels of mental health symptoms were more likely to use medications and nontraditional services, whereas those with greater levels of functional impairment were more likely to use medications and outpatient services. The association of children's level of need for services with greater service utilization suggests that some mental health services are reaching those children in greater need. Moreover, children with prior juvenile justice system involvement were more likely to use inpatient and nontraditional services, which may be related to greater scrutiny received by those who have come to the attention of legal authorities. Finally, children who were members of ethnic and racial minority groups were less likely to use some types of mental health services (medication and outpatient services), which is consistent with findings of previous research (Padgett et al., 1993).

Another study finding was an association between adults' reported levels of strain stemming from caregiving for the child and the child's likelihood of service utilization. Children whose caregivers reported greater strain were significantly more likely than those whose caregivers reported less strain to use inpatient services and medication. Although the design of the study makes it impossible to draw causal inferences, this relationship draws our attention to the service needs of caretakers and to the fact that those under more strain may indeed be caring for children with higher levels of impairment. If this is the case, failure to provide adequate services to the child may have a doubly pernicious effect on the well-being of the caregiver.

In summary, a major finding of this study is that the child's enrollment in state- or county-wide MC programs did not have a major effect on the child's functioning and psychiatric status. However, more research will be needed to assess the long-term effects of MC programs on children's functioning and psychiatric status, especially as they transition into adulthood. The results of this study indicate that future research also could focus on the effects of MC on the mental health of the caregivers and families of children with severe psychiatric symptomatology and functional limitations.

Another major finding of this study is that the MC study condition was significantly and consistently predictive of lower utilization of most services, even controlling for child need, household, and site variations. This finding suggests that more work is needed to ensure that all children with SED receive services that represent best practices, especially under MC. More research is needed into the role of individual child characteristics in predicting different types of services utilization. Research also is needed concerning the role of the families or other caregivers of children with SED in influencing level and type of service utilization under both MC and FFS delivery systems. Finally, additional research might focus on implications of the MC emphasis on traditional outpatient services over other types of services and on the long-term effects on the mental health of children and their families.

We hope that future research studies will explore the generalizability of these findings to other populations of low-income children in other regions of the country.

REFERENCES

Achenbach, T. M., & Edelbrock, C. (1983). *Manual for the Child Behavioral Checklist and Revised Child Behavior Profile.* Burlington: University of Vermont, Department of Psychiatry.

American Managed Behavioral Health Care Association. (1995). *Performance measures for managed behavioral healthcare programs* (PERMS). Washington, DC: Author.

American Psychiatric Association. (1994). *Diagnostic and statistical manual of mental disorders* (4th ed.). Washington, DC: Author.

Attkinson, C. C., Dresser, K., & Rosenblatt, A. (1995). Service systems for youth with severe emotional disorder: System-of-care research in California. In L. Bickman & D. Rog (Eds.), *Children's mental health service systems: Policy, services, and evaluation* (pp. 236–280). Beverly Hills, CA: Sage.

Bird, H., Shaffer, D., Fisher, P., Gould, M., Staghezza, B., Chen, J., & Hoven, C. (1993). The Columbia Impairment Scale (CIS): Pilot findings on a measure of global impairment for children and adolescents. *International Journal of Methods in Psychiatric Research, 3,* 167–176.

Brannan, A. M., Heflinger, C. A., & Bickman, L. (1997). The Caregiver Strain Questionnaire: Measuring the impact on the family of living with a child with serious emotional disturbances. *Journal of Emotional and Behavioral Disorders, 5,* 212–222.

Burns, B. J., Angold, A., Magruder-Habib, K., Costello, E. J., & Patrick, M. K. S. (1996). *Child and Adolescent Services Assessment (CASA) Manual.* Durham, NC: Duke University Medical Center, Developmental Epidemiology Program.

Burns, B. J., Teagle, S. E., Schwartz, M., Angold, A., & Holtzman, A. (1999). Managed behavioral health care: A Medicaid carve-out for youth. *Health Affairs, 18*(5), 214–225.

Collins, H., & Collins, D. (1990). Family therapy in the treatment of child sexual abuse. In M. Rothery & G. Cameron (Eds.), *Child maltreatment: Expanding our concept of helping* (pp. 229–245). Hillsdale, NJ: Erlbaum.

Cook, J. A., Heflinger, C. A., Hoven, C., Kelleher, K., Mulkern, V., Paulson, R., et al. (in press). Effects of Medicaid-funded managed care versus fee-for-service plans on the mental health service utilization of children with severe emotional disturbance. *Journal of Behavioral Health Services & Research.*

Deal, L. W., & Shiono, P. H. (1998). Medicaid managed care and children: An overview. *Children and Managed Health Care, 8*(2), 93–104.

Fox, H. B., Wicks, L. N., McManus, M. A., & Kelly, R. W. (1991). *Medicaid financing for mental health and substance abuse services for children and adolescents.* Washington, DC: Substance Abuse and Mental Health Services Administration, Center for Substance Abuse Treatment.

Heflinger, C. A., & Northrup, D. (1998). Measuring change in mental health services coordination under managed care for children and adolescents. *Research in Community and Mental Health, 9,* 69–88.

Hoberman, H. M. (1992). Ethnic minority status and adolescent mental health services utilization. *Journal of Mental Health Administration, 19*(3), 246–267.

Hurley, R. E., Freund, D. A., & Paul, J. E. (1993). *Managed care in Medicaid: Lessons for policy and program design.* Ann Arbor, MI: Health Administration Press.

Knitzer, J. (1982). *Unclaimed children: The failure of public responsibility to children and adolescents in need of mental health services.* Washington, DC: Children's Defense Fund.

Kutash, K., Rivera, V. R., Hall, K. S., & Friedman, R. M. (1994). Public sector financing of community-based services for children with serious emotional disabilities and their families: Results of a national survey. *Journal of Mental Health Administration, 21*(3), 262–270.

Landgraf, J. M., Abetz, L., & Ware, J. E. (1996). *The CHQ user's manual.* Boston: New England Medical Center, The Health Institute.

Mulkern V. (1998). *SAMHSA managed behavioral health care in the public sector project taxonomy of managed care organizations.* Cambridge, MA: Human Services Research Institute.

Nicholson, J., Young, S. D., Simon, L., Bateman, A., & Fisher, W. H. (1996). Impact of Medicaid managed care on child and adolescent emergency mental health screening in Massachusetts. *Psychiatric Services, 47*(12), 1344–1351.

Padgett, D. K., Patrick, C., Burns, B. J., Schlesinger, H. J., & Cohen, J. (1993). The effect of insurance benefit changes on use of child and adolescent outpatient mental health services. *Medical Care, 31*(2), 96–110.

Panda, A., Shapiro, L. D., & Schaps, M. (1995). *Medicaid managed care and women: Implications of the Illinois MediPlan Plus proposal.* Chicago: Health & Medicine Policy Research Group.

Rosenblatt, A. (1996). Bows and ribbons, tape and twine: Wrapping the wraparound process for children with multi-system needs. *Journal of Child and Family Studies, 5*(1), 101–117.

Saxe, L., & Dougherty, D. (1986). *Children's mental health needs: Problems and services.* Washington, DC: U.S. Government Printing Office, Office of Technology Assistance.

Schlenger, W. E., Ethridge, R. M., Hansen, D. J., Fairbank, D. W., & Onken, J. (1992). Evaluation of state efforts to improve systems of care for children and adolescents with severe emotional disturbances: The CASSP initial cohort study. *Journal of Mental Health Administration, 19,* 131–142.

Shapiro, L. D. (1994). *Analysis of the structure of state Medicaid managed care programs: A preliminary summary of professional literature and interviews with experts on state managed care practices.* Chicago: Chicago Health Policy Research Council.

Stiffman, A. R., Horwitz, S. M., Hoagwood, K., Compton, W., Cottler, L., Bean, D. L., et al. (2000). The Service Assessment for Children and Adolescents (SACA): Adult and Child Reports. *Journal of the American Academy of Child and Adolescent Psychiatry, 39*(8), 1032–1039.

Stroul, B. A. (1996). *Managed care and children's mental health: Summary of the May 1995 state managed care meeting.* Washington, DC: Georgetown University Child Development Center, National Technical Assistance Center for Children's Mental Health, Center for Child and Mental Health Policy.

Stroul, B. A., & Friedman, R. (1986). *A system of care for severely emotionally disturbed children and youth.* Washington, DC: National Institute of Mental Health, CASSP, Technical Assistance Center.

Stroul, B. A., Pires, S. A., Armstrong, M. I., & Meyers, J. C. (1998). The impact of managed care on mental health services for children and their families. *Children and Managed Health Care, 8*(2), 119–133.

U.S. Department of Health and Human Services, Health Care Financing Administration. (1996). *Medicaid national summary statistics.* Baltimore: Authors.

U.S. General Accounting Office.(1994). *Medical prenatal care: States improve access and enhance services, but face new challenges.* Washington, DC: Author.

Ware, J. E., Kosinski, M., & Keller, S. D. (1996). A 12-item short-form health survey. *Medical Care, 34*(3), 220–233.

Weithorn, L. A. (1988). Mental hospitalization of troublesome youth: An analysis of skyrocketing admission rates. *Stanford Law Review, 40,* 773–837.

White House. (1995). *White House Medicaid briefing document.* Washington, DC: Author.

Wickizer, T. M., Lessler, D., & Boyd-Wickizer, J. (1999). Effects of health care cost-containment programs on patterns of care and readmissions among children and adolescents. *American Journal of Public Health, 89*(9), 1353–1358.

Zhang, M., Lancaster, B., Clardy, J. A., & Smith, G. R., Jr. (1999). Mental health capitation for children and adolescents under Medicaid. *Psychiatric Services, 50*(20), 189–191.

Treating Conduct Problems and Strengthening Social and Emotional Competence in Young Children

CHAPTER 25

The Dina Dinosaur Treatment Program

Carolyn H. Webster-Stratton and M. Jamila Reid

Young preschool and early school-age children with early onset conduct problems are at high risk for school dropout, substance abuse, violence, and delinquency in later years. Consequently, developing treatment strategies for reducing conduct problems when aggression is in its more malleable form prior to age 8, and thus interrupting its progression, is of considerable benefit to families and society. This chapter describes a treatment program—Dina Dinosaur's social, emotional, and problem-solving child training program—that was designed specifically with developmentally appropriate teaching methods for young children (ages 4–8 years) and based on theory related to the types of social, emotional, and cognitive deficits or excesses exhibited by children with conduct problems (Webster-Stratton, 1990a). The program emphasizes training children in skills such as emotional literacy, empathy or perspective taking, friendship and communication skills, anger management, interpersonal problem solving, school rules, and how to be successful at school. Emphasis is placed on ways to promote cross-setting generalization of the behaviors that are taught by involving parents and teachers in the treatment. A review of two randomized trials with this treatment approach and long-term results are provided.

Overall, national survey data have suggested that the prevalence of problematic aggressive behaviors in preschool and early school-age children is about 10% and may be as high as 25% for low-income children (Webster-Stratton & Hammond, 1998). Without early intervention, emotional and behavioral problems (e.g., aggression, oppositional behavior, conduct problems) in young children may become crystallized patterns of behavior by age 8 (Eron, 1990), beginning a trajectory of escalating academic problems, school dropout, substance abuse, delinquency, and violence (Snyder, 2001; Tremblay, Mass, Pagani, & Vitaro, 1996). Clearly, treating aggressive behavior in its more malleable form prior to age 8, and thus interrupting its progression, is of considerable benefit to families and society.

Parent training programs have been the single most successful treatment approach for reducing oppositional-defiant disorder (ODD) and conduct disorder (CD) in young children (Brestan & Eyberg, 1998). (Hereafter in this study these ODD/CD problems will be referred to as conduct problems because although most young children with behavior problems meet the criteria for a diagnosis of ODD, many of them also exhibit the aggressive and antisocial features listed as criteria for the diagnoses of CD but are not old enough to exhibit the criminal behaviors.) A variety of parenting programs have resulted in clinically significant and sustained improvements for at least two thirds of young children who are treated for these problems (for reviews, see Brestan & Eyberg, 1998; Taylor & Biglan, 1998). These experimental studies provided evidence supporting the social learning theories that highlight the crucial role that parenting style and discipline effectiveness play in (a) determining children's social competence and (b) reducing conduct problems (Patterson, DeGarmo, & Knutson, 2000).

Despite the clear evidence of the efficacy of parent training as a treatment approach, the approach does have some shortcomings. First, a number of studies have indicated that although parent training results in predictable improvements in child behavior at home, it does not necessarily result in improvements at school and with peers (Taylor & Biglan, 1998). In our own studies, teacher reports indicated that approximately one third of the children with conduct problems whose parents received parent training continued to have clinical levels of peer problems and classroom aggression 3 years after treatment (Webster-Stratton, 1990b). Second, some parents of children with conduct problems cannot, or will not, participate in parent training because of work conflicts, life stresses, personal psychopathology, or lack of motivation. Third, some parents are receptive to parent training but have difficulty implementing or maintaining the strategies taught in parent training programs due to their own interpersonal and family issues or because of their child's difficult temperament (Webster-Stratton, 1990c).

These limitations in parent training have led to a second approach to treating conduct problems, that is, directly training children in social skills, problem solving, and anger management (e.g., Bierman, 1989; Kazdin, Esveldt, French, & Unis, 1987a; Lochman & Dunn, 1993; Shure, 1994). The theory underlying this treatment approach is based on a substantial body of research indicating that children with conduct problems display cognitive and behavioral social skills deficits when interacting with peers (Coie & Dodge, 1998; Dodge & Price, 1994). In a study comparing clinic-referred young children (ages 4–7 years) with conduct problems with a matched group of typically developing children, we found that the former displayed significantly more negative attributions, fewer prosocial problem-solving strategies, and a significant delay in social skills during play interactions with friends than did the latter (Webster-Stratton & Lindsay, 1999).

The ability to form and maintain positive friendships involves a complex interplay of feelings, thoughts, and behaviors. Conversing with other children, solving interpersonal problems, entering into play with groups of peers, and regulating emotional responses to frustrating experiences are skills that contribute to success in making friends (Crick & Dodge, 1994). Socially competent children fairly easily learn strategies for interacting comfortably and positively with others during their everyday experiences at home and at school. Children with a more difficult temperament (e.g., hyperactivity, impulsivity, inattention); with problematic biological factors (learning and language delays); and from disadvantaged family backgrounds of environmental stress, abuse, and conflict may have particular difficulty in learning anger management, social skills, emotional regulation, and friendship skills. Because development of such skills is not necessarily automatic for these children, they need to be identified and targeted for additional intervention (Bredekamp & Copple, 1997).

The preschool and first grades are a strategic time to intervene directly with children who have early onset conduct problems, before negative behaviors crystallize. Research has shown that significant relationships exist among poor peer relationships in early childhood, early-onset conduct problems, and long-term social and emotional maladjustment (Loeber, 1985). In the absence of intervention, child conduct problems intensify after the child begins school, putting him or her at increased risk for peer rejection and poor social skills development (Loeber & Farrington, 2000). Before the middle grades, most children have had at least 5 to 6 years of experience with peer groups. Young children who are aggressive may have already established a pattern of social difficulty in the early elementary years that continues and becomes fairly stable by later elementary school. Many children with conduct problems have already been asked to leave four or five schools or group settings by the time they are 6 years old. By the middle school grades, the aggressive child's negative reputation, peer group rejection, and parental rejection may be well established (Coie, 1990). Even if the child learns appropriate social skills during the middle grades, this pattern of rejection may make it difficult for the child to use these skills to change his or her image. Intervening at a young age thus can help children develop effective social skills early and reduce their aggressive behaviors before these behaviors and reputations develop into permanent patterns.

A number of individual and small-group child treatment programs designed to treat or prevent conduct problems by teaching social skills and problem solving have been evaluated (Bierman, 1989; Lochman & Wells, 1996; Shure, 1994). Thus far, this treatment approach has been promising but less effective than the parent treatment approaches (Asher, Parkhurst, Hymel, & Williams, 1990; Kendall, 1993). Controlled trial evaluations with diagnosed children have demonstrated that teaching social skills, problem-solving, and anger management strategies is effective in reducing conduct problems (Kazdin, Siegel, & Bass, 1992; Webster-Stratton & Hammond, 1997) in the short term (effect sizes ranged from .20 to .67). Some programs appear to be limited in the generalization of changes to other settings (Gresham, 1995; Schneider & Bryne, 1985), however, and long-term effects could not be confirmed in several recent meta-analyses (Beelmann, Pfingste, & Losel, 1994; Gresham, 1998). In fact, these reviews suggested a decrease in effect sizes during follow-up. Most of these studies have been conducted as preventive programs in schools with heterogeneous populations without diagnostic classifications (Kazdin, Esveldt, French, & Unis, 1987b), and less is known about the effects of such programs in mental health clinics with young children with conduct problems. Out of 49 studies reviewed in the Beelmann et al. meta-analyses, only 3 were conducted in a mental health clinic.

The failure of parent and child treatment programs to consistently produce cross-setting generalization and long-term improvements in some children may stem from the intervention's narrow focus on a single risk factor. Most parent programs exclusively focus on training parents to manage children's social behavior at home rather than helping them to address their children's academic problems at school or relationship problems with peers. Parent training programs often fail to involve teachers in the treatment plans. Pull-out treatment groups focusing on children's social skills, on the other hand, do address children's social and emotional deficits but are often delivered without input from, collaboration with, or training for the child's parents or teachers, making generalization of new skills across settings difficult. For generalization across settings or time to occur, treatments must include parents and teachers so that they may take advantage of naturally occurring incidents at home and school to reinforce the appropriate social behaviors. In addition, treatments for young children may not have been effective because either they were too cognitive in orientation (with not enough behavioral practice) and not geared to the developmental level of children in the preoperational phase of cognitive reasoning or they were not tailored to the specific needs of children with a particular diagnosis.

This chapter describes a treatment program specifically designed with developmentally appropriate teaching methods for young children (ages 4–8 years) and with the goals of tailoring the intervention strategies to the particular types of social, emotional, and cognitive deficits or excesses exhibited by children with conduct problems. The small-group treatment Dina Dinosaur social, emotional, and problem-solving child training program (Webster-Stratton, 1990a) was first published in 1989 and emphasizes training children in skills such as emotional literacy, empathy or perspective taking, friendship and communication skills, anger management, interpersonal problem solving, school rules, and how to be successful at school. The intervention utilizes teaching methods that have been shown to be particularly effective for young children, such as puppet and videotape modeling, coaching and reinforcement during structured practice activities, visual imagery, fantasy play, and live role plays. In addition, efforts were made to carefully plan for generalization by asking parents and teachers to help by watching for and reinforcing specific skills whenever they noticed them at home or school.

PARTICIPANTS AND PROGRAM SETTING

Children who participated in the Dina Dinosaur program (Webster-Stratton, 1990a) and its evaluation came from families who requested treatment at the

University of Washington Parenting Clinic, a clinic in a large metropolitan area that is regionally known for its 20-year history of treating young children with conduct problems. Families who requested treatment at the clinic agreed to random assignment to the parent-training, child-training, or wait-list control groups. About half the families seeking treatment were self-referred, and half were referred by professionals in the community. Eligibility criteria were as follows:

- The child was between 4 and 8 years old.
- The child had no history of psychosis and was not receiving any form of psychological treatment at the time of referral.
- The primary referral problem was child conduct problems (e.g., noncompliance, aggression, oppositional behaviors) for at least 6 months.
- The parents reported more than 10 child behavior problems (the recommended cutoff score for screening children for treatment of conduct problems) on the *Eyberg Child Behavior Inventory* (ECBI; Robinson, Eyberg, & Ross, 1980).
- The child met the criteria for either ODD or CD from the *Diagnostic and Statistical Manual of Mental Disorders–Fourth Edition* (*DSM–IV*; American Psychiatric Association, 1994).

An initial phone screening established that the parents reported more than 10 problems on the ECBI. Children meeting the *DSM–IV* criteria for attention-deficit/hyperactivity disorder (ADHD) were also included because of the high co-morbidity of ODD and ADHD. At baseline assessment, 17.4% were classified as ADHD.

The sample consisted primarily of boys (80%) who were Caucasian (86%), with a mean age of 70 months. School level broke down as follows: 26% preschool, 29% kindergarten, 27% first grade, and 29% second grade. The mean number of pretreatment behavior problems according to the mother's ECBI Problem score was 21, indicating that the children were in the clinical range according to Robinson et al. (1980; for the normative sample nonclinic range, $M = 7.1$, $SD = 7.7$). On the ECBI Problem scale, 80.9% of our sample had scores above the 90th percentile of the normative sample (>16). Home observations prior to treatment confirmed the ECBI parent reports, with 51.6% of the children exhibiting one or more deviant and noncompliant behaviors every 3 minutes.

PROGRAM CONTENT AND GOALS

The Dina Dinosaur treatment program targets children with conduct problems, but it is also appropriate for addressing co-morbid problems such as attention problems and peer rejection. The curriculum consists of 18 to 22 weekly 2-hour lessons. It can be delivered by counselors or therapists in a mental health–related field or by early childhood specialists who have experience treating children with conduct disorders or early-onset behavior problems. Therapists receive extensive training in the content and methods of the treatment program. They use comprehensive group leader manuals that describe each session's content, objectives, videotapes to be shown, and small-group activities. Treatment integrity is monitored through session-by-session protocols and unit checklists completed by therapists as well as by supervisor and peer videotape reviews. This program is an ideal companion to the Incredible Years parent programs (Reid & Webster-Stratton, 2001). The 22-session parent group and the child training group may be offered concurrently. (This arrangement also helps with parents' childcare needs, so the parents can attend parent sessions knowing their children are well cared for.) In the material to follow, we provide a brief description of and rationale for each of the treatment components (see Webster-Stratton, 2000).

How To Do Your Best in School (Apatosaurus and Iguanodon Programs)

In working with children with conduct problems, gaining their cooperation and compliance is key to being able to socialize and teach them. Research has indicated that these children are noncompliant about 80% to 90% of the time a request is made of them by parents or teachers (Webster-Stratton & Lindsay, 1999); therefore, one of the first tasks of this treatment program that is somewhat different from other social skills programs is teaching compliance training procedures. Initial group sessions focus on the importance of group rules, such as following directions, keeping hands to selves, raising a quiet hand, using a polite and friendly voice, and so forth. Rules are demonstrated, role-played, and practiced with the children using life-sized puppets. Incentives ("Dinosaur chips") are given to the children for following the rules. The children also learn that a time-out is the consequence for hitting or hurting someone else (two of the most important Dinosaur rules are "using words to express feelings" and "using gentle touch"). Therapists clearly describe the time-out or calm-down procedure for hitting, and the children watch a videotape scene of a child going to time-out and staying calm. Next, the puppets are used to model all the steps involved in taking an appropriate time-out, and the children practice the steps. The children are coached to use positive self-statements while in time-out and are taught to help their friends in time-out by ignoring them until they return to the group. Time-out is framed as time away to think and calm down before trying again. When a child returns to the group after a time-out, the therapists look for the first opportunity to re-engage him or her and offer praise for appropriate behavior. Time-out is conducted in the least restrictive way possible. Children are initially asked to go sit in a time-out or calm-down chair (or turtle chair) that is placed at the back of the group room (low-level whining and wiggly behavior are ignored as long as the child is in close proximity to the time-out chair). Children who will not stay in the chair or who become very disruptive are given one warning before they are escorted to a separate room to complete their time-out.

Understanding and Detecting Feelings (Dina Triceratops Program)

Once the group rules and expectations have been discussed, modeled, practiced, and reinforced, the children are ready to move on to content on emotional literacy. Children with conduct problems often have language delays and a limited vocabulary for expressing their feelings, which contribute to their difficulties in regulating emotional responses (Frick et al., 1991; Sturge, 1982). They may also have negative feelings and thoughts about themselves and others and difficulty perceiving another's point of view or feelings different from their own (Dodge, 1993). They have difficulty reading facial cues and distort or underutilize social cues (Dodge & Price, 1994).

The Triceratops feelings program is designed to help these children learn to regulate their own emotions and to accurately identify and understand others' feelings. The first step in this process is to help children identify their own feelings and be able to accurately label and express these feelings to others. Therapists play a critical role in helping the children learn to manage their feelings of anger or disappointment by helping them to (a) talk about the feelings, (b) think differently about why an event occurred, (c) respond appropriately to situations that cause emotional arousal, such as being teased or left out, and (d) employ self-talk and relaxation strategies to keep themselves calm. Through the use of laminated cue cards and videotapes of children demonstrating various emotions, the children learn how to discuss and understand a wide range of feeling states. The unit begins with basic feelings—sadness, anger, happiness, and fright—and progresses to more complex feelings, such as frustration, excitement, disappointment, loneliness, embarrassment, and forgiveness. The children are helped to recognize their own feelings by checking their bodies and faces for "tight" (tense) muscles, relaxed muscles, frowns, smiles, and sensations in other parts of their bodies (e.g., butterflies in their stomachs). Matching the facial expressions and body postures shown on cue cards helps the children to recognize the cues from their own bodies and to associate a word with these feelings.

Next, the children are guided in using their detective skills to look for clues in another person's facial expression, behavior, or tone of voice to recognize what the person may be feeling and to think about why he or she might be feeling that way. Video vignettes, photos of sports stars and other famous people, and pictures of the children in the group are all engaging ways to provide experience in "reading" feeling cues. Games such as Feeling Dice or Feeling Bingo are played to reinforce these concepts. Nursery rhymes, songs, and children's books provide fun opportunities to talk about the characters' feelings, how they cope with uncomfortable feelings, and how they express their feelings. As the children become more skilled at recognizing feelings in themselves and others, they begin to learn empathy, perspective taking, and emotion regulation.

The children also learn strategies for changing negative (angry, frustrated, sad) feelings into more positive feelings. Wally (a child-sized puppet) teaches the children some of his "secrets" for calming down (take a deep breath, think a happy thought). Games, positive imagery, and activities are used to illustrate how feelings change over time and how different people may react differently to the same event (the metaphor of a "feeling thermometer" is used, and the children practice using real thermometers in hot and cold water to watch the mercury go from "hot and angry" to "cool and calm"). To practice perspective taking, role plays that use scenarios in which the child takes the part of the teacher, parent, or another child who has a problem are employed. The puppets are used to model how to talk about and cope with different feelings. This work on feelings is integrated into and underlies all the subsequent units in this curriculum.

Detective Wally Teaches Problem-Solving Steps (Stegosaurus Program)

Children who are hyperactive, impulsive, inattentive, and aggressive have been shown to have cognitive deficits in key aspects of social problem solving (Dodge & Crick, 1990). Such children perceive social situations in hostile terms, generate fewer prosocial ways of solving interpersonal conflict, and anticipate fewer consequences for aggression (Dodge & Price, 1994). They act aggressively and impulsively, without stopping to think of nonaggressive solutions or of the other person's perspective, and they expect their aggressive responses to yield positive results. There is evidence (Dodge, Pettit, & Bates, 1994) that children who employ appropriate problem-solving strategies play more constructively, are better liked by their peers, and are more cooperative at home and school. Consequently, in this next program of the intervention, therapists teach children to generate more prosocial solutions to their problems and to evaluate which solutions are likely to lead to positive consequences. In essence, these children are provided with a thinking strategy that corrects the flaws in their decision-making process and reduces their risk of developing ongoing peer relationship problems.

Children learn a seven-step problem-solving process:

1. How am I feeling, and what is my problem? (define problem and feelings)
2. What is a solution?
3. What are some more solutions? (brainstorm solutions)
4. What are the consequences?
5. What is the best solution? (Is the solution safe? fair? Does it lead to good feelings?)
6. Can I use my plan?
7. How did I do? (evaluate outcome and reinforce efforts)

A great deal of time is spent on Steps 1, 2, and 3 to help the children increase their repertoire of possible prosocial solutions (e.g., trade, ask, share, take turns, wait, walk away, take a deep breath). In fact, for the 3- to 5-year-olds, these three steps may be the entire focus of the unit. One to two new solutions are introduced in each session, and the children are given multiple opportunities to role-play and practice these solutions with a puppet or another child. Laminated cue cards with pictures of more than 40 solutions are provided in Wally's "detective kit" and are used by the children to generate possible solutions and evaluate whether they will work to solve particular problems. Children role-play solutions to problem scenarios introduced by the puppets, the video vignettes, or the children themselves. In one activity, the children draw or color their own solution cards so that each child has his or her own detective solution kit by the end of the unit. The children are guided to consult their own or the group solution kit when a real-life problem occurs. Activities for this program include writing and acting in a problem-solving play, going "fishing" for solutions (with a magnetized fishing rod), and working as a group to generate enough solutions to join Wally's Problem-Solving Detective Club.

Detective Wally Teaches Problem-Solving Steps (T-Rex Program)

Aggression and inadequate impulse control are perhaps the most potent obstacles children with conduct problems face with regard to effective problem solving and forming successful friendships. Without help, these children are more likely to experience ongoing peer rejection and continued social problems for years afterward (Coie, 1990). Such children have difficulty regulating their negative affect to generate positive solutions to conflict situations. Furthermore, there is evidence that aggressive children are more likely to misinterpret ambiguous situations as hostile or threatening. This tendency to perceive hostile intent in others has been seen as one source of their aggressive behavior (Walker, Colvin, & Ramsey, 1995).

Consequently, once the basic skills for problem solving have been acquired, the children are taught anger management strategies. Anger management programs based on the work of Novaco (1975) have been shown to reduce aggression in aggressive middle and high school students and to maintain gains in problem-solving skills (Lochman & Dunn, 1993). Clearly, children cannot solve problems if they are too angry to think calmly. A new puppet, Tiny Turtle, is used to teach the children a five-step anger management strategy:

1. Recognize anger.
2. Think "stop."
3. Take a deep breath.
4. Go into your shell and tell yourself, "I can calm down."
5. Try again.

Tiny's shell is the basis for many activities: making a large cardboard shell that children can actually hide under, making grocery bag "shells" or vests, molding Play Doh shells for small plastic figures (the children pretend the figures are mad and help them to calm down in the Play Doh shells), and making teasing shields. Each of these activities provides multiple opportunities for the therapist to help the children practice the steps of anger management. Children learn to recognize the clues in their bodies that tell them they are getting angry and to use self-talk, deep breathing, and positive imagery to help themselves calm down. Therapists also use guided imagery exercises with the children (having them close their eyes and pretend to be in a cocoon or turtle shell) to help them experience the feelings of being relaxed and calm.

Videotapes of children handling anger, being teased, or being rejected are used to trigger role plays to practice these calming strategies. In addition, the puppets talk to the children about problems (e.g., a parent or teacher was mad at them for a mistake they made, they were left out of a birthday party, a parent is getting divorced or doing something that disappoints them). The situations that the puppets bring to the group are formulated according to experiences and issues relevant to particular children in the group. For example, if a child in the group is teased at school (and is reacting in an aggressive or angry way), Wally might tell the group that someone at school called him a name and Wally was so mad that he hit the person. Wally would then talk about the consequences of hitting (he felt bad afterward, and he got in trouble). The group would then generate alternative solutions for Wally and would help him practice them. The child who has this same difficulty at school would often be chosen to act out an appropriate solution with Wally.

Throughout the discussion of vignettes and role-play demonstrations, the therapists and puppets help the children to change some of their attributions about events. For example, Molly Manners (Wally's sister) explains, "Maybe he was teasing you because he really wanted to be your friend but didn't know how to ask you nicely" or, "You know, all kids get turned down sometimes when they want to play; it doesn't mean they don't like you," or, "I think that it was an accident that he bumped into you." The Pass the Hat detective game is played to help the children determine when an event might be an "accident" versus when it might be done "on purpose" and how each event could be handled.

Molly Manners Teaches How To Be Friendly (Allosaurus and Brachiosaurus Programs)

Children with conduct problems have particular difficulty in forming and maintaining friendships. Our research, and that of others, has indicated that these children have significantly delayed play skills, including difficulties waiting for a turn, accepting peers' suggestions, offering an idea rather than demanding something, or collaborating in play with peers (Webster-Stratton & Lindsay, 1999). They also have poor conversation skills, difficulty in responding to the overtures of others, and poor group-entry skills. Consequently, in the friendship program we focus on teaching children a repertoire of friendly behaviors, such as sharing, taking turns, asking, making a suggestion, apologizing, agreeing with others, and giving compliments. In addition, the children are taught specific prosocial responses for common peer situations. An example would be entering a group of children who are already playing:

1. Watch from the sidelines and show interest.
2. Continue watching and give a compliment.
3. Wait for a pause.
4. Ask politely to join in and accept the response.

As with other new material, the children see these friendship skills modeled by the puppets or in videotape examples and practice using them in role plays and cooperative games.

PRESENTATION METHOD FOR SMALL-GROUP PROGRAM

Methods and processes for teaching social skills to young children must fit with the children's learning styles, temperaments, and cognitive abilities. Within the 4- to 8-year-old age range, vast differences exist in children's developmental abilities. Some children in a group may be reading fluently, while other children may not read at all. Some children will be able to grasp relatively complicated ideas, such as how to evaluate possible future consequences of an action, while others are operating in the "here and now," with little ability to predict results. The Dina Dinosaur program provides relevant content areas for the preschool to early elementary school group. A skilled therapist will then use developmentally appropriate practices to present the material to the child in any given group according to the goals for that child. The following sections provide guidelines for organizing groups and for tailoring the delivery of the program according to the needs of a particular group.

Selecting Children for Groups

Children's ages within the preschool and early elementary school groups may vary from age 4 to 8 years. We believe this mix is optimal because children who are more mature can model language for the younger children and can participate in leadership and helping roles. It also means that the entire group will not be composed of wiggly, nonverbal children. We suggest selecting pairs of children of similar age (or developmental level) so that each child has at least one peer who is performing at the same level. Mixed-gender groups work well; however, it is important not to have a group with only one girl (many more boys than girls exhibit the conduct problems used to select children for these groups, so most groups will be predominately made up of boys). For practical reasons, we also recommend that groups be composed of children who represent a mix of temperament styles and that each group have no more than 5 to 6 children.

Preparing for the Session

First, therapists plan and prepare each week's session, noting the objectives and tailoring role plays and teaching strategies according to the target goals for each child in the group based on functional assessment procedures, behavior plans, and targeted negative and positive behaviors (Bear, 1998; Wolery, 2000). Therapists also prepare activities that are designed to provide practice opportunities on the new skill for every child. The therapists communicate with their co-leader about which behaviors they will ignore and which they will praise or reward to promote specifically targeted social skills. The therapists think about whether the day's activity needs some adaptation for a child with more or less advanced developmental skills.

Schedule for 2-Hour Session

When children arrive, they share the Dinosaur homework that they have done during the week (and receive compliments and Dinosaur tokens for completing it). The opening discussion lasts 15 to 20 minutes. After this introductory time, new content is presented. Although the Dina Dinosaur curriculum is child focused and individualized for different developmental levels or family situations, it is important that structured learning occur in each session. This learning is interactive, engaging, fun, and paced at the level of the children in the group. The goal is to present new ideas or content so the children begin to increase their repertoire of ideas and responses. This plan to present new material to children in a structured small-group circle time is paired with the idea of taking advantage of teachable moments that occur naturally among the children during the time they are in the group.

The videotapes and puppets are used to present content, which is then processed during discussions, problem solving, role plays, and collaborative learning. After each vignette, the therapist solicits ideas from the children and involves them in the process of problem solving, sharing, and discussing ideas and reactions. To enhance generalization, the scenes selected for each of the units involve real-life situations at school (e.g., playground and classroom) and home. Some vignettes represent children behaving in prosocial ways, such as helping their teachers, playing well with peers, or using problem-solving or anger management techniques. Other vignettes provide examples of children who are having difficulties in conflict situations, such as teasing, arguing, and destructive behavior. The videotapes show children of differing ages, genders, and cultures interacting with adults (parents or teachers) or with other children. After viewing the vignettes, the children discuss their feelings, decide whether the examples are good or bad choices, generate ideas for more effective responses, and role-play alternative scenarios. Although some mild negative videotape examples are shown so that children can show how they would improve the situation, the program uses a far greater number of positive examples than negative examples (about 5 to 1), and the children are coached to help solve or resolve any problems that they see in the vignettes. The children are never asked to act out the inappropriate responses.

After 50 minutes, the children take a snack break, which provides an opportunity for the therapist to coach and praise prosocial behavior and the use of new skills in real life. Therapists also model and coach appropriate social skills as they participate in snack time. After snack time, the children participate in activities related to that session's content. They might work on a cooperative poster or play a board game that involves turn taking and waiting patiently. During the last 10 to 15 minutes of the session, one group leader leaves the group to meet with the parents and give a summary of the session content for the day. Parents are given recommendations for home activities that will reinforce the child's new learning. During this time, another therapist helps the children count their dinosaur chips, which are turned in for prizes from Dina's special box. This is followed by a compliment circle time and a review of homework activities. Each week, the children have Dinosaur homework activities to complete at home with their parents. The parents are asked to sign the home activities so the therapist knows that the parent is being exposed to the content and helping the child with the assignments.

Puppets as Models

The therapists use child-size boy and girl puppets to model appropriate child behavior. There is also a dinosaur puppet (Dina Dinosaur), who is the director of Dinosaur School; she teaches school rules and rewards, and praises the children who are doing well. The puppets, Wally and Molly, help narrate the video vignettes and ask the children for help with common conflict situations they have encountered (based on the problems of the children in the group). Other puppets regularly visit the group (e.g., Oscar the Ostrich hides his head in the sand and has difficulty talking about his problems; Freddy Frog cannot sit still). Particularly when working with diverse populations, a variety of puppets representing the ethnicity and gender of the children in the group are used. The puppets are an integral part of the program's success because they spur the children's imaginations. Young children are enthralled with the puppets and will talk about sensitive or painful issues with a puppet more easily than with adults. The puppets quickly become real to the children and are very effective models.

Live and Videotape Modeling and Role-Playing Methods

In accordance with modeling and self-efficacy theories of learning (Bandura, 1989), children using the program develop their skills by watching (and modeling) videotape examples of key problem-solving and interpersonal skills. Videotape provides a more flexible method of training than didactic instruction or sole reliance on role play; that is, it allows for portrayal of a wide variety of models, situations, and settings for the children to watch and discuss. This flexible modeling approach results in better generalization of the training content and, therefore, better long-term maintenance. Furthermore, it is an engaging method of learning for children who are less verbally oriented, younger children, or children with short attention spans. The program thus makes heavy use of modeling—live modeling, behavioral practice with the puppets, and videotape modeling.

Videotape scenes and puppet role plays serve as stimuli for the children to talk about, demonstrate, and practice different solutions, feelings, or thoughts. Role-playing provides opportunities to practice new skills and experience different perspectives. For example, a difficult situation involving being left out or teased may be role-played with the puppet. The puppet will ask the children how to respond to this feeling or experience. When the children generate suggestions, they are asked to act them out with the puppet. The puppet then demonstrates what he or she has learned from the children to see if he or she has understood it correctly. One activity children play is the Let's Suppose game or the Pass the Detective Hat game. A variety of problems (selected on the basis of issues relevant to the group) are put in a hat, which is passed around the circle. When the music stops, the child holding the hat picks out the problem and suggests a solution. Someone else will try to act out that solution for all to see. For example, a problem situation might be the following: "Suppose you asked to play soccer with some kids and they wouldn't let you play. What would you do?" With children ages 4 to 6, the role-playing can be acted out by a child and the therapist's puppet while the second group leader sits with the remaining children and helps them think of alternative responses. Older children put on skits in pairs, with one therapist acting as a coach.

Practice Activities—Coaching/Cuing/Reinforcing

For each of the sessions, choices can be made from a series of activities for practicing the skills targeted in that session. For example, a friendship session about sharing might be paired with an art project where there are limited supplies and students have to figure out how to share. During a session on cooperation, children might be asked to design a dinosaur that incorporates everyone's ideas. In the problem-solving unit, children might be given a problem and asked to think of as many solutions as they can. The problems might be presented on a colorful cue card or in a problem-solving book. Children who are reading and writing can read the problem and write solutions; nonreaders could dictate or draw a picture of their solutions. Children might also look in the "detective kit" (a box that contains all the solutions that children have learned) for more solutions.

During the activity, children are usually divided into two groups of three children. For some activities, children might be divided along developmental lines, with more advanced children doing a harder version of the same activity than less advanced children. Other times, developmental levels may be mixed so that more advanced children can help the younger children. A therapist sits with each group of students, coaching and commenting on prosocial behavior. We often describe this kind of descriptive commenting as being like a "sports announcer." Dinosaur chips can often be earned for pro-social behaviors during these activities.

Most of the practice activities described in this program help strengthen writing, reading, sequencing, vocabulary, and discrimination skills, enhancing academic and social competence. For example, reading is enhanced through use of the laminated cue cards, the Wally problem-solving detective books, and homework activities books; activities promote communication, language, and writing skills through written stories, pictures of solutions, and play acting. Laminated cue cards are provided for all of the major concepts. These cards show a picture (e.g., sharing or quiet hand up) as well as the words that describe the concept. These picture cue cards are very helpful for children who cannot read and are useful nonverbal cues to remind children of a particular skill on which they might be working. For example, the therapist might point to a picture of Wally sharing to remind a child of the desired behavior in the group, or a child who is beginning to get angry might be prompted to use the Tiny STOP signal or the anger thermometer as a cue to use a self-calming activity. When the children respond to these visual cues, the therapist reinforces their accomplishment. The problem-solving unit provides an opportunity for a discussion of sequencing as the children learn the steps to solving their problems. All of the sessions offer opportunities for promoting effective learning behaviors, such as verbal and nonverbal communication skills that include collaborating, cooperating, listening, attending, speaking up, and asking questions. These are key skills for learning and attaining success in the classroom.

Integration of Cognitive, Affective, and Behavioral Components

Each unit uses this combination of cognitive, affective, and behavioral components to enhance learning. For example, the anger thermometer is used to teach children self-control and to monitor their emotional state. Children decorate the thermometer with pictures of feeling faces from "happy" and "relaxed" in the blue (or cool) section of the thermometer all the way up to "angry" or "stressed out" in the red (or hot) section of the thermometer. The therapist can then ask a child to describe a recent conflict, and together they retrace the steps that led to the angry outburst. The therapist writes down the child's thoughts, feelings, and actions that indicated an escalating anger pattern, for example, "He always takes my toys" (thought), "That really makes me mad" (feeling), "I got so mad that I kicked him" (action). The therapist and the child discuss thoughts, words, and actions that the child can use to reduce his or her anger. As the therapist retraces the steps of the angry outburst, she or he helps the child identify the place where the child was aware that he or she was getting angry. This is marked as the "danger point" on the thermometer.

Once the child has established this danger point, he or she chooses a name that will be the signal for reaching that point (e.g., chill out, cool down, code red, hot engine). This code word will be the teacher and child's signal that anger or stress has reached the threshold and will trigger the use of an agreed-upon calming strategy, such as taking three deep breaths.

Fantasy Play and Instruction

Fantasy play provides the context for this program because a high level of sociodramatic play in early school-age children is associated with sustained and reciprocal verbal interactions and high levels of affective role taking (Connolly & Doyle, 1984). Fantasy play gives children the opportunity to develop intimacy and work out emotional issues (Gottman, 1983). For preschool-age children, sociodramatic play is an important context in which perspective taking, social participation, group cooperation, and intimacy skills develop. This important skill can easily be fostered through the use of the child-sized human puppets.

Promoting Skills Maintenance and Generalization

Because the children are learning these skills in a setting removed from the classroom and home environments, the therapists must do everything they can to promote generalization of skills to other settings. Therapists should look for opportunities to praise and coach prosocial behavior even during less structured times, such as in the waiting room before the group starts, snack time, bathroom breaks, and transitions. For each main intervention component, parents and teachers are sent letters explaining the content of the unit (e.g., expressing feelings, sharing, problem solving) and suggesting ways they can reinforce these behaviors at home and at school. Several times during the program, phone calls are made to parents and teachers to tell them about the children's successes, which behaviors to reinforce, and which ones to ignore. Parents and teachers need to offer praise and reinforcement whenever they see the children using these prosocial behaviors in naturally occurring settings. The homework assignments, which children complete with parents each week, also reinforce these concepts and help parents to learn and understand the same terminology that their children are using in Dinosaur School so that there is cross-setting consistency in responses from therapists and parents.

Group Management

The implementation of the Dina Dinosaur program is dependent on the variety of therapeutic processes and methods described in this article. A final key element of successful group therapy with children who have conduct problems is utilizing research-based group management strategies (e.g., incentives and time-out; Brophy, 1996). To be able to teach these difficult children and provide a safe environment for them, the therapists must manage oppositional and aggressive behaviors extremely well. Research has shown that when children with conduct problems are placed in groups, they may reinforce each other's antisocial behaviors and actually become worse instead of better if their negative behaviors are not managed well (Dishion, McCord, & Poulin, 1999). A well-managed group with consistent rules and limits can provide these children with one of the first opportunities they have ever had to be successful in a learning environment with their peers. In fact, after an initial testing period, most children with conduct problems who participate in these groups enjoy coming to group, follow the rules consistently, and make some of the first positive friendships they have ever had. Group leaders work together, and in consultation with parents and classroom teachers, to develop individual behavior plans for each child in the group. Thus, although all of the children are expected to follow basic group rules, one child may have a special program designed to decrease rude talk, another child might be working on remembering to think before impulsively blurting out answers, and a third child might be working on listening carefully to adult instructions. In this way, the particular issues of each child can be addressed in a group context.

PROGRAM EVALUATION

The Dina Dinosaur treatment program has been shown to have short- and long-term effectiveness with clinic-referred young children (ages 4–8 years) with conduct problems in two randomized control group studies (Webster-Stratton & Hammond, 1997; Webster-Stratton, Reid, & Hammond, 2001, 2004). In the first randomized trial, with 97 clinic-referred children (ages 4–7 years), families were randomly assigned to one of four groups: child training only (CT), parent training only (PT), combined parent and child training intervention (PT + CT), or wait-list control (WLC). Children attended the Dina Dinosaur program in small groups of 6 for 2 hours per week for 18 weeks. Parents in the PT condition attended 22 weekly parenting sessions. Parents in the PT + CT group attended parent groups while their children participated in the child training Dina Dinosaur program. Families in the WLC condition waited 8 to 9 months and then were randomly assigned to one of the three intervention conditions.

Families were assessed at baseline, 2 months after the intervention was completed, and 1 and 2 years posttreatment. Assessments included parent and teacher reports of behavior problems on standardized measures, observations of parent–child interactions at home by observers who did not know what treatment condition families had received, child problem-solving testing, and laboratory observations of children playing with a friend. There were no significant differences among the groups on variables at baseline.

At posttreatment, results showed that the PT + CT training was more effective than the PT and that all three intervention conditions were superior to the control group. The CT program resulted in significant improvements in observed peer interactions, as well as number of different positive solutions on the Wally social problem-solving test (Webster-Stratton, 1990d). Children who had received the Dina Dinosaur curriculum were observed to be significantly more positive and less negative in their social interactions with peers than children whose parents received PT or than controls. Parents in the conditions that included parent training demonstrated significantly more positive parenting behaviors (including praise and positive affect) and parent collaboration, and they reported fewer behavior problems than control families on the *Child Behavior Checklist* (Achenbach & Edelbrock, 1991). These parents also demonstrated significantly more mother praise and parent collaboration than families receiving CT (see Figure 25.1).

One year later, all significant changes noted at posttreatment were maintained. All three treatment groups reported significantly fewer child behavior problems, fewer targeted negative behaviors, less spanking, more positive behaviors, better child problem-solving skills, and lower parenting stress levels compared to baseline. In addition, observers rated all the intervention children as demonstrating significantly less deviance and more positive affect at home, compared to posttreatment, indicating that the children continued to show improvements in the year following treatment. In addition, children in both the CT and PT + CT treatment groups showed maintenance over time in their ability to generate positive social problem-solving strategies in response to hypothetical conflict situations on the Wally test. Analyses of the subsample of children who scored in the abnormal range on teacher reports at baseline ($n = 54$) revealed significant improvements for all treated children at the 1-year follow-up. Analyses of the clinical significance (measured by a 30% reduction in observed total child deviant behaviors at home) revealed that the PT + CT group showed the most sustained effects in child behavior, with 95% of the children demonstrating a clinically significant reduction in deviant behaviors, compared with 74% of the CT condition and 60% of the PT condition (Webster-Stratton & Hammond, 1997). The difference between the PT + CT and PT groups was significant ($p < .01$), indicating the additive effects of CT. Consumer satisfaction continued to be high at follow-up for all treatment conditions, with 95% of mothers and 100% of fathers reporting improvement in their children's behavior.

Despite these positive changes in observed behavioral interactions with peers and in assessments of social problem solving by parents, the behavior changes in the classroom immediately posttreatment were nonsignificant according to teacher reports. This finding may have been due to limited power because only half of the sample of children had clinically significant problems at baseline according to the teachers (thus creating a floor effect). When we looked at the subsample of problem children separately, we did find significant effects. We postulated several other reasons for the teachers' modest effects as well. First, although the teachers were consulted by telephone, sent information about the program, and asked to reinforce specific prosocial behaviors, they received no direct training in behavior management or the curriculum, and they were not monitored in regard to whether they followed through with

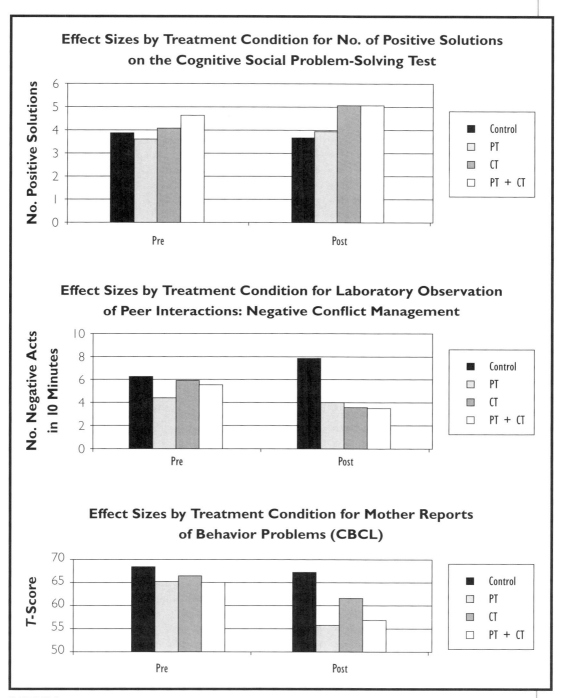

FIGURE 25.1. Graphs based on data from "Treating Children with Early-Onset Conduct Problems: A Comparison of Child and Parent Training Interventions," by C. Webster-Stratton and M. Hammond, 1997, *Journal of Consulting and Clinical Psychology, 65,* pp. 93–109. Effect sizes (d): Top panel: CT versus control, .79 ($p < .05$); PT + CT versus control, .69 ($p < .05$); PT versus control, .25. Middle panel: CT versus control, .58 ($p < .05$); PT + CT versus control, .54 ($p < .05$); PT versus control, .46 ($p < .05$). Bottom panel: CT versus control, .38; PT + CT versus control, .73 ($p < .05$); PT versus control, .89 ($p < .05$). CBCL = *Child Behavior Checklist* (Achenbach & Edelbrock, 1991).

the program suggestions. As we have noted earlier, negative academic and social experiences in the school setting have been shown to contribute to the ongoing development of conduct problems. Teachers with poor classroom management skills and low rates of praise have classrooms with higher levels of aggression and rejection, which in turn have been shown to influence the continued development of individual children's conduct problems (Kellam, Ling, Merisca, Brown, & Ialongo, 1998).

In light of these findings, our next evaluation of the child interventions included a teacher training component (Webster-Stratton & Reid, in press) targeted at specific classroom risk factors (classroom management skills, behavior plans, and collaboration with parents). This teacher training was offered in combination with small-group child social skills training for treating young children with ODD. No studies existed that examined the added benefits of pairing teacher training with child training to treat young children with ODD.

The Incredible Years child and teacher training curricula were evaluated in a randomized trial with 159 clinic-referred families with children (ages 4–8 years) who had been diagnosed with early onset ODD/CD (*DSM–IV*) according to the procedures outlined previously for the first study. Families (85% Caucasian) were randomly assigned to child training only (Dina Dinosaur curriculum, CT), CT combined with teacher training (CT + TT), or a wait-list control (other conditions involving parent training also evaluated in this study are described elsewhere; Reid, Webster-Stratton, & Hammond, 2004; Webster-Stratton et al., 2004). The 18-week child training program was identical to that described previously. The TT component consisted of four full-day workshops offered monthly and a minimum of two school consultations wherein the parents and the child's small-group therapist met with the child's teacher to plan an individual behavior plan. Regular calls were made to teachers to support their efforts and to keep them apprised of the progress of the child. Families in the wait-list control condition waited 8 to 9 months and then were offered treatment.

Assessments were conducted at baseline, 2 months after the intervention was completed, and 1 year and 2 years postassessment. All of the same assessments from the study described earlier were used, along with independent school observations. All of the children were observed at school on four occasions during structured and unstructured times at each assessment phase. Following the 6-month intervention, children in the CT and CT + TT conditions were significantly less negative at home and at school (with teachers and peers) according to parent and teacher reports, as well as independent observations at home and in the classroom at school. Children in the CT and CT + TT groups showed more prosocial skills with peers than did children in the control groups. To our surprise, mothers and teachers of children in both the CT and CT + TT groups were also less critical in their interactions with the children. All TT conditions resulted in teachers who were significantly less critical, more nurturing, and more consistent compared to control teachers (Webster-Stratton et al., 2004). The graphs in Figure 25.1 represent composite scores for several domains of interest. These composite scores contain both report and observational data; consequently, they are a more robust measure of treatment effectiveness than single measures. In all of the results presented, CT and CT + TT are significantly different from control but not from each other (see Figure 25.2). Table 25.1 presents effect size comparisons for CT versus control and CT + TT versus control for all of the domains measured.

In an additional analysis, we combined the sample of children from both these studies to look at how biological risk factors (inattention, impulsivity, hyperactivity), parenting risk factors (critical and physically violent discipline), and family stress risk factors (marital conflict, social class, depression, negative life stress, anger) affected the CT group outcome. The only risk factor related to failure to improve problems of child conduct after CT treatment was negative parenting (i.e., critical statements and reports of physical force; Webster-Stratton et al., 2001).

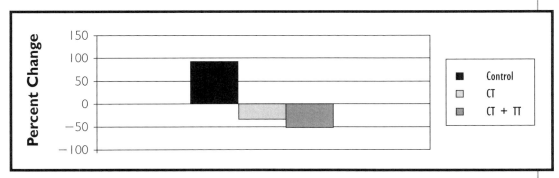

FIGURE 25.2. Percentage of change in classroom observations of aggression from baseline to posttreatment. Data from "Treating Children with Early-Onset Conduct Problems: Intervention Outcomes for Parent, Child, and Teacher Training," by C. Webster-Stratton, M. J. Reid, and M. Hammond, 2004, *Journal of Clinical Child and Adolescent Psychology, 33*(1), pp. 105–124. CT versus control, $d = .50$ ($p < .05$); CT + TT versus control, $d = .66$ ($p < .05$).

TABLE 25.1

Effect Sizes (Cohen's *d*) for CT and
CT + TT Groups Compared to Controls on Composite Scores

Composite Domain	CT vs. Control	CT + TT vs. Control
Mother negative parenting	.51	.51
Child negative at home/mother	.41	.55
Child positive with peers	.35	.29
Child negative at school	.41	.41
Teacher negative	.35	.46

Note. CT = child training only; TT = teacher training; Cohen (1988) $d = .2$, small effect; $d = .5$, moderate effect; $d = .8$, large effect.

SUMMARY

The results of these two studies indicated that of the two single-risk factor interventions, the PT approach was superior to the CT approach in terms of child behavior improvements (as reported by parents), parenting behaviors (as observed by independent raters), and consumer satisfaction. Intervention involving CT was superior to PT in terms of child social problem-solving and conflict management skills with peers (as tested and observed, respectively). Combining PT with CT (the two-risk factors model) produced more significant improvements across a broader range of outcome variables. TT did appear to add significantly to CT in terms of reductions of observed physical aggression in the classroom. For the target child in school 6 hours per day, changes amounted to 25% (CT) to 50% (CT + TT) fewer physically aggressive acts with peers posttreatment, from a mean of 24 acts per day at baseline to 12 per day, whereas control group children increased by 100%. Moreover, one would expect that the trained teachers' responses would affect not only the target child but also other children in the classroom. It was encouraging to find that effects (maintained at the 1-year follow-up) were consistent in the CT condition as well as the PT condition according to parent and teacher reports and independent observations with peers and parents.

These findings related to the CT intervention are of particular interest because they indicate that the CT program not only enhanced parent training outcomes but by itself resulted in sustained improvements in conduct problems and social problem solving across time and settings (moderate effect sizes were found for child negative behavior at home and school). Our data indicate that the social problem-solving skills learned in the program and demonstrated by the children when tested were actually used when the children were faced with real conflict with a friend (effect size = .35). Moreover, improvements in child social skills and conduct problems at home were noted by both mothers and fathers, suggesting that the skills learned in the clinic generalized to the home and were maintained over time. These findings are important in light of earlier reviews of the social skills training literature, which suggested that there is little empirical support for the efficacy of such training in terms of durable gains across situations and over time (Gresham, 1998). We postulate that the efforts in the CT program to link the specific social skills deficits of each child to a particular intervention strategy and to share these strategies with parents and teachers paid important dividends. The significant findings with the CT and TT interventions are also important because it is undeniable that some parents will not be able to participate in parent training, for any number of reasons, and in such cases the CT and TT interventions are the only possible avenue for working with the child.

Finally, we hypothesize that an even more effective model of treatment would be to offer the CT groups in the schools (in conjunction with TT training) rather than pulling out children to meet in a mental health center. In this way, we could take advantage of naturally occurring incidents by having teachers primed to reinforce specific behaviors. Nonetheless, it appears that the best approach is to use CT not as a stand-alone treatment for children with conduct problems but rather as an integral part of an intervention that involves parents and teachers. Although this article focuses on treating small groups of children with diagnosed behavior problems, we are also evaluating a classroom version of the Dina Dinosaur program to be used by teachers. The classroom version is delivered to all children in the classroom, several times per week, throughout the school year. In this way, young children are provided with the language and skills to cope effectively with the emotions and problems that arise in their everyday lives. Preliminary results and experience with the program in more than 40 Head Start, kindergarten, and first-grade classrooms suggests the program is highly regarded by teachers, parents, and children.

Several recent reports, such as the Surgeon General's report on mental health (U.S. Department of Health and Human Services, 1999) and *From Neurons to Neighborhoods: The Science of Early Childhood Development* (National Research Council and Institute of Medicine, 2000), have highlighted the need for the adoption of evidence-based practices that support young children's social and emotional competence and prevent or decrease the occurrences of challenging behavior in early childhood. Research in effective dissemination of empirically supported programs, such as the Dina Dinosaur program, is now needed to understand how to best bring these effective programs into mental health and school settings where children, their families, and teachers will benefit from them.

AUTHORS' NOTES

1. This chapter was previously published in 2003 in the *Journal of Emotional and Behavioral Disorders, 11*(3), 130–143, and is reprinted with permission of the publisher.

2. This research was supported by the National Institute of Health National Center for Nursing Research Grant No. 5 R01 NR01075-11 and Research Scientist Development Award MH00988-10 from the National Institute of Mental Health.

3. Special appreciation is expressed to Lois Hancock, Terry Hollinsworth, Peter Loft, Julie Rinaldi, Aaron Wallis, and Karrin Bianchi for their dedication to the integrity of the child treatment programs.

4. The senior author of this article has disclosed a potential financial conflict of interest because she disseminates these treatments and stands to gain from a favorable report. Because of this, she has voluntarily agreed to distance herself from certain critical research activities (i.e., recruiting, consenting, primary data handling, and analysis), and the University of Washington has approved these arrangements.

REFERENCES

Achenbach, T. M., & Edelbrock, C. S. (1991). *Manual for the Child Behavior Checklist and Revised Child Behavior Profile.* Burlington, VT: University Associates in Psychiatry.

American Psychiatric Association. (1994). *Diagnostic and statistical manual of mental disorders* (4th ed.). Washington, DC: Author.

Asher, S. R., Parkhurst, J. T., Hymel, S., & Williams, G. A. (1990). Peer rejection and loneliness in childhood. In S. R. Asher & J. D. Coie (Eds.), *Peer rejection in childhood* (pp. 253–273). Cambridge, England: Cambridge University Press.

Bandura, A. (1989). Regulation of cognitive processes through perceived self-efficacy. *Developmental Psychology, 25,* 729–735.

Bear, G. G. (1998). School discipline in the United States: Prevention, correction and long-term social development. *School Psychology Review, 2*(1), 14–32.

Beelmann, A., Pfingste, U., & Losel, F. (1994). Effects of training social competence in children: A meta-analysis of recent evaluation studies. *Journal of Abnormal Child Psychology, 5,* 265–275.

Bierman, K. L. (1989). Improving the peer relationships of rejected children. In B. B. Lahey & A. E. Kazdin (Eds.), *Advances in clinical child psychology* (Vol. 12, pp. 53–84). New York: Plenum Press.

Bredekamp, S., & Copple, C. (1997). *Developmentally appropriate practice in early childhood programs.* Washington, DC: National Association for the Education of Young Children.

Brestan, E. V., & Eyberg, S. M. (1998). Effective psychosocial treatments of conduct-disordered children and adolescents: Twenty-nine years, 82 studies, and 5,272 kids. *Journal of Clinical Child Psychology, 27,* 180–189.

Brophy, J. E. (1996). *Teaching problem students.* New York: Guilford Press.

Coie, J. D. (1990). Toward a theory of peer rejection. In S. R. Asher & J. D. Coie (Eds.), *Peer rejection in childhood* (pp. 365–398). Cambridge, England: Cambridge University Press.

Coie, J. D., & Dodge, K. A. (1998). Aggression and antisocial behavior. In W. Damon & N. Eisenberg (Eds.), *Handbook of child psychology: Social, emotional and personality development* (5th ed., Vol. 3, pp. 779–862). New York: Wiley.

Connolly, J. A., & Doyle, A. B. (1984). Relation of social fantasy play to social competence in preschoolers. *Developmental Psychology, 20,* 797–806.

Crick, N. R., & Dodge, K. A. (1994). A review and reformulation of social information processing mechanisms in children's social adjustment. *Psychological Bulletin, 115,* 74–101.

Dishion, T. J., McCord, J., & Poulin, F. (1999). When interventions harm: Peer groups and problem behavior. *American Psychologist, 54,* 755–764.

Dodge, K. A. (1993). Social-cognitive mechanisms in the development of conduct disorder and depression. *Annual Review of Psychology, 44,* 559–584.

Dodge, K. A., & Crick, N. R. (1990). Social information processing bases of aggressive behavior in children. *Personality and Social Psychology Bulletin, 16,* 8–22.

Dodge, K. A., Pettit, G. S., & Bates, J. E. (1994). Socialization mediators of the relation between socioeconomic status and child conduct problems [special issue]. *Child Development, 65*(2), 649–665.

Dodge, K. A., & Price, J. M. (1994). On the relation between social information processing and socially competent behavior in early school-aged children. *Child Development, 65,* 1385–1397.

Eron, L. D. (1990). Understanding aggression. *Bulletin of the International Society for Research on Aggression, 12,* 5–9.

Frick, P., Kamphaus, R. W., Lahey, B. B., Loeber, R., Christ, M. G., Hart, E., et al. (1991). Academic underachievement and the disruptive behavior disorders. *Journal of Consulting and Clinical Psychology, 59,* 289–294.

Gottman, J. M. (1983). How children become friends. *Monographs of the Society for Research in Child Development, 48*(2, Serial No. 201).

Gresham, F. M. (1995). Social skills training. In A. Thomas & J. Grimes (Eds.), *Best practices in school psychology* (Vol. 3, pp. 39–50). Bethesda, MD: National Association of School Psychologists.

Gresham, F. M. (1998). Social skills training: Should we raze, remodel, or rebuild? *Behavioral Disorders, 24,* 19–25.

Kazdin, A. E., Esveldt, D. K., French, N. H., & Unis, A. S. (1987a). Effects of parent management training and problem-solving skills training combined in the treatment of antisocial child behavior. *Journal of the American Academy of Child and Adolescent Psychiatry, 26,* 416–424.

Kazdin, A. E., Esveldt, D. K., French, N. H., & Unis, A. S. (1987b). Problem-solving skills training and relationship therapy in the treatment of antisocial child behavior. *Journal of Consulting and Clinical Psychology, 55*(1), 76–85.

Kazdin, A. E., Siegel, J. C., & Bass, D. (1992). Cognitive problem-solving skills training and parent management training in the treatment of antisocial behavior in children. *Journal of Consulting and Clinical Psychology, 60,* 733–747.

Kellam, S. G., Ling, X., Merisca, R., Brown, C. H., & Ialongo, N. (1998). The effect of the level of aggression in the first grade classroom on the course and malleability of aggressive behavior into middle school. *Development and Psychopathology, 10,* 165–185.

Kendall, P. C. (1993). Cognitive-behavioral therapies with youth: Guiding theory, current status and emerging developments. *Journal of Consulting and Clinical Psychology, 61,* 235–247.

Lochman, J. E., & Dunn, S. E. (1993). An intervention and consultation model from a social cognitive perspective: A description of the anger coping program. *School Psychology Review, 22,* 458–471.

Lochman, J. E., & Wells, K. (1996). A social-cognitive intervention with aggressive children: Prevention effects and contextual implementation issues. In R. D. Peters & R. J. McMahon (Eds.), *Prevention and early intervention: Childhood disorders, substance use, and delinquency* (pp. 111–143). Newbury Park, CA: Sage.

Loeber, R. (1985). Patterns and development of antisocial child behavior. In G. J. Whitehurst (Ed.), *Annals of child development* (Vol. 2, pp. 77–116). New York: JAI.

Loeber, R., & Farrington, D. P. (2000). Young children who commit crime: Epidemiology, developmental origins, risk factors, early interventions, and policy implications. *Developmental Psychopathology, 12,* 737–762.

National Research Council and Institute of Medicine. (2000). *From neurons to neighborhoods: The science of early childhood development.* Committee on Integrating the Science of Early Childhood Development. J. P. Shonkoff & D. A. Phillips (Eds.). Board on Children, Youth, and Families, Commission on Behavioral and Social Sciences and Education. Washington, DC: National Academy Press.

Novaco, R. W. (1975). *Anger control: The development and evaluation of an experimental treatment.* Lexington, MA: D.C. Health.

Patterson, G. R., DeGarmo, D. S., & Knutson, N. (2000). Hyperactive and antisocial behaviors: Comorbid or two points in the same process? *Development and Psychopathology, 12,* 91–106.

Reid, M. J., & Webster-Stratton, C. (2001). The Incredible Years parent, teacher, and child intervention: Targeting multiple areas of risk for a young child with pervasive conduct problems using a flexible, manualized treatment program. *Cognitive & Behavioral Practice, 8*(4), 377–386.

Reid, M., Webster-Stratton, C., & Hammond, M. (2004). Follow-up of children who received the Incredible Years Intervention for Oppositional Defiant Disorder: Maintenance and prediction of 2-year outcome. *Behavior Therapy, 34*(4).

Robinson, E. A., Eyberg, S. M., & Ross, A. W. (1980). The standardization of an inventory of child conduct problem behaviors. *Journal of Clinical Child Psychology, 9,* 22–28.

Schneider, B. H., & Bryne, B. M. (1985). Children's social skills training: A meta-analysis. In K. H. Schneider, K. H. Rubin, & J. E. Ledingham (Eds.), *Children's peer relations: Issues in assessment and intervention* (pp. 175–192). New York: Springer.

Shonkoff, J. P., & Phillips, D. A. (2000). *From neurons to neighborhoods: The science of early childhood development.* Washington, DC: National Academy Press.

Shure, M. (1994). I Can Problem Solve (ICPS): *An interpersonal cognitive problem-solving program for children.* Champaign, IL: Research Press.

Snyder, H. N. (2001). Epidemiology of official offending. In R. Loeber & D. P. Farrington (Eds.), *Child delinquents: Development, intervention, and service needs* (pp. 25–46). Newbury Park, CA: Sage.

Sturge, C. (1982). Reading retardation and antisocial behavior. *Journal of Child Psychology and Psychiatry, 23,* 21–23.

Taylor, T. K., & Biglan, A. (1998). Behavioral family interventions for improving child-rearing: A review for clinicians and policy makers. *Clinical Child and Family Psychology Review, 1*(1), 41–60.

Tremblay, R. E., Mass, L. C., Pagani, L., & Vitaro, F. (1996). From childhood physical aggression to adolescent maladjustment: The Montreal Prevention Experiment. In R. D. Peters & R. J. MacMahon (Eds.), *Preventing childhood disorders, substance abuse and delinquency* (pp. 268–298). Thousand Oaks, CA: Sage.

U.S. Department of Health and Human Services. (1999). *Mental health: A report of the Surgeon General.* Rockville, MD: U.S. Public Health Service.

Walker, H. M., Colvin, G., & Ramsey, E. (1995). *Antisocial behavior in school: Strategies and best practices.* Pacific Grove, CA: Brooks/Cole.

Webster-Stratton, C. (1990a). *Dina Dinosaur's social, emotional and problem-solving curriculum.* (Available from C. Webster-Stratton, 1411 8th Avenue West, Seattle, WA 98119.)

Webster-Stratton, C. (1990b). Long-term follow-up of families with young conduct problem children: From preschool to grade school. *Journal of Clinical Child Psychology, 19,* 144–149.

Webster-Stratton, C. (1990c). Stress: A potential disruptor of parent perceptions and family interactions. *Journal of Clinical Child Psychology, 19,* 302–312.

Webster-Stratton, C. (1990d). *Wally Game: A problem-solving test.* Unpublished manuscript, University of Washington.

Webster-Stratton, C. (2000). *How to promote children's social and emotional competence.* Newbury Park, CA: Sage.

Webster-Stratton, C., & Hammond, M. (1997). Treating children with early-onset conduct problems: A comparison of child and parent training interventions. *Journal of Consulting and Clinical Psychology, 65,* 93–109.

Webster-Stratton, C., & Hammond, M. (1998). Conduct problems and level of social competence in Head Start children: Prevalence, pervasiveness and associated risk factors. *Clinical Child Psychology and Family Psychology Review, 1,* 101–124.

Webster-Stratton, C., & Lindsay, D. W. (1999). Social competence and early-onset conduct problems: Issues in assessment. *Journal of Child Clinical Psychology, 28,* 25–93.

Webster-Stratton, C., & Reid, M. J. (in press). Incredible Years teacher training program: Content, methods and processes. In P. Tolen, J. Szapocznik, & S. Sambrano (Eds.), *Preventing substance abuse ages 3–14.* Washington, DC: American Psychological Association.

Webster-Stratton, C., Reid, M. J., & Hammond, M. (2001). Social skills and problem solving training for children with early-onset conduct problems: Who benefits? *Journal of Child Psychology and Psychiatry, 42,* 943–952.

Webster-Stratton, C., Reid, M. J., & Hammond, M. (2004). Treating children with early-onset conduct problems: Intervention outcomes for parent, child, and teacher training. *Journal of Clinical Child and Adolescent Psychology, 33*(1), 105–124.

Wolery, M. (2000). Behavioral and educational approaches to early intervention. In J. P. Shonkoff & S. J. Meisels (Eds.), *Handbook of early childhood intervention* (2nd ed., pp. 179–203). Cambridge, England: Cambridge University Press.

Author Index

Abbott, R., 481, 501
Abetz, L., 579
Achenbach, T. M., 7, 24, 63, 110, 112, 126, 149, 150, 156, 320, 321, 340, 343, 365, 410, 508, 526, 579, 584, 614, 615
Acker, M. M., 105
Ackerson, T. H., 177
Adair, J., 293
Aday, L., 33
Ageton, S. S., 401
Aiken, L. H., 164
Alarcon, R. D., 278
Alicke, M. D., 146
Allor, J. H., 464
Almeida, D. M., 106, 116
Altschuler, D. M., 378
Alvarez, M., 336
AMBHA. *See* American Managed Behavioral Health Care Association (AMBHA)
Ambrose, D., 378
American Academy of Child and Adolescent Psychiatry, 405
American College of Mental Health Administration, 202–203
American Managed Behavioral Health Care Association (AMBHA), 573
American Psychiatric Association (APA), 8, 289–291, 308, 379, 528, 577, 601
American Psychological Association, 231
Andersen, R., 33
Anderson, D., 290
Anderson, J. A., 457, 458
Anderson, J. C., 26
Andrade, A. R., 16, 79, 80, 226
Andrews, D. W., 485, 552
Anglin, J. P., 283
Angold, A., 7, 10–11, 23, 24, 25, 26, 27, 28, 30, 32, 33, 34, 39, 65, 110, 111, 226, 247, 248, 249, 528, 575, 579
Antil, L. R., 424
Aos, S., 561, 566
APA. *See* American Psychiatric Association (APA)
Armistead, L., 351
Armstrong, B. J., 355–373
Armstrong, K. H., 11

Armstrong, M. I., 576
Armstrong, T. L., 378
Arnold, D. S., 105
Arnold, L. E., 247
Arredondo, P., 297
Ascher, B. H., 25, 26, 248, 268
Asher, S. R., 599
Attkisson, C., 7, 27, 148, 150, 155, 158, 275, 281, 575

Babyak, A. E., 463–464
Bailey, J., 109
Bandura, A., 105, 609
Bank, L., 480, 552
Banks, S. M., 199–224, 230, 234
Barber, C. C., 281, 289
Barkley, R. A., 105, 405
Barnes, T. R., 455
Barnoski, R., 561
Barrish, H. H., 488
Bartko, J. J., 257
Barton, B., 109
Bass, D., 599
Bateman, A., 576
Bates, J. E., 604
Baughman, L., 177, 182, 329, 529
Baum, D. D., 422
Bazron, B. J., 297
Bean, D. L., 256, 263
Bean, R., 469
Bear, G. G., 608
Beard, J. H., 177
Beard, K., 509, 511
Beelmann, A., 600
Behar, L. B., 30, 144, 157, 158, 275
Behn, J. D., 297
Bell, R. Q., 105
Benabarre, A., 111
Bennett, L., 455
Benson, P. L., 132, 134
Benz, M., 377, 378, 382
Berki, S. E., 248
Berlin, L. J., 114
Berlinghoff, D. H., 461, 466
Best, A. M., 59, 281

625

Subject Index

About the Editors

MICHAEL H. EPSTEIN, EdD, is the director of the Center for At-Risk Children's Services and the William E. Barkley Professor of Special Education at the University of Nebraska. He received his doctoral degree in special education from the University of Virginia. He has been employed as a teacher of children with behavior and learning problems, a director of educational programs for students with disabilities, and a university professor. Dr. Epstein has received more than $16 million in external grants, has published more than 220 professional papers, has served as a consultant to various state and federal agencies and foundations, has served as a reviewer for numerous professional journals, and is the founding editor of the *Journal of Emotional and Behavioral Disorders.* He is the author of the *Behavioral and Emotional Rating Scale: A Strength-Based Approach to Assessment* and the *Scale Assessing Emotional Disturbance.* He is the coauthor of *Making Schools Safe and Violence Free.*

KRISTA KUTASH, PhD, is a professor and the deputy director of the Research and Training Center for Children's Mental Health at the University of South Florida in Tampa. She worked as a social worker before joining the center in 1984 to conduct research and training. Her doctorate is in educational measurement and research; she also has an MBA with a specialty in economics. Dr. Kutash has been principal investigator on several grants examining issues related to children who have disabilities and their families. Among her extensive publications is a comprehensive review of the empirical base of the system of care for children who have emotional and behavioral disabilities and their families, as well as more than 100 publications and presentations in the area of improving outcomes for children. Dr. Kutash holds a joint appointment in the Department of Special Education, where she trains doctoral students in program evaluation techniques.

ALBERT J. DUCHNOWSKI, PhD, is a professor of child and family studies and special education (jointly appointed) at the University of South Florida. He serves as deputy director of the Research and Training Center for Children's Mental Health at the Louis de la Parte Florida Mental Health Institute. He has been principal investigator on several grants focusing on training professionals from a multidisciplinary perspective to work with children with disabilities and their families. He has written numerous publications and has co-edited three books on children's mental health services and special education.

In addition to academic experience, Dr. Duchnowski was the director of Pupil Personnel Services and Special Education for 11 years in Gettysburg, Pennsylvania. He has also been a consultant to state directors of special education and children's mental health in 30 states. He is a founding member and past vice president of the Federation of Families for Children's Mental Health.